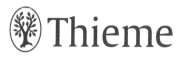

Surgical Decision Making in Acute Care Surgery

Kimberly A. Davis, MD, MBA, FACS, FCCM
Professor of Surgery
Vice Chairman for Clinical Affairs
Chief
Division of General Surgery
Trauma and Surgical Critical Care
Yale School of Medicine
New Haven, Connecticut, USA

Raul Coimbra, MD, PhD, FACS
Surgeon-in-Chief and Director
CECORC–Comparative Effectiveness and Clinical Outcomes Research Center
Riverside University Health System Medical Center
Riverside, California, USA;
Professor of Surgery
Loma Linda University School of Medicine
Loma Linda, California, USA

138 illustrations

Thieme
New York • Stuttgart • Delhi • Rio de Janeiro

Library of Congress Cataloging-in-Publication Data is available with the publisher.

Thieme Publishers New York
333 Seventh Avenue, New York, NY 10001, USA
+1 800 782 3488, customerservice@thieme.com

Georg Thieme Verlag KG
Rüdigerstrasse 14, 70469 Stuttgart, Germany
+49 [0]711 8931 421, customerservice@thieme.de

Thieme Publishers Delhi
A-12, Second Floor, Sector-2, Noida-201301
Uttar Pradesh, India
+91 120 45 566 00, customerservice@thieme.in

Thieme Publishers Rio de Janeiro,
Thieme Publicações Ltda.
Edifício Rodolpho de Paoli, 25º andar
Av. Nilo Peçanha, 50 – Sala 2508,
Rio de Janeiro 20020-906 Brasil
+55 21 3172-2297

Cover design: Thieme Publishing Group
Typesetting by TNQ Technologies, India

Printed in USA by King Printing Company, Inc.   5 4 3 2 1

ISBN 978-1-68420-058-0

Also available as an e-book:
eISBN 978-1-68420-059-7

Important note: Medicine is an ever-changing science undergoing continual development. Research and clinical experience are continually expanding our knowledge, in particular our knowledge of proper treatment and drug therapy. Insofar as this book mentions any dosage or application, readers may rest assured that the authors, editors, and publishers have made every effort to ensure that such references are in accordance with **the state of knowledge at the time of production of the book.**

Nevertheless, this does not involve, imply, or express any guarantee or responsibility on the part of the publishers in respect to any dosage instructions and forms of applications stated in the book. **Every user is requested to examine carefully** the manufacturers' leaflets accompanying each drug and to check, if necessary in consultation with a physician or specialist, whether the dosage schedules mentioned therein or the contraindications stated by the manufacturers differ from the statements made in the present book. Such examination is particularly important with drugs that are either rarely used or have been newly released on the market. Every dosage schedule or every form of application used is entirely at the user's own risk and responsibility. The authors and publishers request every user to report to the publishers any discrepancies or inaccuracies noticed. If errors in this work are found after publication, errata will be posted at www.thieme.com on the product description page.

Some of the product names, patents, and registered designs referred to in this book are in fact registered trademarks or proprietary names even though specific reference to this fact is not always made in the text. Therefore, the appearance of a name without designation as proprietary is not to be construed as a representation by the publisher that it is in the public domain.

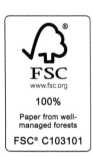

FSC
www.fsc.org
100%
Paper from well-managed forests
FSC® C103101

Contents

Foreword xii

Preface xiii

Contributors xiv

1 The Definition of Acute Care Surgery 1
Robert D. Becher, Raul Coimbra, and Kimberly A. Davis

1.1 Drivers for the Acute Care Surgery Model 1

1.2 Fellowship Training in ACS 3

1.3 Surgeon Satisfaction with ACS 3

1.4 Patient Throughput Improvements with ACS 3

1.5 Care Delivery Models 4

1.6 Standardizing Care: The Development of Grading Systems for EGS Diseases 4

1.7 Improving Patient Outcomes after Emergency General Surgery 4

1.8 Conclusion 6

2 Anatomic and Physiological Considerations 9
Bishwajit Bhattacharya and Kimberly A. Davis

2.1 Introduction 9

2.2 Physiological Effects of Laparoscopy 9

2.2.1 Physiologic Effects of Increased Intra-abdominal Pressure 9

2.2.2 Physiologic Effects of Hypercarbia 10

2.3 Anatomic Considerations 10

2.4 Patient Populations 11

2.4.1 Pediatric Patients 11

2.4.2 Pregnant Patients 11

2.4.3 Geriatric Patients 12

2.5 Other Physiological Considerations of Minimally Invasive Surgery 12

2.6 Future of Minimally Invasive Surgery 12

3 Impact of Acute Surgical Illness on Critical Care Decisions Pre- and Postoperatively 14
Lena M. Napolitano and Jay Doucet

3.1 Preoperative Critical Care 14

3.1.1 Strategies to Optimize Organ Function and Intravascular Volume Preoperatively 14

3.2 Postoperative Critical Care 18

3.2.1 Role of the Surgical Team and Intensivist 18

3.2.2 Resuscitation Goals 19

3.2.3 Transfusion Strategies 20

3.2.4 Management of Sepsis 22

3.2.5 Respiratory Failure/ARDS 24

3.2.6 Acute Kidney Injury 28

3.2.7 Nutrition 28

3.2.8 Pain, Agitation, and Delirium 28

3.2.9 Prevention of Complications/Prophylaxis...... 30

4 Cervical Trauma 34
Aaron Richman and Clay Cothren Burlew

4.1 Penetrating Neck Trauma 34

4.1.1 Tracheal Injury 35

4.1.2 Cervical Esophageal Injury 36

4.1.3 Cervical Vascular Injury 36

4.2 Carotid Artery 37

4.3 Vertebral Artery 38

4.4 Subclavian Artery 38

4.5   **Blunt Neck Trauma** 39

4.5.1   Blunt Cerebrovascular Injury Management 39

5   **Blunt Abdominal Trauma** 46

Morgan Schellenberg and Kenji Inaba

5.1   **Introduction** 46

5.2   **General Approach to Blunt Abdominal Trauma** 46

5.3   **Management of Specific Injuries After Blunt Abdominal Trauma** 47

5.3.1   Solid Organ Injuries 47
5.3.2   Diagnosis 47
5.3.3   Management Strategy 48
5.3.4   Surgical Techniques 48
5.3.5   Complications 50

5.4   **Hollow Viscus Injuries** 50

5.4.1   Diagnosis 50
5.4.2   Management Strategy 51
5.4.3   Surgical Techniques 51

5.5   **Gastroesophageal (GE) Junction Injuries** 51

5.5.1   Stomach 51
5.5.2   Duodenum 52
5.5.3   Small Bowel and Colon 52
5.5.4   Rectum 52
5.5.5   Complications 53

Expert Commentary on Cervical Trauma 45
Timothy C. Fabian

5.6   **Pancreatic Injuries** 53

5.6.1   Diagnosis 53
5.6.2   Management Strategy 53
5.6.3   Surgical Techniques 53
5.6.4   Complications 54

5.7   **Major Vascular Injuries** 54

5.7.1   Diagnosis 54
5.7.2   Management Strategy 54
5.7.3   Surgical Techniques 54
5.7.4   Complications 55

5.8   **Diaphragm Injuries** 55

5.8.1   Diagnosis 55
5.8.2   Management Strategy 55
5.8.3   Surgical Techniques 55
5.8.4   Complications 56

5.9   **Considerations for Abdominal Closure** 56

5.10   **Conclusion** 56

Expert Commentary on Blunt Abdominal Trauma 61
Robert C. Mackersie

6   **Penetrating Abdominal Trauma** 62

Lyndsey E. Wessels, Michael J. Krzyzaniak, and Matthew J. Martin

6.1   **Introduction** 62

6.1.1   A Brief History of Penetrating Abdominal Trauma 62
6.1.2   Epidemiology of Penetrating Abdominal Trauma 62
6.1.3   Abdominal Anatomy 63

6.2   **Basic Principles of Penetrating Abdominal Trauma** 63

6.2.1   Mechanisms of Injury 63
6.2.2   Initial Evaluation 63
6.2.3   Basic Operative Principles 64

6.3   **Evaluation and Management of Abdominal Stab Wounds** 64

6.3.1   Evaluating for "Hard Signs to Operate" 64
6.3.2   Selective Nonoperative Management 65
6.3.3   Operative Principles Unique to Stab Wounds ... 69

6.4   **Evaluation and Management of Gunshot Wounds** 69

6.4.1   Evaluating for "Hard Signs to Operate" 69
6.4.2   Selective Nonoperative Management 70
6.4.3   Operative Principles Unique to Gunshot Wounds 72

6.5   **Laparoscopy in Penetrating Abdominal Trauma** 73

6.6   **Special Scenarios** 73

6.6.1   Penetrating Abdominal Trauma in Pregnancy ... 73

6.7   **Damage Control Surgery** 73

6.7.1   Damage Control Abdominal Procedures 73
6.7.2   Damage Control Resuscitation 75

| 6.8 | Conclusion | 75 |
| | Disclaimer | 75 |

Expert Commentary on Penetrating Abdominal Trauma ... 79
Thomas Scalea

7 Thoracic Trauma ... 80
Benjamin J. Moran, Katherine M. Kelley, and James V. O'Connor

7.1	Introduction	80
7.2	Initial Evaluation	80
7.3	Indications for Operative Intervention	80
7.3.1	Urgent/Emergent	80
7.3.2	Thoracic Damage Control	82
7.3.3	Elective	82
7.4	Video-assisted Thoracoscopic Surgery (VATS)	82
7.4.1	History of VATS	82
7.4.2	Advantages and Indications for VATS	82
7.4.3	VATS Operative Technique	82
7.4.4	VATS Indications	82

7.5	Contraindications and Complications of VATS	83
7.6	Open Thoracic Surgery	83
7.6.1	Operative Exposure	83
7.6.2	Airway Management	85
7.6.3	Operative Techniques	86
7.7	Complications	87
7.8	Cardiac Injuries	87
7.8.1	Presentation and Evaluation	87
7.8.2	Treatment	88

Expert Commentary on Thoracic Trauma ... 93
Gregory J. Jurkovich

8 Vascular Trauma ... 94
Jason Pasley, Megan Brenner, and Raul Coimbra

8.1	Introduction	94
8.2	Diagnostic Testing	94
8.3	Operative Considerations and Approaches	96
8.3.1	Thoracic Aorta and Great Vessels	96
8.3.2	Neck Exposure	98
8.3.3	Carotid Artery	98
8.3.4	Vertebral Artery Exposure	98
8.3.5	Axillary Artery Exposure	98
8.3.6	Brachial Artery	98
8.3.7	Abdominal Aorta and the Inferior Vena Cava (IVC)	99
8.3.8	Celiac Artery	99
8.3.9	Superior Mesenteric Artery (SMA)	99
8.3.10	Inferior Mesenteric Artery (IMA)	99
8.3.11	Portal Vein (PV) and Superior Mesenteric Vein (SMV)	100
8.3.12	Renal Artery and Vein	100
8.3.13	Common Femoral Artery (CFA) and Vein	100
8.3.14	Proximal SFA and Profunda Femoral Artery (PFA)	101
8.3.15	Distal SFA	101
8.3.16	Popliteal Artery	101

8.4	Extremity Injuries	101
8.5	Reconstructive Options	101
8.5.1	Saphenous vein	101
8.5.2	Polytetrafluoroethylene (PTFE)	101
8.5.3	Other Conduits	101
8.6	Venous Injuries	102
8.7	Considerations After Repair of Extremity Injuries	102
8.8	Role of Endovascular Interventions	102
8.8.1	Shunts	105
8.8.2	Tourniquets	105
8.8.3	REBOA	106
8.9	Conclusion	107

Expert Commentary on Vascular Trauma ... 111
David V. Feliciano

9 Appendicitis ... 112
Edward Lineen, Yee Wong, and Nicholas Namias

| 9.1 | Introduction | 112 |
| 9.2 | Epidemiology | 112 |

Contents

9.3 **Pathogenesis** 113

9.4 **Diagnosis** 114

9.4.1 Ultrasound 115
9.4.2 Computed Tomography 116
9.4.3 MRI 118

9.5 **Treatment** 118

9.5.1 Laparoscopic Versus Open Appendectomy 118
9.5.2 Alternative Minimal Invasive Techniques 121

9.5.3 Appendectomy Versus Antibiotics 122
9.5.4 Uncomplicated 122
9.5.5 Complicated Appendicitis 123

9.6 **Appendicitis in the Elderly** 123

9.7 **Pregnancy** 124

Expert Commentary on Appendicitis 131
Purvi P. Patel, Brendan Ringhouse, Christian Renz,
and Fred A. Luchette

10 **Acute Cholecystitis** 132
Giana H. Davidson and Eileen M. Bulger

10.1 **Introduction** 132

10.2 **Diagnostic Evaluation** 132

10.3 **Indications and Timing for Operative**
Intervention 132

10.4 **Symptomatic Gallbladder disease** 133

10.4.1 Acute Cholecystitis 133
10.4.2 Percutaneous Cholecystostomy 133
10.4.3 Chronic Cholecystitis 133

10.5 **Complicated Biliary Disease** 133

10.5.1 Choledocholithiasis 133
10.5.2 Cholangitis 134
10.5.3 Gallstone Pancreatitis 134
10.5.4 Gangrenous Cholecystitis 134
10.5.5 Acalculous Cholecystitis 135
10.5.6 External Compression of the Common Bile Duct:
Mirizzi's and Lemmel Syndrome 135
10.5.7 Hydrops 135
10.5.8 Cholecystenteric Fistula (Gallstone Ileus) 135
10.5.9 Porcelain Gallbladder 136

10.6 **Special Populations** 136

10.6.1 Cholecystitis in Pregnancy 136
10.6.2 Cirrhosis 136
10.6.3 Older population with Cholecystitis 136

10.7 **The Role of Minimally Invasive Surgery** 136

10.7.1 Role Of Intraoperative Cholangiogram (IOC),
Intraoperative Ultrasound, and Indocyanine
Green (ICG) 138

10.8 **Contraindications to an MIS Approach** 139

10.8.1 Open Cholecystectomy 139

10.9 **The Role for Nonoperative Management** 139

10.9.1 Percutaneous Cholecystostomy 139
10.9.2 Perforated Cholecystitis with Hepatic Abscess . . 139

10.10 **The Management of Complications** 139

Expert Commentary on Acute
Cholecystitis 147
Ronald Stewart

11 **Acute Diverticulitis** 148
Maryanne L. Pickett, Joseph P. Minei, and Michael W. Cripps

11.1 **Introduction** 148

11.2 **Indications for Operative Intervention** 148

11.3 **Nonoperative Management** 149

11.4 **Emergent Operation** 149

11.5 **Nonemergent Surgery** 149

11.6 **Role of Minimally Invasive Surgery** 150

11.7 **Contraindications to MIS** 151

11.8 **Open Management Strategies** 152

11.8.1 Hartmann's Procedure 152
11.8.2 Primary Anastomosis (PA), With or Without,
Diverting Loop Ileostomy (DLI) 152

11.9 **Damage Control** 152

11.9.1 Timing of Stoma Reversal 153
11.9.2 Management of Postoperative Complications . . . 153

Expert Commentary on Acute
Diverticulitis 159
Frederick A. Moore

12   A Modern Approach to Complicated Pancreatitis 160

Chris Javadi, Monica Dua, and Brendan Visser

12.1   Terminology Matters 160

12.2   Necrosis and Infection Exist in a Continuum 160

12.3   Indications for Intervention 161

12.4   What is Our Goal? 161

12.5   Evolution of Strategies 161

12.5.1   Open Necrosectomy 161
12.5.2   Laparoscopic Debridement 161

12.5.3   Retroperitoneal Debridement 161
12.5.4   Two Trocar Technique 163
12.5.5   Primary Percutaneous Drainage 164
12.5.6   Transgastric Debridement 164
12.5.7   Endoscopic Transgastric Debridement 164

12.6   Conclusion 166

Expert Commentary on A Modern Approach to Complicated Pancreatitis 171
Peter Fagenholz and George C. Velmahos

13   Inflammatory/Infectious Bowel Disease 172

Cigdem Benlice, Ipek Sapci, and Scott R. Steele

13.1   Crohn's Disease 172

13.1.1   Introduction 172
13.1.2   Indications for Operative Intervention 172
13.1.3   Special Considerations 174
13.1.4   Minimally Invasive Approaches in Crohn's Disease 175
13.1.5   Conclusion 176

13.2   Ulcerative Colitis 176

13.3   Clinical Manifestations 176

13.3.1   Indications for Operative Intervention 177
13.3.2   The Role of Minimally Invasive Surgery 178
13.3.3   Contraindications to an MIS Approach 179
13.3.4   Open Management Strategies 179

13.3.5   The Management of Postoperative Complications 181

13.4   Clostridium Difficile Colitis 181

13.4.1   Indications for Operative Intervention 182
13.4.2   The Role of Minimally Invasive Surgery 182
13.4.3   Contraindications to an MIS Approach 183
13.4.4   Open Management Strategies 183
13.4.5   The Management of Postoperative Complications 183
13.4.6   Conclusion 184

Expert Commentary on Inflammatory/Infectious Bowel Disease 191
Formosa Chen and Clifford Y. Ko

14   Gastroduodenal Ulcers Requiring Surgery 192

Robert D. Winfield and Marie L. Crandall

14.1   Introduction 192

14.2   Risk Factors for Peptic Ulcer Disease 192

14.3   Disease Presentation 192

14.4   Diagnosis 192

14.5   Management of Complicated Peptic Ulcer Disease 193

14.6   Management of Hemorrhagic Peptic Ulcer Disease 197

14.7   Postoperative management of Complicated Peptic Ulcer Disease 198

14.8   Conclusion 200

Expert Commentary on Gastroduodenal Ulcers Requiring Surgery 205
L. D. Britt

15   Intestinal Bowel Obstruction 206

Bishwajit Bhattacharya and Adrian A. Maung

15.1   Introduction 206

15.2   Background 206

15.3   Diagnostic Workup 206

15.4 **Small Bowel Obstruction** 206

15.4.1 Indications for Operative Intervention 206
15.4.2 Minimally Invasive Surgery for Small Bowel
Obstruction 207
15.4.3 Technical Considerations in Minimally Invasive
Surgery for Small Bowel Obstruction. 208
15.4.4 Early Postoperative Obstruction. 209

15.5 **Large Bowel Obstruction** 210

15.5.1 Operative Intervention for Large Bowel
Obstruction 210

15.5.2 Minimally Invasive Surgery for Large Bowel
Obstruction. 210
15.5.3 Technical Considerations in Minimally Invasive
Surgery for Large Bowel Obstruction 210
15.5.4 Endoscopic Management of Large Bowel
Obstruction. 211

**Expert Commentary on Intestinal Bowel
Obstruction** 215
Andrew B. Peitzman

16 **Surgical Management of Incarcerated Hernias** 216
Jessica Koller Gorham and William S. Richardson

16.1 **Introduction** 216

16.2 **Epidemiology** 216

16.3 **Differential Diagnosis** 216

16.4 **Diagnosis** 216

16.5 **Treatment** 216

16.6 **Inguinal Hernia** 217

16.6.1 Examples 217

16.7 **Umbilical Hernia** 218

16.8 **Epigastric, Ventral, and Incisional Hernias** . . . 219

16.9 **Spigelian Hernia** 220

16.10 **Diaphragmatic Hernia** 220

16.11 **Flank Hernia** 222

16.12 **Pelvic Hernia** 222

16.13 **Internal Hernia** 223

**Expert Commentary on Surgical
Management of Incarcerated Hernias** 227
Brent Matthews

17 **Mesenteric Ischemia** 228
James Becker, Todd W. Costantini, and Joseph M. Galante

17.1 **Introduction** 228

17.2 **Anatomy of Mesenteric Circulation** 229

17.3 **Diagnosis of Acute Mesenteric Ischemia** 229

17.3.1 History and Physical Examination 229
17.3.2 Laboratory Analysis 230
17.3.3 Imaging 230

17.4 **Treatment of Acute Mesenteric Ischemia** . . . 232

17.4.1 Resuscitation 232

17.4.2 Operative Exposure of the Mesenteric Vessels . . 232
17.4.3 Thromboembolic Mesenteric Ischemia 233
17.4.4 Veno-occlusive Mesenteric Ischemia 234
17.4.5 Non-Occlusive Mesenteric Ischemia 235

17.5 **Ischemic Colitis** 235

17.6 **Conclusion** 236

Expert Commentary on Mesenteric Ischemia 241
David Spain

18 **Esophageal Emergencies: Emergency Management of Paraesophageal Hernias and
Esophageal Perforations** 242
Geoffrey P. Kohn

18.1 **Introduction** 242

18.2 **Paraesophageal Hernias** 242

18.2.1 Etiology 243
18.2.2 Classification 243

18.2.3 Incarceration and Strangulation 243
18.2.4 Diagnosis 243
18.2.5 Indications for Repair 245
18.2.6 Management of Acute Gastric Obstruction 245
18.2.7 Operative Technique 245

18.3 Esophageal Perforation................... 246

18.3.1 Etiology................................. 246
18.3.2 Investigations........................... 247
18.3.3 Management 248

18.3.4 Outcomes............................... 251
18.3.5 Conclusion.............................. 252

Expert Commentary on Esophageal Emergencies 257
Steven DeMeester

Index 259

Foreword

In the past 15 years, the field of Acute Care Surgery (ACS) and Emergency Surgery has evolved as a surgical subspecialty. Specific journals, texts, handbooks, training curriculum for fellowships, and standards for hospitals (with a verification program) are emerging and define this essential lifesaving care.

Looking at the burden of disease, emergency surgery accounts for at least 20 percent of hospital admissions and 25 percent of costs. Adding trauma and surgical critical care only increases the financial impact of ACS overall.

The foundational contribution of Dr. Kimberly A. Davis and Dr. Raul Coimbra as the editors of this textbook, *Surgical Decision Making in Acute Care Surgery*, has raised the credibility of the field. The contributing authors are the who's who in this surgical discipline.

This textbook covers indications for operative interventions and the operative approach for all the common emergency general surgery and trauma conditions. The role of laparoscopic approaches, the indications for conversion to open approaches, and when open surgery may be most appropriate are all covered in this textbook. Substantially experienced contemporaries define how ACS should be practiced in this evolving field. This book will arm the reader with a thoughtful approach to these challenging problems.

The ultimate *beneficiaries* of this book will be the patients cared for by Acute Care Surgeons. I would like to congratulate the editors for this wonderful contribution. This book fills an important gap in the surgical literature. I wish this book had existed when I started practice 35 years ago.

David B. Hoyt, MD, FACS
Executive Director
American College of Surgeons
Chicago, Illinois, USA

Preface

Acute Care Surgery (ACS), initially proposed in 2003 by the American Association for the Surgery of Trauma (AAST), has rapidly matured in the last decade. This concept evolved to represent a practice standard to meet societal demands for care of those in need of emergent assessments and interventions, be it in emergency general surgery, trauma, or surgical critical care. To support implementation of ACS as a practice paradigm, a well-defined training curriculum was developed.

Concomitant to the creation of this new surgical care delivery paradigm, the landscape of surgery in general was changing dramatically: minimally invasive techniques developed, rapid recovery protocols were implemented in daily practice, economic pressures ensued, and we, general surgeons, dealing with complex surgical emergencies and traumatic injuries had to refocus to be more efficient, decrease costs without compromising quality, avoid complications, and decrease readmissions.

The incorporation of advanced technology in surgery care is here to stay. We must use it to the advantage of our patients in a cost-effective way and with an eye toward high-quality care delivery. The conundrum was a paucity of information presented in a concise way, that was immediately available about when and how to use minimally invasive techniques and advanced technology as opposed to the traditional open approach when dealing with acute surgical emergencies, traumatic or non-traumatic. This is how the book *Surgical Decision Making in Acute Care Surgery* was initially conceived by us.

We are certainly aware of the many excellent textbooks on ACS that are already available in the market. We did not want to write just another textbook. Rather, we want to offer to trainees, junior faculty, and practicing surgeons a source of information they could have at their fingertips regarding the modern practice of ACS, incorporating and embracing minimally invasive approaches, when indicated, which have revolutionized the way we practice surgery in the 21st century. We want to encourage the use of surgical innovation applied to ACS.

We have focused on the indications for operative interventions and operative approaches, including the role of minimally invasive techniques (laparoscopy, thoracoscopy, radiology-based percutaneous techniques, as well as endovascular procedures), the indications for conversion to open approaches, and when open surgery may be most appropriate. The topics span the gamut of both emergency general surgery and trauma. We are certainly indebted to the senior surgeons and their young counterparts, who are the rising stars in American Surgery, for contributing their expertise with chapters and commentaries.

We dedicate this book to all the practicing and trainee surgeons, who provide the best surgical care possible to those affected by surgical emergencies and traumatic injuries.

Kimberly A. Davis, MD, MBA, FACS, FCCM
Raul Coimbra, MD, PhD, FACS

Contributors

Robert D. Becher, MD, MS
Assistant Professor of Surgery
Division of General Surgery, Trauma, and Surgical
  Critical Care
Yale School of Medicine
New Haven, Connecticut, USA

James Becker, MD
Staff Surgeon
Trauma Surgery and Surgical Critical Care
Kaiser Permanente South Sacramento Medical Center
Sacramento, California, USA

Cigdem Benlice, MD
Surgeon
Department of Colorectal Surgery
Digestive Disease and Surgery Institute
Cleveland Clinic
Cleveland, Ohio, USA

Bishwajit Bhattacharya, MD, FACS
Assistant Professor of Surgery
Division of General Surgery, Trauma, and Surgical
  Critical Care
Yale School of Medicine
New Haven, Connecticut, USA

Megan Brenner, MD, MS, RPVI, FACS
Professor of Surgery
University of California Riverside
Director of Surgical Research
Comparative Effectiveness and Clinical Outcomes
  Research Center (CECORC)
Riverside University Health Systems
Moreno Valley, California, USA

L.D. Britt, MD, MPH, FACS, FCCM
Professor and Chair of Surgery
Eastern Virginia Medical School
Norfolk, Virginia, USA

Eileen M. Bulger, MD, FACS
Professor of Surgery
University of Washington
Chief of Trauma
Harborview Medical Center
Seattle, Washington, USA

Clay Cothren Burlew, MD, FACS
Professor of Surgery
Director of Surgical Intensive Care Unit
Program Director-SCC and TACS Fellowships
Denver Health Medical Center
University of Colorado School of Medicine
Denver, Colorado, USA

Formosa Chen, MD, MPH
Assistant Professor of Surgery
Olive View-UCLA Medical Center
Los Angeles, California, USA

Raul Coimbra, MD, PhD, FACS
Surgeon-in-Chief and Director
CECORC–Comparative Effectiveness and Clinical Outcomes
  Research Center
Riverside University Health System Medical Center
Riverside, California, USA;
Professor of Surgery
Loma Linda University School of Medicine
Loma Linda, California, USA

Todd W. Costantini, MD, FACS
Associate Professor of Surgery
Trauma Medical Director
Division of Trauma, Surgical Critical Care, Burns, and Acute
  Care Surgery
Department of Surgery
UC San Diego Health
San Diego, California, USA

Marie L. Crandall, MD, MPH, FACS
Professor of Surgery
Associate Chair for Research
Department of Surgery
Program Director
General Surgery Residency
University of Florida College of Medicine Jacksonville
Jacksonville, Florida, USA

Michael W. Cripps, MSCS, MD
Director
Surgical Critical Care Fellowship
Department of Surgery
University of Texas Southwestern Medical Center
Dallas, Texas, USA

Giana H. Davidson, MD, MPH, FACS
Associate Professor
Department of Surgery
Adjunct Associate Professor
Department of Health Services
Section Chief
Emergency General Surgery
The University of Washington Medical Center
Seattle, Washington, USA

Kimberly A. Davis, MD, MBA, FACS, FCCM
Professor of Surgery
Vice Chairman for Clinical Affairs
Chief
Division of General Surgery
Trauma and Surgical Critical Care
Yale School of Medicine
New Haven, Connecticut, USA

Steven DeMeester, MD
Thoracic and Foregut Surgery
The Oregon Clinic
Portland, Oregon, USA

Jay Doucet, MD, MSc, FRCSC, FACS, RDMS
Professor and Chief
Division of Trauma
Surgical Critical Care, Burns, and Acute Care Surgery
Medical Director
Emergency Management
Surgical Director
Perioperative Services
Department of Surgery
Hillcrest Campus
University of California San Diego Health
San Diego, California, USA

Monica Dua, MD
Clinical Associate Professor
Department of Surgery
Stanford University Medical Center
Stanford, California, USA

Timothy C. Fabian, MD, FACS
Professor Emeritus
Department of Surgery
University of Tennessee Health Science Center
Memphis, Tennessee, USA

Peter Fagenholz, MD
Assistant Professor
Harvard Medical School
Department of Surgery
Massachusetts General Hospital
Boston, Massachusetts, USA

David V. Feliciano, MD
Master Surgeon Educator
American College of Surgeons
Clinical Professor of Surgery
University of Maryland SOM
Attending Surgeon
Department of Surgery
Shock Trauma Center
University of Maryland Medical Center
Baltimore, Maryland, USA

Joseph M. Galante, MD, FACS
Medical Director
Perioperative Services
Division Chief
Trauma and Acute Care Surgery
Trauma Medical Director
Professor of Surgery
Department of Surgery
University of California, Davis
Davis, California, USA

Jessica Koller Gorham, MD
Senior Lecturer
University of Queensland
MIS, Bariatric Surgeon
Associate Program Director
General Surgery Residency
Ochsner Health
New Orleans, Louisiana, USA

Kenji Inaba, MD, FRCSC, FACS
Professor of Clinical Surgery
Division of Acute Care Surgery
LAC+USC Medical Center
University of Southern California
Los Angeles, California, USA

Chris Javadi, MD, PhD
Clinical Instructor
Department of Surgery
Stanford University Medical Center
Stanford, California, USA

Gregory J. Jurkovich, MD, FACS
Professor and Vice Chairman
Lloyd F. and Rosemargaret Donant Chair in Trauma Medicine
Department of Surgery
UC Davis Health
Sacramento, California, USA

Katherine M. Kelley, MD
Visiting Instructor
Department of Surgery
University of Maryland School of Medicine
R Adams Cowley Shock Trauma Center
Baltimore, Maryland, USA

Clifford Y. Ko, MD, MS, MSHS
Professor and Vice Chair
UCLA Department of Surgery
University of California
Los Angeles, California, USA

Geoffrey P. Kohn, MBBS (Hons) MSurg, FRACS, FACS
Upper Gastrointestinal Surgeon
Department of Surgery
Monash University
Melbourne, Australia

Michael J. Krzyzaniak, MD, FACS
Program Director
General Surgery Residency
Department of General Surgery
Naval Medical Center
San Diego, California, USA

Edward Lineen, MD
Assistant Professor of Surgery
Medical Director
Trauma Intensive Care Unit
University of Miami
Miami, Florida, USA

Fred A. Luchette, MD, MSc
Vice Chair
Professor of Surgery
Loyola University Medical Center
Chicago, Illinois, USA
Chief of Surgical Services
Department of Surgery
Edward Hines, Jr. VA Hospital
Hines, Illinois, USA

Robert C. Mackersie, MD
Professor and Vice-Chief of Surgery
Division of General Surgery
Department of Surgery
Zuckerberg San Francisco General
Medical Director
Zuckerberg San Francisco General Trauma Program
San Francisco, California, USA

Matthew J. Martin, MD, FACS
Director of Trauma Research
Professor of Surgery
Scripps Mercy Hospital
San Diego, California, USA

Brent Matthews, MD
Professor and Chair
Department of Surgery
Surgeon-in-Chief
Atrium Health
Charlotte, North Carolina, USA

Adrian A. Maung, MD, FACS, FCCM
Associate Professor
Division of General Surgery, Trauma and Surgical
  Critical Care
Department of Surgery
Yale School of Medicine
New Haven, Connecticut, USA

Joseph P. Minei, MBA, MD
Professor
Department of Surgery
University of Texas Southwestern Medical Center
Dallas, Texas, USA

Benjamin J. Moran, MD
Visiting Instructor
Department of Surgery
University of Maryland School of Medicine
R Adams Cowley Shock Trauma Center
Baltimore, Maryland, USA

Frederick A. Moore, MD, FACS, MCCM
Professor and Chief of Acute Surgery
Department of Surgery
University of Florida College of Medicine
Gainesville, Florida, USA

Nicholas Namias, MD
Chief
Division of Trauma and Acute Care Surgery
Miller School of Medicine
Vice Chair
Quality and Patient Experience
University of Miami
Miami, Florida, USA

Lena M. Napolitano MD, FACS, FCCP, MCCM
Professor of Surgery
Founding Division Chief
Acute Care Surgery
Trauma, Burns, Critical Care, Emergency Surgery
Director
Trauma and Surgical Critical Care
University of Michigan Health System
Ann Arbor, Michigan, USA

James V. O'Connor, MD
Professor of Surgery
University of Maryland School of Medicine
Chief of Thoracic and Vascular Trauma
R Adams Cowley Shock Trauma Center
Baltimore, Maryland, USA

Jason Pasley, DO, FACS
Associate Professor of Surgery
Michigan State University
Trauma Medical Director
McLaren Oakland Hospital
Pontiac, Michigan, USA

Purvi P. Patel, MD
Assistant Professor
Trauma, Surgical Critical Care, and Burns
Loyola University Medical Center
Chicago, Illinois, USA

Andrew B. Peitzman, MD
Mark M. Ravitch Professor of Surgery
Distinguished Professor of Surgery
University of Pittsburgh School of Medicine
Pittsburgh, Pennsylvania, USA

Maryanne L. Pickett, MD
General Surgery Resident
University of Texas Southwestern Medical Center
Dallas, Texas, USA

Christian Renz, BS
Student
Loyola University Maryland
Baltimore, Maryland, USA

William S. Richardson, MD
Professor
University of Queensland
Director
Ochsner Surgical Weight Loss Program
Section Head
General, Laparoscopic, Bariatric, Acute Care, and
   Oncologic Surgery
Ochsner Health
New Orleans, Louisiana, USA

Aaron Richman, MD
Assistant Professor of Surgery
Boston University School of Medicine
Boston, Massachusetts, USA

Brendan Ringhouse, MD
General Surgery Resident
Loyola University Medical Center
Chicago, Illinois, USA

Ipek Sapci, MD
Surgeon
Department of Colorectal Surgery
Digestive Disease and Surgery Institute
Cleveland Clinic
Cleveland, Ohio, USA

Thomas Scalea, MD
Physician in Chief
R Adams Cowley Shock Trauma Center
University of Maryland School of Medicine
Baltimore, Maryland, USA

Morgan Schellenberg, MD, MPH, FRCSC
Assistant Professor of Clinical Surgery
Division of Acute Care Surgery
LAC+USC Medical Center
University of Southern California
Los Angeles, California, USA

David Spain, MD, FACS
David L. Gregg, MD Professor/Chief of Acute Care Surgery
Associate Division Chief of General Surgery
General Surgery Program Director
Department of Surgery
Stanford University
Trauma Medical Director
Stanford Healthcare
Stanford, California, USA

Scott R. Steele, MD, MBA, FACS, FASCRS
Chairman
Department of Colorectal Surgery
Digestive Disease and Surgery Institute
Cleveland Clinic
Cleveland, Ohio, USA

Ronald Stewart, MD
Witten B. Russ Professor and Chair
Department of Surgery
University of Texas Health Science Center at San Antonio
San Antonio, Texas, USA

George C. Velmahos, MD, PhD, MSEd
John F. Burke Professor of Surgery
Harvard Medical School
Chief
Trauma, Emergency Surgery, and Surgical Critical Care
Massachusetts General Hospital
Boston, Massachusetts, USA

Brendan Visser, MD
Associate Professor of Surgery
Hepatobiliary and Pancreatic Surgery
HPB Fellowship Program Director
Medical Director
Cancer Center GI Clinical Care Program
Stanford University School of Medicine
Stanford, California, USA

Lyndsey E. Wessels, MD
General Surgeon
Department of Surgery
Naval Medical Center San Diego
San Diego, California, USA

Robert D. Winfield, MD, FACS
Associate Professor of Surgery
Division Chief
Acute Care Surgery, Trauma, and Surgical Critical Care
Director of Trauma Research
University of Kansas Medical Center
Kansas City, Kansas, USA

Yee Wong, MD
Assistant Professor of Surgery
Department of Surgery
Wright State Physicians
Miami Valley Hospital
Dayton, Ohio, USA

1 The Definition of Acute Care Surgery

Robert D. Becher, Raul Coimbra, and Kimberly A. Davis

Summary

Since 2005, acute care surgery (ACS) has become widely accepted as a distinct surgical specialty and practice paradigm, encompassing three areas of surgical practice: trauma surgery, emergency general surgery, and surgical critical care. The recognition and formalization of the specialty continue to grow, as evidenced by the increasing number of ACS services at institutions throughout the U.S. In this chapter we define ACS, from its inception to today.

Keywords: Acute care surgery, emergency surgical care, surgical critical care, time-sensitive care

1.1 Drivers for the Acute Care Surgery Model

Like many things in medicine, the evolution and development of ACS was born out of necessity and innovation. Over the past three decades, there have been an insufficient number of physicians—including surgeons—participating in emergency call panels, a crisis highlighted by the Institute of Medicine report entitled "Hospital-based emergency care at the breaking point."[1,2,3] Compounding this crisis in access to emergency care is a growing workforce shortage of general surgeons. The American Association of Medical Colleges estimates that a 35% increase in the number of surgeons will be necessary to meet clinical demands by 2032.[4] An aging surgical workforce and increasing surgical subspecialization driven, in part, by technological advances have compounded these shortages, resulting in fewer general surgeons available to take emergency department call.[3] A 2005 survey demonstrated that nearly 75% of emergency department medical directors believed that they had inadequate on-call surgical specialist coverage.[5] Although workforce shortages exist across a range of medical disciplines, they are generally more significant for surgical disciplines. Over the 25-year period between 1981 and 2006, the U.S. population grew 31%, while the number of general surgeons grew by 4%.[6]

The provision of care to critically ill and injured patients challenges not only healthcare providers and medical centers but is straining the healthcare system nationwide.[7,8] According to the National Center for Health Statistics, 36 million people or 11.5% of the population had no health insurance in 2014.[9] From 1993 to 2013, there has been an increase of approximately 44% in the number of patients receiving care in emergency rooms across the country, while the number of emergency departments decreased by 558.[10] This problem is more severe for major teaching institutions, with 79% of their emergency rooms at or exceeding capacity.[11] The nation's emergency medical system is overburdened, underfunded, and highly fragmented.

A "perfect storm" was forming and care delivery to the surgical patient with emergent or urgent conditions could have neverbeen more at risk: few residents were interested in pursuing a career in trauma, there was a crisis in specialty call

coverage, and general surgeons with busy elective practices did not want to provide emergency surgery and trauma care.[12]

To address this multidimensional crisis in emergency care from a surgical patient perspective, in 2003, the surgical leadership of the American College of Surgeons and the American Association for the Surgery of Trauma defined and embraced a new surgical practice paradigm and subspecialty: ACS. In doing so, just as the needs of the injured patient drove the development of the field of trauma surgery, so too did the needs of the emergency general surgery patient drive the development of ACS.[13] The ACS training paradigm enhances the training of young surgeons in the areas of trauma, surgical critical care, and time-sensitive general surgery (▶ Fig. 1.1). This new paradigm begins to respond to the much bigger crises we face in assuring a future emergency surgical workforce.[14]

Although often used interchangeably, "emergency general surgery" and "acute care surgery" have different meanings. Whereas *emergency general surgery* refers to acute general surgical disorders, *ACS* includes surgical critical care and the surgical management of acutely ill patients with a variety of conditions including trauma, burns, surgical critical care, or an acute general surgical condition. The challenges in caring for these patients include round-the-clock readiness for the provision of comprehensive care, often constrained time for preoperative optimization of the patient, and greater potential for intraoperative and postoperative complications due to the emergent nature of care. In managing these patients, acute care surgeons are fulfilling a huge patient care demand as the number of patients with acute surgical disorders is on the rise (▶ Fig. 1.2).[2] Doubling as surgical intensivists, acute care surgeons provide not only a much-needed service but also continuity of care, both operating on the patients with an acute surgical disorder as well as caring for them postoperatively while critically ill in the intensive care unit, which is not matched in any other field.

The unscheduled nature of critical illness, injury, and non-trauma surgical emergencies, combined with the significant resources required to treat these diseases, continues to challenge healthcare providers and medical centers. The introduction of operative emergencies is inherently inefficient and disruptive to the smooth running of an operating room schedule, thereby adding stress to an already strained system and increasing frustration of the surgeons and the staff. In addition, the off-hours nature of most surgical emergencies requires that very costly resources be available 24 hours a day, regardless of utilization.[15]

Concurrently, the trend in patient care has shifted to the outpatient setting whenever possible to reduce costs. Consequently, hospitals have noted an increased acuity of inpatients, while simultaneously dealing with the demands for improved clinical efficiency and quality improvement. Operating rooms are run at maximal efficiency with little slack in the system. Surgeons are increasingly pressured to maximize their productivity as a method of maintaining reimbursement.[16] Almost all surgical specialties contribute positively to the hospital margin and,

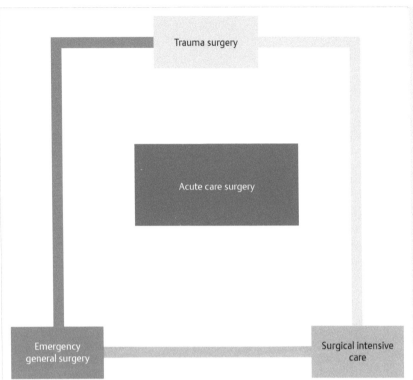

Fig. 1.1 The components of acute care surgery.

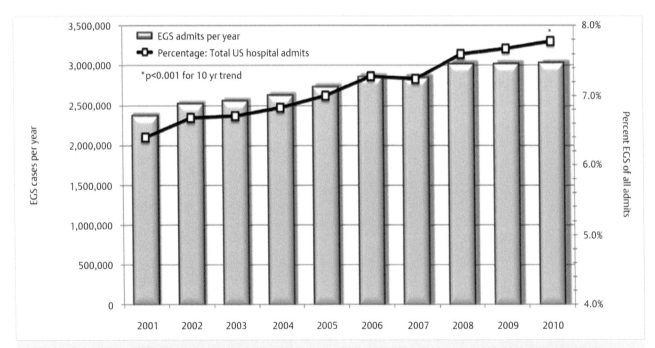

Fig. 1.2 Burden of Disease for Emergency General Surgery—United States. (Reproduced with permission of Gale S, Shafi S, Dombrovskiy V, et al. The public health burden of emergency general surgery in the United States: a 10-year analysis of the nationwide inpatient sample—2001 to 2010. J Trauma Acute Care Surg 2014;77:202–208.)

therefore, to the hospital's overall financial stability.[17] Therefore, it is in the hospital's financial benefit to support surgical activity and utilize a model that will increase that activity such as an ACS model. O'Mara and colleagues demonstrated the sustainability of an ACS model in a nontrauma setting. Evaluating emergency general surgery cases only, they demonstrated lower overall complications, decreased lengths of stay, and lower hospital costs, all attributable to the implementation of an ACS service at their institution.[18] These findings were confirmed by Diaz et al who reported that despite a high severity of illness, overall mortality and hospital lengths of stay would be less when managed by a mature ACS service.[19] Cost modeling analysis of the ACS model, with a dedicated OR, has cost savings potential for the healthcare system without reducing overall surgeon billing.[20] Having dedicated surgeons to this specific field is one hurdle; however, baseline resources like a dedicated operating room is critical.

ACS services must be staffed in such a way as to assure continuity of patient care. A cohesive group of surgeons dedicated to the service will assure accurate handoffs and consistency in patient throughput. There are various ways to implement the ACS model. Given the tripartite missions of ACS, surgeons are often dedicated to either the intensive care unit or a "floor" service, comprising either trauma, emergency general surgery, or some combination thereof. In busier institutions, elective cases are generally reserved for weeks when the ACS surgeon is "off-service," depending on their average volume of emergency and urgent surgery. Some models may incorporate non-ACS surgeons to spread the call out over a larger number of surgeons. This model is attractive to those surgeons who are interested in maintaining their "acute" surgical skills as well as those who wish to augment their elective practice volumes with emergency room referrals.

1.2 Fellowship Training in ACS

The core components of ACS are trauma, surgical critical care, and emergency general surgery. Fellowship training was designed to create a versatile surgeon able to confront a host of acute surgical disease processes. Initially described by the leadership of the American Association for the Surgery of Trauma (AAST), the suggested curriculum focused on both the clinical experience and operative expectations of a trainee. An initial list of "essential and desirable" operative cases was created, which focused on a broad range of predominantly trauma case types divided into anatomic region. This design attempts to ensure that a fully trained acute care surgeon is comfortable with a wide variety of anatomic exposures across all body regions.[21] The goal of the ACS fellowship was to master complex operative procedures in addition to completing an Accreditation Council for Graduate Medical Education (ACGME)-approved surgical critical care fellowship. Like general surgery residency, a case log system (Infotech, San Diego, CA) was created and used to determine if the fellows were receiving the intended operative experience.[21,22] When global deficiencies in training were identified, curricular changes included the identification of a minimum number of operative cases needed in specific body regions and in a manner similar to defined case volumes in general surgery. The desired case volume provides guidance to the fellows, program directors, and subspecialty colleagues with regard to the types of cases deemed important for the fellows' training.[23] Supplementing the operative curriculum required the creation of a comprehensive educational curriculum offering technical tricks needed when conducting complex operative procedures on patients who, due to severity of illness, do not have the luxury of preoperative optimization. The goals of training ACS surgeons would be demonstrated mastery in the field of ACS, above and beyond that learned in a general surgery residency. Unlike most specialty training, this paradigm strives to create a broad-based

surgical specialist, specifically trained in the treatment of acute surgical disease across a wide array of anatomic regions.[23]

As with the addition of any surgical fellowship, there is always a concern for how the current general surgery residents will be impacted. Dinan et al sought to determine if the addition of an ACS fellow negatively impacted the training of the current general surgery residents, comparing ACGME case log data among the general surgery residents before and after the initiation of the AAST-approved ACS fellowship at a level I trauma center. The authors reported that there was no significant change in the number of cases performed by the chief residents. Furthermore, residents were queried about the added value of the ACS fellow. Overall, there was a positive opinion of the fellows as teachers and most agreed that the fellows did not detract from the residents' experience.[24]

1.3 Surgeon Satisfaction with ACS

Several studies have focused on surgeon productivity since the implementation of an ACS model. Barnes et al compared operative productivity before and after the implementation of ACS and demonstrated a 66% increase in operative volume with an ACS service in place. Similarly, there was an increase in evaluation and management (E&M) work Relative Value Unit (wRVU) production as well as a rise in procedural wRVU production for both ACS and nontrauma surgeons. Both ACS surgeons and non-ACS surgeons reported improved job satisfaction with the implementation of an ACS service, stating they would prefer to work in a department that incorporated an ACS model.[16] Other studies have also shown an increase in OR cases and billing as well as an increase in surgeon satisfaction after the implementation of ACS.[25]

Additional studies have focused mainly on resident and surgeon interest and satisfaction with ACS. Recruitment into the field of trauma and critical care surgery was traditionally poor, as demonstrated by approximately 18% of fellowship positions unfilled in 2011. In 2015, this has improved to only 10% of positions going unfilled.[26] In 2012, Coleman et al surveyed residents regarding a career path in ACS which yielded a greater interest and understanding of ACS as a career.[27] Overall, these studies showed much greater interest and understanding of ACS as a career choice, encompassing surgical critical care and emergency surgery.

A Canadian study evaluated surgeons' satisfaction within an ACS model compared to those with a traditional call schedule. Those within the model, on average, had higher satisfaction scores than those surgeons not using an ACS model.[19] As the fellowship matures and acute care surgeons enter the workforce, this will hopefully become a more attractive option for rising surgical residents.

1.4 Patient Throughput Improvements with ACS

Multiple studies in North America, Australia, and Asia have demonstrated the efficiency and utility of an ACS model. Most of these studies analyzed the effectiveness as it pertained to appendectomies, nonelective cholecystectomies, and small bowel obstructions as these are among the most common ACS operations performed. Cubas et al showed a statistically significant decrease in time to surgical consultation, time to the operating room, fewer complications, and a reduced length of stay for appendectomies performed within an ACS model.[28] Fu et al showed a decreased amount of time in the emergency department by approximately 7 hours in Taiwan, and Pillai et al in Australia demonstrated an increase in the proportion of day time procedures.[29,30] Michailidou et al showed similar results when analyzing exclusively nonelective cholecystectomies with 75% of patients undergoing an operation within 24 hours in the ACS group as compared to 59% in the non-ACS group.[31] With the most recent evidence, the ACS model provides an efficient 24-hour coverage for surgical emergencies, providing not only surgical care but postoperative critical care in a timely and efficient fashion.[32]

1.5 Care Delivery Models

There is little data available as to patient care models for the provision of emergency general surgery. To et al used the Michigan Surgical Quality Collaborative to study this question. They found that most of the hospitals (74%) had a general surgery service (GSS) model, 14% had ACS model, and 12% had a hybrid model for emergency general care (EGS) patient care. The hybrid model was defined as a combination of EGS patient care coverage by both ACS and GSS. Most sites (79%) had a 24-hour surgeon call coverage structure for EGS patients. Coverage consisted of a different surgeon on call each night (97%). At half of the sites (58%), surgeons covered both EGS and trauma patients while on call. Only 59% of sites had a backup call system. In more than 50% of the hospitals, the on-call surgeon covered the night and weekend decision-making and the follow-up care for EGS patients. The EGS surgeon mostly had other concurrent responsibilities in addition to the emergency coverage, including teaching/administrative (50%), research (24%), and clinical (65%) responsibilities. This study was the first to demonstrate that an ACS model of care is associated with a 31% reduction in all-cause mortality after EGS.[33]

Daniel et al queried the American Hospital Association (AHA) to identify 3,322 acute care general hospitals providing EGS services. They conducted a survey using a hybrid mail/electronic methodology to determine variations in the delivery of EGS care. Their survey demonstrated that 16% of hospitals used a dedicated clinical team (ACS service) for the delivery of EGS, while 72% of hospitals used a more traditional general surgeon on-call model. Hospitals with ACS services tended to be major teaching institutions and have more than 500 beds.[34]

1.6 Standardizing Care: The Development of Grading Systems for EGS Diseases

EGS cases are a unique set of surgical conditions because they do not always require an urgent surgical intervention (▸ Fig. 1.3). A small subset of EGS conditions comprise 80% of the volume of cases and 74% of the cost associated with care delivery.[35] Unlike traumatic injuries, EGS conditions have historically not been categorized or graded, with few notable exceptions such as acute

pancreatitis[36,37] and colonic diverticulitis.[38,39] The range of patient management options and the lack of uniform risk stratification has made it challenging to study outcomes associated with these diseases and determine the quality of care provided. Furthermore, clear grading scales facilitate adoption by registries. These principles were used to define grades for 16 common EGS conditions (acute appendicitis, breast infections, acute cholecystitis, acute diverticulitis of the colon, esophageal perforation, hernias [internal or abdominal wall], infectious colitis, intestinal obstruction, intestinal arterial ischemia, acute pancreatitis, pelvic inflammatory disease, perirectal abscess, perforated peptic ulcer, pleural space infection, soft tissue infections, and surgical site infections).[40] To date, validation studies for the above grading scales has been performed for small bowel obstruction,[41,42] appendicitis,[43] cholecystitis,[44,45] diverticulitis[46] perforated peptic ulcer,[47] and necrotizing soft tissue infection.[48] It is hoped that formal guidelines for the treatment of EGS diseases will be forthcoming. A gap analysis of EGS guidelines was recently performed to address this issue.[49]

1.7 Improving Patient Outcomes after Emergency General Surgery

Since the 1970s, there has been a tremendous improvement in the outcomes of injured trauma patients in the United States.[50] Two interdependent factors have contributed to advancing the outcomes of injured patients: trauma-systems development and trauma research.[51] Coupled with the creation and advancement of a standardized trauma registry,[52,53,54,55,56] outcomes research has been crucial at defining patterns of injury, benchmarking, understanding and assessing risk-adjusted outcomes, improving trauma systems, and measuring processes of care for quality improvement.[57,58]

Modern-day outcomes research has moved beyond simply predicting mortality, and has become increasingly wide-ranging in its scope, with a mosaic of outcome metrics now analyzed.[58] Accordingly, outcomes research has now completely embraced a more modern definition of health, which is a "state of complete physical, mental, and social well-being and not merely the absence of disease or infirmity."[59]

The specialty of EGS is at a point like that of trauma surgery 45 years ago. The burden of EGS is significant: in 2010, the number of EGS admissions to acute care hospitals outnumbered those of other newly diagnosed common diseases including diabetes, coronary heart disease, cancer, heart failure, stroke, and HIV infection, making EGS a public health concern (▸ Fig. 1.4).[60] There is a lack of understanding about the systems through which EGS care is delivered, and there is a dearth of published studies outlining the determinants of EGS outcomes. For EGS outcomes research to be practice-changing, consistency of patientpopulations across studies and transparency regarding inclusion and exclusion criteria is of paramount importance. Diagnosis-based research was first successfully done at the institutional level[61] and has since been researched at a national level.[62] However, diagnosis-based research does not address the bigger picture of the scope of EGS practice which can be urgent or emergent, elective after a prior admission for an urgent disease process, and with or without serious physiologic derangements, necessitating care in the intensive care unit.

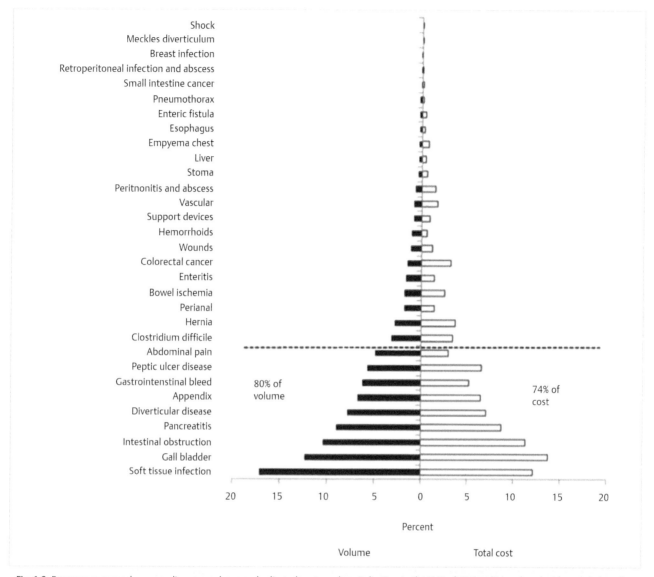

Fig. 1.3 Emergency general surgery diseases: volume and adjusted cost per hospitalization in the United States. (Reproduced with permission of Ogola G and Shafi S. Cost of specific emergency general surgery diseases and factors associated with high-cost patients. J Trauma Acute Care Surg 2016; 80:265–271.)

How best to risk adjust with such patient variability is one major limitation in the EGS outcomes literature to date. Accurate comparisons among disparate patient populations with varying degrees of risk require accurate adjustment strategies. Risk adjustment strategies can be very simple or very complex;[63] the important aspect is that they are valid and validated. This has not yet been done for EGS patients, as the datasets used to study EGS do not allow comprehensive risk adjustment.

A similar issue, also driven by the heterogeneity of the EGS patient population, is benchmarking EGS surgical outcomes and performance. Benchmarks are defined by leading medical and surgical organizations to establish standards of care and ensure surgical quality. Groups defining these measures include the Agency for Healthcare Research and Quality (AHRQ) and the National Quality Forum (NQF). As the discipline of EGS becomes increasingly studied and defined, these measures will be valuable for establishing national norms and standards of care. To date, however, given the poor methodologies at riskadjustment, EGS benchmarking attempts are largely lacking in the literature and have been inconsistent. As a result, despite the known heavy burden of EGS disease, little is known in the way of adjusted risk factors, complication rates, and predictors of EGS outcomes.[64]

The field of EGS is moving to address the need for quality, comprehensive data. Work is underway to create a national EGS data dictionary, and a pilot project has been conducted for an EGS registry modeled after National Surgical Quality Improvement Program (NSQIP).[25,65] This database has the potential to provide the field of EGS a powerful, risk-adjusted, prospective tool for EGS research. It would allow for the creation of metrics unique and specific to EGS: benchmarking, validated severity

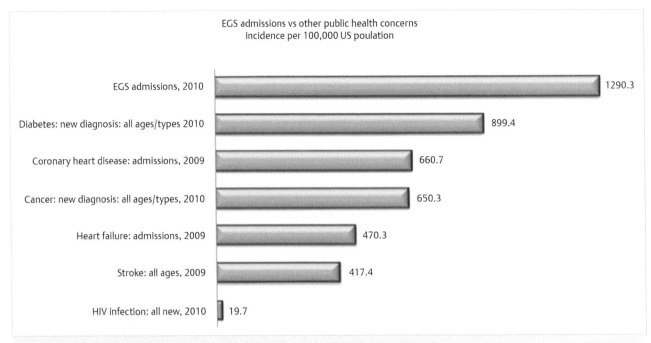

Fig. 1.4 The incidence of admission for emergency general surgery conditions compared with other common public health concerns. (Reproduced with permission of Gale S, Shafi S, Dombrovskiy V, et al. The public health burden of emergency general surgery in the United States: a 10-year analysis of the Nationwide Inpatient Sample—2001 to 2010. J Trauma Acute Care Surg 2014;77:202–208.)

scoring systems, and performance improvement information. The EGS database should also allow for considerable room for growth and advancement in the ability to predict myriad potential outcomes in EGS patients, such as appropriateness of care, cost-utility, patient-reported outcomes, satisfaction with care, functionality, and comparative effectiveness.[66,67,68,69]

1.8 Conclusion

The combination of surgeon shortage and poor access to emergency surgical care drove the creation of the ACS model. Creation of ACS services allow the time-critical delivery of emergent and urgent surgical care in the face of an identified surgeon workforce shortage. Potential pitfalls and initial concerns regarding the implementation of this model and introduction of fellowship training have not come to fruition. Our most critically ill surgical patients appear to have benefited, with improved outcomes, more efficient care, and decreased mortality. Acute care surgeons are uniquely positioned to impact healthcare cost containment and improve care in the United States as mandated by the Affordable Care Act of 2010. Cost savings can be actualized, and the system for care delivery can be focused on throughput as well as the use of standardized, evidence-based, and consistent care. Acute care surgeons stand at the frontline of care delivery for the patients who are most critically ill and for the injured surgical patients with time-sensitive diseases. Getting the right patient to the right venue at the right time is the paramount skill that the acute care surgeon, through training and experience, adds to the value equation.[70,71]

References

[1] Division of Advocacy and Health Policy. A growing crisis in patient access to emergency surgical care. Bull Am CollSurg. 2006; 91(8):8–19

[2] Napolitano LM, Fulda GJ, Davis KA, et al. Challenging issues in surgical critical care, trauma, and acute care surgery: a report from the Critical Care Committee of the American Association for the Surgery of Trauma. J Trauma. 2010; 69(6):1619–1633

[3] Institute of Medicine. The future of emergency care in the United States health system. Hospital based care at the breaking point. 2006

[4] American Association of Medical Colleges. The complexities of physician supply and demand: Projections from 2017 to 2032. Available at: https://aamc-black.global.ssl.fastly.net/production/media/filer_public/31/13/3113ee 5c-a038-4c16-89af-294a69826650/2019_update_-_the_complexities_of_physician_supply_and_demand_-_projections_from_2017-2032.pdf. Accessed April 29, 2020

[5] American College of Emergency Physicians. On-call specialist in U.S. Emergency Departments, ACEP survey of emergency department directors. April 2006

[6] Poley S, Belsky D, Gaul K, Ricketts T, Fraher E, Sheldon G. "Longitudinal trends in the U.S. Surgical Workforce, 1981–2006." Chapel Hill, North Carolina. American College of Surgeons Health Policy Research Institute, May 2009

[7] Jurkovich GJ, et al. Committee to Develop the Reorganized Specialty of Trauma, Surgical Critical Care, and Emergency Surgery. Acute care surgery: trauma, critical care, and emergency surgery. J Trauma. 2005; 58(3):614–616

[8] Moore EE, Maier RV, Hoyt DB, Jurkovich GJ, Trunkey DD. Acute care surgery: Eraritjaritjaka. J Am CollSurg. 2006; 202(4):698–701

[9] National Center for Health Statistics. Available at: https://www.cdc.gov/nchs/. Accessed April 29, 2020

[10] American Association of Medical Colleges. Available at: https://www.aamc.org. Accessed April 29, 2020

[11] American Hospital Association. Available at: https://www.aha.org/. Accessed April 29, 2020

[12] Coimbra R. Challenges, opportunities, unity, and global engagement: The 2017 AAST Presidential Address. J Trauma Acute Care Surg. 2019; 86(1): 62–70

[13] Davis KA, Jurkovich GJ. "An update on acute care surgery: emergence of acute care surgery." ACS Surgery News June 11, 2015

[14] Schwab CW. Crises and war: stepping stones to the future. J Trauma. 2007; 62 (1):1–16

[15] Kaplan LJ, Frankel H, Davis KA, Barie PS. Pitfalls of implementing acute care surgery. J Trauma. 2007; 62(5):1264–1270, discussion 1270–1271

[16] Barnes SL, Cooper CJ, Coughenour JP, MacIntyre AD, Kessel JW. Impact of acute care surgery to departmental productivity. J Trauma. 2011; 71(4): 1027–1032, discussion 1033–1034

[17] Resnick AS, Corrigan D, Mullen JL, Kaiser LR. Surgeon contribution to hospital bottom line: not all are created equal. Ann Surg. 2005; 242(4):530–537, discussion 537–539

[18] O'Mara MS, Scherer L, Wisner D, Owens LJ. Sustainability and success of the acute care surgery model in the nontrauma setting. J Am CollSurg. 2014; 219 (1):90–98

[19] Diaz JJ, Jr, Norris PR, Gunter OL, Collier BR, Riordan WP, Morris JA, Jr. Does regionalization of acute care surgery decrease mortality? J Trauma. 2011; 71 (2):442–446

[20] Anantha RV, Paskar D, Vogt K, Crawford S, Parry N, Leslie K. Allocating operating room resources to an acute care surgery service does not affect wait-times for elective cancer surgeries: a retrospective cohort study. World J EmergSurg. 2014; 9(1):21

[21] Dente CJ, Duane TM, Jurkovich GJ, Britt LD, Meredith JW, Fildes JJ. How much and what type: analysis of the first year of the acute care surgery operative case log. J Trauma Acute Care Surg. 2014; 76(2):329–338, discussion 338–339

[22] Duane TM, Dente CJ, Fildes JJ, et al. Defining the acute care surgery curriculum. J Trauma Acute Care Surg. 2015; 78(2):259–263, discussion 263–264

[23] Davis KA, Dente CJ, Burlew CC, et al. Refining the operative curriculum of the acute care surgery fellowship. J Trauma Acute Care Surg. 2015; 78(1):192–196

[24] Dinan KA, Davis JW, Wolfe MM, Sue LP, Cagle KM. An acute care surgery fellowship benefits a general surgical residency. J Trauma Acute Care Surg. 2014; 77(2):209–212

[25] Davis KA, Cabbad NC, Schuster KM, et al. Trauma team oversight of patient management improves efficiency of care and augments clinical and economic outcomes. J Trauma Inj Infect Crit Care. 2008; 65(6):1236–1242

[26] National Resident Matching Program. Available at: http://www.nrmp.org. Accessed April 29, 2020

[27] Coleman JJ, Esposito TJ, Rozycki GS, Feliciano DV. Acute care surgery: now that we have built it, will they come? J Trauma Acute Care Surg. 2013; 74(2): 463–468, discussion 468–469

[28] Cubas RF, Gómez NR, Rodriguez S, Wanis M, Sivanandam A, Garberoglio CA. Outcomes in the management of appendicitis and cholecystitis in the setting of a new acute care surgery service model: impact on timing and cost. J Am CollSurg. 2012; 215(5):715–721

[29] Fu CY, Huang HC, Chen RJ, Tsuo HC, Tung HJ. Implementation of the acute care surgery model provides benefits in the surgical treatment of the acute appendicitis. Am J Surg. 2014; 208(5):794–799

[30] Pillai S, Hsee L, Pun A, Mathur S, Civil I. Comparison of appendicectomy outcomes: acute surgical versus traditional pathway. ANZ J Surg. 2013; 83 (10):739–743

[31] Michailidou M, Kulvatunyou N, Friese RS, et al. Time and cost analysis of gallbladder surgery under the acute care surgery model. J Trauma Acute Care Surg. 2014; 76(3):710–714

[32] Khalil M, Pandit V, Rhee P, et al. Certified acute care surgery programs improve outcomes in patients undergoing emergency surgery: a nationwide analysis. J Trauma Acute Care Surg. 2015; 79(1):60–63, discussion 64

[33] To KB, Kamdar NS, Patil P, et al. Michigan Surgical Quality Collaborative (MSQC) Emergency General Surgery Study Group and the MSQC Research Advisory Group. Acute care surgery model and outcomes in emergency general surgery. J Am CollSurg. 2019; 228(1):21–28.e7

[34] Daniel VT, Ingraham AM, Khubchandani JA, Ayturk D, Kiefe CI, Santry HP. Variations in the delivery of emergency general surgery care in the era of acute care surgery. JtComm J Qual Patient Saf. 2019; 45(1):14–23

[35] Ogola GO, Shafi S. Cost of specific emergency general surgery diseases and factors associated with high-cost patients. J Trauma Acute Care Surg. 2016; 80(2):265–271

[36] Bradley EL, III. A clinically based classification system for acute pancreatitis. Summary of the International Symposium on Acute Pancreatitis, Atlanta, Ga, September 11 through 13, 1992. Arch Surg. 1993; 128(5):586–590

[37] Banks PA, Bollen TL, Dervenis C, et al. Acute Pancreatitis Classification Working Group. Classification of acute pancreatitis–2012: revision of the Atlanta classification and definitions by international consensus. Gut. 2013; 62(1): 102–111

[38] Hinchey EJ, Schaal PG, Richards GK. Treatment of perforated diverticular disease of the colon. AdvSurg. 1978; 12:85–109

[39] Klarenbeek BR, de Korte N, van der Peet DL, Cuesta MA. Review of current classifications for diverticular disease and a translation into clinical practice. Int J Colorectal Dis. 2012; 27(2):207–214

[40] Tominaga GT, Staudenmayer KL, Shafi S, et al. American Association for the Surgery of Trauma Committee on Patient Assessment. The American Association for the Surgery of Trauma grading scale for 16 emergency general surgery conditions: Disease-specific criteria characterizing anatomic severity grading. J Trauma Acute Care Surg. 2016; 81(3):593–602

[41] Baghdadi YMK, Morris DS, Choudhry AJ, et al. Validation of the anatomic severity score developed by the American Association for the Surgery of Trauma in small bowel obstruction. J Surg Res. 2016; 204(2):428–434

[42] Hernandez MC, Haddad NN, Cullinane DC, et al. EAST SBO Workgroup. The American Association for the Surgery of Trauma Severity Grade is valid and generalizable in adhesive small bowel obstruction. J Trauma Acute Care Surg. 2018; 84(2):372–378

[43] Hernandez MC, Aho JM, Habermann EB, Choudhry AJ, Morris DS, Zielinski MD. Increased anatomic severity predicts outcomes: validation of the American Association for the Surgery of Trauma's Emergency General Surgery score in appendicitis. J Trauma Acute Care Surg. 2017; 82(1):73–79

[44] Hernandez M, Murphy B, Aho JM, et al. Validation of the AAST EGS acute cholecystitis grade and comparison with the Tokyo guidelines. Surgery. 2018; 163(4):739–746

[45] Vera K, Pei KY, Schuster KM, Davis KA. Validation of a new American Association for the Surgery of Trauma (AAST) anatomic severity grading system for acute cholecystitis. J Trauma Acute Care Surg. 2018; 84(4):650–654

[46] Shafi S, Priest EL, Crandall MC, et al. Multicenter validation of American Association for the Surgery of Trauma grading system for acute colonic diverticulitis and its use for emergency general surgery quality improvement program. J Trauma Acute Care Sur. 2016; 80:405–410; discussion 410–411

[47] Hernandez MC, Thorn MJ, Kong VY, et al. Validation of the AAST EGS grading system for perforated peptic ulcer disease. Surgery. 2018; 164(4):738–745

[48] Savage SA, Li SW, Utter GH, et al. The EGS grading scale for skin and soft-tissue infections is predictive of poor outcomes: a multicenter validation study. J Trauma Acute Care Surg. 2019; 86(4):601–608

[49] Schuster K, Davis K, Hernandez M, Holena D, Salim A, Crandall M. American Association for the Surgery of Trauma emergency general surgery guidelines gap analysis. J Trauma Acute Care Surg. 2019; 86(5):909–915

[50] MacKenzie EJ, Rivara FP, Jurkovich GJ, et al. A national evaluation of the effect of trauma-center care on mortality. N Engl J Med. 2006; 354(4): 366–378

[51] Trunkey DD. History and development of trauma care in the United States. ClinOrthopRelat Res. 2000(374):36–46

[52] Champion HR, Copes WS, Sacco WJ, et al. The Major Trauma Outcome Study: establishing national norms for trauma care. J Trauma. 1990; 30(11): 1356–1365

[53] Boyd DR, Lowe RJ, Baker RJ, Nyhus LM. Trauma registry. New computer method for multifactorial evaluation of a major health problem. JAMA. 1973; 223(4):422–428

[54] American College of Surgeons. Trauma Programs: National Trauma Data Bank (NTDB) [Internet]. [cited 2016 Oct 4]. Available at: http://www.facs.org/trauma/ntdb/index.html. Accessed January 21, 2019

[55] Morabito DJ, Proctor SM, May CM. Overview of trauma registries. J AHIMA. 1992; 63(2):39–44, 46, 48

[56] Rutledge R. The goals, development, and use of trauma registries and trauma data sources in decision making in injury. Surg Clin North Am. 1995; 75(2): 305–326

[57] Finlayson EVA, Birkmeyer JD. "Benchmarking Surgical Outcomes" in ACS: Principles and Practice. 6th ed. B.C. Decker; 2007

[58] Kane RL. Understanding Health Care Outcomes Research. 2nd ed. Burlington, MA: Jones & Bartlett Pub; 2005

[59] World Health Organization: WHO constitution. Available at: https://www.who.int/about/who-we-are/constitution. Accessed April 29, 2020

[60] Gale SC, Shafi S, Dombrovskiy VY, Arumugam D, Crystal JS. The public health burden of emergency general surgery in the United States: a 10-year analysis of the Nationwide Inpatient Sample–2001 to 2010. J Trauma Acute Care Surg. 2014; 77(2):202–208

[61] Becher RD, Meredith JW, Chang MC, Hoth JJ, Beard HR, Miller PR. Creation and implementation of an emergency general surgery registry modeled after the National Trauma Data Bank. J Am CollSurg. 2012; 214(2):156–163

[62] Shafi S, Aboutanos MB, Agarwal S, Jr, et al. AAST Committee on Severity Assessment and Patient Outcomes. Emergency general surgery: definition and estimated burden of disease. J Trauma Acute Care Surg. 2013; 74(4): 1092–1097

[63] Iezzoni LI. Risk Adjustment for Measuring Healthcare Outcomes. 3rd ed. Chicago, IL: Health Administration Press; 2003

[64] Shah AA, Haider AH, Zogg CK, et al. National estimates of predictors of outcomes for emergency general surgery. J Trauma Acute Care Surg. 2015; 78: 482–490; discussion 490–491

[65] Yeo H, Bucholz E, Ann Sosa J, et al. A national study of attrition in general surgery training: which residents leave and where do they go? Ann Surg. 2010; 252(3):529–534, discussion 534–536

[66] Lee CN, Ko CY. Beyond outcomes–the appropriateness of surgical care. JAMA. 2009; 302(14):1580–1581

[67] Holtslag HR, van Beeck EF, Lindeman E, Leenen LPH. Determinants of long-term functional consequences after major trauma. J Trauma. 2007; 62(4):919–927

[68] Schluter PJ, Neale R, Scott D, Luchter S, McClure RJ. Validating the functional capacity index: a comparison of predicted versus observed total body scores. J Trauma. 2005; 58(2):259–263

[69] Iglehart JK. Prioritizing comparative-effectiveness research–IOM recommendations. N Engl J Med. 2009; 361(4):325–328

[70] Davis KA, Jurkovich GJ. Fellowship training in acute care surgery: from inception to current state. Trauma Surg Acute Care Open. 2016, May 31; 1(1):e000004

[71] Frankel HL, Butler KL, Cuschieri J, et al. The role and value of surgical critical care, an essential component of acute care surgery, in the Affordable Care Act: a report from the Critical Care Committee and Board of Managers of the American Association for the Surgery of Trauma. J Trauma Acute Care Surg. 2012; 73(1): 20–26

2 Anatomic and Physiological Considerations

Bishwajit Bhattacharya and Kimberly A. Davis

Summary

Minimally invasive surgery has seen an increasing role in the management of several surgical disease processes. This has resulted in the reduction of morbidity for several procedures. However, there are limitations and psychological considerations for the operating surgeon to consider when opting for laparoscopic intervention. In this chapter, we have discussed the unique considerations in a variety of patient populations.

Keywords: Laprascopy, physiology

2.1 Introduction

Over the past three decades, minimally invasive surgery has increasingly been used in the treatment of surgical disease processes, and in many circumstances, it has become the standard of care.[1] Despite the growing acceptability of a minimally invasive approach to surgery, there are anatomic and physiologic limitations to consider. At times, a more traditional open approach may be safer. With technical advances in laparoscopic equipment and growing surgeon familiarity with technique, the ability to perform complex abdominal surgical interventions has increased.[2,3] There are many advantages to a minimally invasive approach including decreased morbidity and improved cosmesis.[4,5] In certain circumstances, the benefits of laparoscopy over laparotomy are debatable.[6] However, an individual's physiology and anatomy must be taken into consideration when opting for a minimally invasive approach.

2.2 Physiological Effects of Laparoscopy

A minimally invasive approach requires the establishment of a working space by insufflation of the abdomen with carbon dioxide. Other gases such as air, oxygen, and nitrogen dioxide have been used in the past but have been discontinued due to concerns with regard to gas embolism, increased abdominal pain, and flammability.[7] Carbon dioxide is the gas of choice due to its high solubility, rapid absorption, elimination, and affordability. ▶ Table 2.1 demonstrates the physiologic effects caused by the combined effects of general anesthesia and intra-abdominal insufflation which are necessary to perform laparoscopy.

The risk of gas embolism with the use of carbon dioxide is estimated at 1:65,000 and more likely in cases of inadvertent venous entry.[8] Operations involving venous dissection such as liver resections are more likely to experience gas embolism. In extreme cases, a large embolus can result in cardiac collapse. Should a gas embolus occur, rapid desufflation of the abdomen should be performed and the patient should be placed in the Trendelenburg position. Pharmacologic cardiac support and, in rare cases, advanced cardiac life support may be required to provide cardiocirculatory support. A central line can be placed to aspirate the embolus.[9]

2.2.1 Physiologic Effects of Increased Intra-abdominal Pressure

Abdominal insufflation leads to hemodynamic and pulmonary effects by two basic mechanisms. First, the intra-abdominal hypertension created by gas insufflation can cause compression of the inferior vena cava (IVC), resulting in decreasing venous return and consequent decreases in cardiac output, displacement of the diaphragm cephalad, and decreased splanchnic blood flow.[10,11] The splanchnic circulation can be directly compromised by the creation of intra-abdominal hypertension during insufflation, a problem that may be mitigated by maintaining the total pressure delivered at less than 15 mm Hg.[12] Patients with preoperative hemodynamic instability may not tolerate abdominal insufflation. In fact, hemodynamic compromise is a relative contraindication to laparoscopy.

Second, the insufflation of the abdomen exerts pressure on the diaphragm and can compromise pulmonary dynamics. Due to the upward pressure on the diaphragm and stiffening of the abdominal part of the chest wall, compliance can decrease by 30 to 40%, which is accompanied by increased pulmonary resistance.[13,14] Patients with normal pulmonary reserve tolerate insufflation well; however, patients with underlying pulmonary insufficiency may have difficulty tolerating pneumoperitoneum. The upward displacement caused by abdominal insufflation can also cause the carina to be shifted cephalad, thus moving a low-lying tracheal tube to an endobronchial position.[7] Insufflation in combination with the Trendelenburg position may increase the risk of aspiration of gastric contents.

Insufflation also causes a neurohormonal response, which has an impact on the cardiovascular system. Plasma norepinephrine, epinephrine, cortisol, vasopressin, atrial natriuretic peptide, renin, and aldosterone levels increase with insufflation.[15] As renal blood supply decreases due to vascular compression, renin and aldosterone levels rise, thereby initially increasing cardiac output. However, with increasing intra-abdominal pressure, cardiac output falls below baseline levels. Abdominal insufflation distends the peritoneum and can increase vagal tone, which can lead to bradycardia and possibly asystole (▶ Fig. 2.1).

Table 2.1 Hemodynamic effects of laparoscopy

	HR	MAP	CO	SVR
Induction of anesthesia	↓	↓	↓	↓
Abdominal insufflation	→	↑	↓	↑
Abdominal desufflation	→↑	↓	↑	↓
Recovery from anesthesia	↑	↑	↑	↑

Abbreviations: CO, cardiac output; HR, heart rate; MAP, mean arterial pressure; SVR, systemic vascular resistance.

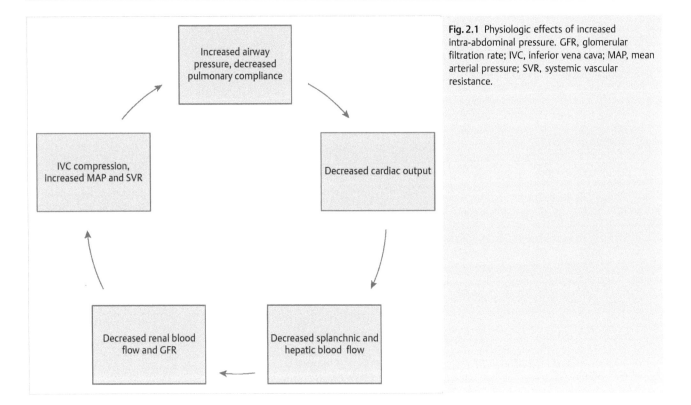

Fig. 2.1 Physiologic effects of increased intra-abdominal pressure. GFR, glomerular filtration rate; IVC, inferior vena cava; MAP, mean arterial pressure; SVR, systemic vascular resistance.

2.2.2 Physiologic Effects of Hypercarbia

Carbon dioxide is also directly absorbed by the peritoneum casing hypercarbia, which may result in systemic acidosis, leading to decreased cardiac contractility and myocardial depression. The resultant acidosis can also impair hemoglobin affinity and oxygen transport. Hypercarbia also causes a centrally mediated sympathetic response, resulting in tachycardia and vasoconstriction that counteracts the vasodilatory effect of the acidosis.[16,17]

Hypercarbia created by carbon dioxide insufflation negatively impacts pulmonary function. Direct effects of hypercarbia include increased pulmonary pressure and pulmonary vascular resistance. These result in pulmonary vasoconstriction. Carbon dioxide insufflation can also result in subcutaneous emphysema in less than 3% of cases. This is usually caused by inadvertent insufflation of the subcutaneous space which dissects through the subcutaneous tissues and retroperitoneum. Subcutaneous emphysema is usually not of clinical significance. However, when emphysema extends into the mediastinum and pleura, it can result in pneumomediastinum or pneumothorax. Usually, the pneumothoraces do not require chest tube decompression as they are reabsorbed quickly.[7]

Visceral perfusion is also impacted by hypercarbia. Diminished cardiac output, due to a combination of decreased venous return and metabolic acidosis, contributes to compromised splanchnic circulation, resulting in decreased hepatic and intestinal pH. The combined effect of these phenomena does not usually cause bowel ischemia in a healthy individual. Similarly, renal perfusion and output can be compromised during laparoscopic surgery, resulting in decreased glomerular filtration rate and oliguria. The presence of acidosis encourages renal proton excretion. Patients with chronic kidney disease are at increased risk of acute kidney injury (▶ Fig. 2.2).[18,19]

2.3 Anatomic Considerations

There are several anatomic considerations when deciding to use a minimally invasive approach. As laparoscopy requires a viable working space, certain anatomic findings and disease-specific anatomic derangements may limit the ability to perform laparoscopically safely.

Port placement should be remote from the anatomic location, requiring intervention to facilitate adequate working space and offer optimal ergonomics for the surgeon. If the surgeon is unsure of the location of the area of pathology, starting with a diagnostic laparoscopy can help in identifying the area of interest before placing additional ports. In the preoperative abdomen, adhesions to the anterior abdominal wall may make abdominal entry difficult. Entrance into the abdomen remote from the patient's prior scar is advisable. Veress needle, open Hasson technique, or optical trocar entry may all be safely used for primary port placement. Previous surgical intervention may create adhesive scar tissue which will limit working space and visualization.[20] Simple adhesions may be taken down laparoscopically, but dense adhesions and prior intraperitoneal mesh increase the likelihood of conversion to an open approach.[21] The patient should be positioned to allow the viscera to fall away from point of interest; however, this may result in respiratory and/or cardiovascular changes that may not be well-tolerated. Patients with a large body habitus may not tolerate an extreme Trendelenburg position due to increased pressure on the diaphragm.[22] Finally, when deciding whether a minimally invasive approach is feasible, the

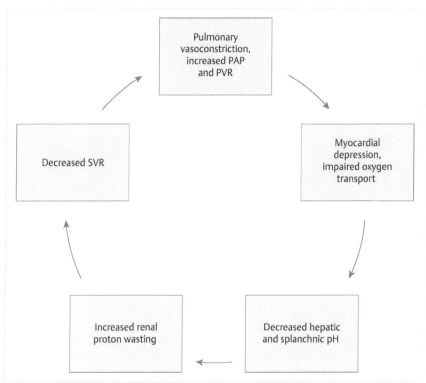

Fig. 2.2 Physiologic effects of hypercarbia. PAP, pulmonary artery pressure; PVR, pulmonary vascular resistance; SVR, systemic vascular resistance.

skill set and comfort of the operating surgeon are important factors to consider. A surgeon who recognizes his/her skill set limitations and opts for an open approach exercises sound judgement.

With the advent of robotic surgery, surgeons are now provided with more dexterity to perform minimally invasive procedures that were previously not feasible or extremely challenging, such as pancreaticoduodenectomy, liver resections, and complex pelvic dissections.[23,24,25]

2.4 Patient Populations

2.4.1 Pediatric Patients

With technological advances in laparoscopic equipment, minimally invasive surgery is now feasible in infants and even neonates. Laparoscopic interventions are performed on a variety of surgical diseases, ranging from common problems such as acute appendicitis and inguinal hernias to less common procedures such as Kasai procedures and abdominal tumor resections.[26,27,28,29,30] In pediatric patients, the creation of a feasible working space can be facilitated by draining the stomach and bladder with catheters to increase abdominal space. In newborn and small infants, pneumoperitoneum can be established with lower pressures (6–8 mm Hg) while higher pressures (8–10 mm Hg) are required in older children. Adolescents can tolerate pressures of 10 to 12 mm Hg.[31] Smaller trocars, 3 to 5 mm in size, are commonly used in pediatric cases. Children maybe more prone to developing trocar site hernia and port sizes greater than 5 mm should be closed.[32,33] The pediatric abdomen is more elastic and thin, thus port site misplacement and inadvertent injury to the underlying viscera are more common.[31] Insufflation causes

pulmonary dynamic changes in infants like adults, but they are not of significant consequence if adequately monitored.[34] Historically, children with cardiac anomalies were excluded from minimally invasive surgery due to concerns related to hemodynamic instability and heart failure. With appropriate perioperative monitoring, these patients can be safely managed during laparoscopy.[35]

2.4.2 Pregnant Patients

It is common for pregnant women to face surgical emergencies, most commonly gallbladder disease and appendicitis.[36] It is estimated that 2% of pregnant patients undergo nonobstetrical surgery in the US.[37] The pregnant patient undergoes many physiological changes, including restrictive pulmonary physiology, due the enlarged uterus and hormone-induced chronic respiratory alkalosis. Cardiac output increases by 30 to 40% by weeks 24 to 28 of gestation, and systemic vascular resistance (SVR) is lowered due to circulating prostacyclin levels. Blood volume increases by 30 to 40% also with a small increase in red blood cell volume, resulting in the physiologic anemia of pregnancy. In addition, pharmacokinetic and pharmacodynamic changes must be considered in the administration of anesthesia, including the possibility of teratogenesis. Minimum alveolar concentration of anesthetics is decreased by 25 to 40%.[38,39]

When creating a pneumoperitoneum, potential physiological changes must be taken into consideration. Insufflation in the pregnant patient can decrease cardiac index and venous return by up to 50%. Positioning the patient in the Trendelenburg can exacerbate these physiologic changes and cause fetal distress.[40]

Insufflation in the presence of a large uterus further limits diaphragm expansion and is associated with a greater increase in peak airway pressure, decrease in functional reserve capacity, increase in ventilation-perfusion mismatch, increase in alveolar-arterial oxygen gradient, decrease in thoracic cavity compliance, and increase in pleural pressure. In combination, these physiologic changes in the pulmonary system increase the risk of maternal hypoxemia and fetal distress. Similarly, carbon dioxide absorbed by the peritoneum can cause maternal hypercapnia, which may potentially affect the fetus.[41]

Despite the potential risks, minimally invasive approaches can be performed in pregnant patients. When feasible, it may be optimal to delay semielective no-obstetric surgery till the second trimester when organogenesis is complete, and the risk of teratogenesis and spontaneous abortions are markedly reduced. Surgery during the third trimester is associated with greater risk of preterm labor and greater difficulty in intra-abdominal visualization due to the presence of the gravid uterus. Pregnant patients undergoing surgical intervention should undergo proper preoperative and postoperative fetal monitoring.[39]

2.4.3 Geriatric Patients

As worldwide life expectancy increases, an increasing number of geriatric patients are undergoing minimally invasive operations, both electively and emergently. Older age is associated with several physiological changes. Cardiac function decreases over time but is dependent upon conditioning. Cardiac output decreases gradually after age 30 and may fall by 50% by age 80.[42] The compliance of the cardiovascular system decreases with stiffening of arteries and cardiac chambers, which make the elderly patient less tolerant to volume changes.[43] Along with changes in compliance, baroreceptors in the elderly have decreased sensitivity, making the patient more prone to hypotension. Pulmonary reserves also decline gradually over time. Vital capacity, FEV_1, and PaO_2 decrease gradually after age 20.[44] Changes in the lung parenchyma cause decreased compliance and increased shunting, reducing efficiency of gas exchange. These changes are also accompanied by a marked suppression of hyperventilation in the presence of hypoxia or hypercapnia, placing these patients at a higher risk of respiratory failure.

Increased intra-abdominal pressure also adds additional pressure on the diaphragm which may further decrease lung compliance, which is already exacerbated by placing the patient in the Trendelenburg position. Insufflation with carbon dioxide can lead to systemic acidosis, resulting in increase in SVR and blood pressure. Patients with decreased pulmonary reserve cannot compensate for the hypercapnia, exacerbating the acidosis. To overcome the increased vascular resistance, patients with adequate cardiopulmonary reserve will compensate by increasing cardiac contractility; however, those with diminished reserve may develop cardiac failure during pneumoperitoneum. There have been case reports of mesenteric ischemia following routine laparoscopic interventions in patients with preexisting cardiovascular, hepatic, and renal compromise.[17]

Despite the potential pitfalls of insufflation, minimally invasive surgery can be safely performed in the elderly. The most common minimally invasive procedures performed in the geriatric population include cholecystectomy, abdominal wall hernia repair, and colon resections. Many studies have demonstrated clear advantages of a minimally invasive approach, not limited to decreased morbidity, mortality, and hospital length of stay among geriatric patients.[45,46] In addition, there may be immunological benefits of laparoscopic surgery which may theoretically reduce postoperative tumor growth.[47]

2.5 Other Physiological Considerations of Minimally Invasive Surgery

A minimally invasive approach to surgery has many other physiological effects that are not apparent to the surgeon immediately in the perioperative setting. Basic science research over the decades has demonstrated many changes in inflammatory and immunological responses during laparoscopic surgery. Compared to conventional invasive operations, laparoscopy imposes a smaller wound burden and stress on the patient. However, the diminished stress and inflammatory response has been shown to be the result of not only a smaller wound burden but many complex beneficial immune responses related to carbon dioxide insufflation into the peritoneum. These include a decreased TNF-α production by peritoneal macrophages as well as a decrease in phagocytosis activity. Several studies have shown a lower level of cytokine and acute phase proteins after a minimally invasive approach compared to open operations. A contributing factor to the decreased adhesion formation after laparoscopic surgery is the inhibition of the plasmin system in the peritoneum which is, in part, attributed to the acidosis created by carbon dioxide insufflation. This beneficial immunological response may confer a benefit in oncological operations by suppressing tumor growth.[47,48]

2.6 Future of Minimally Invasive Surgery

The role of minimally invasive surgery has grown rapidly over the past three decades. In many circumstances, it has been the gold standard in surgical treatment. As minimally invasive surgery evolves with the use of robotic surgery, the physiological and anatomical considerations will also change. Robotic surgery offers the ability to have additional dexterity not afforded by laparoscopic surgery, enabling procedures that were previously too challenging or not feasible to perform. Although in its relatively early stages, robotics is now being used in minimally invasive cardiac surgery, Whipple procedures, and other complex hepatobiliary cases, in addition to complex abdominal wall reconstructions.[23,24,49,50] As these techniques evolve, and surgical experience increases, so will our understanding of potential limitations.

References

[1] Soper NJ, Stockmann PT, Dunnegan DL, Ashley SW. Laparoscopic cholecystectomy. The new 'gold standard'? Arch Surg. 1992; 127(8):917–921, discussion 921 923

[2] Hoogerboord CM, Levy AR, Hu M, Flowerdew G, Porter G. Uptake of elective laparoscopic colectomy for colon cancer in Canada from 2004–05 to 2014–15: a descriptive analysis. CMAJ Open. 2018; 6(3):E384–E390

[3] Jean RA, O'Neill KM, Pei KY, Davis KA. Impact of hospital volume on outcomes for laparoscopic adhesiolysis for small bowel obstruction. J Surg Res. 2017; 214:23–31

[4] Pei KY, Asuzu DT, Davis KA. Laparoscopic colectomy reduces complications and hospital length of stay in colon cancer patients with liver disease and ascites. SurgEndosc. 2018; 32(3):1286–1292

[5] Southgate E, Vousden N, Karthikesalingam A, Markar SR, Black S, Zaidi A. Laparoscopic vs open appendectomy in older patients. Arch Surg. 2012; 147 (6):557–562

[6] Sporn E, Petroski GF, Mancini GJ, Astudillo JA, Miedema BW, Thaler K. Laparoscopic appendectomy–is it worth the cost? Trend analysis in the US from 2000 to 2005. J Am CollSurg. 2009; 208(2):179–85.e2

[7] Gutt CN, Oniu T, Mehrabi A, et al. Circulatory and respiratory complications of carbon dioxide insufflation. Dig Surg. 2004; 21(2):95–105

[8] Root B, Levy MN, Pollack S, Lubert M, Pathak K. Gas embolism death after laparoscopy delayed by "trapping" in portal circulation. AnesthAnalg. 1978; 57 (2):232–237

[9] Kim CS, Kim JY, Kwon JY, et al. Venous air embolism during total laparoscopic hysterectomy: comparison to total abdominal hysterectomy. Anesthesiology. 2009; 111(1):50–54

[10] Odeberg-Wernerman S. Laparoscopic surgery–effects on circulatory and respiratory physiology: an overview. Eur J SurgSuppl. 2000; 166 (585):4–11

[11] Atkinson TM, Giraud GD, Togioka BM, Jones DB, Cigarroa JE. Cardiovascular and Ventilatory Consequences of Laparoscopic Surgery. Circulation. 2017; 135(7):700–710

[12] Hatipoglu S, Akbulut S, Hatipoglu F, Abdullayev R. Effect of laparoscopic abdominal surgery on splanchnic circulation: historical developments. World J Gastroenterol. 2014; 20(48):18165–18176

[13] Pelosi P, Foti G, Cereda M, Vicardi P, Gattinoni L. Effects of carbon dioxide insufflation for laparoscopic cholecystectomy on the respiratory system. Anaesthesia. 1996; 51(8):744–749

[14] Rauh R, Hemmerling TM, Rist M, Jacobi KE. Influence of pneumoperitoneum and patient positioning on respiratory system compliance. J ClinAnesth. 2001; 13(5):361–365

[15] Hirvonen EA, Nuutinen LS, Vuolteenaho O. Hormonal responses and cardiac filling pressures in head-up or head-down position and pneumoperitoneum in patients undergoing operative laparoscopy. Br J Anaesth. 1997; 78(2): 128–133

[16] Feig BW, Berger DH, Dougherty TB, et al. Pharmacologic intervention can reestablish baseline hemodynamic parameters during laparoscopy. Surgery. 1994; 116:733–9; discussion 739–41

[17] Portera CA, Compton RP, Walters DN, Browder IW. Benefits of pulmonary artery catheter and transesophageal echocardiographic monitoring in laparoscopic cholecystectomy patients with cardiac disease. Am J Surg. 1995; 169: 202–206; discussion 206–207

[18] Koivusalo AM, Kellokumpu I, Ristkari S, Lindgren L. Splanchnic and renal deterioration during and after laparoscopic cholecystectomy: a comparison of the carbon dioxide pneumoperitoneum and the abdominal wall lift method. AnesthAnalg. 1997; 85(4):886–891

[19] Dunn MD, McDougall EM. Renal physiology. Laparoscopic considerations. UrolClin North Am. 2000; 27(4):609–614

[20] Nagle A, Ujiki M, Denham W, Murayama K. Laparoscopic adhesiolysis for small bowel obstruction. Am J Surg. 2004; 187(4):464–470

[21] Lujan HJ, Oren A, Plasencia G, et al. Laparoscopic management as the initial treatment of acute small bowel obstruction. JSLS. 2006; 10(4): 466–472

[22] Cunningham AJ. Anesthetic implications of laparoscopic surgery. Yale J Biol Med. 1998; 71(6):551–578

[23] Kornaropoulos M, Moris D, Beal EW, et al. Total robotic pancreaticoduodenectomy: a systematic review of the literature. Surg Endosc. 2017; 31(11): 4382–4392

[24] Di Benedetto F, Magistri P, Halazun KJ. Use of robotics in liver donor right hepatectomy. HepatobiliarySurgNutr. 2018; 7(3):231–232

[25] Lorenzon L, Bini F, Balducci G, Ferri M, Salvi PF, Marinozzi F. Laparoscopic versus robotic-assisted colectomy and rectal resection: a systematic review and meta-analysis. Int J Colorectal Dis. 2016; 31(2):161–173

[26] Canty TG, Sr, Collins D, Losasso B, Lynch F, Brown C. Laparoscopic appendectomy for simple and perforated appendicitis in children: the procedure of choice? J Pediatr Surg. 2000; 35(11):1582–1585

[27] Holcomb GW, III, Olsen DO, Sharp KW. Laparoscopic cholecystectomy in the pediatric patient. J Pediatr Surg. 1991; 26(10):1186–1190

[28] Jessula S, Davies DA. Evidence supporting laparoscopic hernia repair in children. CurrOpinPediatr. 2018; 30(3):405–410

[29] Yamataka A. Laparoscopic Kasai portoenterostomy for biliary atresia. J Hepatobiliary Pancreat Sci. 2013 Jun; 20(5):481–6. J Pediatr Surg. 2014; 49 (11):1544–1548

[30] Warmann SW, Godzinski J, van Tinteren H, Heij H, Powis M, Sandstedt B, et al. Minimally invasive nephrectomy for Wilms tumors in children—data from SIOP 2001. J Pediatr Surg. 2014 Nov; 49(11):1544–1548

[31] Lobe TE. Laparoscopic surgery in children. CurrProblSurg. 1998; 35(10): 859–948

[32] Bloom DA, Ehrlich RM. Omental evisceration through small laparoscopy port sites. J Endourol. 1993; 7(1):31–32, discussion 32–33

[33] Mark SD. Omental herniation through a small laparoscopic port. Br J Urol. 1995; 76(1):137–138

[34] Bannister CF, Brosius KK, Wulkan M. The effect of insufflation pressure on pulmonary mechanics in infants during laparoscopic surgical procedures. PaediatrAnaesth. 2003; 13(9):785–789

[35] Burgmeier C, Schier F, Staatz G. Gastric outlet obstruction in a neonate because of Peutz-Jeghers syndrome. J PediatrSurg. 2012; 47(8):e1–e3

[36] Fatum M, Rojansky N. Laparoscopic surgery during pregnancy. Obstet Gynecol Surv. 2001; 56(1):50–59

[37] Augustin G, Majerovic M. Non-obstetrical acute abdomen during pregnancy. Eur J ObstetGynecolReprodBiol. 2007; 131(1):4–12

[38] Skubic JJ, Salim A. Emergency general surgery in pregnancy. Trauma Surg Acute Care Open. 2017; 2(1):e000125

[39] Shay DC, Bhavani-Shankar K, Datta S. Laparoscopic surgery during pregnancy. AnesthesiolClin North America. 2001; 19(1):57–67

[40] Joris JL, Noirot DP, Legrand MJ, Jacquet NJ, Lamy ML. Hemodynamic changes during laparoscopic cholecystectomy. AnesthAnalg. 1993; 76(5):1067–1071

[41] Steinbrook RA, Brooks DC, Datta S. Laparoscopic cholecystectomy during pregnancy. Review of anesthetic management, surgical considerations. SurgEndosc. 1996; 10(5):511–515

[42] Raymond R. Anesthetic management of the elderly patient. 53rd ASA Annual Meeting Refresher Course Lectures #321. 2002; pp 1–7

[43] Tasch MD. Cardiovascular and autonomic nervous system aging. Syllabus on Geriatric Anesthesiology ASA 2002; pp 1–3

[44] Francis J Jr. Surgery in the elderly. David R Goldman, Frank H Brown, David M Guarneri, eds. Peri-Operative Medicine. 2nd ed. USA: McGraw-Hill, Inc.;1994; 385–94

[45] Stewart BT, Stitz RW, Lumley JW. Laparoscopically assisted colorectal surgery in the elderly. Br J Surg. 1999; 86:938–941

[46] Maxwell JG, Bradford A, Tyler BA, et al. Cholecystectomy in patients aged 80 and older. Am J Surg. 1998; 176:627–631

[47] Sylla P, Kirman I, Whelan RL. Immunological advantages of advanced laparoscopy. Surg Clin North Am. 2005; 85(1):1–18, vii

[48] Buunen M, Gholghesaei M, Veldkamp R, Meijer DW, Bonjer HJ, Bouvy ND. Stress response to laparoscopic surgery: a review. SurgEndosc. 2004; 18(7): 1022–1028

[49] Doulamis IP, Spartalis E, Machairas N, et al. The role of robotics in cardiac surgery: a systematic review. J Robot Surg. 2018

[50] Bittner JG, IV, Alrefai S, Vy M, Mabe M, Del Prado PAR, Clingempeel NL. Comparative analysis of open and robotic transversus abdominis release for ventral hernia repair. SurgEndosc. 2018; 32(2):727–734

3 Impact of Acute Surgical Illness on Critical Care Decisions Pre- and Postoperatively

Lena M. Napolitano and Jay Doucet

Summary

This chapter aims to review optimal patient care, based on the current evidence for acute care surgery critically ill patients. This chapter is separated into preoperative and postoperative management and reviews common care management issues in each of these time periods. The preoperative section reviews appropriate resuscitation strategies, including hemostatic resuscitation in relation to appropriate timing of surgical intervention. Rapid bedside diagnostic imaging, including point of care ultrasonography (POCUS) is reviewed, particularly for differentiation of shock states, comprising hemorrhagic, septic, and cardiogenic shock. Airway management and optimization of respiratory function are important issues. The importance of appropriate monitoring, invasive and noninvasive, and their utility in different shock states are reviewed. The postoperative section covers the optimal role of the surgical and intensive care unit (ICU) teams in the care of the acute care surgery critically ill patients, including the ABCDEF ICU Bundle. Resuscitation goals, transfusion strategies, and prevention and treatment of anemia are important topics as well. The Sepsis-3 new definitions, guidelines, and bundles are reviewed in detail, including new trials for steroids in sepsis that provide consensus management. Treatment and rescue strategies for acute respiratory failure and acute respiratory distress syndrome (ARDS), including new trials for extracorporeal membrane oxygenation (ECMO) and esophageal pressure-guided positive end-expiratory pressure (PEEP) are critically reviewed. Additional topics include nutrition, acute kidney injury, pain/agitation/delirium prevention and management, and prevention of common complications in the ICU.

Keywords: Critical care, critically ill patients, intensive care unit, organ function, organ dysfunction, organ failure, shock, hemorrhage, sepsis, septic shock, resuscitation, transfusion, anemia, respiratory failure, complications

3.1 Preoperative Critical Care

3.1.1 Strategies to Optimize Organ Function and Intravascular Volume Preoperatively

There are two typical scenarios in which critical care is necessary before a major operative procedure. A patient may arrive in the emergency department with evidence of a surgical emergency such as sepsis, ischemia and/or organ failure, and operative intervention is planned immediately upon the patient leaving the emergency room. Alternatively, the patient may already be in an intensive care environment and the decision for surgery is made. In either scenario, surgical critical care, which is part of the acute care surgery (ACS) model, is required to optimize the patient's condition and allow a successful surgical intervention.[1]

Timing of Surgery

Simultaneous Resuscitation and Surgery

Shock is a state of inadequate oxygen delivery to organs that leads to cellular hypoxia, and if not rapidly corrected leads to multiple organ dysfunction and death.[2] Categories of shock that may be present in the ACS patient include hypovolemic shock from hemorrhagic shock, dehydration, fluid losses or shifts. Obstructive shock may be present with patients with tension pneumothorax, cardiac tamponade, abdominal compartment syndrome, and pulmonary or air embolism. Distributive shock may be present in patients with septic shock or those with neurogenic shock, such as after a cervical spinal cord injury. Shock is most obvious in those with hypotension but in the earlier stages it may be subtle and only detectable with modest changes in vital signs, organ function, laboratory results or specific imaging. Simultaneous assessment, resuscitation and initiation are usually required in ACS patients in shock, undergoing emergency surgery, without necessarily having a complete history, imaging or laboratory results. Resuscitation begins immediately and may be necessary throughout the surgical procedure. Excellent teamwork and communication between the surgical and anesthesiology specialties, operating room nurses and technicians is required.

Multiple shock causes may be present in the same ACS patient. For instance, a blunt trauma patient may have hemoperitoneum from a ruptured spleen (hemorrhagic shock), pneumothorax due to fractured ribs (obstructive shock), or spinal cord transection with neurogenic shock (distributive shock). A patient with advanced abdominal sepsis from a perforated viscus may have septic shock from circulating inflammatory mediators (distributive shock), fluid losses from tissue edema and ascites (hypovolemic shock), and poor cardiac performance from sepsis-induced myocardial dysfunction or cardiac ischemia (cardiogenic shock).

Rapid assessment of the preoperative ACS patient with shock includes assessment of vital signs, available preoperative tests, and imaging, especially point of care ultrasonography (POCUS) if there is uncertainty and time, skill and equipment allow.[3,4,5] Vital signs changes include tachycardia, hypertension, and rapid shallow breathing. Hypotension is generally recognized to be a systolic blood pressure of less than 90 mm Hg. In patients with physiologic reserve, increases in peripheral vasoconstriction, cardiac output and regional changes in circulation may delay the onset of hypertension despite significant hypovolemia. Pulse pressure is defined as the difference between the systolic and diastolic pressures. In hypovolemic states, the pulse pressure typically narrows as a result of vasoconstriction before the onset of overt hypotension. A wide pulse pressure, where the difference between systolic and diastolic blood pressures is greater than the diastolic blood pressure, may be a sign of vasodilation, which is seen in early distributive shock states such as septic shock. If time permits, placement of an arterial pressure line allows for immediate assessment of blood pressures and aids performance of blood gas and laboratory tests intraoperatively.

Any available preoperative tests already performed should be reviewed. When the patient is hemodynamically unstable, further testing should be restricted to timely studies that will influence intraoperative decision-making and not place the patient at undue risk of deterioration in inaccessible or poorly monitored settings such as the CT or MRI scanner. Blood gases, including base deficit and lactate, may detect significant respiratory or metabolic acidosis. Complete blood counts may aid in the diagnosis of sepsis and anemia. Electrolytes may be disordered in sepsis or as a result of excess crystalloid administration. Organ ischemia and dysfunction may be detected by cardiac, liver and renal markers.

Rapid bedside imaging can be helpful in differentiating shock states. The chest X-ray can disclose evidence of hypovolemic states from hemorrhagic when a massive hemothorax is detected. While tension pneumothorax is a clinical diagnosis, any simple pneumothorax seen on chest X-ray requires attention, as it may lead to subsequent deterioration, especially after intubation and positive pressure ventilation, and also requires placement of a chest tube. The AP pelvis X-ray detects pelvic fractures which are a potential source of hemorrhagic shock. The kidney, ureter, and bladder (KUB) image can detect free air in the patient with an acute abdomen.

POCUS is a useful skill set for the acute care surgeon, which is also required for the surgical intensivist. POCUS allows differentiation of the shock state.[6,7] POCUS can detect hypovolemia by the presence of a small or collapsible inferior vena cava or poor ventricular filling. It can detect obstructive shock by identifying pneumothorax due to lack of plural sliding on chest views. It can also detect cardiac tamponade via demonstration of a pericardial effusion or right ventricular collapse. Global myocardial dysfunction can be identified in advanced septic shock. Also made obvious is congestive cardiomyopathy with dilated ventricles and poor performance. The abdominal portion of the focused assessment with sonography for trauma (FAST) can detect hemoperitoneum or free abdominal fluid. The gallbladder is best assessed for cholecystitis via ultrasound, and the aorta can be examined for dilation, as in abdominal aortic aneurysm (AAA), or for an intimal flap in the aortic dissection.

The routine placement of the pulmonary artery (PA, Swan-Ganz) catheter in critical care has declined due to lack of evidence in relation to mortality improvement.[8] The PA catheter may still be used by some cases in patients with myocardial dysfunction due to preexisting cardiac ischemic disease, and congestive heart failure, or in patients with acquired myocardial dysfunction such as advanced septic shock.

Immediate Versus Delayed Surgery

Situations in which a life-threatening pathologic process must be stopped by surgery require immediate and rapid assessment, urgent resuscitative maneuvers to correct the detected shock states, expedient transfer to the operating suite, induction of anesthesia and appropriate surgery.

In hypovolemic shock states such as hemorrhage due to trauma, damage control surgery to arrest hemorrhage, preventing contamination of the peritoneum from ruptured hollow viscus injuries, and detecting injuries to be managed after subsequent stabilization, are required before onset of the "lethal triad" of hypothermia, metabolic acidosis and coagulopathy.[9]

Obstructive shock states such as tension pneumothorax or cardiac tamponade require immediate surgical intervention. While a chest tube can be placed quickly to relieve tension pneumothorax, cardiac tamponade due to cardiac injury requires pericardiotomy, usually via median sternotomy, although left anterior thoracotomy may be necessary during cardiac arrest or if sternotomy is not possible.

Septic shock states often require urgent surgery. Necrotizing fasciitis is a condition of high lethality worsened by delays to debridement in the operating room. Rapid source control of sepsis via resection or repair of a necrotic or perforated viscus, drainage of an abscess, or removal of an infected foreign body, may also require rapid operative intervention.

Surgery is usually delayed when possible in patients with cardiogenic shock. This includes cases such as acute myocardial infarction, poorly compensated heart failure, high-grade tachy- or bradyarrhythmias, or severe valvular dysfunction such as severe aortic stenosis or ruptured papillary muscle. A multidisciplinary approach is best, involving the ACS surgeon, intensivist, cardiologist, cardiac surgeon, and anesthesiologist, with the patient and family. The team can then discuss the need, risks and benefits of surgery, timing, and strategies to permit performance or delay of the procedure. Uncorrectable cardiogenic shock is highly lethal and, in such cases, discussion of possible palliative approaches is appropriate.

Airway Management

Induction of anesthesia and intubation are critical steps in the care of the ACS patient. Careful selection of agents and appropriate timing are necessary to avoid exacerbation of shock states and risk of intraoperative cardiac arrest.

Induction agents that have minimal vasodilatory properties, such as etomidate or ketamine, are preferred. Etomidate is known to cause transient adrenocortical suppression and that risk is balanced against the risk of hypotension using conventional agents.[10] Ketamine causes mild myocardial depression and the dose should be reduced in patients with severe shock and possibly depleted adrenergic reserves. While high-opioid dose anesthetics are often used in cardiac surgery due to lack of myocardial effects, this should be avoided in shock states due to patients' dependence on high-catecholamine levels. Propofol should be avoided as it causes arterial and venous vasodilation and decreased cardiac contractility and leads to cardiac arrest after induction in shock states.

Timing of intubation in hypovolemic shock is important and influenced by understanding the effect of increased intrathoracic pressure during a period of inadequate cardiac preload. Patients who are afterload-dependent due to poor left ventricular performance in cardiogenic shock usually tolerate intubation and positive pressure ventilation and PEEP well. However, in patients who are hypovolemic and have reduced preload, intubation and high-airway pressures or high PEEP may precipitate cardiac arrest. Typically, an intravenous fluid bolus is administered prior to induction, intubation and positive pressure intubation. Intubation can often be delayed in shock states in conscious patients until arriving in the OR suite, wherein the optimal combination of team members and equipment is available, adequate time to allow and evaluate fluid resuscitation has passed, and severe hypotension or incipient cardiac arrest can be optimally managed.

Optimizing Respiratory Function

The critically ill ACS patient may present several preoperative challenges in respiratory management. Trauma patients may have thoracic injuries that can affect ventilation and oxygenation. Multiple segmental rib fractures can impair ventilation by creating paradoxical respiratory motion in the flail segment during spontaneous respiration. Hemothorax and pneumothorax can also impair ventilation by reducing available tidal volume and increasing intrathoracic pressures. Pain caused by rib fractures can also impair spontaneous ventilation. Pulmonary contusions can impair oxygenation by direct alveolar injury and regional hypoxic pulmonary vasoconstriction. The primary preoperative tools in the optimization of thoracic injured patients are intubation, mechanical ventilator, and chest drain. Intubation and positive pressure ventilation will stop paradoxical chest wall movement in flail chest and overcome hypoventilation due to pain. Chest tubes can remove air and blood from the pleural space and allow full lung expansion.

Hypoventilation in spontaneously breathing ACS patients can lead to atelectasis, lobar collapse, mucous pugging, hypercarbia, obtundation, aspiration, and respiratory and cardiac arrest. The bedside incentive spirometer is commonly used to encourage deep breathing and make bedside assessments of vital capacity. Chest physiotherapy is commonly used in thoracic trauma patients at risk of pulmonary deterioration.

In intubated patients, monitoring lung performance is performed via arterial blood gas, chest X-ray and ventilator parameters. Thoracic trauma patients may require bronchoscopy to assess for tracheobronchial injury, obtain washings and culture to detect pneumonia, or remove mucous or clots plugging bronchial airways. Video-assisted thoracoscopic surgery may be needed to deal with retained hemothorax despite chest tube drainage.

For ACS patients who are in the intensive care unit (ICU) for several days, hypoxemia may result from acute respiratory distress syndrome (ARDS) or from hospital-acquired pneumonia. ARDS may require advanced ventilatory modes such as pressure-controlled inverse ratio ventilation (PCIRV) or airway pressure release ventilation (APRV), proning, and inhaled broncho-vasodilators such as nitric oxide or extracorporeal membrane oxygenation (ECMO). Such interventions may make surgical procedures difficult or impossible, as many anesthesia machines cannot perform advanced ventilation modes such as PCIRV or APRV, abdominal incisions may preclude proning, and ECMO may require continuous anticoagulation. Small changes in patient position can also precipitate hypoxemia in ARDS patients.

Initial Resuscitation

All trauma and ACS patients who might have gone into a shock state should receive supplemental oxygen. This may counter any hypoventilation and hypoxemia and extends the period of tolerable apnea should intubation become necessary.

Most patients in shock usually initially receive crystalloid boluses of 500 mL or 1000 mL. The bolus can be repeated as needed with certain important exceptions. The optimal fluid is unknown. Lactated Ringer's solution avoids hyperchloremia and resultant metabolic acidosis but contains calcium and is incompatible with transfusion in the same line. Normal saline is compatible with simultaneous or subsequent transfusion in the same line.

Patients with trauma and hemorrhagic shock should be quickly converted to blood products if hypotension does not resolve after 1 liter of crystalloid in adults or 10 mL/kg in children.[11] A 1:1 ratio of packed cells to plasma is maintained. Plateletpheresis units are given every 4 to 6 units. A massive transfusion protocol ensures adequate availability of products, mobilizes resources, and reminds practitioners to test for fibrinolysis, coagulopathies and when to administer calcium, tranexamic acid, fibrinogen, cryoprecipitate, and clotting factors.

Fluid boluses in nonhemorrhagic shock states may be different. In left ventricular dysfunction, small boluses of 500 mL or less are used to avoid increased afterload. Patients with sepsis or right ventricular dysfunction may need 3 to 5 liters of crystalloid before stabilization.

Synthetic colloids (hydroxyethyl starch, dextran, and pentastarch) should be avoided as they have been associated with increased harm in trials. No benefit is associated with the use of intravenous albumin in hemorrhagic shock.

Fluid boluses in nonhemorrhagic shock states may be different. In left ventricular dysfunction, smaller boluses of 500 mL or less are used to avoid excess increases in afterload. Patients with sepsis or right ventricular dysfunction may need cumulative doses of 3 to 5 liters of crystalloid.

Vasopressors may be required preoperatively and intraoperatively in the ACS patient. They are often required to ensure organ perfusion in undifferentiated or nonhemorrhagic shock states but should be avoided in hemorrhagic shock states unless adequate blood and crystalloid administration have failed to correct the shock state.

The optimal vasopressor in ACS patients is unknown.[12] The most commonly used agent is norepinephrine (Levophed) is a potent alpha-adrenergic mediated vasoconstrictor but can cause tachycardia via its beta effects. Early use of norepinephrine in septic shock may be associated with more rapid reversal of hypotension and improve lactate clearance but not lead to improved 28-day mortality.[13] Phenylephrine (NeoSynephrine) is a pure alpha-adrenergic vasoconstrictor which avoids exacerbating tachycardia, although it may cause reflex bradycardia, especially in neurogenic shock. Dopamine (Intropin) is no longer a first-line agent due to its mixed alpha and beta effects and arrhythmogenicity, although in US hospitals, it is the only vasopressor usually immediately available in premixed intravenous bags.

The most commonly used inotrope in ACS patients with acute cardiac decompensation is dobutamine. Its vasodilatory properties may help reduce afterload or produce hypotension, which is often countered by the coadministration of norepinephrine. Titration of vasopressors usually requires the use of an arterial line to provide continuous blood pressure monitoring. Administration of vasopressors typically is done via a central venous catheter due to the risk of tissue necrosis with extravasation at peripheral intravenous sites, although phenylephrine is commonly given via peripheral intravenous sites.

The target blood pressure in preoperative ACS patients is unknown. Higher target mean arterial pressure (MAP) may be associated with decreased need for renal replacement therapy but increased risk of arrhythmia.[14,15] High-doses of vasopressor raise concern for mesenteric ischemia and bowel necrosis. Typically, a MAP of 65 mm Hg is used.[16] Urine output of 0.5 mL/kg is desirable, and decreasing base deficit or lactate on blood gases are evidence of adequate resuscitation.

Monitoring

Standard monitors used preoperatively include the electrocardiograph (EKG), saturation monitor, and blood pressure cuff. End-tidal capnography is useful in intubated patients. Invasive monitoring usually includes intra-arterial line blood pressure monitoring; however, this should not be allowed to delay urgent surgery and can be placed after induction and incision. The arterial line can also allow measurement of pre to postrespiratory variation which can provide stroke volume variation (SVV), stroke volume and calculated cardiac output.[17] An SVV of ≥ 15% implies inadequate preload and fluid responsiveness. The arterial line also facilitates repeat laboratory testing, especially arterial blood gases.

The central venous catheter (CVC) allows measurement of central venous pressure (CVP). Interpretation of the CVP with regard to fluid responsiveness should be performed with caution, as correlation is poor in many scenarios. If the actual need is access for rapid illustration of intravenous fluid, two large bore peripheral IVs that are 18 gauge or larger will generate higher flows than a triple lumen 20 cm 7 French CVC. The CVC can also be used for blood and can obtain superior vena cava oxygen saturation ($S_{cv}O_2$) by venous blood gas sampling or use of an oximetric catheter tip. $S_{cv}O_2$ can be used as a surrogate of oxygen consumption and cardiac output; a $S_{cv}O_2$ greater than 70% is usually considered an indicator of adequate oxygen delivery during resuscitation.

The PA catheter has not been shown to improve survival in critical care but is often used in specific scenarios where cardiac issues predominate such as right ventricular failure, pulmonary hypertension or embolism and acute valvular disease. The PA catheter can measure CVP, right ventricular pressures, pulmonary artery pressures, and pulmonary artery wedge pressure (PAWP) which correlates with left ventricular end diastolic pressure. Thermodilution, either by continuous heated tip or proximal injection of room temperature saline, can allow calculation of cardiac output, systemic vascular resistance (SVR), as well as peripheral vascular resistance. Mixed venous oxygen (MvO_2) blood gas sampling from the pulmonary artery allows determination of oxygen delivery, oxygen consumption, and oxygen extraction ratio. Preload corresponds with PAWP, cardiac muscle function corresponds to cardiac output, afterload corresponds with SVR, and tissue perfusion corresponds with MvO_2. The interaction of these four parameters can then be used to determine the category of shock and desired interventions.

Transesophageal echocardiography (TEE) is increasingly used as an intraoperative monitoring technique in ACS patients.[18,19] Direct visualization and, if desired, measurement of chamber sizes and flows allows rapid differentiation of shock states. Left ventricular diastolic volume (LVEDV) can be measured, which is more readily understood than PAWP, and volume status or preload readily determined. Left or right ventricular function, dilation, global or segmental hypokinesis can be seen. Cardiac output can be calculated by measuring the diameter of the left ventricular outflow tract (LVOT) and integrating the LVOT Doppler flow over a cardiac cycle. Valvular structure and function can be seen. Unlike transthoracic echo, as done in POCUS, TEE views are typically unaffected by pneumothorax, subcutaneous air, wounds, dressings or EKG pads. TEE is usually only performed in the operating room by a trained anesthesiologist and after use requires high-level cleaning like other endoscopic equipment. However, indwelling disposable TEE probes are available which can be placed intraoperatively and left in place postoperatively for up to 72 hours among intubated patients.[20]

The Foley bladder catheter is placed preoperatively, which allows for measurement of urine output and can be reassuring of adequate renal perfusion with 0.5 mL/kg hourly. The Foley catheter can also be equipped with a temperature sensor to provide continuous core body temperature. The sampling port on most Foley catheters can also be used to provide bladder pressures, which can be used to diagnose intrabdominal hypertension and abdominal compartment syndrome.[21]

Management—Hemorrhagic Shock

The primary strategy applied to the ACS patient in hemorrhagic shock involves controlling bleeding and replacing blood losses. Inadequate preload is the principal cause of hypotension. While efforts are underway to control bleeding, judicious intravenous fluid administration is used to increase preload, allow intubation and positive pressure ventilation when ready, and also allow improved organ perfusion. The current standard crystalloid bolus in the Advanced Trauma Life Support (ATLS) program is one liter of crystalloid followed by blood product administration if vital signs are not normalized.[11] Current guidelines recommend a 1:1 packed red cells to plasma ratio.[22] Trials using whole blood, which contains one unit of packed cells, one unit of plasma and one unit of platelets per bag, are underway in prehospital and hospital environments.[23] Fluids should be infused by a warming device to avoid hypothermia. Avoidance of administration of large volumes of crystalloid prevents death and morbidity due to excess tissue edema, pulmonary edema, hypothermia, dilutional coagulopathy, and metabolic acidosis. Careful monitoring is required to avoid excess resuscitation hypervolemia which can result in pulmonary edema, abdominal compartment syndrome, and extremity compartment syndrome. Vasopressors are not used as a substitute for transfusion, although it may be temporarily necessary in the early phases of resuscitation.

Mechanical devices that can be used to reduce blood loss include tourniquets and retrograde balloon occlusion of the aorta (REBOA). Tourniquets have been used in military and civilian prehospital settings to improve survival after extremity hemorrhage, and if effective, it can be left in place until the patient is under anesthesia and proximal arterial vascular control is readily obtainable. Placement of the REBOA balloon via femoral artery above the diaphragm may be an alternative to emergency thoracotomy in patients with severe hypotension due to abdominal hemorrhage prior to arriving in the operating room, but trials have not yet shown a survival advantage.[24,25] It may also play a role in decreasing hemorrhage from pelvic fractures or obstetric hemorrhage when the balloon is placed above the aortic bifurcation.[26]

Management—Septic Shock

The ACS patient with septic shock has significant vasodilation and reduced afterload or SVR. Urgent surgery is frequently required to obtain source control. The initial intervention is intravenous fluid administration, frequently accompanied by vasopressor administration. Intravenous crystalloid and vasopressors are given to obtain a target map of 65. MAP greater than 75 should be avoided as they are associated with increased harm. Typically, boluses of 500 to 1000 mL are used and fluid totals in a short presentation maybe 3 to 5 L. If it alone is not improving the MAP, a vasopressor is started, usually norepinephrine, unless it produces tachyarrhythmias, in which case phenylephrine can be used. If fluids and a first vasopressor is ineffective, vasopressin is typically added at a fixed dose.[27] Using vasopressin as a second vasopressor may reduce the risk or arrhythmia, particularly atrial fibrillation.[28] Although hemodilution can be expected with large volume crystalloid administration, transfusion is deferred unless the hemoglobin level is less than 7 g/dl, as no benefit of higher transfusion thresholds has been shown.[29]

Refractory shock despite intravenous fluids has been managed by a variety of agents. Patients who might have adrenal insufficiency or Addisonian crisis may respond to IV low-dose corticosteroids. Methylene Blue has been used in patients with refractory shock which is thought to be due to vasoplegia caused by pronged cardiopulmonary bypass, sepsis or anaphylaxis, as it reduces guanylyl cyclase and nitric oxide synthase activity, decreasing vessel sensitivity to nitric oxide and increasing SVR.[30,31] Angiotensin II, which is a potent vasoconstrictor that increases blood pressure and reduces catecholamine dose in patients not responsive to norepinephrine or vasopressin, is now available.[32]

Broad-spectrum IV antibiotics should be administered as quickly as possible, as delay is associated with linear increase in mortality, and inadequate regimens may double expected mortality.[33,34,35] If possible, blood cultures should be drawn prior to antibiotic administration to allow later narrowing of the antibiotic spectrum. Necrotizing soft tissue infections are a special case. Acceptable regimens include carbapenem or beta-lactam/beta-lactamase inhibitor plus an antimethicillin-resistant *S. aureus* (MRSA) agent plus clindamycin to reduce toxins from toxin-producing streptococci and staphylococci.

Hyperglycemia and insulin resistance are common in septic shock patients and IV insulin is required to obtain a blood glucose between 140 to 180 mg/dl (7.6–10.1 mmol/l) preoperatively.

Management—Cardiogenic Shock

ACS patients with cardiogenic shock are hypotensive due to failure of their cardiac pump. Initial treatment involves administration of inotropic agents, in order to improve pump performance, and suppression of arrhythmias. Unlike hypovolemic/hemorrhagic shock, or distributive/septic shock, intravenous fluid boluses are avoided, especially if there is evidence of pulmonary edema. Surgery is contraindicated unless there is a reversible life-threatening condition. Advanced forms of other types of shock such as septic shock may be complicated by myocardial dysfunction and cardiogenic shock.

Treatment varies depending on the cause, and acute myocardial infarction is managed with a vasopressor with inotropic properties, usually norepinephrine. SVV monitoring, TEE or PA catheter can be used to determine intravascular volume state and need for fluid administration. Acute left-sided heart failure is managed by reducing preload and afterload, increasing inotropy, and managing arrhythmias. Modestly increased PEEP (≤10 mm Hg) reduces afterload.

Acute right-sided heart failure has high-lethality due to the risk of multi-organ failure. Inotropes and vasodilators such as milrinone or dobutamine are usually attempted, generally in combination with norepinephrine or, to maintain coronary perfusion. Pulmonary artery pressure is reduced by avoiding hypoxia and high-airway pressures or PEEP. Nitric oxide and epoprostenol are used to reduce pulmonary vascular resistance. Very occasionally, mechanical ventricular support devices such as ventricular assist devices (VADs) or venoarterial ECMO are used to manage cardiogenic shock unresponsive to medical therapy in order to allow surgery.

Transport to the Operating Room

ACS patients who require urgent surgery require an organized process to transport the patient and team to the operating room (OR) with appropriate monitoring.[36] Having a dedicated operating room immediately available for surgical emergencies such as trauma cases has been shown to reduce mortality. Trauma centers having a direct to OR capability also have decreased mortality in major trauma victims.[37] Hybrid OR/emergency rooms (ER) with integrated imaging allows simultaneous resuscitation, surgical preparation and operative procedures with a seamless transition between resuscitation and operative teams.[38] A formal handover process between the resuscitation team and the operative team should occur and a senior member of the surgical should be present.

3.2 Postoperative Critical Care

3.2.1 Role of the Surgical Team and Intensivist

Prompt admission of patients with acute surgical illness to the ICU is associated with improved outcomes. It is important to have appropriate ICU admission criteria, and the 2016 ICU Admission, Discharge, and Triage Guidelines provide an excellent framework for implementation in adult ICUs.[39] We strongly recommend ICU admission directly from the OR or emergency department (ED) whenever possible, as it will enable the ICU team to review the patient's clinical issues and physiology, and institute appropriate critical care treatment as soon as possible. It is important to have an appropriate transfer of care from the OR and trauma/ED team to the ICU team which is comprehensive and detailed. Transport of critically ill patients to the postanesthesia care unit (PACU) prior to ICU admission is fraught with many issues related to lack of transition of care from the primary surgical team.

The optimal ICU care model for patients with acute surgical illness is the "semiopen, collaborative care" model in which the ICU is staffed with attending intensivists and an ICU team which is not only responsible for minute-to-minute critical care but also looks into coordination of ICU care and communication with primary surgeons and their teams. The ultimate responsibility for the patient remains with the primary attending surgeon and surgical team, but ICU patient care is a collaborative effort in this model which combines the advantages of critical care expertise for trauma and surgery patients while maintaining primary surgical service responsibility for overall patient management. This is consistent with the Guidelines for the Optimal Care of the Injured Patient recommended by the American College of Surgeons Committee on Trauma for Level 1 Trauma Centers.[40]

ICU Physician Staffing Standard

"High intensity" ICU physician staffing is associated with significantly reduced ICU and hospital mortality, and significantly lower "failure to rescue" rates. A "high-intensity" model not only involves 24/7 dedicated ICU physician staffing and mandatory ICU team involvement with patient management but also includes closed ICUs and most semi-open ICUs. In contrast, "open" units typically utilize "low-intensity" ICU physician staffing. In a meta-analysis of 26 studies, "high-intensity" ICU physician staffing was associated with significantly reduced hospital and ICU mortality (RR 0.71, [95% CI 0.62–0.82] for hospital mortality; RR 0.61, [95% CI 0.5–0.75] for ICU mortality) for both adults and children.[41]

The following ICU physician staffing (IPS) standard by The Leapfrog Group is required for hospitals with adult or pediatric ICUs:

"Hospitals fully meeting the IPS standard will operate adult or pediatric general medical and/or surgical ICUs and neuro ICUs that are managed or comanaged by intensivists who:

- Are present during daytime hours and provide clinical care exclusively in the ICU.
- When not present on site or via telemedicine, return notification alerts at least 95% of the time, (1) within five minutes and (2) arrange for a physician, physician assistant, nurse practitioner, or an FCCS-certified nurse to reach ICU patients within five minutes."[42]

Daily Goals Checklist and ABCDEF Bundle

Daily goals checklists and the ABCDEF Bundle have been documented to improve ICU progress and outcomes. The ICU Liberation Collaborative[43] is a real-world large-scale quality improvement initiative to implement the Society of Critical Care Medicine (SCCM) pain, agitation, delirium (PAD) Guidelines across 76 ICUs using the ABCDEF Bundle (▶ Fig. 3.1).[44]

Implementation of the ABCDEF Bundle in 6064 patients in 7 community hospitals was associated with significantly improved outcomes and significantly increased hospital survival for every 10% increase in total or partial bundle compliance. When ICU patients receiving palliative care were not included, these results were even more striking (12% and 23% higher odds of survival per 10% increase in bundle compliance, respectively, $p < 0.001$). Bundle compliance (total or partial) was also associated with more days alive and free of delirium and coma.[45]

Most recently, a prospective multicenter cohort study (15,226 ICU adult patients, 68 ICUs, 20-month period) from a national quality improvement collaborative reported that complete ABCDEF Bundle performance was associated with lower likelihood of seven outcomes: hospital death within 7 days (adjusted hazard ratio, 0.32; CI, 0.17–0.62), next-day mechanical ventilation (adjusted odds ratio [AOR], 0.28; CI, 0.22–0.36), coma (AOR, 0.35; CI, 0.22–0.56), delirium (AOR, 0.60; CI, 0.49–0.72), physical restraint use (AOR, 0.37; CI, 0.30–0.46), ICU readmission (AOR, 0.54; CI, 0.37–0.79), and discharge to a facility other than home (AOR, 0.64; CI, 0.51–0.80). There was a consistent dose–response relationship between higher proportional bundle performance and improved clinical outcomes (all $p < 0.002$). Significant pain was more frequently reported, as bundle performance proportionally increased ($p = 0.0001$).[46] The ABCDEF Bundle can be challenging to implement, and practical advice regarding bundle implementation is available.[47]

3.2.2 Resuscitation Goals

The primary goal of critical care support among patients with acute surgical illness is restoration of oxygen delivery, hemodynamic stability and maintenance and/or improvement in organ function. It is important to recognize that no single endpoint of resuscitation is optimal in any one ICU patient, and that it is best to assess all potential endpoints with a goal to adequately resuscitate, but NOT over-resuscitate patients, since over-resuscitation is associated with increased pulmonary complications including need for mechanical ventilation.

Hemodynamic endpoints of resuscitation include adequate MAP without vasopressors, transthoracic echocardiography confirming inferior vena cava diameter and compressibility and cardiac function, normal mixed or central venous oxygen saturation, and other monitoring invasive or noninvasive devices, including esophageal Doppler monitor (EDM), pulse contour and pulse pressure variation (FloTrac/Vigileo), transpulmonary thermodilution (PiCCO and LiDCO), and PA catheter.[48]

Laboratory endpoints of resuscitation include normalization of lactate and/or base deficit. However, strict use of these biomarkers may result in over-resuscitation, as the laboratory changes commonly lag behind the physiologic changes in resuscitation of shock patients.

The recent ANDROMEDA Shock Trial 2019[49] randomized 424 septic shock patients into two different resuscitation protocols: Lactate group (normalizing or decreasing lactate levels [>20% per 2 hours]) versus peripheral perfusion group (normalizing capillary refill time [measured in seconds], > 3 sec abnormal). The peripheral perfusion group received less IV fluid in the first 8 hours (2.4 liters) than the lactate group (2.8 liters). There was no difference in 28-day all-cause mortality (43.4% lactate vs. 34.9% peripheral perfusion). Peripheral perfusion-targeted resuscitation was associated with less organ dysfunction at 72 hours (mean SOFA score, 5.6 [SD, 4.3] vs 6.6 [SD, 4.7]; mean difference, − 1.00 [95% CI, − 1.97 to − 0.02]; $p = .045$). There were no significant differences in the other six secondary outcomes. This study also documented fluid responsiveness during the 8-hour resuscitation protocol, and confirmed that at hour zero,

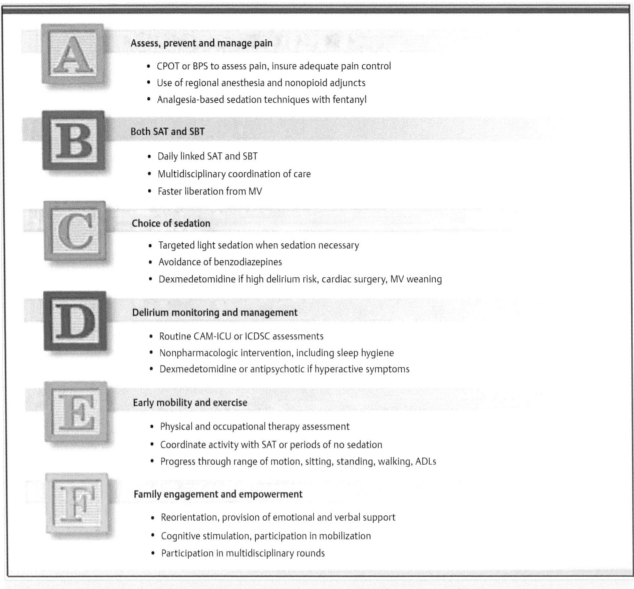

A **Assess, prevent and manage pain**

- CPOT or BPS to assess pain, insure adequate pain control
- Use of regional anesthesia and nonopioid adjuncts
- Analgesia-based sedation techniques with fentanyl

B **Both SAT and SBT**

- Daily linked SAT and SBT
- Multidisciplinary coordination of care
- Faster liberation from MV

C **Choice of sedation**

- Targeted light sedation when sedation necessary
- Avoidance of benzodiazepines
- Dexmedetomidine if high delirium risk, cardiac surgery, MV weaning

D **Delirium monitoring and management**

- Routine CAM-ICU or ICDSC assessments
- Nonpharmacologic intervention, including sleep hygiene
- Dexmedetomidine or antipsychotic if hyperactive symptoms

E **Early mobility and exercise**

- Physical and occupational therapy assessment
- Coordinate activity with SAT or periods of no sedation
- Progress through range of motion, sitting, standing, walking, ADLs

F **Family engagement and empowerment**

- Reorientation, provision of emotional and verbal support
- Cognitive stimulation, participation in mobilization
- Participation in multidisciplinary rounds

Fig. 3.1 The ABCDEF bundle in the intensive care unit.

30% of patients were nonresponders, and this increased significantly over time (72% nonresponders to fluid at hour 2, 85% at hour 4, 86% at hour 6, and 96% at hour 8). Assessment of fluid responsiveness is key to appropriate fluid resuscitation of shock patients. It also demonstrates the important of a personalized critical care approach to the resuscitation of shock patients.

3.2.3 Transfusion Strategies

Many ICU patients (30–50%) receive red blood cell (RBC) transfusions during their ICU stay, with a mean of five units transfused in the ICU.[50,51] The vast majority of these RBC transfusions are for treatment of anemia and not bleeding. It is therefore imperative to understand the appropriate prevention and management of anemia in the ICU and optimal methods for patient blood management.

Restrictive Transfusion Strategies

In general, a restrictive RBC transfusion strategy (consider RBC transfusion when Hb ≤ 7 g/dL) is recommended among critically ill patients. The use of RBC transfusion for the treatment of anemia does not improve outcomes in most critically ill patients, except possibly for patients with acute coronary syndrome. In patients with acute coronary syndrome, consider RBC transfusion when Hb ≤ 8 g/dL. The decision to transfuse RBCs should not be solely based on the hemoglobin level and should include clinical factors, alternative therapies and patient preferences (► Fig. 3.2).[52]

An updated systematic review with trial sequential analysis included 31 trials that compared restrictive versus liberal transfusion strategy in adults or children and included 9813 randomized patients.[53] Compared with liberal strategies, restrictive transfusion strategies were associated with a reduction in the number of RBC units transfused and number of patients

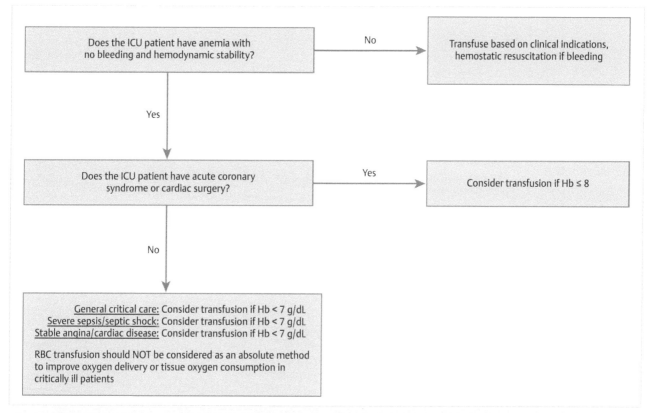

Fig. 3.2 RBC transfusion management of ICU patients with anemia. ICU, intensive care unit; RBC, red blood cell.

Table 3.1 Clinical practice guidelines from AABB, RBC transfusion thresholds and storage

Recommendation 1	A restrictive RBC transfusion threshold in which the transfusion is not indicated until the hemoglobin level is 7 g/dL is recommended for hospitalized adult patients, who are hemodynamically stable, including critically ill patients, rather than when the hemoglobin level is 10 g/dL (strong recommendation, moderate quality evidence).
	A restrictive RBC transfusion threshold of 8 g/dL is recommended for patients undergoing orthopedic surgery, cardiac surgery, and those with preexisting cardiovascular disease (strong recommendation, moderate quality evidence).
	The restrictive transfusion threshold of 7 g/dL is likely comparable with 8 g/dL, but RCT evidence is not available for all patient categories.
	These recommendations do not apply to patients with acute coronary syndrome, severe thrombocytopenia (patients treated for hematological or oncological reasons who are at risk of bleeding), and chronic transfusion-dependent anemia (not recommended due to insufficient evidence).
Recommendation 2	Patients, including neonates, should receive RBC units selected at any point within their licensed dating period (standard issue) rather than limiting patients to transfusion of only fresh (storage length: < 10 days) RBC units (strong recommendation, moderate quality evidence).

Abbreviations: RBC, red blood cell; RCT, randomized control trial.
Source: Adapted from Carson JL, Guyatt G, Heddle NM et al. JAMA. 2016;316(19):2025–2035. doi:10.1001/jama.2016.9185.

transfused, but mortality, overall morbidity, and myocardial infarction were unaltered. Similarly, a review of seven randomized control trials (RCTs) with 5,566 high-risk patients compared restrictive versus liberal transfusion strategy confirming non-inferiority, safety, and a significant reduction in RBC transfusions in the restrictive group.[54]

The Clinical Practice Guidelines from the American Association of Blood Banks (AABB) recommend a restrictive RBC transfusion threshold of 7 g/dL in hemodynamically stable hospitalized adults, including critically ill patients (▶ Table 3.1).[55]

An area of controversy is the optimal hemoglobin target in patients with acute myocardial ischemia and myocardial infarction. A meta-analysis of 10 studies (203,665 participants) confirmed that RBC transfusion was associated with increased all-cause mortality (RR 2.91; 95% CI, 2.46–3.44) and increased risk of subsequent myocardial infarction (RR 2.04; 95% CI, 1.06–3.93). Multivariate meta-regression confirmed that the mortality increase was independent of baseline, nadir, or change in hemoglobin level during the hospital stay.[56] The myocardial ischemia and transfusion (MINT) pilot trial enrolled 110 patients with acute coronary syndrome or stable angina undergoing cardiac catheterization and anemia (Hb < 10 g/dL) and compared a transfusion threshold of < 10 g/dL versus 8.0 g/dL. The predefined primary outcome (composite of death, myocardial infarction, or unscheduled revascularization 30 days post randomization) occurred in six patients (10.9%) in the liberal group and 14 (25.5%) in the restrictive group (risk difference 15.0%; 95% CI 0.7–29.3%; p = .054 and adjusted for age p = .076).[57] The MINT trial is currently ongoing and aiming to enroll 3500 patients randomized to liberal (hemoglobin > 10 g/dL) versus restrictive (hemoglobin 7 g/dL) RBC transfusion strategy. It was initiated in 2017 and its estimated completion year is 2021.[58]

Anemia Management

Anemia is common in all critically ill patients, and is due to anemia of inflammation (high-hepcidin levels resulting in iron-restricted erythropoiesis) and low-erythropoietin levels.[59] Anemia in ICU patients is the result of three main abnormalities related to the host inflammatory response: (1) dysregulation of iron homeostasis due to increased hepcidin concentrations; (2) impaired proliferation of erythroid progenitor cells, and (3) blunted erythropoietin response. Erythropoietin stimulation via erythropoiesis-stimulating agent (ESA) treatment results in decreased hepcidin expression, but the ESA FDA indication is for treatment of anemia due to chronic kidney disease in patients on dialysis and not on dialysis. A new hormone (erythroferrone, ERFE) has been identified, which mediates hepcidin suppression to allow increased iron absorption and mobilization from iron stores. ESA treatment increases ERFE production by erythroblasts and decreases hepcidin expression.

All methods to prevent anemia in the ICU should be implemented, including reduced diagnostic phlebotomy, which is reported to account for 40% of RBC transfusion requirements in the ICU. Blood conservation, with the use of pediatric or low-volume adult blood sampling tubes, is associated with significantly reduced phlebotomy volume also.[60] The use of closed blood conservation devices for arterial and central venous catheters in the ICU is associated with significantly decreased anemia and reduced RBC transfusions in ICU patients.[61]

3.2.4 Management of Sepsis

Sepsis is very common in the surgical ICU, particularly in emergency general surgery patients with abdominal infection. Knowledge of the current evidence-based sepsis guidelines assists with providing optimal care for these critically ill patients.[62]

Sepsis Definitions

Sepsis was previously defined in the Sepsis-2 definition as the presence of a presumed infection in a patient with two or more criteria for the systemic inflammatory response syndrome (SIRS). Severe sepsis included sepsis and one or more organ failures, while septic shock was previously defined as sepsis-induced hypotension and hypoperfusion, refractory to volume replacement and requiring vasopressors.

The new Sepsis-3 definitions include only sepsis and septic shock (▶ Fig. 3.3).[63] **Sepsis** is now defined as life-threatening organ dysfunction caused by a dysregulated host response to infection, suspected or documented infection, and an acute increase of ≥2 SOFA points (proxy for organ dysfunction), which has an associated hospital mortality rate greater than 10%.

Septic shock is now defined as sepsis with persistent hypotension requiring vasopressors to maintain mean arterial pressure ≥ 65 mm Hg and having a serum lactate level > 2 mmol/L (18 mg/dL), despite adequate fluid resuscitation, which has an associated hospital mortality greater than 40%. The Surviving Sepsis Campaign (SSC) 2016 Guidelines and 2018 SSC Bundle provide recommendations to improve outcomes.

Sepsis Guidelines and Sepsis Bundles

The 2016 Surviving Sepsis Campaign Guidelines uses the new Sepsis-3 definitions, and the 3-hour Bundle has been revised to a 1-hour Sepsis Bundle with the intent to begin resuscitation and management immediately (▶ Table 3.2 and ▶ Table 3.3).[64] A significant difference in the new 1-hour Sepsis Bundle is an increase in fluid resuscitation to 30 mL/kg from 20 mL/kg in the 2008 Bundle. But it is clear that this amount of fluid resuscitation may not be appropriate for patients with heart failure or severe hypoxemia, and that vasopressor and cardiotonic medications may be indicated instead.[65]

Another significant change is the removal of early goal-directed therapy (EGDT) recommendations (resuscitation targets CVP ≥ 8, central venous oxygen saturation [ScVO₂] ≥ 70%, and normalization of lactate) in the 6-hour SSC Bundle. This change was based on three large multicenter randomized trials (Protocolized Care for Early Septic Shock [ProCESS] in the United States,[66] Australasian Resuscitation in Sepsis Evaluation [ARISE] in Australia and New Zealand,[67] Protocolised Management in Sepsis [ProMISE] in the United Kingdom[68]) which confirmed no benefit to EGDT in septic shock management, in contrast to the initial single-center EGDT trial which reported a significant reduction in mortality from 46.5 to 30.5% with EGDT.[69]

A trial-level meta-analysis confirmed no overall benefit from EGDT in septic shock.[70] A patient-level meta-analysis of the three trials (3,723 patients) confirmed no difference in 90-day mortality for EGDT (24.9%) versus usual care (25.4%). A subgroup analysis of patients with worse shock (higher lactate, combined hypotension, and high lactate, or higher predicted risk of death) also confirmed that EGDT was not associated with improved survival, but was associated with increased ICU days, cardiovascular support, and higher costs.[71]

Vasopressors in Septic Shock—New Vasopressor

Vasopressor recommendations are unchanged, with norepinephrine as first choice, adding vasopressin or epinephrine if unable to achieve target MAP of 65 mm Hg. But an additional vasopressor (Angiotensin II, Giapreza) is now available based on the ATHOS-3 trial. Adult patients with septic or distributive shock, who remained hypotensive despite fluid resuscitation with standard of care vasopressor therapy, were randomized to angiotensin II versus placebo. The primary endpoint of achievement of target MAP at 3 hours was achieved in 70% of angiotensin II patients compared to 23% of placebo patients.[32] Angiotensin II may preferentially be of benefit in acute kidney injury and ARDS, where the renin–angiotensin–aldosterone system (RAS) is dysregulated.[72]

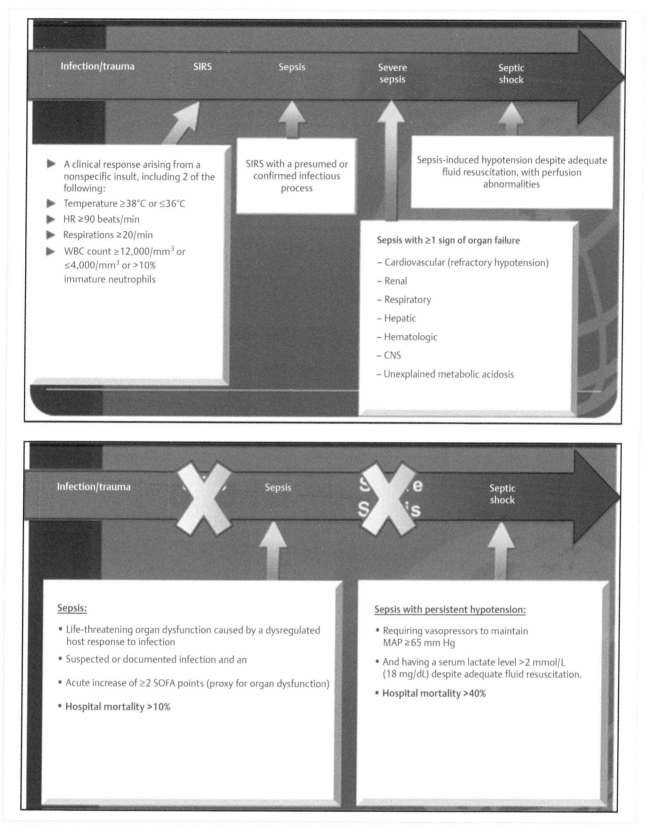

Fig. 3.3 Sepsis-3 new definitions 2016 compared to prior sepsis definitions.

Table 3.2 Surviving sepsis campaign 1-hour bundle

1-hour bundle: initial resuscitation for sepsis and septic shock (begin immediately):
1. Measure lactate.*
2. Obtain blood cultures before administering antibiotics.
3. Administer broad-spectrum antibiotics.
4. Begin rapid administration of 30 mL/kg crystalloid for hypotension or lactate ≥ 4 mmol/L.
5. Apply vasopressors if hypotensive during or after fluid resuscitation to maintain a mean arterial pressure ≥ 65 mm Hg.

* a. Remeasure lactate if initial lactate elevated (> 2 mmol/L).
b. "Time zero" or "time presentation" is defined as the time of triage in the emergency department or, if presenting from another care value, from the earliest chart annotation consistent with all elements of sepsis (formerly severe sepsis) or septic shock ascertained through chart review.

Table 3.3 Sepsis 6-hour bundle: to be completed within 6 hours

In the event of persistent hypotension after initial fluid administration (MAP < 65 mm Hg) or if initial lactate was ≥ 4 mmol/L, reassess volume status and tissue perfusion and document findings with

Either
- Repeat focused examination (after initial fluid resuscitation) by licensed independent practitioner including vital signs, cardiopulmonary, capillary refill, pulse, and skin findings.

or two of the following:
- Measure central venous pressure (CVP).
- Measure central venous oxygen saturation (ScvO₂).
- Bedside cardiovascular ultrasound.
- Dynamic assessment of fluid responsiveness with passive leg raise or fluid challenge.

(3 national and international multicenter trials [ProCESS, ARISE, PROMISE] did not demonstrate superiority of the required use of a central venous catheter to monitor CVP and ScvO₂ in sepsis.)

Abbreviation: CVP, central venous pressure.

Steroids in Septic Shock—Consensus Based on 2 Trials (ADRENAL and APROCCHSS)

Steroid recommendations are unchanged in the 2016 SSC Guidelines—"Consider for patients with septic shock refractory to adequate fluids and vasopressors." But two new large randomized clinical trials have provided consensus for the optimal use of steroids in septic shock.

The APROCCHSS trial (Hydrocortisone plus Fludrocortisone for Adults with Septic Shock) enrolled 1241 ICU patients with septic shock (SOFA score 3–4 for at least two organs and at least 6 hours on vasopressor therapy to maintain mean arterial pressure > 65 mm Hg). Patients were randomized to hydrocortisone (50 mg IV q6 h × 7 days) and fludrocortisone (50 mcg tablet PO × 7 days). Hydrocortisone plus fludrocortisone significantly reduced 90-day all-cause mortality (43 vs. 49%, RR 0.88, 95% CI 0.78–0.99, $p = 0.03$, NNT 17, fragility index 3) and also increased mean vasopressor-free days (17 vs. 15 days, $p < 0.001$).[73]

The ADRENAL (Adjunctive Glucocorticoid Therapy in Patients with Septic Shock) trial enrolled 3658 patients with septic shock requiring vasopressors for ≥ 4 hours and mechanical ventilation. They were randomized to hydrocortisone infusion 200 mg/day for 7 days or ICU discharge versus placebo. Steroids decreased median time to shock reversal (3 vs. 4 days, HR 1.32; 95% CI 1.23–1.41, $p < 0.001$) but did not alter 90-day mortality (27.9 vs. 28.8%).[74]

Based on the findings of these two large RCTs, many ICUs have implemented a quick order for steroid infusion or intermittent dosing (200 mg/day) and fludrocortisone in septic shock patients who continue to require vasopressor therapy for 6 hours or more, with continuation for 7 days or until ICU discharge.

3.2.5 Respiratory Failure/ARDS

Acute respiratory failure is common in adult ICUs. In a study of 2473 patients from 25 ICUs over an 8-week period, 39% required ventilator support (noninvasive or invasive). The 90-day mortality for acute respiratory failure was 31%.[75] In the most recent PReVENT (effect of low vs. intermediate tidal volume strategy on ventilator-free days) trial, 961 patients were randomized to low (6 mL/kg) versus intermediate (10 mL/kg) tidal volumes. It was observed that 90-day mortality was not different (39.1 vs. 37.8%). No difference in ventilator-free days at day 28 (21 vs. 21) or median length of ICU and hospital stay (6 vs. 6) were identified.[76]

Noninvasive Ventilatory Strategies

Not all patients with hypoxemia will require intubation and initiation of invasive mechanical ventilation. Noninvasive ventilation with noninvasive positive pressure ventilation (NIPPV) or heated high-flow nasal cannula (HHFNC) can be used in an attempt to prevent the need for intubation in some patients with hypoxemia. HHFNC is a novel method of oxygen therapy to deliver heated and humidified oxygen at a rate of up to 60 L/min. HHFNC has a widely proven clinical efficacy, easier application, and better patient tolerance in critically ill patients. In a systematic review and meta-analysis of 18 trials with 3881 patients, HHFNC was associated with a lower rate of endotracheal intubation compared to conventional oxygen therapy, and was also a more reliable alternative than NIPPV to reduce the rate of endotracheal intubation due to patient comfort.[77]

ARDS Epidemiology and Outcomes

Some ICU patients with acute respiratory failure will develop hypoxemia and ARDS. Severity of ARDS is classified by degree of hypoxemia as measured by PaO₂/FiO₂ ratios using the Berlin definition[78] of ARDS:
- **Mild ARDS:** PaO₂/FiO₂ 201 to 300.
- **Moderate ARDS:** PaO₂/FiO₂ 101 to 200.
- **Severe ARDS:** PaO₂/FiO₂ ≤ 100.

ARDS patients must also meet the following criteria:
- *Timing*: Within 1 week of a known clinical insult or new/worsening respiratory symptoms.
- *Chest Imaging*: Bilateral opacities not fully explained by effusions, lobar/lung collapse, or nodules.
- *Origin of Edema*: Respiratory failure not fully explained by cardiac failure or fluid overload. Need objective assessment (e.g., echocardiography) to exclude hydrostatic edema if no risk factor is present.

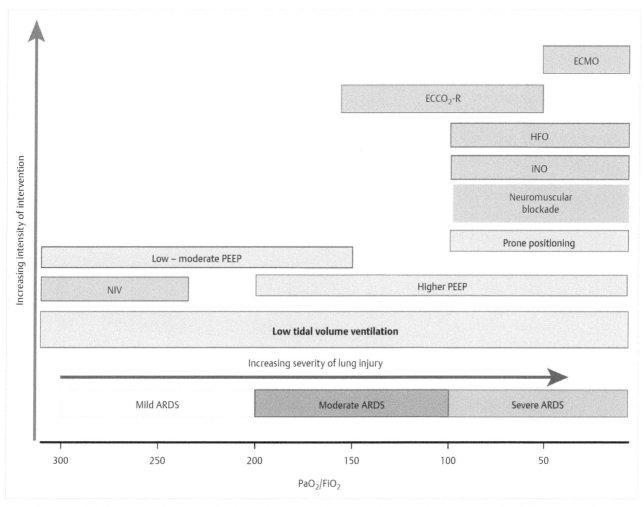

Fig. 3.4 Standard and rescue strategies based on severity of hypoxemia and acute respiratory distress syndrome.

LUNG-SAFE[79] (large observational study to understand the global impact of severe acute respiratory failure) was a multicenter, prospective, observational, 4-week inception cohort global study which enrolled 29,144 patients. ARDS was present in 10.4% of ICU admissions and in 23.4% of ventilated patients with acute respiratory failure. Overall hospital mortality in ARDS patients in the LUNG-SAFE study was as high as 40%. Hospital mortality increased significantly with ARDS severity: mild ARDS (34.9%); moderate ARDS (40.3%); and severe ARDS (46.1%).

Rescue Strategies in ARDS

ARDS treatment includes both "standard" treatment strategies (mechanical ventilation with low-tidal volumes,[80] low-plateau pressures, high PEEP,[81] or restrictive fluid strategy[82]) and "rescue" treatment strategies (neuromuscular blockade, inhaled nitric oxide, prone position, recruitment maneuvers, high-frequency oscillatory ventilation, and extracorporeal membrane oxygenation). Based on the evidence that we possess to date, and using the ARDS Berlin definitions, standard treatment strategies are recommended for all ARDS patients, but rescue treatment strategies are reserved for use

in patients with more severe ARDS and severe hypoxemia, particularly those rescue treatment strategies which are associated with much higher cost (▶ Fig. 3.4). It is useful to have an evidence-based algorithm for ARDS management in the ICU (▶ Fig. 3.5).

The 2017 Clinical Practice Guideline for Mechanical Ventilation in Adult Patients with ARDS has made evidence-based recommendations regarding optimal ICU care of these high-risk patients (▶ Table 3.4), but this guideline was published prior to the ECMO to EOLIA (rescue lung injury in severe ARDS) trial.[83] The EOLIA trial randomized patients with severe ARDS to immediate venovenous ECMO or conventional ARDS treatment. Crossover to ECMO was possible for patients in the control cohort with refractory hypoxemia. It is important to note that after the enrollment of 240 of a projected maximum of 331 patients, the trial was stopped for futility, as per the trial design. Mortality at 60 days was 35% in the ECMO group versus 46% in the control group (RR 0.76, 95% CI 0.55–1.04, $p = 0.09$). Crossover to ECMO occurred in 35 patients (28%) of the control group, with 57% mortality in this cohort. Although 60-day mortality was not different, the relative risk of treatment failure (defined as death by day 60 among patients in the ECMO group, and crossover to ECMO

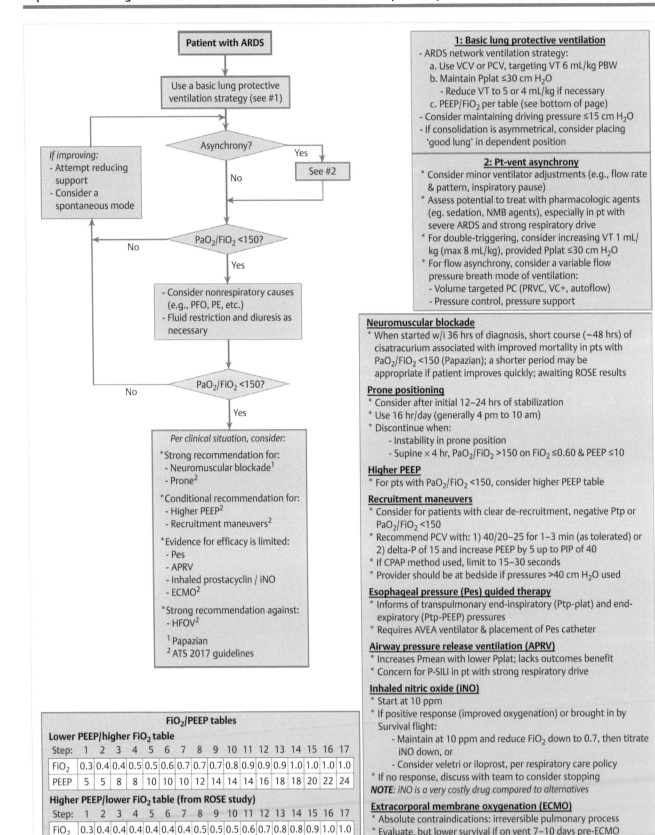

Patient with ARDS

Use a basic lung protective ventilation strategy (see #1)

Asynchrony? → Yes → See #2

No

If improving:
- Attempt reducing support
- Consider a spontaneous mode

PaO₂/FiO₂ <150? → No

Yes

- Consider nonrespiratory causes (e.g., PFO, PE, etc.)
- Fluid restriction and diuresis as necessary

PaO₂/FiO₂ <150? → No

Yes

Per clinical situation, consider:

*Strong recommendation for:
- Neuromuscular blockade[1]
- Prone[2]

*Conditional recommendation for:
- Higher PEEP[2]
- Recruitment maneuvers[2]

*Evidence for efficacy is limited:
- Pes
- APRV
- Inhaled prostacyclin / iNO
- ECMO[2]

*Strong recommendation against:
- HFOV[2]

[1] Papazian
[2] ATS 2017 guidelines

1: Basic lung protective ventilation
- ARDS network ventilation strategy:
   a. Use VCV or PCV, targeting VT 6 mL/kg PBW
   b. Maintain Pplat ≤30 cm H₂O
      - Reduce VT to 5 or 4 mL/kg if necessary
   c. PEEP/FiO₂ per table (see bottom of page)
- Consider maintaining driving pressure ≤15 cm H₂O
- If consolidation is asymmetrical, consider placing 'good lung' in dependent position

2: Pt-vent asynchrony
* Consider minor ventilator adjustments (e.g., flow rate & pattern, inspiratory pause)
* Assess potential to treat with pharmacologic agents (eg. sedation, NMB agents), especially in pt with severe ARDS and strong respiratory drive
* For double-triggering, consider increasing VT 1 mL/kg (max 8 mL/kg), provided Pplat ≤30 cm H₂O
* For flow asynchrony, consider a variable flow pressure breath mode of ventilation:
   - Volume targeted PC (PRVC, VC+, autoflow)
   - Pressure control, pressure support

Neuromuscular blockade
* When started w/i 36 hrs of diagnosis, short course (~48 hrs) of cisatracurium associated with improved mortality in pts with PaO₂/FiO₂ <150 (Papazian); a shorter period may be appropriate if patient improves quickly; awaiting ROSE results

Prone positioning
* Consider after initial 12–24 hrs of stabilization
* Use 16 hr/day (generally 4 pm to 10 am)
* Discontinue when:
   - Instability in prone position
   - Supine × 4 hr, PaO₂/FiO₂ >150 on FiO₂ ≤0.60 & PEEP ≤10

Higher PEEP
* For pts with PaO₂/FiO₂ <150, consider higher PEEP table

Recruitment maneuvers
* Consider for patients with clear de-recruitment, negative Ptp or PaO₂/FiO₂ <150
* Recommend PCV with: 1) 40/20–25 for 1–3 min (as tolerated) or 2) delta-P of 15 and increase PEEP by 5 up to PIP of 40
* If CPAP method used, limit to 15–30 seconds
* Provider should be at bedside if pressures >40 cm H₂O used

Esophageal pressure (Pes) guided therapy
* Informs of transpulmonary end-inspiratory (Ptp-plat) and end-expiratory (Ptp-PEEP) pressures
* Requires AVEA ventilator & placement of Pes catheter

Airway pressure release ventilation (APRV)
* Increases Pmean with lower Pplat; lacks outcomes benefit
* Concern for P-SILI in pt with strong respiratory drive

Inhaled nitric oxide (iNO)
* Start at 10 ppm
* If positive response (improved oxygenation) or brought in by Survival flight:
   - Maintain at 10 ppm and reduce FiO₂ down to 0.7, then titrate iNO down, or
   - Consider veletri or iloprost, per respiratory care policy
* If no response, discuss with team to consider stopping
NOTE: iNO is a very costly drug compared to alternatives

Extracorporal membrane oxygenation (ECMO)
* Absolute contraindications: irreversible pulmonary process
* Evaluate, but lower survival if on vent 7–10 days pre-ECMO

High frequency oscillatory ventilation (HFOV)
* Strong recommendation against routine use; may have benefit if PaO₂/FiO₂ <64; goal is to increase Pmean

---

FiO₂/PEEP tables

Lower PEEP/higher FiO₂ table

Step:	1	2	3	4	5	6	7	8	9	10	11	12	13	14	15	16	17
FiO₂	0.3	0.4	0.4	0.5	0.5	0.6	0.7	0.7	0.7	0.8	0.9	0.9	0.9	1.0	1.0	1.0	1.0
PEEP	5	5	8	8	10	10	10	12	14	14	14	16	18	18	20	22	24

Higher PEEP/lower FiO₂ table (from ROSE study)

Step:	1	2	3	4	5	6	7	8	9	10	11	12	13	14	15	16	17
FiO₂	0.3	0.4	0.4	0.4	0.4	0.4	0.4	0.5	0.5	0.5	0.6	0.7	0.8	0.8	0.9	1.0	1.0
PEEP	5	5	8	10	12	14	16	16	18	20	20	20	20	22	22	22	24

Consider lower PEEP for patients with low PEEP-responsiveness potential (i.e., P/F ≥150);
Higher PEEP if higher PEEP-responsiveness potential (P/F <150) or BMI >35

Fig. 3.5 ARDS mechanical ventilation algorithm, including rescue strategies, used at the University of Michigan. ARDS, acute respiratory distress syndrome.

Table 3.4 Recommendations from the 2017 clinical practice guideline: mechanical ventilation in adult patients with ARDS

Strong recommendations for the following interventions	Mechanical ventilation using lower tidal volumes (4–8 mL/kg predicted body weight) and lower inspiratory pressures (plateau pressure < 30 cm H_2O) *(moderate confidence in effect estimates)*	Prone positioning for more than 12 hours/day in severe ARDS *(moderate confidence in effect estimates)*
Strong recommendations **against** the following interventions	Routine use of high-frequency oscillatory ventilation in patients with moderate or severe ARDS *(high confidence in effect estimates)*	
Conditional recommendations **for** the following interventions	Higher positive end-expiratory pressure in patients with moderate or severe ARDS *(moderate confidence in effect estimates)*	Recruitment maneuvers in patients with moderate or severe ARDS *(low confidence in effect estimates)*
No recommendation	Additional evidence is necessary to make a definitive recommendation for or against the use of ECMO in patients with severe ARDS	

Abbreviations: ARDS, acute respiratory distress syndrome; ECMO, extracorporeal membrane oxygenation.
Source: Adapted from Fan A, DelSorbo L, Goligher EC, et al; on behalf of the American Thoracic Society, European Society of Intensive Care Medicine, and Society of Critical Care Medicine. An Official American Thoracic Society/European Society of Intensive Care Medicine/Society of Critical Care Medicine Clinical Practice Guideline: Mechanical Ventilation in Adult Patients with Acute Respiratory Distress Syndrome. Am J Respir Crit Care Med 2017 May;195(9):1253–1263.

Table 3.5 ARDS net FiO_2 and PEEP titration tables

Lower PEEP/higher FiO_2 table

Step	1	2	3	4	5	6	7	8	9	10	11	12	13	14	15	16	17
FiO_2	0.3	0.4	0.4	0.5	0.5	0.6	0.7	0.7	0.7	0.8	0.9	1.0	1.0	1.0	1.0	1.0	1.0
PEEP	5	5	8	8	10	10	10	12	14	14	14	16	18	18	20	22	24

Higher PEEP/lower FiO_2 table (from ROSE study)

Step	1	2	3	4	5	6	7	8	9	10	11	12	13	14	15	16	17
FiO_2	0.3	0.4	0.4	0.4	0.4	0.4	0.4	0.5	0.5	0.5	0.6	0.7	0.8	0.8	0.9	1.0	1.0
PEEP	5	5	8	10	12	14	16	16	18	20	20	20	20	22	22	22	24

Note: • Consider Lower PEEP table for patients with low lung recruitment potential (P/F ratio ≥ 150).
 • Consider Higher PEEP table for patients with high lung recruitment potential (P/F ratio < 150).
Abbreviations: ARDS, acute respiratory distress syndrome; PEEP, positive end expiratory pressure.

or death in the control group) was significantly lower in the ECMO cohort (RR 0.62, 95% CI 0.47l–0.82, $p < 0.001$).[84] This trial does document the efficacy of ECMO in treatment of severe ARDS, and the significant increased mortality rate when ECMO is provided as a rescue strategy in severe hypoxemia.

The 2017 ARDS Guidelines also did not address recommendations regarding neuromuscular blockade and inhaled nitric oxide. The ACURASYS trial reported that neuromuscular blockade (NMB) with cisatracurium infusion was associated with a significant mortality benefit (hospital mortality decreased 40.7 to 31.6%) and significantly reduced mortality after risk adjustment for baseline P/F ratio, plateau pressure and Simplified Acute Physiology II score (hazard ratio 0.68, 95% CI 0.48–0.98, $p = 0.04$). NMB was associated with increased oxygenation, ventilator-free days, organ-failure-free days, reduced barotrauma (5.1 vs. 11.7%, RR 0.43 [0.20–0.93], $p = 0.03$), and no increased ICU paresis (70.8 vs. 67.5%, p = 0.64).[85]

In contrast to the ACURASYS trial, the 2019 ROSE (re-evaluation of systemic early neuromuscular blockade) trial from The Clinical Trials Network for the Prevention and Early Treatment of Acute Lung Injury (PETAL) documented no difference in 90-day mortality (42.5 vs. 42.8%) in patients with moderate–severe ARDS.[86,87,88] There are significant differences between these trials, with higher PEEP (▶ Table 3.5), lighter sedation, larger sample size (1006 vs. 340) and longer-term

patient outcomes in the ROSE trial.[89] At present, based on the evidence, NMB should only be used as a rescue strategy in ARDS, not as standard of care.

A single-center phase I RCT (n = 61, EPVent1 trial) documented that PEEP adjusted by esophageal pressures to estimate transpulmonary pressure, significantly improved oxygenation, and compliance.[90] Nearly all patients required increased PEEP to maintain a transpulmonary pressure of greater than zero. This trial also documented a trend toward reduced mortality that was maintained at 6 months. The esophageal pressure-guided ventilation 2 (EPVent2) multicenter trial (n = 202) aimed to examine the impact of mechanical ventilation, directed at maintaining a positive transpulmonary pressure in patients with moderate or severe ARDS (P/F ratio ≤ 200).[91,92] The EPVent2 trial differs from the EPVent1 trial with enrollment including patients with moderate or severe ARDS (P/F of 200 or below), control group protocol using a higher PEEP approach, duration of the intervention extending from 3 to 28 days, and the primary endpoint for the current trial being a novel composite measure that combined ventilator-free days and mortality at 28 days, whereas in the EPVent1 trial the primary endpoint was improvement in oxygenation at 72 hours. PEEP titration guided by esophageal pressure resulted in no significant difference in death and days free from mechanical ventilation in the EPVent2 trial.

3.2.6 Acute Kidney Injury

Acute kidney injury (AKI) is a common complication in critically ill patients and is associated with high morbidity and mortality.[93] The etiology of AKI in the ICU is heterogeneous, and can be related to prerenal, renal and postrenal causes. Risk factors for AKI include increased age, heart failure, liver failure, chronic kidney disease, anemia, and exposure to nephrotoxic agents. Sepsis and septic shock are common causes of AKI in critically ill patients and account for more than 50% of cases in the ICU.[94]

Methods to prevent AKI in the ICU include avoidance of nephrotoxic agents, appropriate fluid resuscitation, avoidance of hypovolemic shock, maintenance of adequate mean arterial blood pressure with avoidance of hypotension, and optimization of end-organ perfusion. FeNa and FeUrea can be helpful in determining optimal treatment strategies for early AKI, but are not diagnostically accurate or clinically useful in AKI due to sepsis. Two new biomarkers (urine insulin-like growth factor-binding protein 7 [IGFBP7] and tissue inhibitor of metalloproteinase-2 [TIMP-2]) are now available (NephroCheck) for prediction of AKI risk and the need for renal replacement therapy or persistent renal dysfunction.[95,96,97]

3.2.7 Nutrition

An initial nutrition assessment is very important in all critically ill surgical patients. Not all ICU patients are the same in terms of nutritional status. The NUTRIC (Canadian Nutrition Risk in the Critically Ill) score is one way to accurately quantify nutritional status and risk and can be used to determine optimal nutrition support in ICU patients.

The NUTRIC score (0–10, ▶ Fig. 3.6) is based on age, APACHE II score, SOFA score, comorbidities, pre-ICU hospital length of stay, and blood IL-6 level if available. A high-NUTRIC score is associated with worse outcomes (increased mortality and duration of mechanical ventilation), and these patients benefit the most from aggressive nutrition support. In low-NUTRIC score ICU patients, more nutrition has no benefit, and may have a signal for harm. Defining nutritional risk in individual ICU patients yields the optimal benefit from nutritional therapy in the ICU.

The 2016 ASPEN/SCCM Guidelines[98] suggest starting enteral nutrition within 24 to 48 hours in high-nutritional risk ICU patients (NUTRIC score ≥ 5) with a nutrition goal of 80%, and estimated energy (25–30 kcal/kg/day) and protein (1–2 g/kg/day) goal within 48 to 72 hours. The guidelines also include a "nutrition bundle" (▶ Table 3.6) with additional evidence-based goals for nutrition support in the ICU.

The recent TARGET (The Augmented versus Routine approach to Giving Energy Trial) trial compared energy-dense (1.5 kcal/mL) with routine (1.0 kcal/ml) enteral nutrition at a dose of 1 mL/kg ideal body weight per hour in 3957 ICU patients and concluded that higher calorie delivery had no impact on 90-day mortality, organ support, number of days alive and out of the ICU and hospital or free of organ support.[99] Interestingly, the group receiving high-density feedings had higher need for insulin, more emesis, higher gastric residuals, and receipt of more promotility drugs. These findings are similar to the findings of two other similar studies,[100,101] documenting the overall safety of a low-calorie approach in critical ill patients without malnutrition as long as adequate protein intake (1–2 g/kg/day) is provided.

In most critically ill patients, the use of enteral versus parenteral nutrition has no impact on overall mortality.[102,103,104] For malnourished and long-stay ICU patients, who are usually not included in these clinical trials, additional studies are warranted. Monitoring for refeeding syndrome (hypokalemia, hypophosphatemia) with initiation of nutrition support is very important in ICU patients who meet the criteria for malnutrition.

3.2.8 Pain, Agitation, and Delirium

Pain, agitation, and delirium are very common in ICU patients, and evidence-based management is important in their critical care. The original Pain, Agitation, Delirium (PAD) Guidelines were published in 2013.[105] Agitation in critically ill patients may result from inadequately treated pain, anxiety, delirium and/or ventilator dysynchrony. Detection and treatment of pain, agitation and delirium should be reassessed often in these patients. Light sedation is recommended in ICU patients to prevent delirium. ICU patients should be awake and able to purposely follow commands in order to participate in their ICU care, unless a clinical indication for deeper sedation exists.

The PAD pocket card (▶ Table 3.7) lists the evidence-based recommendations from the original PAD Guidelines, recommending opioids as first-line therapy for treatment of nonneuropathic pain with the use of nonopioid adjuncts to reduce opioid requirements. The use of nonbenzodiazepine sedation (propofol or dexmedetomidine) was recommended in mechanically ventilated adult ICU patients. Delirium assessment should be routinely performed, and early mobility and sleep promotion were recommended.

A recent update in 2018 addressed pain, agitation/sedation, delirium, immobility and sleep disruption (PADIS Guidelines 2018) in adult patients in the ICU.[106] Some new recommendations include consideration of the addition of nefopam and/or ketamine for pain management to reduce opioid requirements. Light sedation and delirium screening are again recommended. For delirium treatment, they "suggest not routinely using haloperidol, an atypical antipsychotic, or a HMG-CoA reductase inhibitor (i.e., a statin) to treat delirium. We suggest using dexmedetomidine for delirium in mechanically ventilated adults where agitation precludes weaning/extubation."

A recent small study documented that the administration of ramelteon, a melatonin-receptor agonist, was associated with a significant reduction in the occurrence rate of delirium (24.4 vs. 46.5%, $p = 0.044$) and duration of delirium (0.78 vs. 1.40 days, $p = -0.048$). A multicenter RCT is ongoing (prophylactic melatonin for delirium in intensive care [Pro-MEDIC]), aiming to enroll 850 patients, and randomized to receive melatonin 4 mg enteral versus placebo once daily at 2100 pm until ICU discharge.[107,108] We commonly use melatonin as a sleep aid in the ICU, given its potential efficacy in prevention of delirium as well.

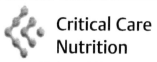

Critical Care
Nutrition

NUTRIC score[1] www.criticalcarenutrition.com

The NUTRIC score is designed to quantify the risk of critically ill patients developing adverse events that may be modified by aggressive nutrition therapy. The score, of 1–10, is based on 6 variables that are explained below in Table 1. The scoring system is shown in Tables 2 and 3.

NUTRIC score variables

Variable	Range	Points
Age	< 50	0
	50 – < 75	1
	≥ 75	2
APACHE II	< 15	0
	15 – < 20	1
	20 – 28	2
	≥ 28	3
SOFA	< 6	0
	6 – < 10	1
	≥ 10	2
Number of co-morbidities	0–1	0
	≥ 2	1
Days from hospital to ICU admission	0 – < 1	0
	≥ 1	1
IL-6	0 – < 400	0
	≥ 400	1

NUTRIC score scoring system: If IL-6 available

Sum of points	Category	Explanation
6–10	High score	➤ Associated with worse clinical outcomes (mortality, ventilation). ➤ These patients are the most likely to benefit from aggressive nutrition therapy.
0–5	Low score	➤ These patients have a low malnutrition risk.

NUTRIC score scoring system: If no IL-6 available*

Sum of points	Category	Explanation
5–9	High score	➤ Associated with worse clinical outcomes (mortality, ventilation). ➤ These patients are the most likely to benefit from aggressive nutrition therapy.
0–4	Low score	➤ These patients have a low malnutrition risk.

*It is acceptable to not include IL-6 data when it is not routinely available; it was shown to contribute very little to the overall prediction of the NUTRIC score.[2]

[1]Heyland DK, Dhaliwal R, Jiang X, Day AG. Identifying critically ill patients who benefit the most from nutrition therapy; the development and initial validation of a novel risk assessment tool. Critical care. 2011;15(6):R268.
[2]Rahman A, Hasan RM, Agarwala R, Martin C, Day AG, Heyland DK. Identifying critically ill patients who will benefit most from nutritional theraphy: Further validation of the "modified NUTRIC" nutritional risk assessment tool. Clin Nutr. 2015. [Epub ahead of print]

Fig. 3.6 NUTRIC score to assess ICU patient nutrition risk. ICU, intensive care unit; NUTRIC, nutrition risk in the critically ill.

Table 3.6 Nutrition bundle and recommendations from the 2016 ASPEN/SCCM guidelines

- Assess patients on admission to the ICU for nutrition risk and calculate both energy and protein requirements to determine goals of nutrition therapy.
  - Calculate the NUTRIC Score (https://www.mdcalc.com/nutrition-risk-critically-ill-nutric-score)
  - Calculate the NRS 2002 score (https://www.mdcalc.com/nutrition-risk-screening-2002-nrs-2002)
- Suggest not using serum markers (albumin, prealbumin, or transferrin) for nutrition assessment in critically ill adults as they are not validated.
- Use indirect calorimetry to determine energy requirements, and if not available, then use published predictive equations or weight-based equation (25–30 kcal/kg/d).
- Initiate enteral nutrition within 24 to 48 hours, following the onset of critical illness and admission to the ICU and increase to goals over the first week of ICU stay.
- For patients who are malnourished or high nutrition risk (NRS or NUTRIC Score 2002 ≥ 5), nutrition support should be advanced toward goal as quickly as possible over 24–48 hours while monitoring for refeeding syndrome.
- Take steps as needed to reduce risk of aspiration or improve tolerance to gastric feeding (use prokinetic agent, continuous infusion, chlorhexidine mouthwash; elevate the head of bed; and divert level of feeding in the gastrointestinal tract from gastric to beyond the ligament of Treitz).
- Implement enteral feeding protocols with institution-specific strategies to promote delivery of enteral nutrition.
- Do not use gastric residual volumes as part of routine care to monitor ICU patients receiving enteral nutrition.
- Start parenteral nutrition early when enteral nutrition is not feasible or sufficient in high-nutrition risk or malnourished patients.

Abbreviations: ICU, intensive care unit; NUTRIC, nutrition risk in the critically ill; NRS, nutrition risk screening.
Source: Adapted from McClave SA, Taylor BE, Martindale RG, et al: Guidelines for the provision and assessment of nutrition support therapy in the adult critically ill patient: Society of Critical Care Medicine (SCCM) and American Society for Parenteral and Enteral Nutrition (A.S.P.E.N.). JPEN J Parenter Enteral Nutr 2016; 40: pp. 159–211.

Table 3.7 Guideline recommendations for treatment of pain, agitation, and delirium

Assess and Treat	Recommendations
Pain	Pain management guided by routine pain assessment Pain should be treated before a sedative agent is considered (analgesia-first sedation), making treating pain a priority Suggest using an assessment-driven, protocol-based, stepwise approach for pain management Suggest using acetaminophen as an adjunct to opioids to decrease pain intensity and opioid consumption in critically ill adults Suggest using nefopam either as adjunct or replacement for opioids Suggest using low-dose ketamine (1–2 ug/kg/hr) as adjunct to opioids in postsurgical adults admitted to the ICU Recommend using neuropathic pain medication (gabapentin, carbamazepine, pregabalin) with opioids for neuropathic pain management Suggest using an NSAID as an alternative to opioids Suggest offering massage, music, cold, or relaxation therapy
Agitation	Suggest using light (vs. deep) sedation in mechanically ventilated adults Suggest using propofol over benzodiazepine for sedation in mechanically ventilated adults after cardiac surgery Suggest using either propofol or dexmedetomidine over benzodiazepines for sedation in mechanically ventilated adults
Delirium	Regular assessment for delirium using a valid tool Suggest not using haloperidol, atypical antipsychotic, dexmedetomidine or ketamine to prevent delirium in all critically ill adults Suggest not using haloperidol or atypical antipsychotic to treat delirium in critically ill adults Suggest using dexmedetomidine for delirium in mechanically ventilated adults where agitation precludes weaning/extubation Suggest using a multicomponent nonpharmacologic intervention focused on reducing modifiable risk factors for delirium Suggest performing rehabilitation/mobilization in critically ill adults

Abbreviation: NSAID, nonsteroidal anti-inflammatory drug.
Source: Adapted from Devlin JW, Skrobik Y, Gelinas C, et al. Clinical practice guidelines for the prevention and management of pain, agitation/sedation, delirium, immobility and sleep disruption in adult patients in the ICU (2018 PADIS Guidelines). Crit Care Med 2018 Sept 46(9):e825–873.

3.2.9 Prevention of Complications/Prophylaxis

One of the important goals of the ICU team is to provide appropriate prophylaxis for prevention of ICU-related complications. Common complications in the ICU include venous thromboembolism (VTE), hyperglycemia, healthcare-associated infections (HAIs), and pressure injuries. Stress ulcers are less common in the ICU than in the past, but stress ulcer prophylaxis is provided for appropriate patients at high risk. The recent stress ulcer prophylaxis in the intensive care unit (SUP-ICU) trial enrolled 3298 patients, randomized to low-dose pantoprazole (40 mg IV daily) or placebo, and found no difference in 90-day mortality. However, in the pantoprazole group, 41 patients (2.5%) had clinically important gastrointestinal bleeding, as compared with 69 (4.2%) in the placebo group, with no difference in pneumonia or C. difficile infection. Therefore, we reserve stress ulcer prophylaxis for patients at high risk for upper gastrointestinal (GI) bleeding, with risk factors of mechanical ventilation and coagulopathy. A checklist using the mnemonic FASTHUG (feeding, analgesia, sedation, thromboembolic prevention, head of the bed elevation, stress ulcer prophylaxis, and glucose control), which is reviewed daily during multidisciplinary ICU rounds to ensure protocol adherence, has been effective.[109]

References

[1] To KB, Kamdar NS, Patil P, et al. Michigan Surgical Quality Collaborative (MSQC) Emergency General Surgery Study Group and the MSQC Research Advisory Group. Acute care surgery model and outcomes in emergency general surgery. J Am Coll Surg. 2019; 228(1):21–28.e7

[2] Vincent JL, De Backer D. Circulatory shock. N Engl J Med. 2013; 369(18): 1726–1734

[3] Kanji HD, McCallum J, Sirounis D, MacRedmond R, Moss R, Boyd JH. Limited echocardiography-guided therapy in subacute shock is associated with change in management and improved outcomes. J Crit Care. 2014; 29(5): 700–705

[4] Shokoohi H, Boniface KS, Pourmand A, et al. Bedside ultrasound reduces diagnostic uncertainty and guides resuscitation in patients with undifferentiated hypotension. Crit Care Med. 2015; 43(12):2562–2569

[5] Ferrada P. Image-based resuscitation of the hypotensive patient with cardiac ultrasound: An evidence-based review. J Trauma Acute Care Surg. 2016; 80 (3):511–518

[6] Bentzer P, Griesdale DE, Boyd J, MacLean K, Sirounis D, Ayas NT. Will This Hemodynamically Unstable Patient Respond to a Bolus of Intravenous Fluids? JAMA. 2016; 316(12):1298–1309

[7] Meisinger QC, Brown MA, Dehqanzada ZA, Doucet J, Coimbra R, Casola G. A 10-year restrospective evaluation of ultrasound in pregnant abdominal trauma patients. Emerg Radiol. 2016; 23(2):105–109

[8] Harvey S, Harrison DA, Singer M, et al. PAC-Man study collaboration. Assessment of the clinical effectiveness of pulmonary artery catheters in management of patients in intensive care (PAC-Man): a randomised controlled trial. Lancet. 2005; 366(9484):472–477

[9] Waibel BH, Rotondo MF. Damage control for intra-abdominal sepsis. Surg Clin North Am. 2012; 92(2):243–257, viii

[10] Bruder EA, Ball IM, Ridi S, Pickett W, Hohl C. Single induction dose of etomidate versus other induction agents for endotracheal intubation in critically ill patients. Cochrane Database Syst Rev. 2015; 1:CD010225

[11] Henry SM. Advanced Trauma Life Support Course Student Manual. 10th ed. Chicago, IL: American College of Surgeons; 2018

[12] Gamper G, Havel C, Arrich J, et al. Vasopressors for hypotensive shock. Cochrane Database Syst Rev. 2016; 2:CD003709

[13] Permpikul C, Tongyoo S, Viarasilpa T, Trainarongsakul T, Chakorn T, Udompanturak S. Early Use of Norepinephrine in Septic Shock Resuscitation (CENSER). a randomized trial. Am J Respir Crit Care Med. 2019; 199(9): 1097–1105

[14] Poukkanen M, Wilkman E, Vaara ST, et al. FINNAKI Study Group. Hemodynamic variables and progression of acute kidney injury in critically ill patients with severe sepsis: data from the prospective observational FINNAKI study. Crit Care. 2013; 17(6):R295

[15] Hylands M, Moller MH, Asfar P, et al. A systematic review of vasopressor blood pressure targets in critically ill adults with hypotension. Can J Anaesth. 2017; 64(7):703–715

[16] Rochwerg B, Hylands M, Møller MH, et al. CCCS-SSAI WikiRecs clinical practice guideline: vasopressor blood pressure targets in critically ill adults with hypotension and vasopressor use in early traumatic shock. Intensive Care Med. 2017; 43(7):1062–1064

[17] Jozwiak M, Monnet X, Teboul JL. Pressure Waveform Analysis. Anesth Analg. 2018; 126(6):1930–1933

[18] Porter TR, Shillcutt SK, Adams MS, et al. Guidelines for the use of echocardiography as a monitor for therapeutic intervention in adults: a report from the American Society of Echocardiography. J Am Soc Echocardiogr. 2015; 28 (1):40–56

[19] Reeves ST, Finley AC, Skubas NJ, et al. Council on Perioperative Echocardiography of the American Society of Echocardiography and the Society of Cardiovascular Anesthesiologists. Special article: basic perioperative transesophageal echocardiography examination: a consensus statement of the American Society of Echocardiography and the Society of Cardiovascular Anesthesiologists. Anesth Analg. 2013; 117(3):543–558

[20] Maltais S, Costello WT, Billings FT, IV, et al. Episodic monoplane transesophageal echocardiography impacts postoperative management of the cardiac surgery patient. J Cardiothorac Vasc Anesth. 2013; 27(4): 665–669

[21] Kirkpatrick AW, Sugrue M, McKee JL, et al. Update from the Abdominal Compartment Society (WSACS) on intra-abdominal hypertension and abdominal compartment syndrome: past, present, and future beyond Banff 2017. Anaesthesiol Intensive Ther. 2017; 49(2):83–87

[22] Holcomb JB, Tilley BC, Baraniuk S, et al. PROPPR Study Group. Transfusion of plasma, platelets, and red blood cells in a 1:1:1 vs a 1:1:2 ratio and mortality in patients with severe trauma: the PROPPR randomized clinical trial. JAMA. 2015; 313(5):471–482

[23] Spinella PC, Gurney J, Yazer MH. Low titer group O whole blood for prehospital hemorrhagic shock: it is an offer we cannot refuse. Transfusion. 2019; 59(7):2177–2179

[24] Joseph B, Zeeshan M, Sakran JV, et al. Nationwide analysis of resuscitative endovascular balloon occlusion of the aorta in civilian trauma. JAMA Surg. 2019; 154(6):500–508

[25] Doucet J, Coimbra R. REBOA: is it ready for prime time? J Vasc Bras. 2017; 16 (1):1–3

[26] Ordoñez CA, Manzano-Nunez R, Parra MW, et al. Prophylactic use of resuscitative endovascular balloon occlusion of the aorta in women with abnormal placentation: A systematic review, meta-analysis, and case series. J Trauma Acute Care Surg. 2018; 84(5):809–818

[27] Russell JA, Walley KR, Singer J, et al. VASST Investigators. Vasopressin versus norepinephrine infusion in patients with septic shock. N Engl J Med. 2008; 358(9):877–887

[28] McIntyre WF, Um KJ, Alhazzani W, et al. Association of vasopressin plus catecholamine vasopressors vs catecholamines alone with atrial fibrillation in patients with distributive shock: a systematic review and meta-analysis. JAMA. 2018; 319(18):1889–1900

[29] Dupuis C, Sonneville R, Adrie C, et al. Impact of transfusion on patients with sepsis admitted in intensive care unit: a systematic review and meta-analysis. Ann Intensive Care. 2017; 7(1):5

[30] McCartney SL, Duce L, Ghadimi K. Intraoperative vasoplegia: methylene blue to the rescue! Curr Opin Anaesthesiol. 2018; 31(1):43–49

[31] Lo JC, Darracq MA, Clark RF. A review of methylene blue treatment for cardiovascular collapse. J Emerg Med. 2014; 46(5):670–679

[32] Khanna A, English SW, Wang XS, et al. ATHOS-3 Investigators. Angiotensin II for the treatment of vasodilatory shock. N Engl J Med. 2017; 377(5):419–430

[33] Leibovici L, Paul M, Poznanski O, et al. Monotherapy versus beta-lactam-aminoglycoside combination treatment for gram-negative bacteremia: a prospective, observational study. Antimicrob Agents Chemother. 1997; 41 (5):1127–1133

[34] Liu VX, Fielding-Singh V, Greene JD, et al. The timing of early antibiotics and hospital mortality in sepsis. Am J Respir Crit Care Med. 2017; 196(7): 856–863

[35] Sherwin R, Winters ME, Vilke GM, Wardi G. Does early and appropriate antibiotic administration improve mortality in emergency department patients with severe sepsis or septic shock? J Emerg Med. 2017; 53(4):588–595

[36] Warren J, Fromm RE, Jr, Orr RA, Rotello LC, Horst HM, American College of Critical Care Medicine. Guidelines for the inter- and intrahospital transport of critically ill patients. Crit Care Med. 2004; 32(1):256–262

[37] Deree J, Shenvi E, Fortlage D, et al. Patient factors and operating room resuscitation predict mortality in traumatic abdominal aortic injury: a 20-year analysis. J Vasc Surg. 2007; 45(3):493–497

[38] Watanabe H, Shimojo Y, Hira E, et al. First establishment of a new table-rotated-type hybrid emergency room system. Scand J Trauma Resusc Emerg Med. 2018; 26(1):80

[39] Nates JL, Nunnally M, Kleinpell R, et al. ICU Admission, Discharge, and Triage Guidelines: a framework to enhance clinical operations, development of institutional policies, and further research. Crit Care Med. 2016; 44(8): 1553–1602

[40] Resources for Optimal Care of the Injured Patient. 2014

[41] Pronovost PJ, Angus DC, Dorman T, Robinson KA, Dremsizov TT, Young TL. Physician staffing patterns and clinical outcomes in critically ill patients: a systematic review. JAMA. 2002; 288(17):2151–2162

[42] The Leapfrog Group. Available at: https://www.leapfroggroup.org/sites/default/files/Files/2018%20IPS%20Fact%20Sheet.pdf. Accessed March 24, 2020

[43] Society of Critical Care Medicine. Available at: www.iculiberation.org. Accessed March 24, 2020

[44] Ely EW. The ABCDEF Bundle: science and philosophy of how ICU liberation serves patients and families. Crit Care Med. 2017; 45(2):321–330

[45] Barnes-Daly MA, Phillips G, Ely EW. Improving hospital survival and reducing brain dysfunction at seven California community hospitals: implementing PAD Guidelines Via the ABCDEF Bundle in 6,064 patients. Crit Care Med. 2017; 45(2):171–178

[46] Pun BT, Balas MC, Barnes-Daly MA, et al. Caring for critically ill patients with the ABCDEF Bundle: Results of the ICU Liberation Collaborative in over 15,000 adults. Crit Care Med. 2019; 47(1):3–14

[47] Balas MC, Pun BT, Pasero C, et al. Common challenges to effective ABCDEF Bundle implementation: the ICU Liberation Campaign Experience. Crit Care Nurse. 2019; 39(1):46–60

[48] Huygh J, Peeters Y, Bernards J, Malbrain ML. Hemodynamic monitoring in the critically ill: an overview of current cardiac output monitoring methods. F1000Res. 2016:5. pii: F1000 Faculty Rev-2855. eCollection 2016. (Open access)

[49] Hernández G, Ospina-Tascón GA, Damiani LP, et al. The ANDROMEDA SHOCK Investigators and the Latin America Intensive Care Network (LIVEN). Effect of a resuscitation strategy targeting peripheral perfusion status vs serum lactate levels on 28-day mortality among patients with septic shock: the ANDROMEDA-SHOCK Randomized Clinical Trial. JAMA. 2019; 321(7): 654–664

[50] Napolitano LM. Anemia and red blood cell transfusion: advances in critical care. Crit Care Clin. 2017; 33(2):345–364

[51] Shehata N, Forster AJ, Lawrence N, et al. Transfusion patterns in all patients admitted to the intensive care unit and in those who die in hospital: a descriptive analysis. PLoS One. 2015; 10(9):e0138427

[52] Napolitano LM, Kurek S, Luchette FA, et al. EAST Practice Management Workgroup, American College of Critical Care Medicine (ACCM) Taskforce of the Society of Critical Care Medicine (SCCM). Clinical practice guideline: red blood cell transfusion in adult trauma and critical care. J Trauma. 2009; 67 (6):1439–1442

[53] Holst LB, Petersen MW, Haase N, Perner A, Wetterslev J. Restrictive versus liberal transfusion strategy for red blood cell transfusion: systematic review of randomised trials with meta-analysis and trial sequential analysis. BMJ. 2015; 350:h1354

[54] Spahn DR, Spahn GH, Stein P. Evidence base for restrictive transfusion triggers in high-risk patients. Transfus Med Hemother. 2015; 42(2):110–114

[55] Carson JL, Guyatt G, Heddle NM, et al. Clinical Practice Guidelines From the AABB: red blood cell transfusion thresholds and storage. JAMA. 2016; 316 (19):2025–2035

[56] Chatterjee S, Wetterslev J, Sharma A, Lichstein E, Mukherjee D. Association of blood transfusion with increased mortality in myocardial infarction: a meta-analysis and diversity-adjusted study sequential analysis. JAMA Intern Med. 2013; 173(2):132–139

[57] Carson JL, Brooks MM, Abbott JD, et al. Liberal versus restrictive transfusion thresholds for patients with symptomatic coronary artery disease. Am Heart J. 2013; 165(6):964–971.e1

[58] ClinicalTrials.gov. Available at: https://clinicaltrials.gov/ct2/show/NCT-02981407. Accessed March 24, 2020

[59] Cherry-Bukowiec JR, Engoren M, Wiktor A, Raghavendran K, Napolitano LM. Hepcidin and anemia in surgical critical care: a prospective cohort study. Crit Care Med. 2018; 46(6):e567–e574

[60] Dolman HS, Evans K, Zimmerman LH, et al. Impact of minimizing diagnostic blood loss in the critically ill. Surgery. 2015; 158(4):1083–1087, discussion 1087–1088

[61] Mukhopadhyay A, Yip HS, Prabhuswamy D, et al. The use of a blood conservation device to reduce red blood cell transfusion requirements: a before and after study. Crit Care. 2010; 14(1):R7

[62] Napolitano LM. Sepsis 2018: Definitions and Guideline Changes. Surg Infect (Larchmt). 2018; 19(2):117–125

[63] Singer M, Deutschman CS, Seymour CW, et al. The Third International Consensus Definitions for Sepsis and Septic Shock (Sepsis-3). JAMA. 2016; 315(8):801–810

[64] Levy MM, Evans LE, Rhodes A. The Surviving Sepsis Campaign Bundle: 2018 Update. Crit Care Med. 2018; 46(6):997–1000

[65] Dellinger RP, Schorr CA, Levy MMA. A Users' Guide to the 2016 Surviving Sepsis Guidelines. Crit Care Med. 2017; 45(3):381–385

[66] Yealy DM, Kellum JA, Huang DT, et al. ProCESS Investigators. A randomized trial of protocol-based care for early septic shock. N Engl J Med. 2014; 370 (18):1683–1693

[67] Peake SL, Delaney A, Bailey M, et al. ARISE Investigators, ANZICS Clinical Trials Group. Goal-directed resuscitation for patients with early septic shock. N Engl J Med. 2014; 371(16):1496–1506

[68] Mouncey PR, Osborn TM, Power GS, et al. ProMISe Trial Investigators. Trial of early, goal-directed resuscitation for septic shock. N Engl J Med. 2015; 372 (14):1301–1311

[69] Rivers E, Nguyen B, Havstad S, et al. Early Goal-Directed Therapy Collaborative Group. Early goal-directed therapy in the treatment of severe sepsis and septic shock. N Engl J Med. 2001; 345(19):1368–1377

[70] Angus DC, Barnato AE, Bell D, et al. A systematic review and meta-analysis of early goal-directed therapy for septic shock: the ARISE, ProCESS and ProMISe Investigators. Intensive Care Med. 2015; 41(9):1549–1560

[71] Rowan KM, Angus DC, Bailey M, et al. PRISM Investigators. Early, goal-directed therapy for septic shock—A patient-level meta-analysis. N Engl J Med. 2017; 376(23):2223–2234

[72] Bussard RL, Busse LW. Angiotensin II: a new therapeutic option for vasodilatory shock. Ther Clin Risk Manag. 2018; 14:1287–1298

[73] Annane D, Renault A, Brun-Buisson C, et al. CRICS-TRIGGERSEP Network. Hydrocortisone plus fludrocortisone for adults with septic shock. N Engl J Med. 2018; 378(9):809–818

[74] Venkatesh B, Finfer S, Cohen J, et al. ADRENAL Trial Investigators and the Australian–New Zealand Intensive Care Society Clinical Trials Group. Adjunctive glucocorticoid therapy in patients with septic shock. N Engl J Med. 2018; 378(9):797–808

[75] Linko R, Okkonen M, Pettilä V, et al. FINNALI-study group. Acute respiratory failure in intensive care units. FINNALI: a prospective cohort study. Intensive Care Med. 2009; 35(8):1352–1361

[76] Simonis FD, Serpa Neto A, Binnekade JM, et al. Writing Group for the PReVENT Investigators. Effect of a low vs intermediate tidal volume strategy on ventilator-free days in intensive care unit patients without ARDS: a randomized clinical trial. JAMA. 2018; 320(18):1872–1880

[77] Ni YN, Luo J, Yu H, et al. Can high-flow nasal cannula reduce the rate of endotracheal intubation in adult patients with acute respiratory failure compared with conventional oxygen therapy and noninvasive positive pressure ventilation? A systematic review and meta-analysis. Chest. 2017; 151 (4):764–775

[78] Ranieri VM, Rubenfeld GD, Thompson BT, et al. ARDS Definition Task Force. Acute respiratory distress syndrome: the Berlin Definition. JAMA. 2012; 307 (23):2526–2533

[79] Bellani G, Laffey JG, Pham T, et al. LUNG SAFE Investigators, ESICM Trials Group. Epidemiology, patterns of care, and mortality for patients with acute respiratory distress syndrome in intensive care units in 50 countries. JAMA. 2016; 315(8):788–800

[80] Brower RG, Matthay MA, Morris A, Schoenfeld D, Thompson BT, Wheeler A, Acute Respiratory Distress Syndrome Network. Ventilation with lower tidal volumes as compared with traditional tidal volumes for acute lung injury and the acute respiratory distress syndrome. N Engl J Med. 2000; 342(18): 1301–1308

[81] Briel M, Meade M, Mercat A, et al. Higher vs lower positive end-expiratory pressure in patients with acute lung injury and acute respiratory distress syndrome: systematic review and meta-analysis. JAMA. 2010; 303(9): 865–873

[82] Wiedemann HP, Wheeler AP, Bernard GR, et al. National Heart, Lung, and Blood Institute Acute Respiratory Distress Syndrome (ARDS) Clinical Trials Network. Comparison of two fluid-management strategies in acute lung injury. N Engl J Med. 2006; 354(24):2564–2575

[83] Fan E, Del Sorbo L, Goligher EC, et al. American Thoracic Society, European Society of Intensive Care Medicine, and Society of Critical Care Medicine. An Official American Thoracic Society/European Society of Intensive Care Medicine/Society of Critical Care Medicine Clinical Practice Guideline: mechanical ventilation in adult patients with acute respiratory distress syndrome. Am J Respir Crit Care Med. 2017; 195(9):1253–1263

[84] Combes A, Hajage D, Capellier G, et al. EOLIA Trial Group, REVA, and ECMONet. Extracorporeal membrane oxygenation for severe acute respiratory distress syndrome. N Engl J Med. 2018; 378(21):1965–1975

[85] Papazian L, Forel JM, Gacouin A, et al. ACURASYS Study Investigators. Neuromuscular blockers in early acute respiratory distress syndrome. N Engl J Med. 2010; 363(12):1107–1116

[86] Huang DT, Angus DC, Moss M, et al. Reevaluation of Systemic Early Neuromuscular Blockade Protocol Committee and the National Institutes of Health National Heart, Lung, and Blood Institute Prevention and Early Treatment of Acute Lung Injury Network Investigators. Design and rationale of the reevaluation of systemic early neuromuscular blockade trial for acute respiratory distress syndrome. Ann Am Thorac Soc. 2017; 14(1): 124–133

[87] ClinicalTrials.gov. Available at: https://clinicaltrials.gov/ct2/show/NCT-02509078. Accessed March 24, 2020

[88] Petal Network. Available at: http://petalnet.org/. Accessed March 24, 2020

[89] Moss M, Huang DT, Brower RG, et al. National Heart, Lung, and Blood Institute PETAL Clinical Trials Network. Early neuromuscular blockade in the acute respiratory distress syndrome. N Engl J Med. 2019; 380(21): 1997–2008

[90] Talmor D, Sarge T, Malhotra A, et al. Mechanical ventilation guided by esophageal pressure in acute lung injury. N Engl J Med. 2008; 359(20): 2095–2104

[91] ClinicalTrials.gov. Available at: https://clinicaltrials.gov/ct2/show/NCT01681225?term=epvent2&rank=1. Accessed March 24, 2020

[92] Beitler JR, Sarge T, Banner-Goodspeed VM, et al. EPVent-2 Study Group. Effect of Titrating Positive End-Expiratory Pressure (PEEP) with an esophageal pressure-guided strategy vs an empirical high PEEP-Fio2 strategy on death and days free from mechanical ventilation among patients with acute respiratory distress syndrome: a randomized clinical trial. JAMA. 2019; 321(9): 846–857

[93] Bellomo R, Ronco C, Mehta RL, et al. Acute kidney injury in the ICU: from injury to recovery: reports from the 5th Paris International Conference. Ann Intensive Care. 2017; 7(1):49

[94] Uchino S, Kellum JA, Bellomo R, et al. Beginning and Ending Supportive Therapy for the Kidney (BEST Kidney) Investigators. Acute renal failure in critically ill patients: a multinational, multicenter study. JAMA. 2005; 294 (7):813–818

[95] Kashani K, Al-Khafaji A, Ardiles T, et al. Discovery and validation of cell cycle arrest biomarkers in human acute kidney injury. Crit Care. 2013; 17(1):R25

[96] Bihorac A, Chawla LS, Shaw AD, et al. Validation of cell-cycle arrest biomarkers for acute kidney injury using clinical adjudication. Am J Respir Crit Care Med. 2014; 189(8):932–939

[97] Vijayan A, Faubel S, Askenazi DJ, et al. American Society of Nephrology Acute Kidney Injury Advisory Group. Clinical use of the urine biomarker [TIMP-2] × [IGFBP7] for acute kidney injury risk assessment. Am J Kidney Dis. 2016; 68(1):19–28

[98] Taylor BE, McClave SA, Martindale RG, et al. Society of Critical Care Medicine, American Society of Parenteral and Enteral Nutrition. Guidelines for the provision and assessment of nutrition support therapy in the adult critically ill patient: Society of Critical Care Medicine (SCCM) and American Society for Parenteral and Enteral Nutrition (A.S.P.E.N.). Crit Care Med. 2016; 44(2):390–438

[99] Chapman M, Peake SL, Bellomo R, et al. TARGET Investigators, for the ANZICS Clinical Trials Group. Energy-dense versus routine enteral nutrition in the critically ill. N Engl J Med. 2018; 379(19):1823–1834

[100] Arabi YM, Aldawood AS, Haddad SH, et al. PermiT Trial Group. Permissive underfeeding or standard enteral feeding in critically ill adults. N Engl J Med. 2015; 372(25):2398–2408

[101] Rice TW, Wheeler AP, Thompson BT, et al. National Heart, Lung, and Blood Institute Acute Respiratory Distress Syndrome (ARDS) Clinical Trials Network. Initial trophic vs full enteral feeding in patients with acute lung injury: the EDEN randomized trial. JAMA. 2012; 307(8):795–803

[102] Harvey SE, Parrott F, Harrison DA, et al. CALORIES Trial Investigators. Trial of the route of early nutritional support in critically ill adults. N Engl J Med. 2014; 371(18):1673–1684

[103] Elke G, van Zanten ARH, Lemieux M, et al. Enteral versus parenteral nutrition in critically ill patients: an updated systematic review and meta-analysis of randomized controlled trials. Crit Care. 2016; 20(1):117

[104] Lewis SR, Schofield-Robinson OJ, Alderson P, Smith AF. Enteral versus parenteral nutrition and enteral versus a combination of enteral and parenteral nutrition for adults in the intensive care unit. Cochrane Database Syst Rev. 2018; 6:CD012276

[105] Barr J, Fraser GL, Puntillo K, et al. American College of Critical Care Medicine. Clinical practice guidelines for the management of pain, agitation, and delirium in adult patients in the intensive care unit. Crit Care Med. 2013; 41 (1):263–306

[106] Devlin JW, Skrobik Y, Gélinas C, et al. Clinical practice guidelines for the prevention and management of pain, agitation/sedation, delirium, immobility and sleep disruption in adult patients in the ICU (2018 PADIS Guidelines). Crit Care Med. 2018; 46(9):e825–e873

[107] ANZCTR. Available at: https://www.anzctr.org.au/Trial/Registration/TrialReview.aspx?id=369434. Accessed March 24, 2020

[108] Martinez FE, Anstey M, Ford A, et al. Prophylactic Melatonin for Delirium in Intensive Care (Pro-MEDIC): study protocol for a randomised controlled trial. Trials. 2017; 18(1):4

[109] Vincent WR, III, Hatton KW. Critically ill patients need "FAST HUGS BID" (an updated mnemonic). Crit Care Med. 2009; 37(7):2326–2327, author reply 2327

4 Cervical Trauma

Aaron Richman and Clay Cothren Burlew

Summary

As with all traumatic injuries, the wide variation in presentation and management of cervical trauma presents a significant challenge to the trauma surgeon. The spectrum of injury ranges from obviously life-threatening injuries, which necessitate immediate operative treatment, to subtle injuries with more indolent courses. The potential for concomitant aerodigestive tract and vascular injury can result in catastrophic neurologic injury or death if not recognized early and managed properly.

Penetrating tracheal injuries depend on skilled and appropriate airway management. Smaller injuries may be managed expectantly; however, larger lesions will demand surgical repair. Esophageal injuries can be difficult to detect but can lead to significant morbidity and mortality. Appropriate surgical management is focused on debridement, tension-free repair, and drainage. Vascular injuries resulting from penetrating neck trauma require effective utilization of various imaging modalities and detailed knowledge of vascular anatomy, and solid surgical skills are crucial to success. Rapid restoration of vessel continuity is key and can be achieved via open surgical techniques. Novel endovascular therapies have begun to emerge but require further study.

Blunt cerebrovascular injury (BCVI) is increasingly recognized as a cause of catastrophic neurologic injury. Patients with BCVI often present with a seemingly innocuous examination. Therefore, a high-level of suspicion is required with regard to these injuries. Evidence-based screening protocols have not only led to better recognition of BCVI but also allowed for early medical and procedural intervention, yielding improved outcomes.

Keywords: Cervical trauma, penetrating neck injury, carotid artery, vertebral artery, blunt cerebrovascular injury, esophagus, trachea

4.1 Penetrating Neck Trauma

Given the location of critical aerodigestive, vascular, and neurologic structures, management of penetrating neck trauma (PNT) presents a significant challenge to trauma surgeons. Although relatively rare, representing between 1 and 11% of trauma cases in the United States, mortality is as high as 10% in some series.[1] The recommendations for evaluation of injury and subsequent management have evolved significantly in the past few decades.

The neck is divided into three zones. Zone 1, also known as the thoracic outlet, extends from a line below the midpoint of the clavicles down to the chest. Zone 2 extends from the line at the midpoint of the clavicles up to the angle of the mandible. Zone 3 covers the angle of the mandible superiorly to the base of the skull. Zone 2 injuries are the most common, most clinically apparent, and most surgically accessible. Zones 1 and 3 injuries are relatively more difficult to access, given the overlying skeletal structures.[2,3]

Initial evaluation and management of patients presenting with PNT should follow standard advanced trauma life support (ATLS) guidelines. Given the potential for laryngotracheal trauma, care should be taken in evaluating and managing the airway to avoid exacerbating an injury. Active hemorrhage from penetrating injury to the neck is best controlled with direct digital pressure. Hemodynamically unstable patients or those with uncontrollable hemorrhage should proceed immediately to the operating room for exploration. Foley balloon tamponade can be used to manage bleeding in patients en route to definitive management and is discussed in detail below. Stable patients or those who can be temporized with volume resuscitation should be carefully evaluated to help guide further management.[4]

Physical examination remains key to effective workup and treatment of PNT. Obvious signs and symptoms of major vascular or aerodigestive injuries, also known as "hard signs," require urgent surgical intervention (▶ Table 4.1). The choice of incision depends on the location of the likely injury. Surgical management of the various injuries is discussed below.[3,4,5]

Patients presenting with less overt findings, also known as "soft signs," necessitate a more comprehensive diagnostic workup (▶ Table 4.2). For decades, algorithms guiding the trauma surgeon in cases of symptomatic PNT utilized the zones of the neck to dictate evaluation and management. Historically, operative exploration was mandated for all patients with platysmal violation in zone 2. More recent studies have demonstrated that outcomes from selective management of zone 2 resulted in fewer negative explorations.[6,7,8] In addition, the external wound may be in a different zone from the deeper injury. Diagnostic evaluation is currently based on physical examination and symptoms.[6,7,8]

Hemodynamically, normal patients without signs or symptoms indicative of injury can be safely observed with lose monitoring. If the overall suspicion for injury is low, observation and serial examination has been shown to reliably detect clinically significant occult injuries while avoiding unnecessary or invasive studies.[3,7]

Table 4.1 Hard signs

- Airway compromise
- Massive subcutaneous emphysema or air bubbling through wound
- Active bleeding, expanding, or pulsatile hematoma
- Shock
- Neurologic deficit
- Hematemesis

Table 4.2 Soft signs

- Dysphagia
- Hoarseness or voice change
- Hemoptysis
- Widened mediastinum
- Subcutaneous emphysema

Multidetector computed tomographic angiography (MD-CTA) has emerged as the most broadly useful imaging modality for cervical trauma patients. MD-CTA is readily available at most centers and can be rapidly obtained and reviewed by surgeons or radiologists. In addition, unlike ultrasound or angiography, CT image quality is not operator-dependent. Studies evaluating CTA detection of cervical vascular injuries have found sensitivity of 90% or greater and specificity of 98 to 100%.[1,9] Subsequent series have found high-sensitivity for aerodigestive injuries as well.[9,10,11,12] MD-CTA is recommended as standard evaluation for patients with zone 1 or 3 penetrating trauma. Zone 2 management continues to be debated. Although some authors recommend mandatory exploration of all patients with symptoms of vascular or aerodigestive injuries, we recommend that all symptomatic patients, without the need for emergent surgical intervention, undergo CTA.[3,4,13] The amount of information available from axial imaging will help guide management and assist with operative planning.[7,8,14]

Suspicion of aerodigestive injury found on CT is further evaluated based on symptoms and clinical signs. Patients with injuries traversing zones 1 and 2 in the area of the trachea or esophagus should be evaluated with contrast esophagography or esophagoscopy and flexible bronchoscopy. For a definitive diagnosis of esophageal injury, combining contrast esophagography with flexible esophagoscopy yields a sensitivity of 90 to 100%.[15] Endoscopic evaluation is particularly critical in the evaluation and management of tracheobronchial injuries to ensure appropriate positioning and selection of incision in the operating room.[12,15] Zone 3 aerodigestive injuries are not well-characterized by contrasted swallow studies, and these patients should be evaluated with video laryngoscopy or flexible endoscopy.[16] Intraoperative endoscopy of the trachea and esophagus should be performed for patients with other injuries requiring surgical control.

The assessment of penetrating neck trauma remains a challenge. Improvements in axial imaging have allowed for rapid assessment of vascular and aerodigestive injuries with good sensitivity and specificity. Algorithm-based patient resuscitation and diagnostic evaluation have helped to speed detect injury while preventing unnecessary operative morbidity. Despite these ongoing improvements, variations in patient presentation, local resources, and capabilities need to be considered. The trauma surgeon's physical examination and clinical decision-making remain key to effective treatment, and surgical repair of identified injury remains the standard of care.

4.1.1 Tracheal Injury

As with all trauma patients, airway management is first and foremost in patients with tracheal injury. Literature regarding the management of the airway in PNT is varied and conflicting with some authors finding good success rates with orotracheal intubation, while others describe airway catastrophes.[5,17] Due to the heterogeneity of this population, no standard algorithm for management of the airway is possible. Patients who present with hoarseness, stridor, subcutaneous emphysema, or sucking or bubbling neck wound are concernedabout an aerodigestive injury; the presence of any such symptoms does not correlate to the severity of injury or likelihood of

decompensation.[17] In patients with airway compromise, orotracheal intubation performed by an experienced provider is successful in the majority of cases; however, there is potential for avulsion of incomplete injuries, false-passage intubation, and respiratory arrest.[5,17] If readily available, awake fiberoptic intubation can avoid the loss of muscle tone, which is associated with rapid sequence intubation, and ensure entry into the appropriate lumen. Regardless of the technique selected, providers should be ready to perform a surgical airway immediately should orotracheal intubation fail.[5,17,18,19]

When there is an obvious disruption of laryngotracheal anatomy, surgical control of the airway is preferred. Attempts at orotracheal intubation may exacerbate existing airway compromise in these patients. A vertical incision through the skin and subcutaneous tissue is recommended, with entry into the airway, at least, one tracheal ring below the site of injury. For larger wounds, intubation directly through the injury can also be used for temporary access until a definitive surgical airway can be established.[4,5,17,18]

Small tracheal injuries in otherwise stable patients may be managed nonoperatively although definitive criteria are not well-established. The lesions should be less than one-third the diameter of the trachea, well-approximated, and without significant tissue loss. These patients should be closely monitored for respiratory distress, worsening subcutaneous emphysema, or signs of sepsis, which would indicate a need for surgical intervention. Primary surgical repair remains the preferred management strategy in most cases.[4,20]

The majority of tracheal injuries occur in zone 2 of the neck. For isolated laryngotracheal injuries in this region, a cervical collar incision provides good access for evaluation and repair. A right thoracotomy is often necessary for access to the distal portion of the trachea, as anterior exposure is limited by the aortic arch and great vessels. Minimal debridement of the trachea is performed to ensure sufficient tissue for closure. Simple lacerations can be repaired with simple interrupted absorbable sutures. For more complicated or extensive lesions, circumferential resection and end-to-end anastomosis arepreferred. Lateral dissection around the trachea should be avoided to preserve the segmental blood supply. Simple interrupted absorbable sutures are used to minimize stenosis and correct any sizemismatch. Gaps of 2 to 3 cm are typically reapproximated without difficulty. Wider spans require more extensive mobilization maneuvers. Pretrachealfascial dissection and suprahyoid laryngeal release can yield an additional 1 to 2 cm of mobility each. Maintaining postoperative neck flexion can minimize tension on the repair and allow for healing. Complex tracheal repairs and those associated with vascular or esophageal injuries should be buttressed with a pedicled muscle flap. Definitive tracheostomy may be required in some patients who are hemodynamically unstable or with injuries too extensive for immediate repair.[4,20,21]

Postoperative anastomotic complications such as dehiscence or restenosis occur in roughly 5% of patients. In these patients, definitive airway management takes precedence and subsequent airway reconstruction by a specialist should be performed in a delayed fashion.[22]

4.1.2 Cervical Esophageal Injury

Penetrating injury to the esophagus is relatively rare, occurring in 5 to 10% of cases. The majority of trauma to the esophagus is iatrogenic. Many of the guidelines for management of external trauma to the esophagus are derived from this experience.[1,13,23]

Stabilization of the patient with an esophageal injury should follow the standard ATLS principles. Given the proximity of the trachea and the esophagus, it is imperative to ensure the patient's airway is appropriately controlled. Appropriate resuscitation with blood products and fluids for bleeding patients is key to maintain perfusion and provide time to fully evaluate the patient's injuries. Broad-spectrum antibiotics with coverage of both aerobes and anaerobes should be started immediately in all patients with suspected aerodigestive tract injuries. Antifungal coverage for candida is controversial but should be considered in patients with a history of prolonged proton pump inhibitor usage.[5,13,24]

Nonoperative management of cervical esophageal injuries may be offered to selected patients.[25] Hypopharyngeal lacerations, contusions/partial thickness lacerations (Grade 1), and lacerations involving less than 50% of the circumference (Grade 2) with well-contained perforations can be safely observed, provided there are no other injuries requiring intervention. These patients should be treated with broad-spectrum antibiotics, and maintained nil per os, with enteral nutrition via feeding tube or total parenteral nutrition. They should be monitored closely for signs of sepsis or hemodynamic instability that would indicate a need for urgent surgical intervention. Interventional radiology can aid in percutaneous drainage of collections that develop in these patients. Despite success rates greater than 90% with nonoperative management in some series, delays in treatment more than 24 hours have been repeatedly found to increase mortality in patients requiring surgical management.[26,27,28]

Patients with hemodynamic instability, evidence of sepsis, or uncontained esophageal injury should be managed surgically. Surgical exposure of the esophagus is typically approached through a longitudinal incision along the left sternocleidomastoid muscle. A collar incision or an apron incision may also be used if a bilateral neck exploration is required. The sternocleidomastoid is mobilized laterally, exposing the carotid sheath and deep cervical fascia. The anterior belly of the omohyoid muscle can be divided to improve exposure. The carotid sheath and its contents are retracted laterally, and the middle layer of the deep cervical fascia is incised to allow entry into the retropharyngeal/paraesophageal space. The inferior thyroid artery should be ligated to prevent traction injury to the recurrent laryngeal nerve. The esophagus is then dissected circumferentially away from the prevertebral fascia and the posterior wall of the trachea. Careful dissection around the trachea should prevent injury to the thin membranous portion of the trachea. A Penrose drain placed around the esophagus can aid with manipulation and retraction.[24,29]

Management of esophageal injury depends on the extent of the injury and timing of diagnosis. Primary repair is possible in a majority of cases with nondestructive lesions.[23,28] The injury should be fully explored with debridement of all devitalized tissue. The healthy margins are then closed in a single-layer, tension-free fashion. Some authors advocate the use of a 46-french Bougie dilator to prevent narrowing of the lumen. A vascularized muscle flap should buttress the esophageal repair to prevent fistulization to the trachea or breakdown of associated vascular repairs from ongoing esophageal leaks. A portion of strap muscle or the sternocleidomastoid muscle can be swung over the repair and sutured in place. It is important to remember the blood supply for the strap muscles originates cephalad and so the muscle must be divided at its distal insertion. Closed-suction drains should be placed in the field to control the effluent from a leak should it occur. A nasogastric tube should be placed across the injury during the repair to ensure safe enteral access for immediate initiation of enteral nutrition while the injury heals. A swallow study to ensure patency of the esophagus without leak is performed prior to starting oral feeds.[24,26,30]

Higher grade injuries involving more than 50% of the esophageal circumference or those with segmental destruction preventing primary repair may require a staged approach to repair if one is technically unable to perform a primary repair. Exposure and debridement proceed similarly to primary repair. The esophagus is then mobilized sufficiently to bring it up to the skin of the neck. To prevent ongoing contamination, a side or loop cervical esophagostomy is created. The distal lumen can be left open and used as a conduit for access to the stomach or closed with absorbable suture. End-cervical esophagostomy and distal closure can be performed but should be avoided. Diversion of the esophagus while maintaining esophageal continuity avoids a more complex exploration and reconstruction later. Once the patient has recovered, the side or loop esophagostomy can be closed by freeing the stoma from the surrounding skin, closing the esophageal mucosa transversely and dropping the esophagus back into the neck. A swallow study performed a few days postoperatively verifies patency and evaluates for leak prior to restarting oral feeds.[4,8,24,31]

Despite appropriate management, esophageal injuries remain quite morbid. Infectious complications like abscess, mediastinitis, and empyema occur in up to 40% of patients. Delays in diagnosis and management appear to increase morbidity and mortality, and so all efforts should be made to expedite administration of antibiotics, source control, and definitive management after initial resuscitation and evaluation.[7,8,13,24,27]

4.1.3 Cervical Vascular Injury

Vascular structures are the most commonly injured structures in PNT, occurring in about 25% of patients.[1,10] Despite the increasingly standardized evaluation of penetrating cervical injury, management of the vascular injury is still highly dependent on the zone of the neck and the vascular structure involved.

As with all trauma patients, hemodynamic instability with signs of hemorrhage is an indication for immediate surgical intervention. Control of bleeding in an exsanguinating patient with a neck injury can most often be achieved with direct digital pressure. In cases where this is not sufficient to control hemorrhage, particularly in zones 1 and 3, an inflated 18-french Foley catheter balloon can be used to provide extrinsic tamponade. The catheter is inserted with a finger and directed to the site of bleeding. The balloon is then inflated with sterile water until the bleeding stops or resistance is felt. A clamp is then applied to the catheter just above the wound, and the soft tissue defect sutured close to prevent migration and close the space.[5,32] Patients who are sufficiently stable after this intervention can undergo CTA to enhance operative planning. If operative intervention is not necessary based on imaging, the catheter can remain in place for 24 to 48 hours to allow smaller arteries and veins to thrombose. Indeed, for some patients experiencing difficulty in accessing isolated venous injury, this technique can provide definitive control.[25]

4.2 Carotid Artery

The right and left common carotid arteries (CCAs) originate from the brachiocephalic artery and aorta, respectively, before following symmetrical oblique courses cephalad and posterior to the sternocleidomastoid within the carotid sheath. The CCA splits into the internal carotid (ICA) and external carotid (ECA) at about the level of the thyroid cartilage or the fourth cervical vertebra. The ECA travels anteriorly to provide blood supply to the pharynx and face, while the ICA remains in the carotid sheath and enters the skull via the foramen lacerum in the temporal bone. The carotid artery is divided into zones that match the corresponding zones of the neck.[2,33,34]

Operative exposure of the carotid artery requires a wide surgical field that includes the entirety of the neck and chest to ensure proximal and distal control. Preparation of the thigh in an uninjured leg is recommended should a vein graft be required. If possible, the patient's head should be turned away from the side of the injury to facilitate exposure higher in the neck. As with brachiocephalic and proximal subclavian artery injuries, injuries to the proximal common carotid artery may necessitate a median sternotomy. This incision can be continued along the anterior border of the sternocleidomastoid to access the carotid from its origin to the skull base. The incision also provides excellent access to the cervical esophagus and trachea.[33,35,36]

Proximal or zone 1 injuries can be difficult to manage due to the many crossing structures in this junctional zone. The thymus and brachiocephalic veins are encountered first after entry into the mediastinum via a sternotomy. The aortic arch is uncovered via superior and medial retraction of the left brachiocephalic vein. The origins of the brachiocephalic artery, left CCA, and left subclavian artery can then be exposed and controlled. If necessary for exposure or control of hemorrhage, the jugular or brachiocephalic veins can be ligated and divided. The left recurrent laryngeal and vagus nerves should be identified and protected during dissection. The vagus nerve runs through the carotid sheath between the ICA and ECA, then posterolateral to the carotid artery, before moving posteriorly to lay along the esophagus. The left recurrent laryngeal nerves branch off of the left vagus nerve at the aortic arch and wraps around the arch anterior to posterior. The right recurrent laryngeal branches off of the right vagus nerve at the right subclavian artery and wraps behind it. Both recurrent laryngeal nerves travel superiorly to the larynx in their respective trachea-esophageal grooves.[33,35,36,37]

The carotid sheath is encountered deep to the anterior border of the sternocleidomastoid. Incising the sheath longitudinally and retracting the jugular vein laterally will expose zone 2 of the carotid artery. Care should be taken to avoid injuring the vagus nerve within the sheath and the hypoglossal nerve more distally during exposure. The facial vein joins the internal jugular vein at the level of the carotid bifurcation and should be ligated and divided to allow more lateral retraction of the internal jugular vein.

Exposure of the carotid artery in distal zone 2 through zone 3 is one of the most challenging procedures in trauma surgery. The artery is reached by extending the longitudinal sternocleidomastoid incision cephalad and posterior to the ear. To enhance the exposure of the distal portion of the carotid artery one may divide the posterior belly of the digastric muscle and ligate the occipital artery arising from the external carotid artery. The retromandibular position of the artery in zone 3 limits higher access, requiring manipulation of the mandible. Anterior subluxation requires preoperative planning and nasotracheal intubation to be successful but can expand the base of the operative field by up to 2 cm. Intraoral wires are placed around the 1st and 2nd lower molars on the injured side and tied to wires placed around the upper incisor and molar on the contralateral side, holding the mandible in an anterior position. A mandibular osteotomy can expand the operative field but it requires more involved dissection as well as risking injury to the marginal mandibular and inferior alveolar nerves and so it is not recommended. These techniques can expose the ICA almost at its entry to the base of the skull. Even with full exposure in this area, distal control may be difficult; intraluminal balloon occlusion may be necessary and can be accomplished with a Pruitt–Inahara shunt or a small Fogarty balloon.[33,35,38]

Once proximal and distal control have been established, exposure and repair of the injured arterial segment can proceed. Flushing with heparinized saline or small balloon-tipped catheter can be used to clear the vessel lumen of clot and debris. In addition, careful inspection of the lumen should be performed to ensure any associated intimal flaps are debrided and repaired. Definitive management of the injured vessel is determined by the nature of the injury. Smaller injuries without significant tissue destruction may be amenable to lateral arteriorraphy or patch angioplasty. Short segments (1–2 cm) of the ICA can also be excised, and the proximal and distal ends mobilized and reanastomosed. For longer injuries, a graft may be needed to span the excised segment. Both autogenous and prosthetic grafts are acceptable. Although prosthetic grafts have been shown to be safe in contaminated fields, most authors advocate the use of a vein graft in the presence of aerodigestive injuries. Injuries to the carotid bulb or proximal ICA can be repaired with an ECA-to-ICA transposition. The ECA is ligated and divided a few centimeters from its origin and the proximal stump anastomosed with the distal ICA stump.[13,14,33,37,39]

Temporary intravascular shunting should be used during repair of injuries involving the carotid bifurcation and ICA to ensure adequate cerebral perfusion. Patients with backbleeding from the ICA or stump pressures greater than 40 mm Hg may not necessitate shunt placement; delaying definitive management in any acutely ill trauma patient for shunting does not seem warranted. Systemic heparinization should be initiated, if not contraindicated by other injuries, to minimize the risk of embolization and limit potential areas of cerebral infarct. Due to the collateral flow through the ECA and circle of Willis, CCA repairs do not require routine placement of a shunt.[4,33,39,40]

Given the difficult operative exposure, distal ICA injuries at the base of the skull care are optimally managed using endovascular techniques. Stents may be used to cover a disrupted vessel wall with associated hemorrhage, pseudoaneurysm, or arteriovenous fistula. Effective endovascular management of these lesions ensures flow is maintained through the vessel while also correcting the lesion. While the procedural success rates of these techniques are well-established, the long-term patency is less defined. Often, concomitant injuries may limit the use of antiplatelet agents and anticoagulation that are necessary to prevent early stent thrombosis. Although promising, further studies are needed to define the indications and postprocedural management of endovascular techniques for vascular injuries.[2]

4.3 Vertebral Artery

The vertebral arteries are the first branch of the subclavian artery. The paired arteries course anteriorly to the transverse processes of C 7 before ascending vertically through the transverse foramina of the C 1–C 6 vertebrae. After passing through the foramen transversarium of C 1, the suboccipital vertebral arteries continue in a groove along the posterior arch of the atlas before entering the cranial cavity through the foramen magnum. The left and right arteries run along the medulla before uniting at the pons to form the basilar artery. The left vertebral artery arises directly from the aortic arch in approximately 6% of people. These arteries are divided into four anatomic zones, the cervical segment, or V1, which spans from the origin until the entry into the C 6 transverse foramen. The vertebral segment, or V2, extends from C 6 until the exit at the C 2 transverse foramen. V3, or the suboccipital segment, which begins at the exit from C 2 and ends at the foramen magnum. The cranial segment, or V4, extends from the foramen magnum until the confluence at the basilar artery. A plexus of veins runs an antiparallel course to the arteries coalescing into a singular vertebral vein around the lower cervical vertebrae. This vein drains into the subclavian vein adjacent to the internal jugular vein.[2,30,41]

The management of vertebral artery injury depends primarily on the patient's physiology and the type of injury. Most penetrating vertebral artery injuries present with extensive vessel damage, often complete transection. However, less than 20% of patients with a vertebral artery injury require open surgical management and it is rare for a unilateral vertebral artery injury to present with neurological symptoms.[30,42] The unique redundancy of the vertebral system permits ligation or endovascular embolization of a bleeding vessel without significant sequelae.

Should operative exposure or repair be necessary, the anatomic zone of injury determines the optimal approach. V1 injuries can be approached through an anterior cervical incision along the sternocleidomastoid or through a transverse supraclavicular incision. The longitudinal cervical incision provides more mobility for exposure of injuries to V2 and of concomitantly injured structures such as the carotid artery or esophagus. The sternocleidomastoid is retracted laterally, the omohyoid muscle divided, and the carotid sheath rotated medially to expose the longus cervicalis colli and anterior longitudinal ligament of the spine. The anterior longitudinal ligament is incised laterally, and a periosteal elevator used to reflect the ligament and the underlying longus colli muscle, laterally exposing the vertebral body and transverse processes. The bony canal is entered by resecting the anterior component of the transverse process, exposing the artery within the transverse foramen. Bleeding from the venous plexus here can be avoided with careful dissection of the underlying fascia or be controlled using pressure or commercially available hemostatic agents. Care should be taken to avoid injury to the cervical spinal nerves which are located posterior and lateral to the transverse foramen.[30,35,43]

Much like zone 3 of the carotid artery, exposure of the V3 segment of the vertebral artery is quite challenging. This area requires a posterior auricular extension of the cervical incision. The sternocleidomastoid is detached off of the mastoid and retracted laterally. Transection of the splenius capitus muscle off the mastoid may also be necessary. The spinal accessory nerve runs in this plane and should be identified and preserved. The prevertebral fascia of C 1 and C 2 can then be incised, exposing the vertebral artery before it enters the skull. The V4 segment exposure requires a craniotomy and should be performed with the assistance of a neurosurgeon.[30,35,43]

Surgical management of the injured vertebral artery injury generally consists of proximal and distal ligation. Repair of the vertebral is rarely indicated and subsequent neurologic complications are rare.[5,44] Ligation for control of the distal end of the vessel high in the neck can be difficult and some authors have advocated utilizing intravascular balloon catheters for both temporary tamponade and definitive thrombosis. A number 3 balloon-tipped Fogarty catheter is inserted in to the vessel, advanced just distal to the injury, and inflated with saline until backbleeding ceases. The catheter is then crimped onto itself and secured in place with sutures. The catheter is then trimmed and left in the wound. The proximal end is ligated, and the incision closed. The wound is reexplored 3 to 7 days later and the catheter removed with the distal vessel thrombosed.[38]

Endovascular techniques are the preferred modality for managing vertebral artery injuries that do not necessitate an emergent operative approach. Angiographic evaluation of the vertebral system can further assess the nature of the injury as well as the patency and resiliency of the uninjured circulation. Stents can be used to preserve the injured dominant vertebral artery, hemorrhage and pseudoaneurysms can be controlled with coils or hemostatic agents, and arteriovenous fistulae can be excluded with proximal and distal embolization. Patients will require, at least, a short course of antiplatelet agents or anticoagulation following these injuries or interventions to prevent further thrombosis or embolization. The safety of these agents in the context of the patient's other injuries should be considered when deciding upon an interventional technique. Given the difficult access and the multiple interventional options available, open surgical techniques should be reserved for those patients with active, uncontrollable hemorrhage or those who have failed endovascular management.[13,14,41,42,45,46,47,48]

4.4 Subclavian Artery

The left subclavian artery originates from the posterior aspect of the aortic arch just distal to the left CCA. The right subclavian artery arises from the brachiocephalic artery. The subclavian artery extends from its origin to the lateral border of the first rib and is divided into three segments based on the relationship of the anterior scalene muscle. Segment 1, from the vessel origin to the medial border of the anterior scalene muscle, gives rise to the most important branches, including the vertebral artery, internal mammary artery, and thyro-cervical trunk. Segment 2 lies posterior to the anterior scalene and gives off the costocervical trunk. The short third segment extends from the lateral border of the anterior scalene muscle to the lateral edge of the first rib, where it becomes the axillary artery. The phrenic nerve runs either directly over or medial to the anterior scalene muscle and can be injured during exposure of the first and second segments of the artery. Through its course, the artery lies posterior to the subclavian vein, vertebral vein, anterior scalene muscle, and thoracic duct on the left.[35,49]

Due to the physical limitations of the rib cage and the divergent pathways of vessels in the area, effective access to the vasculature in zone 1 requires appropriate positioning and incisions. Exposure of the aortic arch is often necessary for proximal control and so the operative field should allow for either a median sternotomy or anterolateral thoracotomy. An uninjured leg should be included in the operative field should there be a need to utilize saphenous vein in the repair. The ultimate incision needed will depend on the wound trajectory and the involved vessels.

A median sternotomy provides the most versatile exposure in patients with zone 1 injuries. The incision allows access to the heart, entire aortic arch, and its branches for proximal control and repair. Median sternotomy provides the best approach for brachiocephalic artery and vein and bilateral CCAs. In addition, the exposure can be easily extended laterally along the supraclavicular fossa to access the more distal subclavian vessels, and cephalad along the sterno-cleidomastoid to allow access to the distal carotid artery. In cases where the extent of injury is not well-established, the median sternotomy is an excellent place to start. If the exact injury is well-defined, a more targeted incision can be performed. For hemodynamically unstable patients, a left anterolateral thoracotomy may be a more appropriate initial incision.[4,33,35]

The subclavian artery is often a challenge to access as it requires mobilization or resection of the clavicle. The standard s-shaped incision begins at the sternoclavicular junction, extends laterally along the superior border of the clavicle, then crosses the middle of the clavicle, and curves downward along the deltopectoral groove. As noted before, this incision can be extended with a median sternotomy for more proximal access. For left-sided injuries, some authors advocate a "trap-door" incision rather than a full sternotomy by combining the supraclavicular incision with an upper median sternotomy and an anterior thoracotomy at the third or fourth intercostal space. However, given the increased risk of bleeding and postoperative morbidity of the "trap-door," the incremental improvement in visualization does not appear to justify routine use of this approach.[35,46,50,51]

Full exposure of the subclavian vessels requires mobilization or resection of the clavicle. Although the clavicle can be released from its proximal joint to the sternum and reflected

laterally, resection of the middle portion of the bone may be less prone to procedural misadventures or postoperative morbidity.[49,51] Resection of the medial portion of the clavicle appears to offer the best exposure without introducing significant functional deficits. The attachments of the platysma, sternocleidomastoid, subclavian, and pectoralis muscles are stripped off using a combination of electrocautery and periosteal elevators. The clavicle can then be divided and retracted, or the middle portion resected to visualize the retroclavicular space.[35,50] Care should be taken to avoid injury to the vagus nerve, phrenic nerve, and subclavian vein during dissection as they lie anterior to the proximal portion of the artery in this space. The brachial plexus also courses through this region and is intimately associated with the artery; injury to nerves here can cause significant disability and should be avoided. The thoracic duct crosses the first portion of the left subclavian artery and terminates at the junction of the left internal jugular and subclavian veins. Extending the incision and dissection more distally can allow for identification of the axillary artery in cases where transected vessel ends have retracted or overlying hematoma hamper visualization.[50]

As with all arterial injuries, management of subclavian artery injuries should focus on restoration of flow. Stab wounds or other low-energy penetrating mechanisms can often be treated by simple suture repair or debridement with end-to-end anastomosis. Higher energy mechanisms with more tissue destruction often cannot be repaired primarily without tension; in such cases, interposition grafts with autologous vein or prosthetic material are acceptable. If necessary, these grafts can utilize the carotid, proximal brachiocephalic artery, or aorta for inflow. Given the extensive collaterals in the shoulder and neck, ligation of the subclavian artery is acceptable for patients in extremis or with injuries not amenable to repair. Temporary shunting may offer a better solution than ligation in many cases and can allow for delayed repair.[13,39,51,52]

Given the proximity to other structures, concomitant venous and nerve injury is common. Brachial plexus injury can accompany subclavian artery injury in up to 30% of cases. This injury can lead to significant functional decrement. Intraoperative consultation with a hand surgeon should be considered if one is available and the patient's physiology allows it.[51,52,53] Associated injuries to the subclavian or brachiocephalic veins should be managed with lateral suture venorraphy if possible. Alternatively, ligation is well-tolerated for patients presenting with more extensive or complex venous injury. Elevation of the ipsilateral extremity is recommended to help manage edema while the venous system collateralizes.[36,49]

4.5 Blunt Neck Trauma

4.5.1 Blunt Cerebrovascular Injury Management

Blunt injuries to the carotid or vertebral arteries, also known as blunt cerebrovascular injury (BCVI), can present significant difficulties in management. The overall incidence of BCVI is low,

Table 4.3 BCVI screening criteria

- High-energy transfer mechanism
- Displaced midface fracture (LeFort II or III)
- Mandible fracture
- Complex skull fracture/basilar skull fracture/occipital condyle fracture
- SevereTBI with GCS < 6
- Near hanging with anoxic brain injury
- Scalp degloving
- Cervical spine fracture, subluxation, or ligamentous injury at any level
- Clothesline type or seat belt injury with significant swelling, pain, or altered mental status
- TBI with thoracic injuries
- Thoracic vascular injuries
- Blunt cardiac rupture
- Upper rib fractures

Abbreviations: GCS, Glasgow coma scale; TBI, traumatic brain injury.

Table 4.4 Grading scale for BCVI

Grade	Description
I	Luminal irregularity or dissection with <25 % luminal narrowing
II	Dissection or intramural hematoma with >25 % luminal narrowing, intraluminal thrombus, or raised intimal flap
III	Pseudoaneurysm
IV	Occlusion
V	Transection with free extravasation

occurring in roughly 1 to 3% of patients admitted for blunt traumatic injury.[54,55] Although rare, mortality rates from unrecognized or untreated BCVI are as high as 31% and permanent neurologic morbidity rates of up to 58% have been reported in some series.[56,57]

As with all trauma, mechanism and examination should guide the initial assessment and diagnostic workup. Blunt trauma patients presenting with cervicofacial hemorrhage, expanding cervical hematoma, cervical bruit, or lateralizing neurologic deficit incongruous with head CT findings should be considered to have BCVI. Cervical hyperextension or hyperflexion mechanisms with rotation, as well as direct anterior cervical trauma, account for the majority of injuries. Early studies found specific injury patterns consistent with these mechanisms have been demonstrated as reliable indicators to screen for BCVI. These early screening criteria included LeFort II or III fracture, cervical–spine fractures, basilar skull fracture with carotid canal involvement, petrous bone fracture, diffuse axonal injury with Glasgow Coma Score (GCS) less than 6, and near hanging with anoxic brain injury. Use of these criteria captured roughly 80% of BCVI.[58,59] To capture the approximately 20% of injuries missed with the standard criteria, an additional group of high-risk injuries were identified: scalp degloving, mandibular fractures, complex skull fractures, thoracic vascular injury, and skeletal injuries to the upper chest. These expanded criteria captured the vast majority of the previously missed injuries. However, injury mechanism should still prompt imaging in patients deemed to be at risk by the trauma team. To ensure early diagnosis of BCVI and expedite management, decisions regarding diagnostic imaging should follow these expanded criteria (▶ Table 4.3).[58,59,60]

A grading scale for BCVI was described in 1999 to risk stratify patients and guide management (▶ Table 4.4). Lesions are characterized as nonhemodynamically significant intimal injuries with < 25% intimal stenosis (grade I), potentially hemodynamically significant dissections and hematomas with > 25% intimal stenosis (grade II), pseudoaneurysms (grade III), occlusions (grade IV), and vessel transections (grade V). Higher grade

injuries have been reliably demonstrated to confer higher risk of stroke and mortality, particularly for carotid artery injury.[61]

Nonoperative treatment with antithrombotic agents is the mainstay of treatment for BCVI. Systemic anticoagulation has been shown to improve rates of resolution of the lesion, neurologic outcome, and overall mortality. Continuous heparin infusion with a goal partial thromboplastin time (PTT) of 40 to 50 seconds is the best studied regimen and is considered the standard of care.[2,54,56,57,62] Antiplatelet therapy including full-strength aspirin and clopidogrel have also been evaluated and appear to have similar efficacy with regard to stroke prevention.[55,62] Heparin remains the preferred agent in the acute setting as it is reversible.[60,62,63] Patients who managed nonoperatively, particularly those with low-grade lesions, are reimaged with CTA 7 to 10 days after initiating therapy to assess for either resolution or progression that would alter long-term management.[54,64]

Operative management of BCVI is challenging. Vertebral lesions are particularly difficult to access due to the surrounding bony and nervous anatomy. Carotid lesions are often high in zone 3 and involve the base of the skull precluding open repair.[54] Nevertheless, surgical repair should be considered for accessible Grade II or higher injuries and operative exposure follows the same principles described for penetrating injury.[60] Grade V BCVI commonly occurs with other injuries that require operative management and present significant neurologic deficit. Revascularization does not improve neurologic recovery in these patients and ligation is recommended. For patients with high-grade injuries and minor or no neurologic symptoms, repair improves mortality and should be considered.[37,60,64]

Endovascular therapy for high-grade lesions in both surgically accessible and inaccessible regions has become increasingly common over the last few years.[48,65] Options include stenting, temporary or permanent embolization, and recanalization depending on the lesion.[66] Initial studies evaluating the use of stents suggested higher rates of occlusion when compared to antithrombotic therapy alone; however, more aggressive use of antiplatelet agents appears to ameliorate this risk. Indeed, in most other regions of the body, use of aspirin or clopidogrel is critical in preventing thrombosis or embolism after endovascular intervention.[37,42,47,62,63,65,67] However, even in these high-grade injuries, pharmacologic antithrombotic therapy has demonstrated similar efficacy in stroke prevention without associated increased in rupture.[63,68] Stenting should be considered only for symptomatic or markedly expanding grade III pseudoaneurysms.

References

[1] Saito N, Hito R, Burke PA, Sakai O. Imaging of penetrating injuries of the head and neck: current practice at a level I trauma center in the United States. Keio J Med. 2014; 63(2):23–33

[2] Ray CE, Jr, Spalding SC, Cothren CC, Wang W-S, Moore EE, Johnson SP. State of the art: noninvasive imaging and management of neurovascular trauma. World J EmergSurg. 2007; 2(1):1

[3] Sperry JL, Moore EE, Coimbra R, et al. Western Trauma Association critical decisions in trauma: penetrating neck trauma. J Trauma Acute Care Surg. 2013; 75(6):936–940

[4] Feliciano DV. Penetrating cervical trauma: "current concepts in penetrating trauma", IATSIC Symposium, International Surgical Society, Helsinki, Finland, August 25–29, 2013. World J Surg. 2015; 39(6):1363–1372

[5] Burgess CA, Dale OT, Almeyda R, Corbridge RJ. An evidence based review of the assessment and management of penetrating neck trauma. Clin Otolaryngol. 2012; 37(1):44–52

[6] Ibraheem K, Khan M, Rhee P, et al. "No zone" approach in penetrating neck trauma reduces unnecessary computed tomography angiography and negative explorations. J Surg Res. 2018; 221:113–120

[7] Nowicki JL, Stew B, Ooi E. Penetrating neck injuries: a guide to evaluation and management. Ann R CollSurgEngl. 2018; 100(1):6–11

[8] Shiroff AM, Gale SC, Martin ND, et al. Penetrating neck trauma: a review of management strategies and discussion of the 'No Zone' approach. Am Surg. 2013; 79(1):23–29

[9] Inaba K, Branco BC, Menaker J, et al. Evaluation of multidetector computed tomography for penetrating neck injury: a prospective multicenter study. J Trauma Acute Care Surg. 2012; 72(3):576–83; discussion 583–4; quiz 803–4

[10] Demetriades D, Theodorou D, Cornwell E, et al. Evaluation of penetrating injuries of the neck: prospective study of 223 patients. World J Surg. 1997; 21 (1):41–47, discussion 47–48

[11] Schroeder JW, Ptak T, Corey AS, et al. Expert Panels on Neurologic and Vascular Imaging. ACR Appropriateness Criteria Penetrating Neck Injury. J Am CollRadiol. 2017; 14 11S:S500–S505

[12] Madsen AS, Oosthuizen G, Laing GL, Bruce JL, Clarke DL. The role of computed tomography angiography in the detection of aerodigestive tract injury following penetrating neck injury. J Surg Res. 2016; 205(2):490–498

[13] Weinberg JA, Moore AH, Magnotti LJ, et al. Contemporary management of civilian penetrating cervicothoracic arterial injuries. J Trauma Acute Care Surg. 2016; 81(2):302–306

[14] Tisherman SA, Bokhari F, Collier B, et al. Clinical practice guideline: penetrating zone II neck trauma. J Trauma. 2008; 64(5):1392–1405

[15] Soliman AMS, Ahmad SM, Roy D. The role of aerodigestive tract endoscopy in penetrating neck trauma. Laryngoscope. 2014; 124 Suppl 7:S1–S9

[16] Ahmed N, Massier C, Tassie J, Whalen J, Chung R. Diagnosis of penetrating injuries of the pharynx and esophagus in the severely injured patient. J Trauma. 2009; 67(1):152–154

[17] Schaefer SD. Management of acute blunt and penetrating external laryngeal trauma. Laryngoscope. 2014; 124(1):233–244

[18] Tallon JM, Ahmed JM, Sealy B. Airway management in penetrating neck trauma at a Canadian tertiary trauma centre. CJEM. 2007; 9(2):101–104

[19] Bell RB, Osborn T, Dierks EJ, Potter BE, Long WB. Management of penetrating neck injuries: a new paradigm for civilian trauma. J Oral Maxillofac Surg. 2007; 65(4):691–705

[20] Altinok T, Can A. Management of tracheobronchial injuries. Eurasian J Med. 2014; 46(3):209–215

[21] Lyons JD, Feliciano DV, Wyrzykowski AD, Rozycki GS. Modern management of penetrating tracheal injuries. Am Surg. 2013; 79(2):188–193

[22] Wright CD, Grillo HC, Wain JC, et al. Anastomotic complications after tracheal resection: prognostic factors and management. J Thorac Cardiovasc Surg. 2004; 128(5):731–739

[23] Zenga J, Kreisel D, Kushnir VM, Rich JT. Management of cervical esophageal and hypopharyngeal perforations. Am J Otolaryngol. 2015; 36(5):678–685

[24] Petrone P, Kassimi K, Jiménez-Gómez M, Betancourt A, Axelrad A, Marini CP. Management of esophageal injuries secondary to trauma. Injury. 2017; 48(8): 1735–1742

[25] Madsen AS, Bruce JL, Oosthuizen GV, Bekker W, Laing GL, Clarke DL. The Selective Non-operative Management of Penetrating Cervical Venous Trauma is Safe and Effective. World J Surg. 2018; 42(10):3202–3209

[26] Onat S, Ulku R, Cigdem KM, Avci A, Ozcelik C. Factors affecting the outcome of surgically treated non-iatrogenic traumatic cervical esophageal perforation: 28 years experience at a single center. J CardiothoracSurg. 2010; 5(1):46

[27] Asensio JA, Chahwan S, Forno W, et al. American Association for the Surgery of Trauma. Penetrating esophageal injuries: multicenter study of the American Association for the Surgery of Trauma. J Trauma. 2001; 50(2): 289–296

[28] Madsen AS, Oosthuizen GV, Bruce JL, Bekker W, Laing GL, Clarke DL. Selective nonoperative management of pharyngoesophageal injuries secondary to penetrating neck trauma: A single-center review of 86 cases. J Trauma Acute Care Surg. 2018; 85(3):541–548

[29] Komanapalli C. James Cohen MS.Exposure of the cervical esophagus | CTSNet. Available at: https://www.ctsnet.org/article/exposure-cervical-esophagus. Published 2010. Accessed July 15, 2018

[30] Roberts LH, Demetriades D. Vertebral artery injuries. SurgClin North Am. 2001; 81(6):1345–1356

[31] Koniaris LG, Spector SA, Staveley-O'Carroll KF. Complete esophageal diversion: a simplified, easily reversible technique. J Am CollSurg. 2004; 199 (6):991–993

[32] Evans C, Chaplin T, Zelt D. Management of major vascular injuries: neck, extremities, and other things that bleed. Emerg Med Clin North Am. 2018; 36 (1):181–202

[33] Kumar SR, Weaver FA, Yellin AE. Cervical vascular injuries: carotid and jugular venous injuries. SurgClin North Am. 2001; 81(6):1331–44

[34] Sidawy AN, Perler BA. Rutherford's Vascular Surgery and Endovascular Therapy. 9th ed. Philadelphia: Elsevier; 2019

[35] Hoyt DB, Coimbra R, Potenza BM, Rappold JF. Anatomic exposures for vascular injuries. SurgClin North Am. 2001; 81(6):1299–330

[36] Demetriades D, Asensio JA, Velmahos G, Thal E. Complex problems in penetrating neck trauma. SurgClin North Am. 1996; 76(4):661–683

[37] Karaolanis G, Maltezos K, Bakoyiannis C, Georgopoulos S. Contemporary strategies in the management of civilian neck zone II vascular trauma. Front Surg. 2017; 4(September):56

[38] Feliciano DV, Burch JM, Mattox KL, Bitondo CG, Fields G. Balloon catheter tamponade in cardiovascular wounds. Am J Surg. 1990; 160(6):583–587

[39] Tisherman SA. Management of Major Vascular Injury: Open. OtolaryngolClin North Am. 2016; 49(3):809–817

[40] Reva VA, Pronchenko AA, Samokhvalov IM. Operative management of penetrating carotid artery injuries. Eur J VascEndovascSurg. 2011; 42(1):16–20

[41] Mwipatayi BP, Jeffery P, Beningfield SJ, Motale P, Tunnicliffe J, Navsaria PH. Management of extra-cranial vertebral artery injuries. Eur J VascEndovascSurg. 2004; 27(2):157–162

[42] Herrera DA, Vargas SA, Dublin AB. Endovascular treatment of traumatic injuries of the vertebral artery. AJNR Am J Neuroradiol. 2008; 29(8):1585–1589

[43] George B, Blanquet A, Alves O. Surgical exposure of the vertebral artery. Oper Tech Neurosurg. 2001; 4(4):182–194

[44] Reid JD, Weigelt JA. Forty-three cases of vertebral artery trauma. J Trauma. 1988; 28(7):1007–1012

[45] Sinha S, Patterson BO, Ma J, et al. London Trauma Network: systematic review and meta-analysis of open surgical and endovascular management of thoracic outlet vascular injuries. J VascSurg. 2013; 57(2):547–567.e8

[46] O'Brien PJ, Cox MW. A modern approach to cervical vascular trauma. Perspect Vasc Surg Endovasc Ther. 2011; 23(2):90–97

[47] Almazedi B, Lyall H, Bhatnagar P, et al. Endovascular management of extra-cranial supra-aortic vascular injuries. CardiovascInterventRadiol. 2014; 37 (1):55–68

[48] Reuben BC, Whitten MG, Sarfati M, Kraiss LW. Increasing use of endovascular therapy in acute arterial injuries: analysis of the National Trauma Data Bank. J VascSurg. 2007; 46(6):1222–1226

[49] Demetriades D, Chahwan S, Gomez H, et al. Penetrating injuries to the subclavian and axillary vessels. J Am CollSurg. 1999; 188(3):290–295

[50] Demetriades D, Asensio JA. Subclavian and axillary vascular injuries. SurgClin North Am. 2001; 81(6):1357–73

[51] Sobnach S, Nicol AJ, Nathire H, Edu S, Kahn D, Navsaria PH. An analysis of 50 surgically managed penetrating subclavian artery injuries. Eur J Vasc Endovasc Surg. 2010; 39(2):155–159

[52] Carrick MM, Morrison CA, Pham HQ, et al. Modern management of traumatic subclavian artery injuries: a single institution's experience in the evolution of endovascular repair. Am J Surg. 2010; 199(1):28–34

[53] Gilani R, Tsai PI, Wall MJ, Jr, Mattox KL. Overcoming challenges of endovascular treatment of complex subclavian and axillary artery injuries in hypotensive patients. J Trauma Acute Care Surg. 2012; 73(3):771–773

[54] Biffl WL, Ray CE, Jr, Moore EE, et al. Treatment-related outcomes from blunt cerebrovascular injuries: importance of routine follow-up arteriography. Ann Surg. 2002; 235(5):699–706, discussion 706–707

[55] Miller PR, Fabian TC, Croce MA, et al. Prospective screening for blunt cerebrovascular injuries: analysis of diagnostic modalities and outcomes. Ann Surg. 2002; 236(3):386–393, discussion 393–395

[56] Biffl WL, Moore EE, Ryu RK, et al. The unrecognized epidemic of blunt carotid arterial injuries: early diagnosis improves neurologic outcome. Ann Surg. 1998; 228(4):462–470

[57] Fabian TC, Patton JH, Jr, Croce MA, Minard G, Kudsk KA, Pritchard FE. Blunt carotid injury. Importance of early diagnosis and anticoagulant therapy. Ann Surg. 1996; 223(5):513–522, discussion 522–525

[58] Emmett KP, Fabian TC, DiCocco JM, Zarzaur BL, Croce MA. Improving the screening criteria for blunt cerebrovascular injury: the appropriate role for computed tomography angiography. J Trauma. 2011; 70(5):1058–1063, discussion 1063–1065

[59] Geddes AE, Burlew CC, Wagenaar AE, et al. Expanded screening criteria for blunt cerebrovascular injury: a bigger impact than anticipated. Am J Surg. 2016; 212(6):1167–1174

[60] Biffl WL, Cothren CC, Moore EE, et al. Western Trauma Association critical decisions in trauma: screening for and treatment of blunt cerebrovascular injuries. J Trauma. 2009; 67(6):1150–1153

[61] Biffl WL, Moore EE, Offner PJ, Brega KE, Franciose RJ, Burch JM. Blunt carotid arterial injuries: implications of a new grading scale. J Trauma. 1999; 47(5):845–853

[62] Edwards NM, Fabian TC, Claridge JA, Timmons SD, Fischer PE, Croce MA. Antithrombotic therapy and endovascular stents are effective treatment for blunt carotid injuries: results from long-term follow-up. J Am CollSurg. 2007; 204(5):1007–1013, discussion 1014–1015

[63] Shahan CP, Sharpe JP, Stickley SM, et al. The changing role of endovascular stenting for blunt cerebrovascular injuries. J Trauma Acute Care Surg. 2018; 84(2):308–311

[64] Bromberg WJ, Collier BC, Diebel LN, et al. Blunt cerebrovascular injury practice management guidelines: the Eastern Association for the Surgery of Trauma. J Trauma. 2010; 68(2):471–477

[65] DuBose J, Recinos G, Teixeira PGR, Inaba K, Demetriades D. Endovascular stenting for the treatment of traumatic internal carotid injuries: expanding experience. J Trauma. 2008; 65(6):1561–1566

[66] Scalea TM, Sclafani S. Interventional techniques in vascular trauma. SurgClin North Am. 2001; 81(6):1281–1297

[67] McNeil JD, Chiou AC, Gunlock MG, Grayson DE, Soares G, Hagino RT. Successful endovascular therapy of a penetrating zone III internal carotid injury. J VascSurg. 2002; 36(1):187–190

[68] Burlew CC, Biffl WL, Moore EE, et al. Endovascular stenting is rarely necessary for the management of blunt cerebrovascular injuries. J Am CollSurg. 2014; 218(5):1012–1017

**Expert Commentary on
Cervical Trauma by
*Timothy C. Fabian***

Expert Commentary on Cervical Trauma

Timothy C. Fabian

I begin by congratulating the authors on a thorough and well-written treatise, detailing the management of blunt and penetrating cervical injuries. A great strength of this work is the precise detailing of the anatomy of the region. This especially applies to their description of surgical exposures of aerodigestive and vascular structures. Indeed, the chapter provides a nice primer for surgeons seeking a quick review prior to going to the operating room.

The diagnostic approaches are classical. Emphasis is directed at physical examination which, in turn, is aimed at "hard and soft signs" that are provided in the tables. Adjunctive measures of endoscopy and esophagoscopy are used for suspicion of tracheal and esophageal injuries. They rightly point out that CT angiography, in recent years, has become an indispensable diagnostic tool for vascular injuries.

There are a few areas in which I take some different approaches. I emphasize "different," not necessarily "better." These considerations begin with the management of esophageal injuries. The authors suggest that lacerations involving less than 50% of the circumference (Grade 2) with well-contained perforations can be safely observed, provided there are no other injuries requiring intervention. That strategy requires treatment with broad-spectrum antibiotics, and nil per os (NPO) maintenance with enteral nutrition via feeding tube or total parenteral nutrition. They note that close monitoring for signs of sepsis or hemodynamic instability would indicate a need for urgent surgical intervention, and that interventional radiology can aid in percutaneous drainage of collections that develop. While that is all true, I believe immediate operative repair is preferable. I think the length of hospital stay and costs are less as is the risk of serious morbidity.

I also manage esophageal repair differently. They describe closing esophageal wounds in one layer. I repair the injury in two layers, taking care to close the mucosa separately, as the first layer followed by the muscular layer. I believe the separate mucosal closure reduces the risk of dehiscence of the repair.

While they recommend using closed-suction drains, I believe those foreign bodies promote repair failure. In that scenario, the drains may provide a self-fulfilling prophecy.

The left subclavian artery can prove to be a tricky problem. The brachiocephalic, left common carotid, and left subclavian arteries are the large branches of the aortic arch. While the first two come off the arch anteriorly and are relatively easily dissected following sternotomy, the left subclavian is far posterior and very difficult to get to via sternotomy, especially in a pool of clot and audible hemorrhage. If the wounding location or preoperative study indicates injury to the first portion, I prefer a high anterolateral thoracotomy to secure control of the origin of the left subclavian; this may follow a sternotomy. As the authors point out, trap-door incisions are rarely necessary. However, that approach provides exceptional exposure for repair of a proximal first segment wound. One other subclavian caveat is as follows: those vessels are rather "buttery" in consistency and must be handled very carefully.

Toward the end of the discussion of managing penetrating vertebral artery injuries, the authors emphasize the importance of angiographic and endovascular approaches. I can only say amen to that. Exposing those vessels makes the left subclavian look like a walk in the park. Throughout most of their course, the vertebral arteries are extremely deep and surrounded by bone. Proximal and distal control are somewhat theoretical. They are also larger than commonly appreciated. As a result, when injured, they hemorrhage profusely from that deep chasm after the clot is knocked off by the well-intentioned surgeon (I speak from unpleasant experience). I would strongly advocate for rapid transport to the angiography suite rather than clot disruption, or rapid transport following the use of balloon tamponade, as suggested by the authors when faced with ongoing hemorrhage.

The only slight quibble I have with blunt cerebrovascular injury (BCVI) management with regard to stent treatment of internal carotid injuries. In addition to the authors' suggestion that stents are appropriate for enlarging pseudoaneurysms, I believe they should also be considered for significant stenoses (greater than 70%) that have progressed since initial diagnosis.

All in all, I thoroughly enjoyed the chapter and enthusiastically recommend it to all surgeons who provide care for the injured.

5 Blunt Abdominal Trauma

Morgan Schellenberg and Kenji Inaba

Summary

Blunt abdominal trauma is an important cause of morbidity and mortality worldwide. There are a number of structures in the abdomen that can be injured following blunt trauma, including the aorta, inferior vena cava, and their branches or tributaries; solid organs, comprised of the liver, kidneys, and spleen; the pancreas; the gastrointestinal tract; and the diaphragm. This chapter provides a discussion of the initial approach to resuscitation and assessment of the undifferentiated blunt trauma patient. This is followed by an in-depth review of the diagnostic work-up and management of blunt abdominal injuries.

Keywords: Hemorrhage control, blunt hollow viscus injury, nonoperative management of blunt solid organ injury, retrohepatic caval injury

5.1 Introduction

Unintentional injury is the leading cause of death among people between the ages of 1 to 44 years in the United States and is one of the most frequent causes of death among those ≥ 45 years of age.[1] Motor vehicle collisions (MVCs), auto versus pedestrian collisions (AVPs), and falls are common blunt mechanisms of injury. The leading causes of death after blunt trauma are traumatic brain injury (TBI) and exsanguination.[2]

The abdomen contains multiple structures at risk for hemorrhage after trauma and therefore blunt abdominal trauma is an important contributor to morbidity and mortality. Contemporary advances in imaging techniques, particularly computed tomography (CT) scan, over the past several decades have improved our ability to diagnose and manage intra-abdominal injuries successfully nonoperatively. Angioembolization has also represented an important step forward in the management of blunt trauma patients, as it allows for nonoperative hemorrhage control, particularly for blunt solid organ injury. In appropriately selected patients, angioembolization has several benefits over operative management, including organ preservation and avoidance of exploratory laparotomy and general anesthesia. Although laparoscopic surgery represents a minimally invasive option for the surgical management of many general surgery conditions, it has yet to gain widespread acceptance in the management of patients with blunt abdominal trauma.

In this chapter, blunt abdominal trauma will be explored in detail. A general approach to the patient with blunt abdominal trauma will be presented first. This is followed by an in-depth discussion of the diagnosis, management strategy, surgical techniques, and complications of solid organ, hollow viscus, pancreatic, major vascular, and diaphragm injuries following blunt abdominal trauma.

5.2 General Approach to Blunt Abdominal Trauma

The initial assessment of any trauma patient begins in the same way; with a rapid evaluation of the airway, breathing, and circulation (ABCs) for life-threatening injuries.[3] The general approach to patients with blunt abdominal trauma is best considered based on the patient's hemodynamic stability.

Unstable blunt trauma patients can be challenging to manage. The primary goal must be rapid identification of the body cavity that contains the potentially lethal injury. The old adage that hemorrhagic shock results from bleeding into at least one of five places (the chest, abdomen, pelvis, large muscular compartments, and externally) remains useful. Routine evaluation of the abdomen for the potential source of instability after blunt trauma consists of a physical examination and focused abdominal sonography for trauma (FAST). On physical examination, peritonitis indicates a surgical abdomen, which constitutes an indication for immediate laparotomy. Although peritonitis caused by hollow viscus injury is unlikely to trigger hemodynamic instability in the immediate period, hemoperitoneum can also cause peritonitis and is a common cause of hypotension after blunt trauma.

FAST is the rapid ultrasonographic evaluation of the abdomen and pericardium for hemoperitoneum and hemopericardium, respectively. It consists of three abdominal views (right upper quadrant, left upper quadrant, and pelvis) and a subxiphoid view of the heart and pericardium. FAST allows for the rapid bedside identification of hemoperitoneum.[4] Regardless of the specific source of intraperitoneal bleeding, the right upper quadrant is where blood is most likely to accumulate.[5]

FAST is highly sensitive and specific for hemoperitoneum. Early studies examining the accuracy of FAST found a sensitivity and specificity approaching 100% among hypotensive blunt trauma patients.[6,7] The true diagnostic yield of FAST in clinical practice, when the examination is performed in emergency settings by nonradiologists or by those who are less experienced, still demonstrates a sensitivity that approaches 100%.[8] A positive FAST in an unstable blunt trauma patient is an indication for immediate laparotomy.

A negative FAST in an unstable blunt trauma patient poses more of a diagnostic dilemma. Particularly if chest and pelvis X-rays do not reveal a potential source for the patient's hypotension, such as hemopneumothorax or open-book pelvic fracture, concern may persist for an intra-abdominal source of hypotension. We find two techniques helpful in this situation: repeating the FAST examination or performing a diagnostic peritoneal aspirate (DPA).

The rationale for repeating the FAST examination is that several hundred cc's of blood must accumulate in the abdomen before it can be detected with ultrasound.[9] This means that among patients who arrive to the emergency department immediately after injury, for example in urban centers with short transport times, sufficient blood may not have yet accumulated in the abdomen to produce a positive FAST despite the presence of significant intraperitoneal bleeding. A FAST examination repeated several minutes later may then be able to detect hemoperitoneum after more blood is shed. Repeat FAST examination among stable blunt trauma patients has been shown to increase its sensitivity.[10]

An alternative to repeated FAST examination is a DPA. DPA is a bedside technique used to identify intraperitoneal blood. DPA represents an evolution of the diagnostic peritoneal lavage (DPL), in which saline is instilled into the peritoneal cavity through a catheter inserted percutaneously and then withdrawn to check for bloody discoloration.[11,12] DPL was an early technique for the detection of hemoperitoneum that has been supplanted by FAST. DPA, on the other hand, is a modified DPL in which a catheter is inserted blindly into the peritoneal cavity and any underlying blood or fluid is aspirated out with a syringe. Removal of any amount of blood is considered a positive DPA and is an indication for laparotomy in the appropriate clinical setting. Because DPA can safely and accurately diagnose hemoperitoneum with a sensitivity and specificity that approach that of the FAST examination,[13] at most centers, DPA is used as a confirmatory test in unstable patients with a negative or equivocal FAST.

Stable patients who have sustained blunt abdominal trauma should undergo CT scan with intravenous contrast. Although oral and rectal contrast can be useful in specific situations, they should not be used routinely in the acute setting. CT scan allows complete assessment of the abdomen for injury. Although there is a subset of trauma patients who can be observed for injury instead of undergoing CT scan, this patient population is not safely delineated by the current literature and physician judgement must be used. Particularly in the adult trauma population, we favor liberal CT scan after significant traumatic mechanisms or when injury is suspected based on physical examination, in order to avoid missing injuries.

5.3 Management of Specific Injuries After Blunt Abdominal Trauma

5.3.1 Solid Organ Injuries

The abdominal solid organs consist of the liver, spleen, and kidney. Injuries to these structures have both similarities and differences in their diagnosis and management, which are highlighted here.

5.3.2 Diagnosis

Solid organ injuries are diagnosed at laparotomy or on CT scan of the abdomen with IV contrast. The American Association for the Surgery of Trauma (AAST) provides a grading system for the severity of solid organ injuries, with splenic and renal injuries graded from I to V and liver injuries from grades I to VI (▶ Table 5.1; ▶ Fig. 5.1).[14] This classification serves a number of useful purposes. First, it serves as a communication tool between trauma surgeons, emergency room physicians, radiologists, and interventionalists to describe the severity of the injury. Second, the success of nonoperative management decreases with increasing AAST grade, so it can be useful for prognostication.[15] Importantly, while higher grades of injury are more likely to fail in nonoperative management and require delayed intervention, surgical intervention is never mandated based on the grade of injury alone. An assessment of a patient's

Table 5.1 AAST grading of solid organ injuries

AAST Grade	Liver	Spleen	Kidney
I	Subcapsular hematoma, <10%	Subcapsular hematoma, <10%	Microscopic or gross hematoma with normal urologic studies (contusion)
	Capsular tear, <1 cm	Capsular tear, <1 cm	
			Subcapsular hematoma, nonexpanding without parenchymal laceration
II	Subcapsular hematoma, 10–50%	Subcapsular hematoma, 10–50%	Nonexpanding perirenal hematoma confined to renal retroperitoneum
	Intraparenchymal hematoma, <10 cm	Intraparenchymal hematoma, <5 cm	
	Capsular tear, 1–3 cm	Capsular tear, 1–3 cm	Laceration, <1 cm without urinary extravasation
III	Subcapsular hematoma, >50%	Subcapsular hematoma, >50% or expanding	Laceration, >1 cm without urinary extravasation or collecting system rupture
	Intraparenchymal hematoma, >10 cm	Ruptured subcapsular/parenchymal hematoma	
	Laceration, >3 cm		
		Intraparenchymal hematoma =5 cm or expanding	
		Laceration, >3 cm or involving trabecular vessels	
IV	Parenchymal disruption involving 25–75% of hepatic lobe or 1–3 Couinaud's segments	Laceration of segmental/hilar vessels producing devascularization >25% of spleen	Parenchymal laceration through renal cortex, medulla, and collecting system
			Main renal artery or vein injury with contained hemorrhage
V	Parenchymal disruption involving >75% of hepatic lobe or >3 Couinaud's segments within a single lobe	Completely shattered spleen	Completely shattered kidney
		Hilar vascular injury which devascularizes spleen	Avulsion of renal hilum which devascularizes kidney
	Retrohepatic vena caval injuries		
VI	Hepatic avulsion	—	—

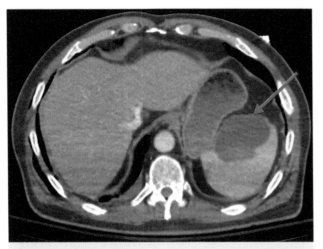

Fig. 5.1 AAST grade III splenic injury on CT scan with IV contrast (portal venous phase). A 7 cm (> 50 %) subcapsular hematoma of the spleen is demonstrated (*arrow*). AAST, American Association for the Surgery of Trauma.

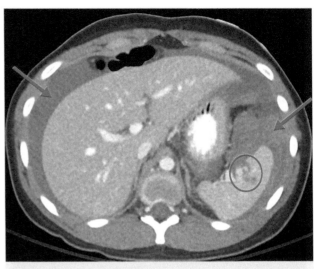

Fig. 5.2 AAST grade IV splenic injury on CT scan with contrast blush (*circle*) and moderate volume of associated hemoperitoneum (*arrows*). AAST, American Association for the Surgery of Trauma.

hemodynamics and overall injury burden must be taken into consideration as well as the type and grade of solid organ injury before a management plan is decided.

5.3.3 Management Strategy

The management options for blunt solid organ injuries are nonoperative, angioembolization, and surgical. Nonoperative management with or without angioembolization is only an option among hemodynamically normal patients. Patients with hemodynamic instability are managed operatively.

Nonoperative management consists of close clinical monitoring and serial hemoglobin measurements. The only clear contraindications to nonoperative management are hemodynamic instability or other indications for immediate laparotomy such as peritonitis. Factors that increase the risk of failure of nonoperative management, however, are older age,[16,17] volume of associated hemoperitoneum > 300 cc,[18] need for blood transfusion,[18] presence of multiple (≥ 2) solid organ injuries,[19] associated traumatic brain injury,[20] and increasing grade of injury.[15] For example, one large study from the Eastern Association for the Surgery of Trauma (EAST) demonstrated failure rates of blunt splenic trauma managed nonoperatively to be 5% for grade I injuries, 10% for grade II, 20% for grade III, 33% for grade IV, and 75% for grade V.[15] Identification of risk factors for failure, careful consideration of the patient's overall injury burden, and an assessment of the patient's physiologic capacity to tolerate ongoing blood loss should be balanced against the benefits of organ preservation and avoidance of laparotomy.

Patients with solid organ injury managed nonoperatively must undergo close clinical monitoring, with frequent vital sign recordings, serial abdominal exams, and trending of their hemoglobin levels. Patients who become hemodynamically unstable should undergo immediate laparotomy. Patients with a downtrending hemoglobin, particularly to the point of requiring transfusion, should be considered for laparotomy, angioembolization, repeat imaging, or continued observation, according to the patient's overall clinical picture and the surgeon's judgement.

Angioembolization is a useful adjunct to nonoperative management among hemodynamically stable patients with blunt solid organ injury. Especially among patients with a contrast blush (▶ Fig. 5.2) or pseudoaneurysm (▶ Fig. 5.3) seen on CT scan, angioembolization decreases the risk of failure of nonoperative management.[21,22] It can also be considered for patients with high-grade injuries. For operative liver injuries, angioembolization can also be a useful adjunct immediately following damage control surgery.

There are no universally accepted minimally invasive approaches to the surgical management of solid organ trauma. Hemodynamically unstable patients with blunt solid organ injury should undergo immediate exploratory laparotomy. After the successful nonoperative management of a solid organ injury associated with a significant amount of free intra-abdominal blood, laparoscopy may be used to evacuate the hemoperitoneum.

5.3.4 Surgical Techniques

Spleen and Kidney

Blunt injuries to the spleen and kidney can be considered together. For both structures, organ preservation is desirable. Particularly in the young patient, splenic preservation to maintain immune function is preferable. Kidney mass should be preserved whenever possible to maintain renal function and avoid need for dialysis. However, both organs are expendable and can be removed quickly if necessary. In the unstable, bleeding trauma patient, injuries to the spleen or kidney are treated with expeditious splenectomy or nephrectomy, respectively. Attempts at repair or partial resection are appropriate if the patient responds well to resuscitation intraoperatively and the surgeon's skill set allows. For a patient *in extremis*, rapid removal of the hemorrhaging organ should be performed without hesitation.

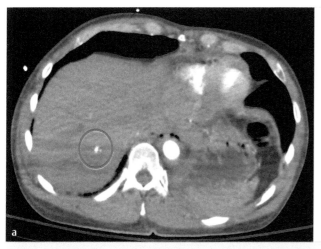
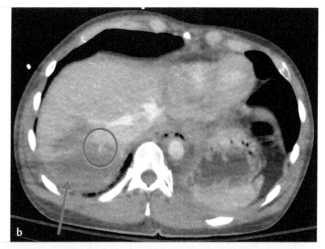

Fig. 5.3 AAST grade IV liver injury on CT scan with 9 cm laceration of the right hepatic lobe (*arrow*) and a pseudoaneurysm (*circles*) in segment 7. **(a)** arterial phase. **(b)**, portal venous phase. AAST, American Association for the Surgery of Trauma.

Prior to nephrectomy, the classic teaching is to palpate for a contralateral kidney before removing the injured one. Although leaving grossly normal kidney mass *in situ* can be reassuring prior to performing a contralateral nephrectomy, practically the presence or absence of the contralateral kidney is irrelevant as attempts at kidney preservation should never be performed while the patient exsanguinates.

Liver

Liver injuries must be considered distinctly from spleen and kidney injuries, because while it has been described,[23] hepatectomy is neither expeditious nor survivable unless a transplant is rapidly secured. Furthermore, hemorrhage from the liver is more challenging to control because it does not have a single vascular pedicle. For these reasons, the approach to a bleeding liver differs significantly.

Blunt liver injuries causing hemodynamic instability should first be managed with vectored packing via exploratory laparotomy. After entry into the peritoneal cavity, the falciform ligament is rapidly taken down. A hand is reached above the dome of the liver to break its suction against the diaphragm and allow for packs to be placed between the liver and the diaphragm. Additional packs are then placed below the liver to compress the injured hepatic parenchyma between packs. In the vast majority of cases, this staunches bleeding and allows for continued resuscitation and an organized plan of attack.

Superficial blunt liver injuries will stop with appropriately placed packs. Other options include topical hemostatic agents applied to the surface of the injured liver or the placement of chromic sutures to reapproximate hepatic parenchyma. These sutures should incorporate liver capsule to give strength to the repair. If there is a devascularized segment, nonanatomic resection of the injured portion should be quickly performed.

If packing is successful at stopping the bleeding, avoid the temptation to remove the packs and fiddle with the injury. If bleeding persists despite attempts at appropriate packing, this is a significant problem and an organized and expeditious approach to the injury should ensue. The first step is to improve exposure. Typically, a right subcostal incision will suffice. If concern for retrohepatic caval injury exists, heralded by brisk dark bleeding from behind the liver that worsens when the liver is tipped anteriorly, a right thoracotomy can be added and connected to the laparotomy incision. Division of the right diaphragm will further improve this exposure.

The next step is achieving at least partial vascular control to allow for visualization of the injury and repair. A Pringle maneuver is accomplished by bluntly creating an aperture in the avascular portion of the lesser omentum and encircling the porta hepatis through the foramen of Winslow. Occlusion of the inflow through the portal vein and proper hepatic artery can first be accomplished with a finger and then replaced with a vascular clamp, vessel loop, or Rummel tourniquet. This may slow the bleeding enough to allow visualization of an injured vessel through a crack in the liver, which can then be oversewn.

A Pringle maneuver occludes the porta hepatis but does nothing to control the inflow from the IVC. If application of a Pringle maneuver does not slow the bleeding from a deep liver laceration, a retrohepatic caval injury should be suspected. These patients infrequently survive to the operating room and when they do, there is little time to arrest the bleeding before the patient expires. The two options for retrohepatic caval injuries that are not controlled with packing are total hepatic vascular exclusion and placement of a Schrock shunt.

Total hepatic vascular exclusion involves four points of vascular occlusion: the aorta, the porta hepatis, and both the infra- and suprahepatic IVC. The aortic clamp must be applied prior to occluding the IVC. Removing the venous return below the diaphragm dramatically drops the cardiac preload and this will induce cardiac arrest unless the heart needs only to circulate blood to the upper body, head, and neck. Aortic control is best achieved via supraceliac clamp. Infrahepatic IVC occlusion is achieved by encircling the cava above the renal veins. Suprahepatic IVC control can be achieved above the liver, immediately below the diaphragm, but this is technically challenging and difficult to obtain in an emergency. It is much simpler to encircle the intrapericardial segment of the IVC from within the chest through a median sternotomy or clamshell thoracotomy. Achieving total hepatic vascular exclusion will provide a short period of hemorrhage control during which to mobilize the liver, expose the injury, and repair it. If this cannot be accomplished quickly, the patient will arrest.

While rarely employed successfully, a Schrock shunt excludes blood flow through the injured segment of retrohepatic cava to allow visualization and repair of the injury. If repair is impossible, the patient can be made anhepatic and listed for liver transplant after creating a mesocaval shunt to allow for venous drainage of the gastrointestinal (GI) tract. Placement of a Schrock shunt first involves preparation of the shunt. A chest tube or endotracheal tube can be used. A hole must be cut in the tube over the portion that will sit in the right atrium, to allow unloading of blood from the lower body into the right atrium. A clamp is also needed on the proximal end of the tube to ensure blood is returned to the patient via the right atrium and not exsanguinated onto the floor. Once the shunt is ready, a pursestring suture is placed into the right atrial appendage. The shunt is then inserted through an atriotomy in the center of the pursestring suture and passed inferiorly through the right atrium and into the IVC. This is advanced through the retrohepatic past the injury. The Schrock shunt is secured above the renal veins and affixed to prevent dislodgement or embolization. Repair of the injury or total hepatectomy is then attempted. It should be noted that any suspected retrohepatic venous injury that is contained or controlled with packing should be left undisturbed followed by a temporary abdominal closure.

5.3.5 Complications

Complications vary according to the management strategy and time from injury. After nonoperative management with or without angioembolization, in the immediate period, ongoing bleeding is the primary concern and is discussed above under management strategies. Other complications include delayed bleeding and abscess. Delayed bleeding can occur as a result of a ruptured pseudoaneurysm not appreciated on the index CT scan or because of a ruptured subcapsular hematoma. Although evidence concerning these complications is limited, we generally repeat a CT scan with IV contrast prior to discharge among patients who are symptomatic or who have a solid organ injury of grade III or higher. If a pseudoaneurysm is detected, we pursue angioembolization. Abscess as a result of tissue necrosis following nonoperative management is suggested clinically by the presence of tachycardia, fever, increased abdominal tenderness, or leukocytosis, and is confirmed with CT scan. Treatment consists of antibiotics with or without percutaneous drainage, depending on the size and location of the abscess as well as the physiologic condition of the patient.

Following surgical management of blunt solid organ injury, there are general as well as organ-specific complications that should be considered. As with any postoperative patient, patients should be monitored for wound infection or dehiscence. Long-term complications include adhesive small bowel obstruction and incisional hernias. A recent study demonstrated that approximately 10% of patients who undergo single look laparotomy for trauma are readmitted to the hospital for a surgery-related complication, of which small bowel obstruction and hernia are the most common.[24]

Following splenectomy, overwhelming postsplenectomy infection (OPSI) is an established risk. Asplenic individuals are susceptible to infection by encapsulated bacteria. When this results in fulminant sepsis, the clinical condition is termed OPSI. The risk of OPSI following trauma splenectomy is much lower than that after an elective splenectomy, potentially because of abdominal splenosis following splenic bleeding.[25] Although OPSI is exceedingly rare following trauma splenectomy (0.21/100 person years),[26] it is an important reason to consider organ preservation whenever feasible as mortality rates following OPSI are 50 to 70%.[25]

Following trauma nephrectomy, there is a theoretically increased risk of chronic renal failure, necessitating dialysis as a result of the single kidney state. Data are extremely limited, but one study postulated that the lifetime risk of long-term dialysis following trauma nephrectomy is only approximately 0.5% and thus the concern for this complication may be overstated.[27]

Regardless of management strategy, patients with blunt liver injury are at risk of bile leak. This is a frequent complication and occurs in up to 20% of patients.[28] Clinical suspicion for bile leak should arise in the setting of increased right upper quadrant tenderness and hyperbilirubinemia. CT scan is a useful initial imaging modality and may demonstrate a biloma amenable to percutaneous drainage. This is often all that is needed as most bile leaks are self-limited. Laparoscopy can be considered for bilomas that are not amenable to percutaneous drainage. Persistent or large bile leaks can be further evaluated with hydroxyiminodiacetic acid (HIDA) scan or magnetic resonance cholangiopancreatography (MRCP) and may require percutaneous transhepatic cholangiogram (PTC) or endoscopic retrograde cholangiopancreatography (ERCP) with stenting for management.

5.4 Hollow Viscus Injuries

5.4.1 Diagnosis

Hollow viscus injuries are diagnosed in one of two ways: on physical examination or on CT scan. Although free air under the diaphragm on an upright abdominal X-ray (AXR) after blunt trauma would also indicate hollow viscus perforation, this image series is rarely performed immediately following blunt trauma.

On physical examination, patients with hollow viscus perforation can present with peritonitis, diaphoresis, tachycardia, and fever. Patients with hollow viscus injury and short transport times to hospital may not have time to manifest these signs and may present with abdominal tenderness alone. A high degree of suspicion for injury must be maintained.

On CT scan, hollow viscus injuries can present in a number of different ways. Free intraperitoneal air represents a hollow viscus injury until proven otherwise. Free intraperitoneal fluid also commonly represents hollow viscus injury. The density of the fluid can be checked to distinguish between water, indicating hollow viscus perforation, and blood. Although a small amount of free fluid is physiologic in women of reproductive age, even trace free fluid can represent a hollow viscus injury in the appropriate clinical context. In patients without free air or fluid, bowel wall thickening can reflect hematoma or ischemia and may indicate partial thickness injury.

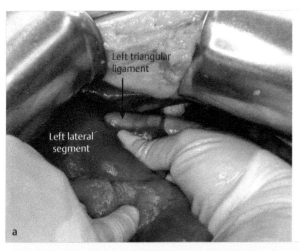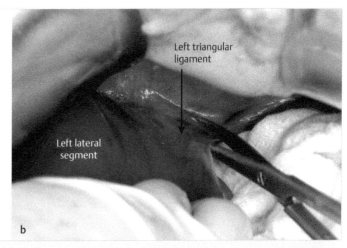

Fig. 5.4 To expose the gastroesophageal (GE) junction, take down the left lateral segment of the liver by identifying (**a**) and dividing (**b**) the left triangular ligament. (Reproduced with permission of Schellenberg M, Schlitzkus LL, Inaba K. Gastrointestinal Tract. In: Atlas of Surgical Techniques in Trauma. Demetriades D, Inaba K, Velmahos G, eds. 2nd ed. Cambridge: Cambridge University Press; 2019.[33])

5.4.2 Management Strategy

Patients with trace free fluid on CT scan or other subtle signs of hollow viscus injury, who lack clinical suggestion of GI tract perforation, may undergo a period of close clinical observation with serial abdominal examinations, close monitoring of vital signs, and repeated laboratory draws. Worsened abdominal tenderness, peritonitis, fever, tachycardia, and leukocytosis all herald hollow viscus injury and should be considered indications for laparotomy in these patients. This period of observation is typically for 24 hours after injury.

In general, blunt hollow viscus injuries are managed operatively. Low-grade blunt hollow viscus injuries, i.e., contusions, hematomas, and partial thickness injuries, do not routinely require intervention. All other hollow viscus injuries, with the exception of extraperitoneal rectal injuries, require repair or resection according to the extent of injury. The remainder of this section will describe the surgical management of full-thickness hollow viscus injuries.

The operative approach to identification and management of hollow viscus injuries is generally through an exploratory laparotomy. The role of laparoscopic surgery in these patients remains highly controversial. Although some surgeons with extensive experience in minimally invasive surgery at highly specialized centers report improved outcomes and few missed injuries when using laparoscopy to evaluate and manage blunt hollow viscus injuries,[29,30,31] there is no evidence that these results are generalizable on a large scale.

5.4.3 Surgical Techniques

Blunt hollow viscus injuries are typically managed with resection. Although primary repair is theoretically an option, these injuries tend to be sufficiently destructive and warrant resection. Due to regional variations in GI tract anatomy, surgical techniques in blunt hollow viscus injury are best considered by anatomic structure.

5.5 Gastroesophageal (GE) Junction Injuries

Blunt GE junction injuries are extremely rare.[32] They are often associated with other abdominal injuries and are therefore approached initially through a laparotomy. The GE junction can be exposed by dividing the left triangular ligament in order to mobilize the left lateral segment of the liver and then taking down the avascular portion of the gastrohepatic ligament (▶ Fig. 5.4a, b). Application of downward traction on the stomach will deliver the distal intrathoracic esophagus into the abdomen, if this is required to fully expose the injury. Division of the left crus will facilitate this exposure.

Blunt GE junction injuries tend to be extensive and require resection with reconstruction. As associated injuries are common, especially to critical structures such as the liver, heart, and aorta, this often requires a staged approach. At the index operation, the injured GE junction can be rapidly resected using staplers, thereby controlling contamination. The GE junction is then left in discontinuity, with reconstruction planned for 24 to 48 hours later if the patient survives. The proximal segment of the GE junction should be tacked to the diaphragm after division to avoid retraction into the chest, which will complicate attempts at reconstruction. Reconstruction may require the addition of a thoracotomy and can be performed with a stapled or handsewn anastomosis. Although routine surgical placement of a jejunal feeding tube is unnecessary after GE junction injuries, it is prudent after a blunt GE junction injury requiring resection and reconstruction.

5.5.1 Stomach

Gastric injuries following blunt trauma are rare. To assess the stomach for injury at laparotomy, both the anterior and posterior walls must be completely visualized. The posterior stomach is exposed via the lesser sac by dividing the gastrocolic ligament. This is facilitated by retracting the stomach cephalad and the transverse colon caudally to place the gastrocolic ligament on tension. After division of the gastrocolic ligament through a relatively avascular segment, placing two wide malleable retractors deep into the lesser sac and then slowly withdrawing them allows for inspection of the posterior aspect of the stomach.

Even after blunt trauma, gastric injuries can typically be managed with a two-layer primary repair or a stapled wedge resection of the injured segment. Notably, wedge resection cannot be used for injuries to the pylorus or any other location where luminal stenosis may occur as a result. Destructive gastric injuries require partial gastrectomy and reconstruction.

5.5.2 Duodenum

If concern for duodenal injury exists, either due to preoperative imaging or a hematoma seen in the retroperitoneum, the duodenum should be mobilized and thoroughly inspected. To do this, the hepatic flexure must first be mobilized. Although the first and part of the second portions of the duodenum are intraperitoneal, the remainder are retroperitoneal and a Kocher maneuver must be performed to free the duodenum completely from its retroperitoneal attachments.

Injuries to the duodenum can be difficult to manage due to challenges in exposure and concomitant injuries to adjacent structures such as the pancreas, IVC, and portal vein. After excluding a full-thickness component, duodenal hematomas do not require intervention. Full-thickness duodenal injuries, even if extensive, should be managed with primary repair if this can be accomplished without stenosis.[34,35] There is no need for routine pyloric exclusion.[36] Destructive duodenal injuries require resection and Roux-en-Y reconstruction.

5.5.3 Small Bowel and Colon

Bowel injuries after blunt trauma can occur by way of three different mechanisms: direct injury, perforation after a closed loop obstruction (wherein entrapment of the bowel at two points causes a sudden increase in intraluminal pressure), and bucket handle injury (in which a mesenteric injury occurs without initial injury to the bowel itself) (▶ Fig. 5.5). To inspect for injury, the entire small bowel must be run from the ligament of Treitz to the ileocecal valve. The intraperitoneal segments of the colon, that is, the transverse and sigmoid colons, are inspected circumferentially. The retroperitoneal segments of the colon, that is, the ascending and descending colons, do not need to be mobilized for inspection unless a hematoma is noted or there is suggestion of injury based on preoperative CT scan.

Blunt small and large bowel injuries that encompass < 50% of the circumference of the bowel can be considered for a two-layer primary repair after debriding to clean edges; otherwise, resection is required. Handsewn and stapled anastomoses are both appropriate and the decision should be based largely on surgeon preference, since the available literature suggests outcomes are similar between the two techniques.[37] In some hands, a stapled anastomosis is more expedient. On edematous bowel, conversely, a handsewn anastomosis may be a more prudent choice. Bowel discontinuity should be reserved only for profoundly unstable patients. In all others, even during damage control laparotomy, a rapid reanastomosis should be performed.

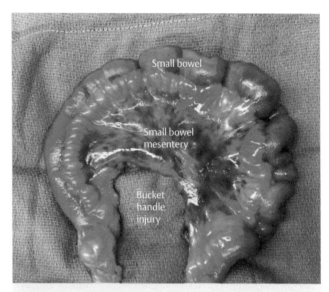

Fig. 5.5 Intraoperative specimen photograph of a bucket handle injury to the small bowel mesentery, necessitating small bowel resection.

When serosal injuries to the bowel are encountered, they should be imbricated with Lembert sutures to avoid conversion to full-thickness injury.

The role of proximal diversion or end colostomy after colon resection is controversial. In practice, these techniques are infrequently required. We generally reserve diversion for patients with poor tissue quality and who are at high-risk of anastomotic leak. This includes patients left in discontinuity at the index operation and whose bowel integrity remains questionable after restoration of continuity. Proximal diversion is also prudent for patients among whom an anastomotic leak would likely be catastrophic, such as elderly, comorbid patients. It must be remembered that if stoma creation and laparotomy closure are not occurring at the same operation, the stoma should not be placed through the rectus muscle as described in elective operations. Instead, the stoma should be sited more laterally. The laparotomy incision tends to retract away from the midline as the abdomen is left open. If a stoma is placed too medially, it will complicate both abdominal closure and fecal diversion.

5.5.4 Rectum

The first step in management of a rectal injury is identification and determination of its location relative to the peritoneal reflection. The combination of rigid proctoscopy and CT scan is typically sufficient to identify these injuries.[38] Defining a rectal injury as intra- or extraperitoneal is critical as these injuries are managed differently according to their anatomic location. Intraperitoneal rectal injuries are managed as colon injuries. Primarily seen after penetrating injury, extraperitoneal rectal injuries are managed either with proximal diversion or primary transanal repair. Primary repair is more common for penetrating extraperitoneal rectal injuries as blunt injuries to the extraperitoneal rectum tend to be destructive. Presacral drains and distal rectal washout, while commonly used in the past, are now considered unnecessary and potentially harmful.[39] If the location of the rectal injury is questionable, diagnostic laparoscopy can be performed as the first step in management to exclude an intra-peritoneal component.

5.5.5 Complications

Many complications after surgical management of hollow viscus injury are the same as those following operative management of solid organ injury, such as the long-term risks of adhesive small bowel obstruction and incisional hernia. Other long-term risks after hollow viscus injury repair include anastomotic stricture which requires revision of the anastomosis.

One complication after management of hollow viscus injury that merits specific consideration is the development of an ischemic stricture. This occurs after a bucket handle injury to the small bowel mesentery. Although ischemia of the associated segment of small bowel may not be immediately apparent, over time this segment becomes ischemic as a result of reduced blood supply. Frank necrosis and perforation can result, or the segment will stricture and present as a mechanical small bowel obstruction. In either case, the management concerns resection of the segment involved with anastomosis. Ischemic strictures following bucket handle injuries can be avoided by resecting the associated segment of small bowel at the index operation. If the mesenteric injury is small and the associated small bowel is viable, closure of the mesenteric defect, and reinspection of the small bowel in 24 to 48 hours for viability, may allow salvage of that segment and avoidance of an anastomosis.

5.6 Pancreatic Injuries

5.6.1 Diagnosis

The optimal diagnostic workup of patients with suspected pancreatic injury remains elusive. Pancreatic injuries are infrequent and tend to occur in conjunction with severe, frequently lethal injuries due to the proximity of the pancreas to major vascular structures including the aorta and IVC. This makes them a challenge to study. While CT scan is the most frequently used cross-sectional imaging modality to screen blunt trauma patients for injury, its sensitivity in diagnosing pancreatic injuries varies from 47 to 76%,[40,41,42,43] rendering it insufficient to exclude injury.

Because of the pitfalls of CT scanning after pancreatic injury, other imaging modalities as well as laboratory tests have been investigated to aid in diagnosis. Serum amylase has limited utility due to lack of both sensitivity and specificity. The value of a single serum lipase value is similarly limited, but an elevated or rising serum lipase >6 hours postinjury is highly sensitive and specific for pancreatic injury.[44]

Magnetic resonance cholangiopancreatography (MRCP) and endoscopic retrograde cholangiopancreatography (ERCP) are excellent imaging modalities to assess the pancreatic duct for injury. After blunt trauma, MRCP accurately identifies the AAST grade of pancreatic injury and pancreatic duct injury in 93% and 92% of patients, respectively.[45] However, MRCP and ERCP are costly and necessitate patient transport for prolonged periods, which is of particular concern for severely injured blunt polytrauma patients; in addition, ERCP is invasive.

Taking into consideration the available evidence, our approach to the stable trauma patient at risk of pancreatic injury is to begin with a CT scan. If this raises concerns for pancreatic duct injury, we proceed with MRCP. Because of the invasive nature of ERCP, we reserve it for management, and not diagnostic, purposes. In patients with a CT scan negative for pancreatic injury but, who are at high risk of pancreatic injury, such as those with a handle bar injury to the abdomen or with associated duodenal or L1/L2 fracture, we order serial serum lipase measurements. Rising serum lipase or worsening abdominal pain in these patients prompts MRCP for further investigation.

Unstable patients with concerns for pancreatic injury are brought in for immediate laparotomy. Various methods have been described to intraoperatively assess the pancreatic duct for injury, including visual inspection as well as various methods of intra-operative pancreatography, either using on-table ERCP or via cannulation through a duodenotomy or cholecystotomy. Some early studies emphasized thorough visual inspection of the gland, with pancreatic duct injury heralded by direct visualization of duct injury, complete transection or disruption of >50% of the pancreas, central perforation, or severe maceration.[46] Other early work argued in favor of the liberal use of intraoperative pancreatography.[47] Modern studies have demonstrated that visual inspection of the pancreas at laparotomy is sufficient to rule in or out a pancreatic duct injury and that there should be a very limited role for intraoperative pancreatography.[40,48,49]

5.6.2 Management Strategy

The management of pancreatic injuries is dependent upon the AAST grade of injury, wherein grades I and II injuries do not involve disruption of the pancreatic duct; grade III injury involves distal duct disruption; grade IV involves proximal duct disruption; and grade V is massive pancreatic head disruption. Grades I and II injuries can be managed nonoperatively if they are diagnosed on imaging.[41] If discovered intraoperatively, closed-suction drain placement is prudent, especially if associated injuries are present to avoid spillage of pancreatic secretions onto adjacent repaired viscera.

Grade III and higher pancreatic injuries require intervention. This usually consists of surgical resection, as delineated under Surgical Techniques. For patients with no other indication for laparotomy or those who are diagnosed in a delayed fashion, ERCP and stenting may be a viable option for these injuries. Laparoscopic pancreatic resection is not routinely performed in the trauma patient but may be an option in select circumstances.

5.6.3 Surgical Techniques

Grade III pancreatic injuries are generally managed with distal pancreatectomy. The spleen is often removed with the distal pancreas, even if the spleen is uninjured, to increase the expediency of the operation. There exists evidence to support a spleen-preserving distal pancreatectomy for young blunt trauma patients with a relatively minor burden of overall injuries.[50] In all other patients, or if the surgeon's skill set does not allow for a safe and swift spleen-preserving distal pancreatectomy, the spleen should be removed with the distal pancreas. Closed-suction drains are typically left in the surgical bed.

High grade (grades IV–V) pancreatic injuries are often managed using a staged approach. Because of the force required to disrupt the pancreas to this extent as well as the proximity of the head of the pancreas to major structures including the aorta, IVC, portal vein, liver, and duodenum, patients with high-grade pancreatic injuries tend to sustain severe associated injuries which are often present *in extremis*. Consequently, they are managed with a damage control approach, with high-grade pancreatic injuries drained or resected at the index operation followed by a staged approach to reconstruction.

The decision to resect the injured pancreatic head versus simply placing drains over the injury at the initial damage control operation is left to the surgeon's judgement and is based upon the patient's overall burden of injuries, physiologic status, and status of the duodenum. In general, if there is an associated duodenal injury that cannot be reconstructed, a pancreaticoduodenectomy will be required. Regardless of the approach taken, the index operation should be expedient and limited to controlling hemorrhage and spillage from the GI tract. Once the patient's status has improved, a second look laparotomy is performed. Any remaining devitalized pancreas can be resected and reconstruction is performed. If the patient's status remains tenuous, the pancreaticoduodenectomy can be completed at this stage and reconstruction attempted at a subsequent 24- to 48-hour interval.

5.6.4 Complications

A number of complications can ensue following pancreatic injury, including pancreatic leaks, fistulization, abscesses, and pancreatic insufficiency. Pancreatic leaks can occur from the injured gland itself or from a staple or suture line following resection; many are self-limited. Particularly if a drain was left intraoperatively, this is often all that is required until the leak spontaneously closes. If the leak is high-volume or persists, ERCP with stenting is indicated. Fistulization, for example to the pleura, can occur if leaks are allowed to persist uncontrolled. These can be extremely difficult to treat and therefore early attempts to control pancreatic leaks are prudent. Pancreatic abscesses are managed with antibiotics and drainage. Pancreatic insufficiency after resection for trauma is rare.[51] Only 10 to 15% of the pancreatic mass is required in order to preserve normal endocrine and exocrine pancreatic functions.

5.7 Major Vascular Injuries

5.7.1 Diagnosis

Injuries to the major abdominal vasculature, that is, the abdominal aorta, IVC, and their branches or tributaries, are diagnosed on CT scan or laparotomy. As with any blunt trauma patient, the physical examination may be consistent with hemorrhage, tachycardia, hypotension, and/or positive abdominal views on FAST, if there is associated injury to the retroperitoneum with free bleeding into the abdomen. However, due to the retroperitoneal nature of the major abdominal vasculature, bleeding from these structures is not well-assessed on FAST.

On CT scan, injuries to the major abdominal vasculature appear as hematomas, vessel wall abnormalities, contrast extravasation, or a lack of filling with contrast, depending on the nature of the injury. On laparotomy, these injuries present as retroperitoneal hematomas.

The retroperitoneum is divided into four zones. Zone I is located medially and travels from the aortic hiatus in the diaphragm to the aortic bifurcation at the pelvic inlet. It includes the abdominal aorta, celiac trunk, both the superior and inferior mesenteric arteries (SMA, IMA), as well as the inferior vena cava. Zone II is located lateral to Zone I bilaterally and includes the kidneys and renal arteries and veins. Zone III consists of the pelvis, containing the common, internal, external iliac arteries and veins, as well as the presacral venous plexus. Zone IV comprises the retrohepatic vena cava.

5.7.2 Management Strategy

The management of blunt retroperitoneal hematomas hinges upon the hemodynamic status of the patient. Blunt retroperitoneal hematomas, without evidence of ongoing bleeding, that are discovered on CT scan may be managed nonoperatively, with close clinical observation for ongoing bleeding if the patient is hemodynamically normal and without evidence of ischemia.

Although there are no laparoscopic options for the management of retroperitoneal hematomas, minimally invasive approaches to these injuries can be considered in the form of angioembolization or endovascular interventions. Angioembolization is an option for a number of different clinical scenarios. First, it can be considered for patients with a retroperitoneal hematoma on CT scan and suggestion of ongoing bleeding, including contrast extravasation, large hematomas, or associated hemoperitoneum if the vessel can be safely occluded. In addition, for renal injuries, demonstration of a pseudoaneurysm or contrast blush on CT scan is an indication for embolization, as discussed above under solid organ injuries. Endovascular intervention can be considered for patients with blunt aortic injuries or injuries to the major abdominal aortic branches.

Patients with retroperitoneal hematomas on CT scan who become unstable, should be taken for laparotomy. One possible exception to this principle is patients with pelvic bleeding. If angioembolization is an appropriate treatment option but interventional radiology requires additional time to arrive to hospital, resuscitative endovascular balloon occlusion of the aorta (REBOA) can be used as a bridge to angioembolization.

The management of blunt retroperitoneal hematomas discovered at laparotomy depends upon the zone of injury and the characteristics of the hematoma. All blunt zone I hematomas should be explored. Retroperitoneal hematomas in Zones II and III need only be explored if the hematoma is large, pulsatile, or expanding. Zone IV hematomas should only be explored if brisk bleeding refractory to packing occurs. This is detailed above under the management of high-grade liver injuries.

5.7.3 Surgical Techniques

Exploration of zones I and II is accomplished via a medial visceral rotation on the side of the hematoma, which involves division of the white line of Toldt and rotation of the colon medially, off of the retroperitoneum. Suspected injuries to the infrahepatic IVC are explored with a Cattell Braasch maneuver, which consists of a right medial visceral rotation, Kocherization of the duodenum, and division of the peritoneum overlying the small bowel mesentery from the right lower quadrant to the ligament of Treitz. This fully mobilizes the viscera off of the right side of the retroperitoneum.

Blunt pelvic bleeding, that is, zone III hematomas, infrequently needs to be explored operatively as it is often self-contained or controlled with angioembolization. When bleeding requires surgical control, there are a litany of options: preperitoneal pelvic packing, intraperitoneal packing, and bilateral internal iliac artery ligation. Each has evidence supporting its use and the selection of one technique over another is largely a matter of institutional or surgeon preference.

Once vascular exposure is achieved in any of the zones of the retroperitoneum, the options for hemorrhage control are simple. For a patient *in extremis*, damage control consists of ligation or shunting. The aorta and SMA cannot be ligated, while the celiac trunk and IMA can be. The renal artery may be ligated if loss of the ipsilateral kidney is accepted. Ligation of the infrarenal IVC is acceptable if repair would result in > 50% stenosis of the lumen. If the injury to the IVC occurs above the renal veins, reconstitution of flow must be achieved. Definitive repair of a major vascular injury, either at the index case if the patient responds to resuscitation or at the second look, involves a standard vascular repair or bypass.

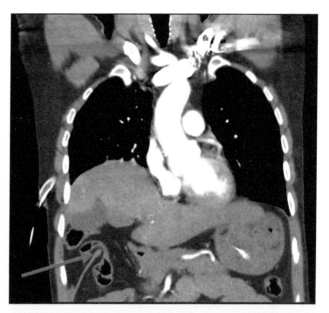

Fig. 5.6 Blunt injury to the right diaphragm (*arrow*) with herniation of liver and bowel as seen on CT scan.

5.7.4 Complications

After repair of injury to the aorta or its major branches, the patient should be monitored to ensure adequate perfusion distal to the injury. If the SMA was reconstructed, for example, the surgeon should monitor the patient closely in the postoperative period for signs of small bowel ischemia. If the distal abdominal aorta was repaired, pulses in the patient's lower extremity should be monitored.

After repair of an IVC injury, any degree of luminal stenosis will place the patient at increased risk of venous thromboemboli (VTE). The patient should be started on VTE prophylaxis as soon as is feasible and the clinician should maintain a high-degree of suspicion for VTE in these patients. In the case of IVC ligation, edema of the lower extremities can prove to be a serious sequela. These patients should have the lower extremities wrapped with compression bandages and elevated to help reduce edema. The extremities should be monitored closely for signs and symptoms of compartment syndrome postoperatively.[52]

5.8 Diaphragm Injuries

5.8.1 Diagnosis

Blunt diaphragm injuries are exceedingly rare (< 0.1% of all blunt trauma patients)[53] and are less common than penetrating diaphragm injuries by a ratio of approximately 1:3.[54] These injuries are more commonly left-sided due to protection of the right diaphragm by the liver. Because of the blunt force necessary to disrupt the diaphragm, these injuries tend to occur after a high-force mechanism of injury. Clinical signs and symptoms that may be observed in these patients include chest pain, shortness of breath, decreased breath sounds, and low-oxygen saturation. Because all of these features may also be seen with a pneumothorax, a rapid chest X-ray (CXR) in the trauma bay is needed to discriminate between the two pathologies. The distinction is

critical because chest tube insertion into a diaphragmatic hernia containing abdominal viscera can be harmful.

Although penetrating diaphragmatic injuries can be radiographically subtle, even on cross-sectional imaging, blunt injuries to the diaphragm tend to be large and therefore easier to detect radiographically. In addition, herniation is common in the acute setting following blunt, but not penetrating, diaphragmatic injury, which further facilitates radiographic diagnosis.[55] If a blunt trauma patient does not receive a CXR in the trauma bay, the diagnosis of a blunt diaphragm injury can be made intraoperatively or on CT scan (▸ Fig. 5.6). CT findings tend to be more subtle with right-sided injuries.[56]

5.8.2 Management Strategy

Most blunt diaphragm injuries require repair. Extrapolation from the penetrating trauma literature may lead some surgeons to manage a small, right-sided diaphragm injury nonoperatively, but this has not been formally studied. Even a small, right-sided injury should likely be closed in the presence of a concomitant liver injury because bile leakage can spill into the chest.

While the laparoscopic management of penetrating diaphragmatic injuries is arguably the only well-accepted indication for laparoscopy in trauma, repair via laparotomy remains the standard of care for blunt diaphragmatic injuries. Some injuries will require a combined approach via laparotomy and thoracotomy if extensive or diagnosed in a delayed fashion.[57]

5.8.3 Surgical Techniques

Once the peritoneal cavity is entered via laparotomy, the left upper quadrant viscera are gently retracted caudally to allow visualization and inspection of the diaphragm. If there is herniation through the diaphragmatic defect, the contents are gently reduced by applying careful downward pressure.

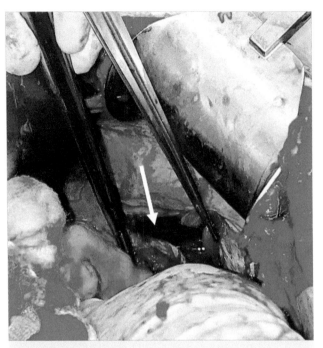

Fig. 5.7 Blunt injury to the left diaphragm (*arrow*) as seen intraoperatively. Placement of Allis clamps along the edge of the defect as shown here can help to elevate the injury into the surgical field and facilitate repair.

After reduction of the hernia contents, if any, repair of the defect is facilitated by placing long Allis clamps along the edges (▶ Fig. 5.7). This allows the surgeon to pull the defect into the surgical field to increase ease of suture placement. A nonabsorbable suture such as 0 prolene can be used to close the defect in an interrupted fashion.

The vast majority of diaphragm injuries can be closed primarily, even if the defect is large. On rare occasions with especially destructive injuries, or in situations where the diaphragm has been avulsed off of the chest wall, transposition of the diaphragm up a few intercostal spaces will allow reconstitution of the diaphragm when primary repair is not feasible. While very rare, mesh-based reconstruction also remains an option.

5.8.4 Complications

The major complication related to diaphragm injuries is a missed diagnosis, the rates of which are difficult to capture in epidemiologic studies due to lack of trauma patient follow-up. These patients can present weeks, months, or years after the inciting trauma with typical signs of organ herniation. The diagnosis is secured on CT scan or intraoperatively. Operative reduction of the hernia contents and repair of the defect should ensue immediately. These delayed or chronic diaphragmatic hernias are often best approached first through a thoracotomy, rather than a laparotomy,[58] unlike diaphragmatic hernias in the acute setting, where associated intra-abdominal injuries must be ruled out.

5.9 Considerations for Abdominal Closure

Many patients can have their laparotomy closed at the index operation. This is typically done with a running absorbable suture to the fascia and staples to the skin. After closing a laparotomy incision following repair of a hollow viscus injury, the skin is generally left open to mitigate the risk of a surgical site infection. Placement of a negative pressure wound therapy dressing can be considered.

Drain placement is left to the surgeon's discretion. After splenectomy, a closed-suction drain placed near the tail of the pancreas is prudent if there is any concern about injury during the dissection. Drain placement to the surgical bed can also be considered after splenectomy or nephrectomy to avoid hematoma accumulation. After liver injury, especially those that are high-grade, placement of drains above and below the liver can be helpful in controlling postoperative bile leakage, a common complication of hepatic injury.

Patients undergoing damage control surgery, such as temporary packing of a liver injury, are left open with planned return to the operating room within 24 hours of the index operation or sooner if the patient deteriorates. These patients are temporarily closed using a commercial negative pressure therapy device or by creating one with towels, plastic drapes, and closed-suction drains.

5.10 Conclusion

Blunt abdominal trauma can be challenging to diagnose and manage due to the multitude of viscera at risk for injury. Patients who are hemodynamically abnormal or who have peritonitis are brought in for immediate laparotomy. Patients without these signs undergo CT scan of the abdomen as the initial cross-sectional imaging modality of choice. Knowledge of the appropriate diagnostic workup, management strategy, and surgical techniques relevant to each organ system will allow for safe and expedient care of blunt trauma patients.

References

[1] Centers for Disease Control and Prevention. Ten Leading Causes of Death and Injury. National Center for Injury Prevention and Control. 2019. Available at: https:// www.cdc.gov/injury/wisqars/LeadingCauses.html. Accessed March 1, 2019

[2] Oyeniyi BT, Fox EE, Scerbo M, Tomasek JS, Wade CE, Holcomb JB. Trends in 1029 Trauma Deaths at a Level I Trauma Center. Injury. 2017; 48(1):5–12

[3] American College of Surgeons Committee on Trauma. Advanced Trauma Life Support (ATLS), 10th ed. Chicago: Hearthside Publishing Services; 2018

[4] Rozycki GS, Ochsner MG, Jaffin JH, Champion HR. Prospective evaluation of surgeons' use of ultrasound in the evaluation of trauma patients. J Trauma. 1993; 34(4):516–526, discussion 526–527

[5] Rozycki GS, Ochsner MG, Feliciano DV, et al. Early detection of hemoperitoneum by ultrasound examination of the right upper quadrant: a multicenter study. J Trauma. 1998; 45(5):878–883

[6] Kirkpatrick AW, Simons RK, Brown R, Nicolaou S, Dulchavsky S. The hand-held FAST: experience with hand-held trauma sonography in a level-I urban trauma center. Injury. 2002; 33(4):303–308

[7] Rozycki GS, Ballard RB, Feliciano DV, Schmidt JA, Pennington SD. Surgeon-performed ultrasound for the assessment of truncal injuries: lessons learned from 1540 patients. Ann Surg. 1998; 228(4):557–567

[8] Kim J, Schellenberg M, Inaba K. Calculated decisions: focused assessment with sonography for trauma (FAST). Emerg Med Pract. 2018; 18 Suppl 3:1–3

[9] Von KuenssbergJehle D, Stiller G, Wagner D. Sensitivity in detecting free intraperitoneal fluid with the pelvic views of the FAST exam. Am J Emerg Med. 2003; 21(6):476–478

[10] Blackbourne LH, Soffer D, McKenney M, et al. Secondary ultrasound examination increases the sensitivity of the FAST exam in blunt trauma. J Trauma. 2004; 57(5):934–938

[11] Gumbert JL, Froderman SE, Mercho JP. Diagnostic peritoneal lavage in blunt abdominal trauma. Ann Surg. 1967; 165(1):70–72

[12] Root HD, Hauser CW, McKinley CR, Lafave JW, Mendiola RP, Jr. Diagnostic peritoneal lavage. Surgery. 1965; 57:633–637

[13] Kuncir EJ, Velmahos GC. Diagnostic peritoneal aspiration–the foster child of DPL: a prospective observational study. Int J Surg. 2007; 5(3):167–171

[14] Moore EE, Cogbill TH, Malangoni MA, et al. Organ injury scaling. Surg Clin North Am. 1995; 75(2):293–303

[15] Peitzman AB, Heil B, Rivera L, et al. Blunt splenic injury in adults: multi-institutional study of the Eastern Association for the Surgery of Trauma. J Trauma. 2000; 49(2):177–187, discussion 187–189

[16] Trust MD, Teixeira PG, Brown LH, et al. Is It safe? Nonoperative management of blunt splenic injuries in geriatric trauma patients. J Trauma Acute Care Surg. 2018; 84(1):123–127

[17] Harbrecht BG, Peitzman AB, Rivera L, et al. Contribution of age and gender to outcome of blunt splenic injury in adults: multicenter study of the eastern association for the surgery of trauma. J Trauma. 2001; 51(6):887–895

[18] Velmahos GC, Toutouzas KG, Radin R, Chan L, Demetriades D. Nonoperative treatment of blunt injury to solid abdominal organs: a prospective study. Arch Surg. 2003; 138(8):844–851

[19] Malhotra AK, Latifi R, Fabian TC, et al. Multiplicity of solid organ injury: influence on management and outcomes after blunt abdominal trauma. J Trauma. 2003; 54(5):925–929

[20] Velmahos GC, Zacharias N, Emhoff TA, et al. Management of the most severely injured spleen: a multicenter study of the Research Consortium of New England Centers for Trauma (ReCONECT). Arch Surg. 2010; 145(5):456–460

[21] Davis KA, Fabian TC, Croce MA, et al. Improved success in nonoperative management of blunt splenic injuries: embolization of splenic artery pseudoaneurysms. J Trauma. 1998; 44(6):1008–1013, discussion 1013–1015

[22] Schurr MJ, Fabian TC, Gavant M, et al. Management of blunt splenic trauma: computed tomographic contrast blush predicts failure of nonoperative management. J Trauma. 1995; 39(3):507–512, discussion–512–513

[23] Plackett TP, Barmparas G, Inaba K, Demetriades D. Transplantation for severe hepatic trauma. J Trauma. 2011; 71(6):1880–1884

[24] Bowie JM, Badiee J, Calvo RY, et al. Outcomes after single-look trauma laparotomy: a large population-based study. J Trauma. 2018:Epub ahead of print

[25] Okabayashi T, Hanazaki K. Overwhelming postsplenectomy infection syndrome in adults: a clinically preventable disease. World J Gastroenterol. 2008; 14(2):176–179

[26] Cullingford GL, Watkins DN, Watts AD, Mallon DF. Severe late postsplenectomy infection. Br J Surg. 1991; 78(6):716–721

[27] Dozier KC, Yeung LY, Miranda MA, Jr, Miraflor EJ, Strumwasser AM, Victorino GP. Death or dialysis? The risk of dialysis-dependent chronic renal failure after trauma nephrectomy. Am Surg. 2013; 79(1):96–100

[28] Croce MA, Fabian TC, Menke PG, et al. Nonoperative management of blunt hepatic trauma is the treatment of choice for hemodynamically stable patients. Results of a prospective trial. Ann Surg. 1995; 221(6):744–753, discussion 753–755

[29] Di Saverio S, Birindelli A, Podda M, et al. Trauma laparoscopy and the six w's: why, where, who, when, what, and how? J Trauma Acute Care Surg. 2019; 86(2):344–367

[30] Cirocchi R, Birindelli A, Inaba K, et al. Laparoscopy for trauma and the changes in its use from 1990 to 2016: a current systematic review and meta-analysis. SurgLaparoscEndoscPercutan Tech. 2018; 28(1):1–12

[31] Mandrioli M, Inaba K, Piccinini A, et al. Advances in laparoscopy for acute care surgery and trauma. World J Gastroenterol. 2016; 22(2):668–680

[32] Schellenberg M, Inaba K, Bardes JM, et al. Defining the gastroesophageal junction in trauma: epidemiology and management of a challenging injury. J Trauma Acute Care Surg. 2017; 83(5):798–802

[33] Schellenberg M, Schlitzkus LL, Inaba K. Gastrointestinal tract. In: Atlas of Surgical Techniques in Trauma. Demetriades D, Inaba K, Velmahos G, eds. 2nd ed. Cambridge: Cambridge University Press; 2019

[34] Aiolfi A, Matsushima K, Chang G, et al. Surgical trends in the management of duodenal injury. J GastrointestSurg. 2019; 23(2):264–269

[35] Ferrada P, Wolfe L, Duchesne J, et al. Management of duodenal trauma: a retrospective review from the Panamerican Trauma Society. J Trauma Acute Care Surg. 2019; 86(3):392–396

[36] DuBose JJ, Inaba K, Teixeira PG, et al. Pyloric exclusion in the treatment of severe duodenal injuries: results from the National Trauma Data Bank. Am Surg. 2008; 74(10):925–929

[37] Witzke JD, Kraatz JJ, Morken JM, et al. Stapled versus hand sewn anastomoses in patients with small bowel injury: a changing perspective. J Trauma. 2000; 49(4):660–665, discussion 665–666

[38] Trust MD, Veith J, Brown CVR, et al. AAST Contemporary Management of Rectal Injuries Study Group. Traumatic rectal injuries: is the combination of computed tomography and rigid proctoscopy sufficient? J Trauma Acute Care Surg. 2018; 85(6):1033–1037

[39] Brown CVR, Teixeira PG, Furay E, et al. AAST Contemporary Management of Rectal Injuries Study Group. Contemporary management of rectal injuries at Level I trauma centers: the results of an American Association for the Surgery of Trauma multi-institutional study. J Trauma Acute Care Surg. 2018; 84(2):225–233

[40] Schellenberg M, Inaba K, Bardes JM, et al. Detection of traumatic pancreatic duct disruption in the modern era. Am J Surg. 2018; 216(2):299–303

[41] Ho VP, Patel NJ, Bokhari F, et al. Management of adult pancreatic injuries: a practice management guideline from the Eastern Association for the Surgery of Trauma. J Trauma Acute Care Surg. 2017; 82(1):185–199

[42] Phelan HA, Velmahos GC, Jurkovich GJ, et al. An evaluation of multidetector computed tomography in detecting pancreatic injury: results of a multicenter AAST study. J Trauma. 2009; 66(3):641–646, discussion 646–647

[43] Velmahos GC, Tabbara M, Gross R, et al. Blunt pancreatoduodenal injury: a multicenter study of the Research Consortium of New England Centers for Trauma (ReCONECT). Arch Surg. 2009; 144(5):413–419, discussion 419–420

[44] Mahajan A, Kadavigere R, Sripathi S, Rodrigues GS, Rao VR, Koteshwar P. Utility of serum pancreatic enzyme levels in diagnosing blunt trauma to the pancreas: a prospective study with systematic review. Injury. 2014; 45(9):1384–1393

[45] Panda A, Kumar A, Gamanagatti S, et al. Evaluation of diagnostic utility of multidetector computed tomography and magnetic resonance imaging in blunt pancreatic trauma: a prospective study. ActaRadiol. 2015; 56(4):387–396

[46] Berni GA, Bandyk DF, Oreskovich MR, Carrico CJ. Role of intraoperative pancreatography in patients with injury to the pancreas. Am J Surg. 1982; 143(5):602–605

[47] Jones RC, Shires GT. Pancreatic trauma. Arch Surg. 1971; 102(4):424–430

[48] Sharpe JP, Magnotti LJ, Weinberg JA, et al. Impact of a defined management algorithm on outcome after traumatic pancreatic injury. J Trauma Acute Care Surg. 2012; 72(1):100–105

[49] Patton JH, Jr, Lyden SP, Croce MA, et al. Pancreatic trauma: a simplified management guideline. J Trauma. 1997; 43(2):234–239, discussion 239–241

[50] Schellenberg M, Inaba K, Cheng V, et al. Spleen-preserving distal pancreatectomy in trauma. J Trauma Acute Care Surg. 2018; 84(1):118–122

[51] Mansfield N, Inaba K, Berg R, et al. Early pancreatic dysfunction after resection in trauma: an 18-year report from a Level I trauma center. J Trauma Acute Care Surg. 2017; 82(3):528–533

[52] Schellenberg M, Chong V, Cone J, Keeley J, Inaba K. Extremity compartment syndrome. CurrProblSurg. 2018; 55(7):256–273

[53] Mahamid A, Peleg K, Givon A, Alfici R, Olsha O, Ashkenazi I, Israeli Trauma Group. Blunt traumatic diaphragmatic injury: a diagnostic enigma with potential surgical pitfalls. Am J Emerg Med. 2017; 35(2):214–217

[54] Fair KA, Gordon NT, Barbosa RR, Rowell SE, Watters JM, Schreiber MA. Traumatic diaphragmatic injury in the American College of Surgeons National Trauma Data Bank: a new examination of a rare diagnosis. Am J Surg. 2015; 209(5):864–868, discussion 868–869

[55] Hammer MM, Raptis DA, Mellnick VM, Bhalla S, Raptis CA. Traumatic injuries of the diaphragm: overview of imaging findings and diagnosis. AbdomRadiol (NY). 2017; 42(4):1020–1027

[56] Sprunt JM, Brown CVR, Reifsnyder AC, Shestopalov AV, Ali S, Fielder WD. Computed tomography to diagnose blunt diaphragm injuries: not ready for prime time. Am Surg. 2014; 80(11):1124–1127

[57] Lim KH, Park J. Blunt traumatic diaphragmatic rupture: single-center experience with 38 patients. Medicine (Baltimore). 2018; 97(41):e12849

[58] Sattler S, Canty TG, Jr, Mulligan MS, et al. Chronic traumatic and congenital diaphragmatic hernias: presentation and surgical management. Can Respir J. 2002; 9(2):135–139

Expert Commentary on Blunt Abdominal Trauma by *Robert C. Mackersie*

Expert Commentary on Blunt Abdominal Trauma

Robert C. Mackersie

The approach to the diagnosis and management of blunt abdominal trauma has undergone major change over the last 15 to 20 years through a combination of improved imaging, interventional and minimally invasive techniques, and a better understanding of risk stratification for the nonoperative management of solid organ injuries. Drs. Shellenberg and Inaba have provided a nicely written, concise summary of this large and complex topic area, incorporating many of the changes that have occurred. Abdominal injuries are central to the overall management of the critically injured patient, with delayed diagnosis and missed injuries historically accounting for the most common cause of preventable death, even in organized trauma systems. Despite gains in knowledge and technical methods, management errors continue to occur. The diagnostic priorities in the management of blunt abdominal trauma have not changed substantially and include the immediate operative management of life-threatening hemorrhage, identification and control of hemorrhage amenable to nonoperative management, and accurate and timely diagnosis of injuries to the gastrointestinal (GI) system.

The authors have described the techniques of the focused assessment with sonography for trauma (FAST) examination and diagnostic peritoneal aspiration (DPA) and their utility as bedside methods capable of accurately diagnosing life-threatening intra-abdominal hemorrhage. The classic conundrum of the patient with profound (systolic BP < 90) unexplained hypotension with negative FAST and/or negative DPA continues to present a challenge. Not all studies of these techniques have reproduced the high-sensitivity described in this chapter (Rowell SE, Trauma Surg Acute Care Open, 2019, Kuncir EJ, Int J Surg, 2007), and strong consideration should still be given to operative exploration in this setting. The FAST examination remains an operator-dependent test, and its accuracy should be carefully assessed, and relied upon accordingly, at each trauma center.

Computed tomography (CT) imaging has long been the diagnostic study of choice for blunt abdominal injury, and as the speed, accuracy, and resolution of these scanners have improved, the CT scanner has become known in some centers as the "answer machine." While the old dictum of "death begins in radiology" provided an important warning to clinicians taking hypotensive patients off through the back corridors of the hospital to a remote CT scanner, the increasing speed and access to these scanners, some of which are located in the trauma resuscitation area or hybrid operating rooms, has acted to increase their utilization even in hypotensive patients. The safety and efficacy of this approach, however, remains to be fully demonstrated.

As the experience and skill level of surgeons with laparoscopy has increased, so has the potential utilization of this technique in the trauma patient. For stable patients with suspected but not proven blunt intestinal or diaphragmatic injury, laparoscopy offers an accurate, minimally invasive means of assessment and reduces the risk of missed injury. Blunt intestinal injuries of these patients are typically not subtle and an experienced laparoscopist can examine both small and large bowel reliably enough to either exclude significant blunt intestinal injury or reveal findings that will trigger a full exploratory laparotomy.

The optimal management of pelvic fracture hemorrhage is another area that has historically been the source of some controversy. The immediate reduction of displaced pelvic ring fractures has evolved from the use of external fixators and emergency 'C' clamps to the use of pelvic binding. The exposure of pelvic (zone III) retroperitoneal hematomas was historically regarded as dangerous due to the risk of creating uncontained hemorrhage. As a result of several European studies followed by American studies, pelvic packing has now not only become an important element in the control of major pelvic hemorrhage but has also been incorporated into pelvic fracture management guidelines by major trauma organizations (EAST & Western Trauma Association). This reflects the increasing awareness that early death from massive pelvic injuries generally occurs from venous bleeding and not so much from arterial bleeding. Immediate pelvic packing can be lifesaving in these situations. An important adjunct to packing of both pelvic and hepatic injuries is the use of kaolin-impregnated packs (e.g., Quik Clot). Their ability to activate factor XII and absorb water promotes faster and more durable coagulation; also, it appears to work even in the setting of anticoagulants.

Perhaps the most important development in the management of massive intra-abdominal injuries involves an understanding of the pathophysiology of the intra-abdominal compartment syndrome and the utilization of the open abdomen and "damage-control" laparotomy. However, like most things, once the perception that "if a little is good, then more is better" takes hold, the pendulum swings, and increasingly the open abdomen gets overutilized. The use of the open abdomen as an approach to damage control should have a clearly defined rationale—more than just "there is a lot of injury." The inability to complete a definitive operation secondary to the need for pelvic or intra-abdominal/hepatic packing; the need to terminate an operation quickly due to refractory acidosis, hypothermia, and coagulopathy; the need to leave bowel in discontinuity out of concern for additional injury, terminate an operation as quickly as possible, or the physical inability to close the abdomen constitute legitimate reasons for utilizing "damage control" with delayed fascial closure.

The philosophical approach to intra-abdominal injuries as it should be with most traumatic injuries is "management according to worst reasonable case scenario"—taking no chances and making no optimistic (and unwarranted) assumptions about the presumed absence of a given injury. The immediate operative control of major hemorrhage for transient and nonvolume responders in shock, comprehensive diagnosis using CT and other imaging, targeted nonoperative control of both hollow or solid organ in pelvic hemorrhage, and use of other risk-reduction maneuvers, as nicely outlined in this chapter, may allow the goal of eliminating preventable deaths from abdominal injury to be achieved.

6 Penetrating Abdominal Trauma

Lyndsey E. Wessels, Michael J. Krzyzaniak, and Matthew J. Martin

Summary

Evaluating and managing penetrating abdominal trauma is a central skill to the acute care surgeon. These injuries vary in complexity based on mechanism, trajectory, and patient characteristics. Whereas, traditional teaching guides every patient to the operating room if the abdominal fascia is violated, more recent data suggests a nonoperative approach that can be applied in select patients. In this chapter, we have discussed different patterns of injury based on mechanism, key diagnostic maneuvers, basic operative principles, and special circumstances that arise in the care of these patients. We have also examined the role of damage control surgery and resuscitation. Discussion of the management as they pertain to specific intra-abdominal organs is outside the scope of this chapter.

Keywords: Penetrating, abdominal trauma, gunshot, stab, nonoperative management, damage control surgery

6.1 Introduction

6.1.1 A Brief History of Penetrating Abdominal Trauma

In ancient medicine, the abdominal cavity was regarded with fear and mystery. It represented an internal world where the treatment of ailments or injuries was based on superstition and misconception rather than anatomy and physiology. Surgical exploration was uniformly fatal and considered malpractice of the highest order. The oldest known text that describes treatment of traumatic injury, *The Edwin Smith Papyrus,* contains 48 trauma cases and their treatment with no mention of abdominal trauma or surgery. This is likely because surgical exploration of the abdomen was uniformly fatal prior to the era of anesthesia, antiseptics, and antibiotics. Patients with penetrating abdominal trauma largely succumbed to their injuries due to either bleeding, gastrointestinal spillage, or subsequent infections. As both the field of anesthesia and antiseptic technique developed in the latter half of the 19th century, surgeons could now work in the abdomen with a reasonable expectation of doing more good than harm.

Once these advances took place, it soon became standard for all penetrating wounds to result in laparotomy. This change, largely taking place in the first half of the 20th century, occurred in parallel with major military conflict. Hippocrates has been quoted as saying "He who wishes to be a surgeon should go to war." Prior to World War I (1914–1918), most penetrating abdominal injuries were treated expectantly. However, during World War II (1939–1945) and the Korean War (1950–1953), the sheer number of cases allowed for an acceleration of experience and knowledge in penetrating injury. Laparotomy for penetrating wounds was met with improved survival rates, as surgeons developed a better understanding of fluid shifts and proper use of antibiotics. As is often the case, the most pivotal transformations in the field of surgery came from the dire circumstances of war.

Penetrating abdominal injury is overall decreasing in incidence in the United States, with blunt mechanism being far more common. Only a small number of high-volume urban trauma centers continue to see overall rates of penetrating injury above 40%, with most modern trauma centers reporting a penetrating trauma incidence of 10% or less. However, the most recent global conflicts, including the Gulf War (1990–1991), Operation Iraqi Freedom (2003–2011), Operation Enduring Freedom and Resolute Support (2001–present) along with domestic mass casualty events, continue to result in refinement to the approach of the penetrating abdominal injury. Both civilian and military trauma surgeons have embraced and continue to refine the practice of damage control laparotomy over the past several decades. During this time, the risks and morbidity associated with nontherapeutic trauma laparotomy have also become more evident. This was recognized as early as the 1960s when the ubiquity of trauma laparotomy for all penetrating abdominal wounds was called into question.[1] Contemporary research is aimed at defining patients with penetrating injuries who can safely avoid the operating room. This research is discussed in detail in the proceeding sections.

6.1.2 Epidemiology of Penetrating Abdominal Trauma

Penetrating abdominal trauma is less common than blunt mechanism with the overall majority consisting of stab and gunshot wounds. Given this, the intent of injury is most often violence or self-harm. Overall, penetrating trauma accounts for less than 10% of trauma cases at most centers, with rates above 20% seen only at a select few, high-volume urban institutions.[2] This number sinks as low as 1 to 12% at rural centers based on the data from the National Center for Injury Prevention and Control. Most patients are male, constituting 70 to 90% of all cases with predominant race (i.e., Caucasian, African American, Hispanic, etc.) affected by rurality. Urban centers see more non-Hispanic African Americans, while suburban and rural centers see more non-Hispanic Caucasians. Data from the 2016 National Trauma Databank Bank report found 4.2% of all trauma-related admissions were due to firearm injury, with 4.1% attributed to stab wounds. This varies according to region, with the southern US seeing the highest proportion of firearm-related injuries at 5.4%, whereas the northeast accounts for most stab-related injuries at 4.8%. The case-fatality rate has proven much higher for gunshot wounds in comparison to stab wounds at 15.3% and 2.2%, respectively.

The injury patterns with penetrating trauma are also significantly different versus blunt abdominal trauma. The most commonly injured organs in penetrating cases are small intestine and colon, whereas the larger solid organs (spleen, liver, kidney) are most commonly injured by blunt trauma. The overall trend is a decreasing amount of penetrating abdominal wounds in the face of increasing incidence of blunt injury. These trends have resulted in significantly decreased exposure to penetrating abdominal trauma, and emergent open abdominal exploration, for most surgeons. Therefore, it is even more critical for surgeons and surgical trainees to understand the key anatomy, physiology, and patient management and evaluation strategies to ensure rapid and safe decision-making along with evidence-based interventions.

6.1.3 Abdominal Anatomy

A working knowledge of abdominal anatomy is key in determining the evaluation and treatment approach to penetrating abdominal wounds. For this purpose, the abdomen can be divided into anterior, flank, back, and thoracoabdominal zones. Identifying the trajectory of a penetrating object or missile within or across each of these areas can be helpful in guiding the workup and interventions but should not be considered in isolation. The anterior abdomen is defined as the area between the axillary lines, extending cephalad from the costal margins to the bilateral groin creases caudally. This is a highly vulnerable area with most penetrating abdominal wounds occurring in this region. Intraperitoneal organs are at risk in this area to include the small bowel, stomach, transverse colon, liver, and spleen. The flank is defined as the area from the inferior costal margins to the iliac crest. It is bordered laterally by the posterior and anterior axillary lines. The back is the area from the inferior costal margins to the iliac crests and bordered laterally by the posterior axillary lines. Wounds in these areas should prompt investigation into injury to retroperitoneal structures, which include the kidneys, ureters, adrenal glands, pancreas, duodenum, ascending and descending colon, rectum, and major abdominal vessels. The thoracoabdominal area is defined by its cephalad border as the region from the fourth intercostal space (also the nipple line) anteriorly to the seventh intercostal space (tip of the scapulae) posteriorly, with the caudal border being the inferior costal margin. Injuries in this area prompt suspicion for intrathoracic, mediastinal, and diaphragmatic injury.

6.2 Basic Principles of Penetrating Abdominal Trauma

6.2.1 Mechanisms of Injury

Penetrating abdominal wounds can occur via a variety of methods, but they are most often categorized as either a stab wound or gunshot wound. Each mechanism has its own characteristic pattern of injury as does the specific weapon used. Stab wounds are low-velocity and cause injury by direct contact, laceration, and devascularization of tissue. This leads to a narrow wound tract which, even with peritoneal violation, may have no other intra-abdominal injury. Kitchen knives will typically lead to a wound that is wide at the entrance with narrowing of the tract internally. Objects that are rotated, pivoted, or have jagged irregular edges, will result in more injury due to increased surface area contact with tissue in its path. Despite a seemingly minor entrance wound, internal damage may be significant.

Gunshot wounds are often more devastating as a property of the increased kinetic energy is dispersed to adjacent tissues upon contact, leading to significantly longer wound tracts that can cross multiple cavities. The most commonly utilized broad classification of projectile injuries is based on the velocity, with most civilian firearms being in the low-velocity category. High-velocity is typically defined as greater than 1000 to 2000 feet per second and is characteristic of military weaponry and select civilian firearms (typically rifles). High-velocity rounds in general have a much greater potential for both size and degree of tissue injury, although this will vary depending on the type of tissue and several other important factors. The projectile may fragment upon impact, causing many smaller ballistic injuries or a much larger area of diffuse tissue injury. Size and velocity of the bullet play a role in determining the severity of damage. These properties contribute to the "temporary cavity," which is the displacement of tissue as the object travels through a structure, transmitting waves of energy through tissue interfaces. This has the potential to cause injury to intraperitoneal structures even if the bullet tract is completely outside the peritoneum. Several additional properties of the missile play a key role in determining the level of damage. These include its physical characteristics such as the amount of spin and yaw, deformities, jacketing and trajectory capabilities. Where it was once thought velocity and size were the most important factors determining the level of injury, these additional properties are now proving to be the most influential.[3]

6.2.2 Initial Evaluation

Receiving a trauma patient with a penetrating abdominal injury can be an anxiety-provoking experience due to the higher likelihood of requirement of emergent intervention as well as the decreasing experience levels of most surgeons with regard to penetrating trauma. It is in these circumstances that it is most important to remain systematic in approach. Consistent adherence to the Advanced Trauma Life Support (ATLS) primary survey is mandatory, but with an expedited focus, looking for only the immediately life-threatening or emergent problems that require intervention. Providers should avoid the temptation to focus solely on the ballistic wound, abdominal evisceration, or other distracting issues, without first assessing the patient's airway, breathing and circulation.

An organized trauma team will have enough assets to care for the multiply injured patient such that all members of the team should have a clearly defined role. As the patient arrives, dedicated team members will secure the airway, while another obtains IV access. Additional team members are physically ensuring the initiation of resuscitation (if needed); simultaneously, another team member assists in maneuvering and exposing the patient, while the provider performs the primary survey, focused evaluation of the truncal wounds, and any point of care bedside imaging (X-ray and/or ultrasound). A dedicated team member should also be gathering information from the prehospital team. Important questions to ask in the case of penetrating abdominal trauma include: were the vital signs unstable for any period prior to arrival? Was there loss of consciousness prior to arrival? How much blood loss occurred at the scene? Can you provide a description of the weapon? Were there any impaled objects removed prior to arrival? In the case of a gunshot wound, how many shots were heard? The answers to these questions frame the scenario, assist in risk stratification, and may raise your index of suspicion for other injuries.

6.2.3 Basic Operative Principles

Although there has been a trend in nonoperative management for penetrating abdominal trauma, there are cases when emergent laparotomy is completely necessary and unavoidable. Indications will be discussed in subsequent sections of this chapter; however, there are several basic operative principles worth mentioning at this point. The adept trauma surgeon will constantly be anticipating his or her next move, never venturing into the operating room without a plan. Most importantly, the surgeon must be in constant communication with the anesthesiologist to ensure the highest likelihood of success. Positioning needs to be discussed. Patients are almost always positioned supine to maximize options and extensions, and they should be prepped and draped from clavicles to knees. If there is time and resources to place an external fixator for a concomitant orthopedic injury, special positioning, prepping, and draping should be quickly decided with the orthopedic surgical team. In a volume-depleted patient, induction may result in circulatory collapse. The surgeon must know the status of resuscitation and the availability of additional blood products prior to induction. If ventilation is proving difficult, consider a diaphragm injury or pneumothorax, or if one is known prior to intubation, it should be clearly communicated with the anesthesiologist. If a large amount of hemoperitoneum is suspected, consider the possibility that it has created a tamponade of additional bleeding. Premature incision into the peritoneum before the anesthesiologist can adequately resuscitate the patient, or has blood products on hand, will release tamponade that could result in catastrophic bleeding.

After these important issues have been addressed, the laparotomy can proceed in typical fashion with the two immediate goals of hemorrhage control and identification/control of gastrointestinal spillage or contamination. A large midline incision is made, fluid is evacuated, and the four quadrants of the abdomen are packed if massive hemoperitoneum is encountered. In the case of penetrating abdominal trauma, all four quadrants are packed and the packing is sequentially removed to investigate for bleeding. The supra- and inframesocolic compartments are interrogated, while retroperitoneal exploration is limited and guided based on clinical suspicion, presence of hematomas, and trajectory of the wound. If the patient is hemodynamically stable, or a transient responder, it is reasonable to pursue computed tomography (CT) of the abdomen with IV contrast to assist in determination of the extent of injury.[4] It is the opinion of the authors that exploring a retroperitoneal hematoma in the absence of known injury can lead to a high-incidence of iatrogenic injury. To be clear, this is in the absence of an expanding hematoma that is enlarging in front of the operating surgeon's field of view. A left-sided medial visceral rotation (Mattox maneuver) is performed to visualize the suprarenal aorta and proximal branch vessels. A right-sided medial visceral rotation (including Kocherization of the duodenum) will provide excellent exposure and access to the duodenal and inferior vena cava (IVC) as well as the inframesolic aorta, depending on how extensive of a maneuver is performed. The anterior portion of the stomach is investigated for injury from gastroesophageal junction to the pylorus; thereafter,the lesser sac is opened by dividing the gastrocolic omentum to inspect the posterior surface and pancreas. If a Kocher maneuver has been performed, all surfaces of the duodenum can be examined. The small bowel is visualized in 360-degree fashion from the ligament of Treitz to the terminal ileum. The colon is also examined in entirety. To the extent possible, solid organs are not only inspected visually but also palpated for nonvisualized segments to identify an abnormal contour. The pelvis is interrogated for additional injury to genitourinary organs or the rectum. Finally, the diaphragm is inspected. Depending on the overall status of the patient and the type and severity of injuries, the decision for damage control interventions only versus definitive repair will be made. Damage control surgery will be discussed further at the end of this chapter.

6.3 Evaluation and Management of Abdominal Stab Wounds

6.3.1 Evaluating for "Hard Signs to Operate"

All trauma care regardless of injury begins with the ATLS primary survey, the elements of which have been discussed already. Patients with stab wounds must be fully exposed to properly identify all wounds. These wounds are easily missed in the groin, axilla, perineum, and skin folds. Interrogation, especially in these troublesome areas, must be thorough. The decision algorithm for treating abdominal stab wounds focuses on the immediate decision to operate or trial nonoperative management. There is a subset of patients for which operating immediately without extensive imaging or other evaluations is most appropriate. These patients have "hard signs" to operate. They include hemodynamic instability, peritonitis, and evisceration. Hemodynamic instability represents inadequate end-organ perfusion and, in the case of penetrating abdominal trauma, is likely due to massive hemorrhage. The definition of true hypotension in a trauma patient is, however, nuanced. It depends on the patient's age, comorbidities, mental status, and response to initial fluid resuscitation. Furthermore, there is benefit to allowing "permissive hypotension" in penetrating truncal trauma, so as not to potentially increase hemorrhage prior to surgical control. Generally, sustained systolic blood pressures below 80 to 90 mm Hg with fluid resuscitation, or recurrent hypotension after fluid challenge (transient responders), should undergo prompt abdominal exploration. Peritonitis represents peritoneal irritation likely due to intra-abdominal solid or viscus organ injury. Notably, peritonitis is difficult to assess in many clinical situations where altered mental status exists. This includes head injury, intoxication, in the intubated patient, etc. You cannot rely on detection of peritonitis in these patients and further investigative studies or mandatory surgical exploration are warranted to avoid missed injuries and delays to critical interventions. Evisceration (see ▶ Fig. 6.1) always requires restoration of contents to the abdominal cavity, but is also often a harbinger for other operative intra-abdominal injury and should prompt exploration.[5,6,7] Other less common findings that require immediate operative intervention include hematemesis, gross blood in gastric aspirate or per rectum, or impalement with the penetrating object still in place. The factors found to have the highest positive predictive value for therapeutic laparotomy include development of hypotension after normotension (86%), shock on presentation (83%), and generalized peritonitis (81%).[8]

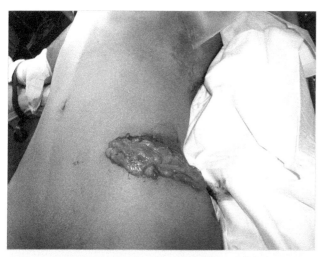

Fig. 6.1 Anterior abdominal stab wound with omental evisceration.

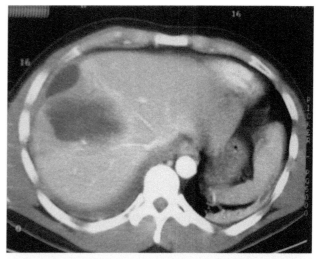

Fig. 6.2 CT scan after anterior abdominal stab wound demonstrating an isolated liver injury successfully managed nonoperatively.

6.3.2 Selective Nonoperative Management

In the absence of hard signs mandating surgical intervention, patients are increasingly being managed nonoperatively. This approach has led to a significant decrease in the number of nontherapeutic laparotomies without creating additional morbidity or preventable mortality.[9,10,11,12] In 2009, Biffl et al demonstrated the safety of close observation and operation for patients without hard clinical signs of injury in a multicenter prospective observational study that enrolled 359 patients.[13] A simplified algorithm for this approach was then studied in a follow-up multicenter trial with 211 patients and confirmed the safety of selective nonoperative management. These studies need to be interpreted with caution; however, as there was a 49% deviation from study protocol, it highlighted the fact there is no "one size fits all" approach. Furthermore, generalizability is limited as these studies only enrolled patients with anterior abdominal wounds and the algorithm was based largely on local wound exploration (LWE) which is not applicable in all types of penetrating injury.

The benefit of a selective nonoperative approach lies in the avoidance of a negative or nontherapeutic laparotomy. In the era of liberal laparotomy, this occurred in up to 30 to 50% of patients. The selective approach has decreased rates of nontherapeutic laparotomy to 5 to 10%.[14] The most significant concern is missing an operative injury and delaying intervention until the patient has developed a life-threatening illness. Research has shown that only about 4% of patients selectively managed nonoperatively go on to require laparotomy, with morbidity and mortality rates mirroring those of patients requiring immediate laparotomy.[2] However, the caveat to this approach is that the patients must be closely observed, have serial examinations and evaluations performed by an experienced team, and undergo immediate reevaluation or operation for any signs of deterioration.

Selective or nonoperative management can only be performed if a patient can participate in serial examinations of the abdomen.

A Glasgow coma scale (GCS) score of 13 or higher is generally considered examinable, but that determination is made on an individualized basis. If a patient cannot be reliably examined, adjunctive measures are typically used upfront to evaluate for peritoneal violation. These include LWE, focused assessment with sonography for trauma (FAST) examination, cross-sectional imaging, and diagnostic laparoscopy. Patients with depressed levels of consciousness have historically been excluded from much of the research investigating nonoperative management, making directive statements regarding the best course of action difficult. Some trauma surgeons may elect to take these patients for exploration routinely. However, in the absence of hard signs, it is also appropriate to perform additional studies and extend nonoperative management to those patients, albeit with a very low threshold for surgical exploration. LWE interrogates the wound tract to identify penetration of the anterior rectus fascia. It is useful when clearly negative, however, when positive or equivocal additional imaging may be needed to help guide decision-making. This is because violation of the anterior fascia does not necessarily correlate to intra-abdominal injury. There is no mandate to explore the abdominal cavity in the presence of fascial violation in a hemodynamically normal patient, but that patient must either undergo additional evaluations or be admitted for serial examinations. Conversely, the FAST examination is most useful when clearly positive, although there is ongoing debate about the role of FAST examination in penetrating abdominal trauma. Negative or equivocal examinations do not preclude significant injury and may need to be further investigated with additional diagnostic modalities or serial examinations. It is also important to remember FAST is highly operator-dependent and is poor at identifying diaphragm and hollow viscus injury.[15] CT has proven more useful in these scenarios with fine, 3 mm intervals optimizing injury detection (see ▶ Fig. 6.2). A triple-contrast CT imaging study (oral, intravenous, and rectal contrast) has extraordinarily high sensitivity and accuracy (100% and 98% respectively) for identifying injuries requiring operative intervention.[16,17,18] However, good results have also been reported with double or intravenous contrast only.[19,20,21]

Fine cuts to recreate the stab wound tract, the so-called "CT-tractography," should be attempted when possible as it may provide valuable information. Reliability is limited, however, and this should not be used as the sole criteria for ruling out peritoneal violation.[22,23] Diagnostic laparoscopy is highly accurate for ruling out peritoneal violation.[10] This approach will be discussed in detail later in the chapter. These decisions are often case-specific. For example, in the case of a patient with concomitant severe traumatic brain injury, the threshold for operative exploration in the face of equivocal findings might be lower than for a patient who is only temporarily intoxicated. In the former, a missed injury could fester for days leading to devastating consequences; however, in the latter, the injury will likely be picked up on examination within hours and result in no additional morbidity.

In the case of an examinable patient, an upright chest X-ray should be performed during the initial trauma evaluation, as it can rapidly provide immediately actionable information. If free intra-abdominal air is present, the patient should likely be taken to the operating room for exploration. However, in instances of low suspicion for hollow viscus injury or questionable amount of free air and otherwise benign examination, it is not unreasonable to opt for observation and/or additional diagnostic imaging. The chest X-ray may also identify thoracic pathology such as hemothorax, pneumothorax, or diaphragmatic hernia, which will require some form of intervention. It is critical to remember that hemo- or pneumothorax on chest X-ray in a patient with an abdominal stab wound is also diagnostic of a diaphragm injury which usually requires operative repair.

In patients who have not demonstrated an operative indication up to this point, the clinical pathway to follow now depends largely on location of injury. Stab wounds to the abdomen are classified as anterior, thoracoabdominal, and back or flank. For most purposes of evaluation and management, the flank and back locations can be grouped together, while anterior stab wounds will follow a somewhat different algorithm.

The anterior abdomen is the most common location for stab wounds, as it is highly exposed in violent scenarios where the victim is facing the offender. Wounds can occur anywhere on the anterior trunk, but are more commonly seen on the left side, as most assailants are right-handed. Several clinical pathways exist as viable options for selective nonoperative management of injuries in this location. Decision on what specific pathway is most appropriate to follow is highly dependent on the clinical situation as well as local resources and expertise. The recently published algorithm on abdominal stab wounds from the Western Trauma Association (see ▶ Fig. 6.3) provides an evidence-based and highly flexible strategy for the evaluation and management of these patients that can be adapted to a wide variety of settings.[13] Furthermore, the Eastern Association for the Surgery of Trauma (EAST) has also published practice management guidelines for selective nonoperative management of trauma.[10] These guidelines are summarized in ▶ Table 6.1.

LWE is an attempt to identify penetration of the anterior fascia of the rectus muscle. If present, this historically is interpreted as high-likelihood for peritoneal penetration and would prompt an exploratory laparotomy. However, this maneuver is now appreciated as more of a sensitive examination for ruling out an abdominal injury, but not specific enough to rule it in. A positive or equivocal examination should not necessarily equate to

laparotomy. Instead, the winner-take-all (WTA) advocates for continued serial examinations or additional diagnostic imaging, especially in the patient with an otherwise benign abdominal exam. Furthermore, although this is usually a good initial test to rule out peritoneal violation, not all stab wounds are amenable to LWE. For example, long tangential wound tracts, very narrow ice pick wounds, multiple stab wounds, or the obese patient with a significant layer of subcutaneous fat represent wounds difficult to fully and accurately explore at the bedside. In addition, this technique is not advisable in a noncooperative or combative patient. These patients should begin a selective nonoperative pathway, utilizing an alternative strategy to LWE.

Instead of LWE, surgeons can choose admission with serial clinical examinations (SCEs) or elect to obtain additional diagnostic imaging. Serial clinical examinations should be performed only in well-resourced settings, and ideally when the same provider or team can perform the examination, or where there is adequate turnover to covering providers. SCE consists of serial abdominal examinations watching for the development of peritonitis as well as monitoring vital signs and laboratory values to identify possible ongoing hemorrhage or signs of hollow viscus perforation. Using SCE alone has demonstrated a decrease of nontherapeutic laparotomy from 52% to 12% at one center.[24] The safety of this approach has been demonstrated in several studies, with reported failure rates of only 2 to 10%, and with no added morbidity among the subgroup that failed a period of initial SCEs.[9,25,26,27] Although the exact optimal duration of SCE is not well-validated, most centers continue for 24 to 48 hours before discharging the patient. The WTA algorithm recommends a minimum of 24 hours, although there is data that supports shorter periods of 8 to 12 hours in highly select patients.

Alternatively, selective nonoperative management can begin with diagnostic imaging. CT scan, including all suspected areas of injury, has clearly become the study of choice in these patients. As previously discussed, this should be performed in 3 mm or finer cuts and with radio-opaque markers placed at the external sites of the wound or wounds to help assess the wound tract and trajectory. There is generally agreement that intravenous contrast should be used routinely, but there is significant debate over the utility and indications for using additional contrast such as oral, rectal, or even injection of contrast into the wound tract. For anterior abdominal stab wounds, there is little utility to adding oral or rectal contrast. Instead, IV contrast is the only preferred initial screening study. The addition of oral contrast, rectal contrast, or both (aka the "triple contrast CT") is recommended primarily for flank and back stab wounds, but this will vary based on the local practices and experience of the managing surgeon and radiologists. It is also important to remember that pathways that began with LWE or SCE may cross over to the diagnostic imaging pathway, depending on evolving findings and local practices. If there are signs of operative injury on the CT scan (or other diagnostic study), the patient obviously should be taken for immediate surgical exploration. However, there are many injuries identified on imaging that are well-suited for nonoperative management, like their blunt trauma counterparts. In the case of an identified solid organ injury from a penetrating mechanism, the patient can be followed

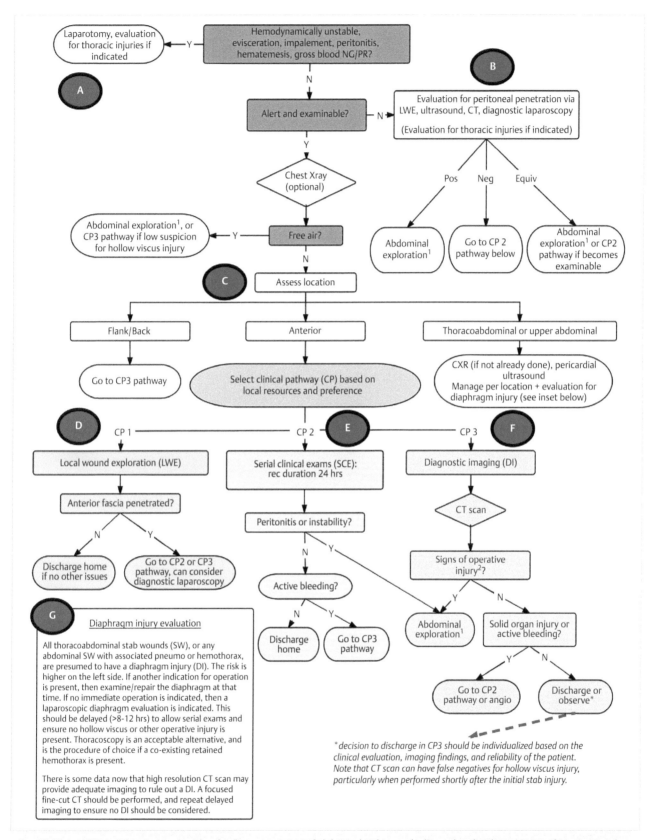

Fig. 6.3 Western Trauma Association algorithm for the management of abdominal stab wounds. (Reproduced with permission of Martin MJ, Schatz DV, Brown CVR, et al. Evaluation and management of abdominal stab wounds: A Western Trauma Association critical decisions algorithm. *J Trauma Acute Care Surg.* 2018;85(5):1007–1015. doi:10.1097/TA.0000000000001930.)

Table 6.1 Summary of EAST practice management guidelines for selective nonoperative management of penetrating abdominal trauma[10]

Recommendation	Level of evidence	Comments/tips
1. Hemodynamically unstable or peritonitis should proceed to the OR	I	Variable definitions of "unstable" are utilized, and response to initial resuscitation should also be considered. For peritonitis, look for pain and rebound tenderness in the quadrant furthest from the stab wound
2. Hemodynamically stable patients with underlying reasons for an unreliable examination should undergo further diagnostic workup or an exploratory surgery	I	Should consider not only current status and reason for a compromised examination, but also the expected duration of incapacity. Most patients should have further diagnostic studies, or diagnostic laparoscopy, rather than exploratory laparotomy
3. Routine laparotomy not indicated in stable patients without peritonitis	II	Laparotomy based only on presence of stab wound or positive local wound exploration has high negative/nontherapeutic rate
4. Routine laparotomy not indicated in stable gsw patients with tangential wounds and no peritonitis	II	Initial evaluation should focus on examination for peritonitis and hemodynamics, as well as examination of wounds and likely trajectory. Mandatory laparotomy is not required if experienced provider/team and close serial monitoring available
5. Serial physical examination by experienced provider is reliable at detecting significant injury in penetrating abdominal trauma patients	II	Preferable to have serial examinations done by the same person or team, clearly documented, and swift action taken if any change or deterioration in clinical status or examination
6. Abdominal/pelvic ct should be strongly considered for patients undergoing nonoperative management	II	CT scan with fine cuts through area of wound or wound tract helpful for both identifying injuries and evaluating trajectory. Weaknesses are decreased sensitivity for bowel injury and diaphragm injury
7. Penetrating injury to the right upper quadrant may be managed nonoperatively if the patient is stable and no peritonitis	III	No different than injury to other quadrants, but the right upper quadrant has lower chance of a hollow-viscus injury due to the presence of the liver
8. Most patients managed nonoperatively can be discharged after 24 hours of observation	III	Some data supports shorter intervals of 8 to 12 hours, particularly if a CT scan was entirely negative
9. Consider laparoscopy in evaluation of diaphragmatic laceration and peritoneal violation	II	Laparoscopy should be performed for signs of diaphragm injury or left thoracoabdominal/upper abdominal penetrating wounds. Is being used by some to evaluate for peritoneal penetration, but there is little advantage to this over serial examinations

with SCE, providing there is no concern for associated operative injuries. If active bleeding is noted, the patient may be taken to the operating room or angiography can be considered when appropriate and feasible. If no significant injury is seen on CT, then discharge may be considered. However, it is important to note that CT can have false negatives, especially in the case of hollow viscus injury and when performed at a very short interval from the injury. For this reason, it is important to also consider the reliability and ability of the patient to follow-up after discharge.

Comprehensive assessment of injuries to the flank and back should include a CT scan of the abdomen and pelvis. Specific injuries of concern are those to the duodenum, colon, kidneys/ureters, spleen, pancreas, and major blood vessels of the retroperitoneum. LWE is not appropriate in these situations, as fascial penetration has even less significance than in the anterior abdominal location. It is also important to recognize that retroperitoneal injuries are less likely to have clinical examination findings; therefore, risking underappreciation for many injuries that could be life-threatening.

Wounds to the upper abdomen (above the umbilicus) or the thoracoabdominal region should yield a higher index of suspicion for thoracic or mediastinal injury. All patients in this scenario warrant a chest X-ray as part of their initial ER workup, preferably performed in the sitting upright or the reverse Trendelenburg position. The abdominal portion of the FAST examination has questionable utility in penetrating trauma, but the pericardial view is of critical importance for injuries in this location and should be performed immediately after patient arrival. Patients who have clear evidence of pericardial fluid, with or without the signs or symptoms of cardiac tamponade, should proceed directly to median sternotomy. Those with an equivocal ultrasound or no concerning symptoms can be further evaluated with either higher quality imaging (CT or echocardiography) or subxiphoid pericardial window.

As mentioned earlier, traumatic diaphragm injury (TDI) should always be considered in the evaluation process of any upper abdominal stab wound or abdominal stab wound with an associated hemo- or pneumothorax. TDI must also be identified early due to the morbidity associated with the sequelae of a missed injury. Incidence of missed injury as high as 40% has been reported and is often attributed to its clinically silent nature.[28,29,30] TDI most commonly occurs on the left side, representing up to 75% of all cases, but detecting it may be difficult.[28] They are typically 2 cm or less and, in the absence of herniated contents, often missed on the initial X-rays or conventional CT scans. A debate currently exists as to whether modern multidetector scanners have enough sensitivity and specificity to act as the definitive study for TDI. Unfortunately, no clear conclusion has been made. Although any diagnosed TDI should undergo operative repair, the timing of repair should also take into consideration the possible associated injuries and timing from the initial injury. For patients with an identified or suspected TDI, who are undergoing SCEs, we recommend delaying exploratory laparoscopy and repair of the diaphragm injury until enough time has lapsed (8–12 hours) to confidently rule out the presence of an associated abdominal hollow viscus injury. The alternative is to perform an immediate TDI exploration, but in that case the entire abdomen should be explored to rule out any other associated injuries that were not identified during the initial evaluation. Laparoscopy has become the technique of choice for both diagnosis and intervention in upper abdominal stab wounds with suspicion of TDI. Definitive repair is often achievable with this modality if the surgeon is facile, with minimally invasive suturing techniques or using assistive suturing devices to facilitate an adequate TDI repair. Alternatively, video-assisted thoracoscopy (VATS) can be utilized and possesses an equivalent accuracy for identifying TDI. We primarily recommend VATS be used if there is a retained hemothorax, some other indication for a thoracic approach, or a contra-indication to the first-line abdominal approach.

6.3.3 Operative Principles Unique to Stab Wounds

Basic operative principles for emergent laparotomy have been previously discussed. However, there are several operative principles unique to stab wounds worth mentioning. Upon entering the abdominal cavity, the surgeon may opt to go directly to the area of penetration in order to look for injury as opposed to packing all four quadrants. However, this approach is ill-advised as it may lead to tunnel vision and miss other injuries. Stab wounds are considered low-velocity, creating a narrow tract from which the path of injury can be inferred. However, if the specifics of the weapon are unknown, multiple stab wounds are present and/or the weapon may have been rotated internally a wider zone of injury is possible. Unless an injury is easily identifiable upon entry into the abdomen, the trauma surgeon should proceed with standardized exploration of the abdomen.

Patients with impaled objects into the abdominal cavity should only have them removed in the controlled setting of the operating room. By nature of the injury, nonoperative management is inappropriate. That said, if hemodynamics are stable for preoperative imaging, it may be of benefit, allowing the surgeon to map the path of impaled object and tailor the operative plan accordingly. Broad-spectrum antibiotics and tetanus prophylaxis should be given as all impaled objects are considered contaminated. Myriad case reports on management of impalement injuries exist in the literature, highlighting the basic treatment principles of minimal prehospital manipulation, a multidisciplinary approach to preoperative and operative planning, as well as specialized wound care.[31,32,33,34] The placement of the impaled object may make positioning difficult in the operating room. When necessary, the protruding object may be shortened to optimize patient positioning. Depending on the nature of the impaled object, extensive debridement of wound edges may be necessary to control contamination.

The safety of a trial of nonoperative management in patients with multiple stab wounds is not well-described. In the setting of an otherwise stable patient, we advocate for additional imaging with a low threshold to proceed to the operating room for inconclusive findings. Although diagnostic peritoneal lavage has largely been abandoned and has little role in most trauma centers, it may be useful for guiding the decision to operate or observe in highly select cases, including the patient with multiple stab wounds and an equivocal examination/imaging or who is not examinable.[35] In these cases, the value is mainly in

looking for evidence of hollow viscus injury, characterized by fluid analysis with an elevated white blood cell count > 500/mL, elevated amylase/alkaline phosphatase/bilirubin, or enteric bacteria or food particles.

6.4 Evaluation and Management of Gunshot Wounds

6.4.1 Evaluating for "Hard Signs to Operate"

Gunshot wounds are associated with a significantly higher case-fatality rate than stab wounds, but the initial evaluation still begins with the primary survey and focuses on identifying immediately life-threatening pathology. It is important to recognize that, due to the larger spread of kinetic energy across tissue interfaces and resultant nontangential path of travel through the body, gunshot wounds have a much higher likelihood of injury. This had previously led to the common practice of most abdominal gunshot wounds undergoing exploratory laparotomy versus a more selective approach with abdominal stab wounds. However, recent experience and data have clearly demonstrated that selective nonoperative management can safely be applied to both gunshot and stab wounds.

Outside of the ATLS primary survey, many of the same tenants regarding initial evaluation of stab wounds holds true for gunshot wounds. It is vital to fully expose the patient to interrogate for all ballistic wounds. As in the case with stab wounds, areas notorious for missed injury are the groin, axilla, perineum, and skin folds. In patients with lower abdominal wounds, rectal and genitourinary examinations are crucial as the first step in identifying colorectal and pelvic injury. In addition, the chest is examined, palpated, and auscultated in the search for pneumothorax and/or hemothorax as well as mediastinal injury. The focus of investigation for additional injury should not narrow to areas where ballistic wounds are easily identified. The projectile's path can be nonlinear, and in the case of multiple gunshot wounds becomes even more convoluted. If imaging is possible, CT scan is most useful in identifying injuries and can be helpful in reconstructing the trajectory and tract of the ballistic in three-dimension.

The indications for immediate laparotomy for gunshot wounds mirror those for abdominal stab wounds. That is, when peritonitis, hemodynamic instability, and/or evisceration of intra-abdominal contents are present, further study is not necessarily warranted. These patients should be taken directly to the operating room for exploration. Once again, the unexaminable patient (psychiatric illness, intoxication, intubated, etc.) presents a difficult situation. Depending on the overall clinical picture and the local resources/experience, the trauma surgeon may have a lower threshold to operate regardless of the presence of other hard signs of injury.

In the case of hemodynamic instability, the presumed source should always be the abdomen, but it is important to rule out any extra-abdominal sources of bleeding prior to laparotomy. Specifically, sequestering of fluid within the chest needs to be examined, and this can quickly be achieved with either a portable chest X-ray or with an extended ultrasound examination including both the pericardial view and assessment for pneumothorax on both sides of the chest. In the patient who is hemodynamically unstable secondary to noncompressible torso hemorrhage, there have been few effective interventions that can be performed outside of the operating room setting. Resuscitative endovascular balloon occlusion of the aorta (REBOA) is a relatively new and emerging technology that can be used to mitigate blood loss in the setting of noncompressible torso hemorrhage and provide a window of hemodynamic stability to allow for transport to the operating room.[36] At centers with expertise in this technique, it can be considered as a temporary measure to stabilize perfusion to the myocardium and brain, while measures are being taken to get to the operating room for exploration. In a patient who has lost vital signs completely, and in centers not using REBOA, emergency resuscitative thoracotomy should be considered as a final maneuver to restore signs of life and act as a bridge to the operating room. There is limited data arguing whether resuscitative thoracotomy has any role in exsanguinating hemorrhage causing traumatic arrest within the abdominal cavity. In the absence of any other therapeutic modality in a patient that loses vital signs from exsanguinating intra-abdominal hemorrhage, resuscitative thoracotomy is a reasonable approach to undertake.[37] Other less common signs mandating operative exploration include hematemesis, gross blood in gastric aspirate, or gross blood per rectum.

6.4.2 Selective Nonoperative Management

In the absence of hard signs to operate, prior additional imaging in order to determine an operative plan is favored. As in the case of stab wounds, several options exist depending on injury location, clinical parameters, and hospital resources. LWE is typically not successful in this cohort of patients as it is nearly impossible to follow the wound tract completely. However, in the very rare case the wound is superficial, with the entire pathway able to be visualized, this course of action is a viable option for ruling out deeper injury. Often with these extraperitoneal injuries, the diagnosis can be made by palpating the ballistic tract, which will be painful along the entire course of the missile.

More commonly, additional imaging is pursued. In the era of multidetector computed tomography (MDCT), diagnostic peritoneal lavage is rarely used due to its invasive nature and lag time in laboratory results. It can be useful in resource-limited settings when the decision to transfer the patient needs to be made. Most centers will opt to begin with a FAST examination followed by plain film abdominal X-ray and/or MDCT. The utility of FAST in penetrating trauma is debatable, given the low-sensitivity for identifying peritoneal penetration, and concerns over the false-negative rate. However, the FAST examination can be helpful in identifying patients who clearly have abdominal hemorrhage (versus other sources), and for assessing the pericardium to rule out cardiac injury and/or tamponade. If a patient is hypotensive from a penetrating abdominal injury, requiring blood product resuscitation, or otherwise not stable enough for CT, the FAST examination has little utility and the patient should proceed immediately to the operating room.

The FAST examination is useful for examining multiple compartments quickly for fluid, including posterior to the bladder (pouch of Douglas) and the pericardium. As mentioned in the section on stab wounds, it not useful in detecting diaphragm and hollow viscus injury. Plain films are most useful in the case of a single gunshot with single ballistic wound. When external radiopaque surface markers are placed at the wound site and two views obtained, the trajectory of the bullet can often be determined with relatively good accuracy. This guides clinical suspicion to further injury, based on the organs and structures within the bullet's path. It is significantly more challenging to determine trajectory with multiple gunshot wounds. However, estimating trajectory by using external markers on wound sites still has utility.

Availability, sensitivity, and accuracy make MDCT the preferred modality for investigating operative injury in gunshot wounds at most modern centers (see ▶ Fig. 6.4). Obtaining results is quick and the provider can image all needed body compartments with great anatomic detail. The option exists for triple, double, or rectal contrast; however, IV contrast alone has demonstrated 90% sensitivity and 96% specificity for detecting operative injury in prospective observational study.[38] Using MDCT in the decision-making for selective nonoperative management, another prospective study demonstrated its safety in 41 such patients, of which 24 had initially negative CT scans. One patient in this group went on to have a nontherapeutic laparotomy based on clinical findings. The other 17 who initially had positive findings on CT were all managed nonoperatively based on their specific injuries with only one nontherapeutic laparotomy.[39] The WTA has developed a simplified algorithm for the management of abdominal gunshot wounds (see ▶ Fig. 6.5), based largely on utilizing MDCT, to guide management in the case of an examinable patient with no hard indications to operate. Evaluation of this approach is ongoing, and this algorithm may not be applicable or appropriate in all centers or for all scenarios.

Following the WTA algorithms for abdominal stab wounds and gunshot wounds mandates attention to several key features. First, anatomic location, although difficult to determine solely for ballistic wounds, will guide clinical suspicion for injury to certain organs and adjunctive imaging. Any trajectory involving the upper abdomen or thorax should prompt investigation for diaphragm, lung, and mediastinal injury. Suspicion for injury to

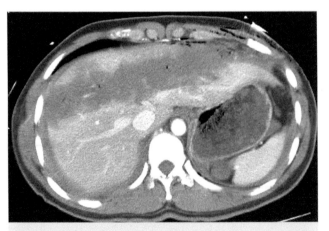

Fig. 6.4 CT scan demonstrating gunshot wound to the abdomen with tangential path through liver successfully managed nonoperatively.

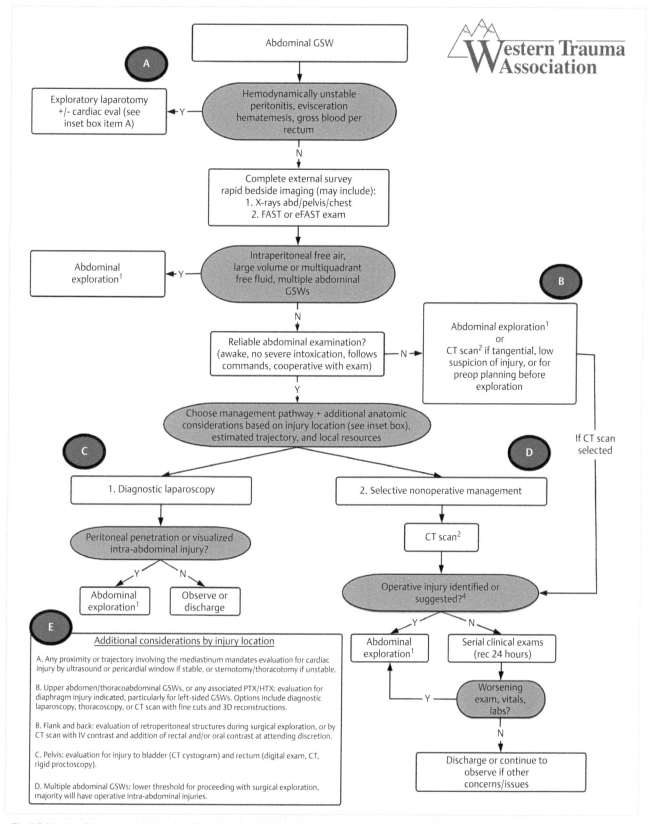

Fig. 6.5 Western Trauma Association algorithm for the management of abdominal gunshot wounds.

retroperitoneal structures exist in the case of flank and back wounds. MDCT is often the best choice as these injuries often have few findings on examination and may be delayed in presentation. In lower abdominal involvement, consider injury to the pelvic structures, including the bladder, ureters, uterus, rectum, etc., to evaluate accordingly. Special consideration should be given to performing delayed imaging (approximately 8 min postcontrast bolus) to look for renal collecting systems injuries once contrast is excreted by the kidneys.

Another aspect of this algorithm is the increasing use of diagnostic laparoscopy to evaluate for peritoneal violation, diaphragm injury, and intra-abdominal organ or bowel injury. This approach is like stab wounds such that patients who can otherwise tolerate an operation benefit from the avoided radiation and consternation over equivocal findings. Specific technique will be discussed in subsequent sections of this chapter. The degree of injury is likely to be greater in gunshot wounds and, unless very adept at laparoscopy, most surgeons will be more comfortable exploring via a laparotomy. Also, previously mentioned, posterior diaphragm and retroperitoneal injuries are technically very challenging to manage via this technique.

Finally, a word of caution in determining when it is appropriate to discharge patients with negative findings on complete workup. The WTA algorithm for managing stab wounds advocates for a minimum of 24 hours of observation with clinical examinations approximately every four hours.[14] It is not unreasonable to extend this approach in the case of gunshot wounds. However, one study performed at a busy urban trauma center demonstrated relative safety of discharging patients with a negative workup after six hours of observation.[40] These patients had local wound exploration, CT scan, and serial abdominal examinations. The 66% who were available for follow-up had no severe morbidity or mortality. Although several series have suggested that shorter observation periods of 8 to 12 hours may be safe, we recommend the more cautious 24-hour admission, as data justifying shorter duration is limited and of low quality.

Like stab wounds, there is no evidence to support the relatively common practices of keeping the patient nil per os or giving routine prophylactic antibiotics for nonoperative injuries. All patients need tetanus vaccine update, and follow-up should be determined by initial findings during the evaluation. That is, if other nonoperative injuries were discovered on imaging (e.g., hepatic parenchymal injury), follow-up visits and imaging are in accordance with the specific injury.

6.4.3 Operative Principles Unique to Gunshot Wounds

When comparing operative principles in lower velocity (stab) to moderately higher velocity (handgun) and high-velocity (rifle rounds), it is intuitive that as the amount of energy increases, so should the index of suspicion of more extensive injury and the need for operative intervention (see ▸ Fig. 6.6). Whether a patient is stable for imaging or needs immediate operative intervention is determined by the clinical parameters seen at the time of the initial patient evaluation versus any general rule about the type of penetrating trauma. Similarly, damage control surgery is more dependent on clinical factors than specific injuries caused by the type of weapon that inflicts injury.

The single most important factor in correlating to amount of tissue destruction with ballistic injuries is the velocity of the round.[3] Higher velocity rounds create a pressure wave and temporary cavity that inflicts far greater injury beyond the permanent cavity created by the missile. This cavitation is seen largely in high-velocity hunting or military-grade rifles. Very few handguns fire rounds at enough velocity to cause cavitation injury. Although velocity is a widely recognized as an important factor, there are other factors that may be equally important in the ultimate amount and severity of resultant tissue injury. These include the pitch and yaw of the round, any "tumbling" that occurs after entry, any fragmentation of the bullet, and the type of external jacketing of the ballistic. Another special category that may be evaluated and managed differently are shotgun wounds. Wounds inflicted by shotgun rounds are heavily dependent on the distance from the muzzle. Closer proximity creates injury more consistent with blast wounds, and with greater distance, multiple small wounds are seen with

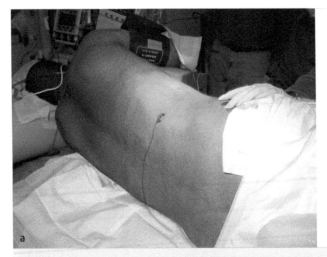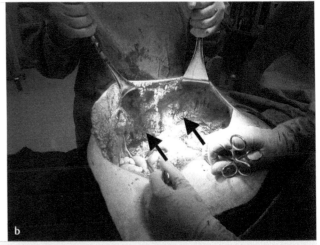

Fig. 6.6 Low-velocity gunshot wound to the right flank **(a)** compared to intraoperative view of a high-velocity gunshot wound to the anterior abdomen **(b)** with a large cavitary wound (*black arrows*).

varying degrees of tissue penetration. Close-proximity wounds from a shotgun need to be thoroughly explored. Metallic fragments within the wound can be seen with radiographic imaging. However, the shotgun wad is radiolucent and its presence within a wound should be suspected.

6.5 Laparoscopy in Penetrating Abdominal Trauma

Laparoscopy in penetrating abdominal trauma is undertaken as a diagnostic tool, a therapeutic maneuver, or combination of both. It is helpful in identifying peritoneal violation in stab wounds, evaluating left-sided thoracoabdominal gunshot wounds, and with confirming suspected extraperitoneal trajectory.[41] It can also be used as a tool for diagnosing solid organ, visceral injury and diaphragmatic injury. Currently, it is contraindicated in the hemodynamically unstable, head-injured patients requiring swift intervention to minimize the risk of secondary brain injury, and in patients with known operative retroperitoneal injuries.

Laparoscopic skill among trauma surgeons can be highly variable. Traditionally, laparoscopy has been avoided due to the risk of missed injury, especially to the small bowel and retroperitoneal structures. One nonrandomized but prospective analysis demonstrated, with a standardized approach to laparoscopy in trauma, missing these injuries can be avoided.[42] Patients undergoing diagnostic laparoscopy with equivocal findings for intra-abdominal injury were converted to laparotomy. Specifically, if there was identifiable small bowel injury, lesions to areas poorly visualized with laparoscopy, retroperitoneal hematoma that warranted exploration, injuries to segments VI or VII of the liver, or injuries to the posterior area of the spleen were indications to convert to an open procedure. This approach based on specific criteria achieved an excellent diagnostic degree of accuracy and nontherapeutic laparotomies were avoided in 73% of patients.

Two recent systematic reviews have been completed to compare outcomes between laparoscopy and laparotomy.[43,44] In general, laparoscopy has been linked to decreased postoperative wound infections, pneumonia, and length of hospital stay. Operative costs are higher but long-term costs appear to be decreased. Sensitivity ranges from 66 to 100% with improved results in more recent studies. Results are difficult to interpret because included studies were often of poor quality with high amounts of heterogeneity between them. For example, rates of missed injury ranged from 0 to 20%, likely representing variable skill level among surgeons and selection bias. Overall, it appears there may be an advantage to laparoscopy in penetrating abdominal trauma in specific circumstances in the hands of surgeons experienced with minimally invasive techniques, who also follow a systematic approach and specific criteria for conversion to laparotomy.

6.6 Special Scenarios

6.6.1 Penetrating Abdominal Trauma in Pregnancy

Penetrating abdominal trauma occurring in pregnancy does not necessarily change the central tenets of care for these patients. However, interpreting the overall status of the patient needs to be done in the context of the physiologic changes which happen in pregnancy. Specifically, the determination of shock and, therefore, the goals of resuscitation are different. Abdominal anatomy varies according to gestational age and therefore suspicion of injury may be different based on this. Although the managing physician should be cognizant that there are "two patients" to evaluate, the primary evaluation and interventions should focus on the mother.

During pregnancy, blood plasma volume increases with only modest increase in actual red blood cells. Hematocrit in the range of 31 to 35% is normal in late pregnancy. Cardiac output increases 1 to 1.5 L/min and the placenta is receiving 20% by the third trimester. Pregnant women can lose up to 1200 to 1500 mL of blood before demonstrating symptoms of hypovolemia. Knowledge of these changes is vital during the initial evaluation of these patients.

Intra-abdominal anatomy varies with each trimester as the uterus enlarges. The uterus remains within the pelvis until approximately the 12th week of gestation. Between weeks 12 to 20, its position is between the pubic symphysis and the umbilicus. After 20 weeks, the uterus gradually makes its way to near the costal margins. It is initially thick-walled until near term when it thins significantly. With growth of the uterus, the bowel moves cephalad. Once the uterus is out of the pelvis, many intra-abdominal organs are protected by it from penetrating trauma. However, in cases of penetrating injury to the upper abdomen in the later stages of pregnancy, there should be higher suspicion for injury to the bowel. As the uterus and fetus enlarge, special consideration should be made for positioning. Supine placement can lead to catastrophic decrease in cardiac output due to compression of the IVC.

Care for the mother is always prioritized over the fetus. Hemorrhage control and resuscitation lead to increased survival for both the mother and fetus. In circumstances of ongoing uterine hemorrhage, the fetus can be delivered via a cesarean section. This may allow definitive control of hemorrhage; however, in rare cases, it may be necessary to perform a hysterectomy. Regarding the fetus, most state laws require fetal resuscitation to be attempted after delivery at 24 weeks gestation and beyond. This requirement does vary by state and trauma surgeons should be aware of their state's laws. Probability of survival for the infant is based on the likelihood of a good neurologic outcome. Neurologic outcome varies with infant weight because this is the factor deciding if the newborn is a candidate for extracorporeal membrane oxygenation. We recommend a multidisciplinary approach with the obstetrics team in all cases of penetrating abdominal trauma to help guide resuscitation goals and assist intraoperatively, if needed.

6.7 Damage Control Surgery

6.7.1 Damage Control Abdominal Procedures

Damage control surgery (DCS) is an approach meant to expeditiously control hemorrhage and contamination in the unstable trauma patient without providing definitive repair. Longer operating times perpetuate the lethal triad of hypothermia, coagulopathy, and acidosis, increasing morbidity and mortality. Improved outcomes following DCS were originally reported in the 1990s and attributed to decreased time in the operating room.[45] DCS is now embraced internationally as the management strategy of choice for operative patients in extremis. Various forms of DCS exist across specialists who engage in trauma care. In the case of penetrating abdominal trauma, it consists largely of packing the abdomen, ligating bleeding vessels or placing temporary vascular shunts, and closing or resecting damaged mesentery and bowel to control gastrointestinal spillage. Vascular or bowel anastomoses are usually avoided to minimize operative time, avoid worsening of the lethal triad, and focus on restoration of normal physiology. The objective is control of hemorrhage and contamination, therefore ▶ Table 6.2 describes operative maneuvers that can be performed for specific injuries.[46]

Temporary abdominal closure is also a staple of DCS. It helps to avoid abdominal compartment syndrome as well as easily regain access to the abdomen in order to reassess injury. There are multiple existing devices that are available to facilitate temporary abdominal closure, but this can also be performed with existing basic OR supplies. Previous methods of temporary closure would simply utilize some type of dressing or impermeable barrier sewn to the fascia or the skin, but these caused significant problems with control and evacuation of fluid as well as protection of the underlying bowel. Current practice mainly uses some type of negative-pressure vacuum dressing systems that both protect the bowel and allow for egress of intra-abdominal fluid or blood. These systems may also help keep fascia approximated by controlling abdominal pressure and maintain some degree of medial tension to prevent retraction of fascial edges. Sedation with intubation are often continued until the abdomen is closed; however, emerging data supports the safety of extubating select patients with an open abdomen.[47,48] We advocate for aggressive attempts at early fascial closure, at the first takeback if at all possible. Patients should usually be kept intubated and sedated during this process. If fascial closure cannot be performed and will likely require multiple subsequent takebacks, then extubation can be attempted if there are no other factors requiring mechanical ventilation.

Although this approach is nearly ubiquitous in the sickest of trauma patients, its overuse has come into question. A Cochrane systematic review concluded the evidence demonstrating

Table 6.2 Operative principles of damage control surgery

	Operative maneuvers	Pearls	Pitfalls
Liver	• Packing above and below liver • Clamp and ligate small bleeding vessels • Foley balloon into small projectile holes to tamponade bleeding • Pringle maneuver	• Rapid control of bleeding depends on quick identification of the source • Persistent bleeding despite Pringle maneuver suggests a retrohepatic IVC injury	• Prolonged exploration and delayed hemorrhage control
Spleen	• Splenectomy • Splenic packing	• Rapid splenectomy usually procedure of choice • Packing alone with later splenectomy/splenorrhaphy also an option	• Inappropriate splenic preservation • Failing to give vaccinations
Kidney	• Nephrectomy is warranted in the presence of major active bleeding	• Nonpulsatile, nonexpanding hematomas can be observed	• Inappropriate attempts at renal salvage
Vascular	• Clamp and ligate small vessels • Temporary shunts placed in named/critical vessels	• Ligation is acceptable of the IMA, hypogastric arteries, tributaries of the SMA or SMV, celiac axis, and infrarenal IVC • Consider shunting major associated vein injuries	• Ligating the SMA, SMV portal vein, suprarenal IVC, or iliac arteries
Pancreas	• Clamp and ligate tributaries from SMA and SMV • Temporary packing and closed-suction drainage if ductal injury	• Distal pancreatectomy and drain for body/tail injuries • Proximal injury with ductal involvement should be widely drained	• Attempting complex reconstruction in damage control setting
Duodenal	• Quickly control gross spillage • If damage is < 50 % circumference, then repair primarily • If damage is > 50 %, bowel is multiply damaged or viability questionable, provide wide drainage until second look	• Primary repair performed with single layer of interrupted sutures • Perform resections with a stapler, if available • Duodenal injuries not amenable to resection can be repaired with a duodenojejunostomy • Consider pyloric exclusion or gastric diversion	• Attempting advanced maneuvers for reanastomosis or resection • Failing to assess for ampulla or pancreas injury
Bowel	• Quickly control gross spillage • If damage is < 50 % circumference then repair primarily • If damage is > 50 % circumference, bowel is multiply damaged or devascularized, resect and reconstruct later	• Stapled resection, if available, is more efficient than a hand-sewn maneuver	• Attempting reanastomosis or stoma formation during damage control surgery

Abbreviations: CT, computed tomography; GSW, gunshot wounds; IMA, inferior mesenteric artery; IVC, inferior vena cava; OR, operating room; SMA, superior mesenteric artery; SMV, superior mesenteric vein.

improved outcomes over traditional laparotomy was limited.[49] DCS has been linked to increased rates of ventral hernia, enteroatmospheric fistulae, and stressing the capability of hospital resources. Current research is focused on identifying long-term outcomes and defining who can safely avoid DCS.

6.7.2 Damage Control Resuscitation

Damage control resuscitation (DCR) occurring in conjunction with DCS has demonstrated a survival advantage.[50] DCR attempts to correct the "lethal triad" of trauma which consists of hypothermia, coagulopathy, and acidosis. Patients undergo balanced resuscitation with blood products; however, permissive hypotension (systolic blood pressure 80s–90s) is permitted in an attempt not to dislodge helpful clot prior to the operating theater. Resuscitation goals have been difficult to fully define. In general, base deficit of less than 2 and normal blood lactate levels serve as a surrogate for determining adequate end-organ perfusion. Vasopressors play limited role in the setting of hypovolemic shock; however, they may be utilized if sepsis is suspected. In hypovolemic shock, priority of restoring circulating blood volume via component therapy should be given over temporizing measures like vasoactive agent administration. Bicarbonate as an attempt to improve acid/base balance should also avoided as it does not address the underlying problem of hypovolemia and anaerobic respiration. Once physiology is restored, patients can proceed with definitive repair and closure, typically within 24 to 48 hours. However, if lactic acidosis, coagulopathy and/or hypotension persist in the face of aggressive resuscitation, it is likely there is an uncontrolled operative injury that needs to be addressed.

6.8 Conclusion

The appropriate evaluation and management of penetrating abdominal trauma requires a strict focus on rapid identification of life-threatening pathology and other injuries that require immediate operative intervention. These patients should usually be immediately transported to the operating room to undergo prompt surgical exploration, identification of injuries, and appropriate repair or temporizing maneuvers. This is of particular importance to centers and surgeons that see a lower incidence of penetrating trauma and have less comfort and familiarity with these issues. An algorithmic and evidence-based approach should be followed to minimize any delays to definitive intervention among patients with significant intra-abdominal injury, and to identify those patients who can be safely managed with a selective nonoperative approach.

Disclaimer

The views expressed herein are the author's own and do not necessarily reflect the official policy or position of the Department of the Navy, Department of the Army, Department of Defense, or the U.S. Government.

References

[1] Shaftan GW. Indications for operation in abdominal trauma. Am J Surg. 1960; 99(5):657–664

[2] Martin MJ, Rhee PM. Nonoperative management of blunt and penetrating abdominal injuries. In: Current Therapy of Trauma and Surgical Critical Care; Asensio J. and Trunkey D. (eds): 2008:352–362

[3] Rhee PM, Moore EE, Joseph B, Tang A, Pandit V, Vercruysse G. Gunshot wounds: a review of ballistics, bullets, weapons, and myths. J Trauma Acute Care Surg. 2016; 80(6):853–867

[4] Cook MR, Holcomb JB, Rahbar MH, et al. An Abdominal CT may be safe in selected hypotensive trauma patients with positive FAST exam. Am J Surg. 2016; 209(5):834–840

[5] Yücel M, Özpek A, Yüksekdağ S, et al. The management of penetrating abdominal stab wounds with organ or omentum evisceration: The results of a clinical trial. Ulus Cerrahi Derg. 2014; 30(4):207–210

[6] Nicholson K, Inaba K, Skiada D, et al. Management of patients with evisceration after abdominal stab wounds. Am Surg. 2014; 80(10):984–988

[7] Doll D, Matevossian E, Kayser K, Degiannis E, Hönemann C. Eviszeration von Darm nach Stichverletzung des Abdomens: Häufigkeit und klinische Aspekte des klinischen Schockraummanagements. Unfallchirurg. 2014; 117(7):624–632

[8] Leppäniemi AK, Voutilainen PE, Haapiainen RK. Indications for early mandatory laparotomy in abdominal stab wounds. Br J Surg. 1999; 86(1):76–80

[9] Dayananda K, Kong VY, Bruce JL, Oosthuizen GV, Laing GL, Clarke DL. Selective non-operative management of abdominal stab wounds is a safe and cost effective strategy: A South African experience. Ann R Coll Surg Engl. 2017; 99(6):490–496

[10] Como JJ, Bokhari F, Chiu WC, et al. Practice management guidelines for selective nonoperative management of penetrating abdominal trauma. J Trauma. 2010; 68(3):721–733

[11] Hulzinga W, Baker L, Mtshali Z. Selective management of abdominal and thoracic stab wounds with established peritoneal violation: the eviscerated omentum. Am J Surg. 1987; 152:564–568

[12] Rothschild PD, Treiman RL. Selective management of abdominal stab wounds. Am J Surg. 1966; 111(3):382–387

[13] Biffl WL, Kaups KL, Cothren CC, et al. Management of patients with anterior abdominal stab wounds: a Western Trauma Association multicenter trial. J Trauma. 2009; 66(5):1294–1301

[14] Martin MJ, Brown CVR, Shatz DV, et al. Evaluation and management of abdominal stab wounds: A Western Trauma Association critical decisions algorithm. J Trauma Acute Care Surg. 2018; 85(5):1007–1015

[15] Beck-Razi N, Gaitini D. Focused Assessment with Sonography for Trauma (FAST) Examination. Assoc. Med Ultrasound. 2014:1–10

[16] Pham TN, Heinberg E, Cuschieri J, et al. The evolution of the diagnostic work-up for stab wounds to the back and flank. Injury. 2009; 40(1):48–53

[17] Albrecht RM, Vigil A, Schermer CR, Demarest GB, III, Davis VH, Fry DE. Stab wounds to the back/flank in hemodynamically stable patients: evaluation using triple-contrast computed tomography. Am Surg. 1999; 65(7):683–687, discussion 687–688

[18] Hauser CJ, Huprich JE, Bosco P, Gibbons L, Mansour AY, Weiss ARS. Triple-contrast computed tomography in the evaluation of penetrating posterior abdominal injuries. Arch Surg. 1987; 122(10):1112–1115

[19] Kirton OC, Wint D, Thrasher B, Windsor J, Echenique A, Hudson-Civetta J. Stab wounds to the back and flank in the hemodynamically stable patient: a decision algorithm based on contrast-enhanced computed tomography with colonic opacification. Am J Surg. 1997; 173(3):189–193

[20] Fletcher TB, Setiawan H, Harrell RS, Redman HC. Posterior abdominal stab wounds: role of CT evaluation. Radiology. 1989; 173(3):621–625

[21] Meyer DM, Thal ER, Weigelt JA, Redman HC. The role of abdominal CT in the evaluation of stab wounds to the back. J Trauma. 1989; 29(9):1226–1228, discussion 1228–1230

[22] Bansal V, Reid CM, Fortlage D, et al. Determining injuries from posterior and flank stab wounds using computed tomography tractography. Am Surg. 2014; 80(4):403–407

[23] Sarici İS, Kalayci MU. Is computed tomography tractography reliable in patients with anterior abdominal stab wounds? Am J Emerg Med. 2018; 36(8):1405–1409

[24] Mason JH. The expectant management of abdominal stab wounds. J Trauma. 1964; 4:210–218

[25] Biffl WL, Kaups KL, Pham TN, et al. Validating the Western Trauma Association algorithm for managing patients with anterior abdominal stab wounds: a Western Trauma Association multicenter trial. J Trauma. 2011; 71(6):1494–1502

[26] Plackett TP, Fleurat J, Putty B, Demetriades D, Plurad D. Selective nonoperative management of anterior abdominal stab wounds: 1992–2008. J Trauma. 2011; 70(2):408–413, discussion 413–414

[27] Breigeiron R, Breitenbach TC, Zanini LAG, Corso CO. Comparison between isolated serial clinical examination and computed tomography for stab wounds in the anterior abdominal wall. Rev Col Bras Cir. 2017; 44(6):596–602

[28] Hanna WC, Ferri LE. Acute traumatic diaphragmatic injury. Thorac Surg Clin. 2009; 19(4):485–489

[29] Mjoli M, Oosthuizen G, Clarke D, Madiba T. Laparoscopy in the diagnosis and repair of diaphragmatic injuries in left-sided penetrating thoracoabdominal trauma: laparoscopy in trauma. Surg Endosc. 2015; 29(3):747–752

[30] Murray JA, Demetriades D, Cornwell EE, III, et al. Penetrating left thoracoabdominal trauma: the incidence and clinical presentation of dia-phragm injuries. J Trauma. 1997; 43(4):624–626

[31] Eachempati SR, Barie PS, Reed RL, II. Survival after transabdominal impale-ment from a construction injury: a review of the management of impalement injuries. J Trauma. 1999; 47(5):864–866

[32] Gölder SK, Friess H, Shafighi M, Kleeff JH, Büchler MW. A chair leg as the rare cause of a transabdominal impalement with duodenal and pancreatic involvement. J Trauma. 2001; 51(1):164–167

[33] Mohan R, Ram DU, Baba YS, Shetty A, Bhandary S. Transabdominal impalement: absence of visceral or vascular injury a rare possibility. J Emerg Med. 2011; 41(5):495–498

[34] Angelopoulos S, Mantzoros I, Kyziridis D, et al. A rare case of a transabdominal impalement after a fall from a ladder. Int J Surg Case Rep. 2016; 22:40–43

[35] Whitehouse JS, Weigelt JA. Diagnostic peritoneal lavage: a review of indications, technique, and interpretation. Scand J Trauma Resusc Emerg Med. 2009; 17(13):13

[36] DuBose JJ, Scalea TM, Brenner M, et al. AAST AORTA Study Group. The AAST prospective Aortic Occlusion for Resuscitation in Trauma and Acute Care Sur-gery (AORTA) registry: data on contemporary utilization and outcomes of aortic occlusion and resuscitative balloon occlusion of the aorta (REBOA). J Trauma Acute Care Surg. 2016; 81(3):409–419

[37] Biffl WL, Fox CJ, Moore EE. The role of REBOA in the control of exsanguinating torso hemorrhage. J Trauma Acute Care Surg. 2015; 78(5):1054–1058

[38] Velmahos GC, Constantinou C, Tillou A, Brown CV, Salim A, Demetriades D. Abdominal computed tomographic scan for patients with gunshot wounds to the abdomen selected for nonoperative management. J Trauma. 2005; 59(5): 1155–1160, discussion 1160–1161

[39] Chiu WC, Shanmuganathan K, Mirvis SE, Scalea TM. Determining the need for laparotomy in penetrating torso trauma: a prospective study using triple-contrast enhanced abdominopelvic computed tomography. J Trauma. 2001; 51(5):860–868, discussion 868–869

[40] Conrad MF, Patton JH, Jr, Parikshak M, Kralovich KA. Selective management of penetrating truncal injuries: is emergency department discharge a reasonable goal? Am Surg. 2003; 69(3):266–272, discussion 273

[41] Simon RJ, Rabin J, Kuhls D. Impact of increased use of laparoscopy on negative laparotomy rates after penetrating trauma. J Trauma. 2002; 53(2):297–302, discussion 302

[42] Kawahara NT, Alster C, Fujimura I, Poggetti RS, Birolini D. Standard examination system for laparoscopy in penetrating abdominal trauma. J Trauma. 2009; 67(3): 589–595

[43] O'Malley E, Boyle E, O'Callaghan A, Coffey JC, Walsh SR. Role of laparoscopy in penetrating abdominal trauma: a systematic review. World J Surg. 2013; 37 (1):113–122

[44] Hajibandeh S, Hajibandeh S, Gumber AO, Wong CS. Laparoscopy versus lapa-rotomy for the management of penetrating abdominal trauma: a systematic review and meta-analysis. Int J Surg. 2016; 34:127–136

[45] Rotondo MF, Schwab CW, McGonigal MD, et al. 'Damage control': an approach for improved survival in exsanguinating penetrating abdominal injury. J Trauma. 1993; 35(3):375–382, discussion 382–383

[46] Rodriguez A, Elliot D. Damage control laparotomy. In: Cameron J, Cameron A, eds. Current Surgical Therapy. 12th ed. Philadelphia: Elsevier; 2017: 1210–1216

[47] Taveras LR, Imran JB, Cunningham HB, et al. Trauma and emergency general surgery patients should be extubated with an open abdomen. J Trauma Acute Care Surg. 2018; 85(6):1043–1047.–E-pub ahea–d of print

[48] Sujka JA, Safcsak K, Cheatham ML, Ibrahim JA. Trauma patients with an open abdomen following damage control laparotomy can be extubated prior to abdominal closure. World J Surg. 2018; 42(10):3210–3214

[49] Cirocchi R, Montedori A, Farinella E, Bonacini I, Tagliabue L, Abraha I. Damage control surgery for abdominal trauma. Cochrane Database Syst Rev. 2013; 28 (3):CD007438

[50] Duchesne JC, Kimonis K, Marr AB, et al. Damage control resuscitation in com-bination with damage control laparotomy: a survival advantage. J Trauma. 2010; 69(1):46–52

Expert Commentary on Penetrating Abdominal Trauma by *Thomas Scalea*

Expert Commentary on Penetrating Abdominal Trauma

Thomas Scalea

In the past, all patients with transperitoneal trajectory underwentdiagnostic laparotomy. In fact, laparotomy was often advocated for anyone in whom there was a suspicion of intra-abdominal injury. As diagnostic testing and technology improved, and the complications of nontherapeutic laparotomy were recognized, surgeons adopted a more selective approach.

Serial physical examination, ultrasound (focused assessment with sonography for trauma [FAST]), computed tomography (CT) scanning, and diagnostic laparoscopy all have a place in the management of hemodynamically stable patients without peritonitis. Selective management is likely best practiced at centers with real expertise in trauma and those that have house staff and operating rooms available 24/7. In other venues, it is likely safer to explore questionable patients in order to avoid the serious complications associated with the missed injury.

Physiology should drive most decisions about care. Even if blood pressure is normal, other signs of shock such as tachycardia, thready pulse on examination, or metabolic acidosis, should prompt strong consideration for early operation. Diagnostic exploration should be carried out through a large incision. This is no time to struggle. The surgeon must be able to fully evaluate all abdominal structures. Solid organs such as the liver, spleen, or kidney must be mobilized up to the abdominal wall to allow good visualization.

The abdominal contents are in intimate proximity to retroperitoneal and thoracic structures. The surgeon must be prepared to deal with injury in either of these locations. A wide prep to include the thorax, abdomen, and thighs is essential. Additional incisions may be necessary when other injuries are discovered at the time of exploration.

Damage control laparotomy (DCL) was first described for use in patients with severe penetrating abdominal trauma. In our practice, penetrating trauma is still the most frequent indication for the use of DCL. The principles of rapid hemorrhage control and control of contamination followed by a decision as to whether definitive care is feasible are important today as they were in 1993 when Mike Rotondo wrote his seminal paper. However, the overuse of DCL can worsen outcomes. Younger surgeons or surgeons with less experience likely use DCL more often than more experienced clinicians. When faced with complex decision-making, younger surgeons should phone a more experienced colleague for help.

Several new adjuncts can be very helpful in patients with penetrating abdominal trauma. Transfemoral aortic balloon occlusion (REBOA) can be helpful in obtaining temporary inflow control in patients with significant intra-abdominal hemorrhage. REBOA is only a temporizing measure. Patients still require an immediate operation. Other catheter techniques such as embolization can be useful adjuncts. The decision to use these innovative techniques should be based on expertise, availability of resources, and patient stability.

Penetrating abdominal trauma is relatively rare. However, every surgeon is likely to encounter it at least a few times during his/her career. The principles described in this well-written chapter by Matthew J. Martin and his colleagues should prove valuable. I congratulate the authors on a wonderful job.

7 Thoracic Trauma

Benjamin J. Moran, Katherine M. Kelley, and James V. O'Connor

Summary

This chapter discusses the evaluation of the patient with chest trauma, indications for surgery, damage control, and the role of video-assisted procedures. Detailed information is provided on operative exposure and surgical techniques used to manage lung, cardiac, and vascular injuries.

Keywords: Lung injury, cardiac injury, airway management, damage control, operative indications, surgical techniques

7.1 Introduction

Thoracic pathology and injury contribute significantly to patient morbidity and mortality. Nearly 50% of all trauma-related deaths in patients under 40 years of age are due to thoracic injury, making chest trauma a common presentation seen in any trauma center.[1,2] Minimally invasive approaches for the diagnosis and treatment of surgical conditions have evolved and grown in precision and technology over the past decade. While these treatment options have become the standard of care in the elective setting, these minimally invasive techniques have been more slowly adopted in the acute and emergent surgical settings. The skill set involved in treating acute thoracic problems relies on a prompt accurate diagnosis, knowledge of anatomy, refined clinical judgment, and technical proficiency. This chapter will focus on indications for thoracic surgery and discuss operative decision-making with regard to thoracoscopic and open thoracic surgery.

7.2 Initial Evaluation

Patients presenting following thoracic injury should undergo the standard evaluation for any trauma patient following advanced trauma life support (ATLS) guidelines and the well-described airway, breathing, and circulation (ABCs). Life-threatening external hemorrhage must be controlled. Particular care must be exercised in assessing the airway in the thoracic trauma patient, as a tracheobronchial injury may be present. If intubation is indicated, a rapid evaluation for signs of airway injury must be performed. The presence of stridor, hoarseness, subcutaneous emphysema, persistent pneumothorax, or large continuous air leak following chest tube insertion should alert the clinician about the possibility of a tracheobronchial injury. If care is not taken in securing the airway, a partial tracheobronchial injury can be converted to a total transaction with catastrophic consequences. The use of video laryngoscopy and fiberoptic intubation are extremely useful in safely securing the airway. If the airway cannot be secured by these methods, then a surgical airway is established.

Once the airway is secured, breath sounds should be evaluated. Absence or decreased breath sounds may represent a hemothorax, pneumothorax, or hemopneumothorax. The presence of these findings can be confirmed by the focused assessment with sonography in trauma (FAST) examination. Chest tube insertion is warranted in these situations. Evaluation of the circulation and adequacy of tissue perfusion can be accomplished by palpating the patient's foot. A warm foot with a palpable pedal pulse is indicative of adequate peripheral perfusion. On the contrary, a cool foot with an absent pulse is a marker for inadequate tissue perfusion and the clinical presence of shock. Relying on vital signs alone to assess shock can be misleading. In a study of patients undergoing a damage control thoracotomy, the admission median systolic blood pressure was 118 mm Hg; however, the mean pH and base deficit were 7.07 and 11.1 mmol/L, respectively.[3] These findings emphasize the degree of hemodynamic compensation present in profound shock, especially in the young trauma patient. Physiologic markers, including lactate and arterial blood gas, are invaluable in determining the presence of shock, its depth and degree of compensation. In addition, an arterial blood gas yields important information regarding the adequacy of oxygenation and ventilation, which are especially relevant with a chest injury.

A rapid, thorough physical examination is performed. The absence of an upper extremity pulse may indicate a subclavian arterial injury and limb viability should be assessed. In addition to the standard laboratory studies, a thromboelastogram is ordered as indicated. Point of care laboratory testing will reduce the time within which results are reported. It is the authors' practice to include an admission arterial blood gas on all patients with significant thoracic injury. Plain radiographs of the chest and pelvis are part of the evaluation as is ultrasonography. The extended focused assessment with sonography for trauma (eFAST) provides pertinent information regarding lung sliding, hemopericardium, and hemoperitoneum.

Following an expeditious initial evaluation, the first pivotal decision must be made; is an emergency operation indicated? Shock, large volume chest tube output, and hemopericardium are the principle indications for emergent surgical intervention. For those patients who do not require immediate operative intervention, additional imaging studies are quite helpful. The standard is a computed tomography angiogram (CTA) of the chest which defines the anatomy as well as the location and extent of any intrathoracic injury. If an aerodigestive injury is suspected, further evaluation with bronchoscopy, esophagoscopy, and esophagram will define the presence, location, and extent of aerodigestive injury.

7.3 Indications for Operative Intervention

7.3.1 Urgent/Emergent

Indications for emergent operation include shock, hemorrhage, persistent chest tube output, clinical evidence of tamponade or hemopericardium on FAST, and aerodigestive injury. Initial chest drainage of 1,500 mL or persistent chest tube drainage greater than 200 mL per hour for 2 hours are indications for surgery in patients who are not on anticoagulants. There are several important points when evaluating chest tube output, as it may underestimate the degree of hemorrhage. Following the initial chest tube output, there be may be a large retained hemothorax, which may prompt urgent intervention (▶ Fig. 7.1). Also, the clinician should not conclude that decreased chest tube output implies cessation of intrathoracic bleeding. Ongoing bleeding may not be apparent if the chest tube is malpositioned or clotted; therefore, a chest radiograph is obtained following chest tube placement and when chest tube output decreases or stops.

With precordial wounds, a cardiac injury must be excluded. Clinical and/or ultrasound evidence of cardiac tamponade demands immediate operative intervention. eFAST is an invaluable modality that reliably diagnoses hemopericardium (▶ Fig. 7.2). One important caveat: it is unreliable if there is a concomitant hemothorax. In this instance, or if the FAST results are equivocal, a pericardial window is indicated for diagnosis.

Subcutaneous emphysema, persistent pneumothorax following chest drain placement, large continuous air leak, or significant pneumomediastinum suggests an aerodigestive injury (▶ Fig. 7.3). Typically, esophageal injures result in less subcutaneous emphysema and pneumomediastinum than tracheobronchial trauma. A

large continuous air leak or persistent pneumothorax following chest tube placement requires further evaluation to rule out tracheobronchial injury (▶ Fig. 7.4). Esophagogastroduodenoscopy or esophagoscopy, with or without an esophagram, will reliably exclude an esophageal injury. For optimal visualization, the endoscopy should be performed prior to the contrast study. Possible airway injuries are evaluated by bronchoscopy. It is imperative that the surgeon performs the endoscopy, evaluating the location and extent of the injury; the location of the injury will dictate the operative approach.

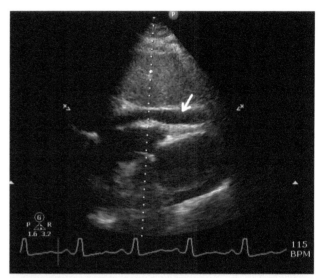

Fig. 7.2 Hemopericardium. An eFAST image of a hemopericardium (*arrow*) in a patient with a precordial stab wound. eFAST is very reliable in diagnosing hemopericardium, except if a hemothorax is present. eFAST, extended, focused assessment with sonography in trauma.

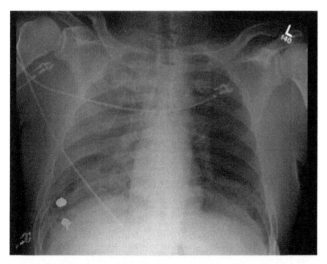

Fig. 7.1 Retained hemothorax. Portable supine chest radiograph demonstrates a retained right hemothorax. The diffusely hazy right hemithorax is the result of blood layering posteriorly with the patient supine. Ballistic fragments are noted.

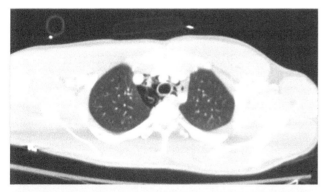

Fig. 7.3 Pneumomediastinum. An axial image of a CTA with obvious pneumomediastinum. This finding should prompt an evaluate of the aerodigestive tract. The combination of a normal endoscopy and contrast studies essentially excludes an aerodigestive injury. CTA, computed tomography angiography.

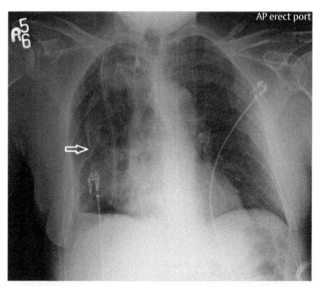

Fig. 7.4 Persistent pneumothorax. A persistent right pneumothorax (*arrow*) after chest tube insertion is seen on this portable supine chest X-ray. This finding or a large continuous air leak may indicate a tracheobronchial injury. Bronchoscopy is the diagnostic modality of choice.

An absent upper extremity pulse, with or without shock, indicates a subclavian injury. Emergent exploration is warranted in the presence of shock, and additional imaging with CTA is useful for those not in shock. Imaging studies, the patient's overall clinical condition, and limb viability will influence the management: nonoperative, open repair, or endovascular approach.

7.3.2 Thoracic Damage Control

The principles of damage control are well-established and include rapid hemorrhage control, minimizing contamination, resuscitation in the intensive care unit, and a delayed, definitive repair.[4] This approach, originally utilized in physiologically depleted patients with penetrating abdominal injuries, has expanded to vascular trauma, but is of only limited use for thoracic injuries.[5,6] Extreme acidosis, hypothermia, coagulopathy, massive transfusion requirement, protracted operative time, and significant extra-thoracic injuries all influence the decision to perform thoracic damage control. Techniques for expeditious hemorrhage control include tractotomy, stapled nonanatomic lung resection, and use of temporary vascular shunts.[7] Drains are positioned in the pleural spaces and, if opened the mediastinum, the chest is packed with laparotomy pads and a temporary closure applied. Concerns that packing the chest results in cardiopulmonary compromise are unjustified.[7] Following restoration of normal physiology, the chest is closed, generally within 3 days.

7.3.3 Elective

The most common indications for nonemergent operation are: retained hemothorax, persistent pneumothorax, chest wall instability, and posttraumatic empyema.

7.4 Video-assisted Thoracoscopic Surgery (VATS)

7.4.1 History of VATS

The first thoracoscopic surgery is frequently attributed to Hans Christian Jacobaeus in 1910; however, there are earlier reports of Francis Cruise using an endoscope to evaluate a patient's thoracic cavity as early as 1866.[8] The technological advances in video and instruments for laparoscopic and thoracoscopic surgery combined with the widespread adoption of laparoscopy for cholecystectomies led to increased interest in VATS for advanced thoracic procedures including lobectomies. The first major meeting to discuss the use of VATS was held at the annual Society of Thoracic Surgeons meeting in San Antonio, Texas, in 1992.[9] From that time, VATS has become increasingly sophisticated and utilized.

7.4.2 Advantages and Indications for VATS

VATS allows access to and visualization of the thoracic cavity through significantly smaller incisions than traditional thoracotomy. Compared with thoracotomy, patients undergoing VATS have fewer complications, decreased narcotic requirements, are more likely to resume their normal lifestyle, have an earlier return to normal activity, and are happier with their health and scars.[10]

There are several diagnoses that lend themselves to a VATS approach. Common applications include retained hemothorax, recurrent spontaneous pneumothorax or persistent pneumothorax after trauma, and posttraumatic empyema. VATS can also be used to treat ongoing intrathoracic hemorrhage in a hemodynamically stable patient and assess for diaphragmatic injury. Less common applications include thoracic duct ligation, foreign body removal, and diagnosis of cardiac and mediastinal injuries.[11,12]

7.4.3 VATS Operative Technique

The patient is intubated with a double lumen endotracheal tube, allowing single lung ventilation and then placed in lateral decubitus position. The bed is flexed to open the rib spaces. The patient should be prepped and draped for possible conversion to open procedure. The initial camera port is placed in the 4th intercostal space in the midaxillary line. This port can be placed through prior chest tube insertion site if appropriately located or placed under direct visualization using sharp dissection and electrocautery. Prior to port placement, digital inspection should be performed to ensure there are no adjacent adhesions. Two additional ports are placed under thoracoscopic guidance triangulated to the area of interest within the thoracic cavity. At the conclusion of the procedure, hemostasis should be achieved and chest tubes placed.

7.4.4 VATS Indications

Retained Hemothorax

Retained hemothorax after trauma is a frequently encountered problem. VATS is an accepted part of the treatment algorithm. In the AAST multicenter prospective observational trial of retained hemothorax by Dubose et al, VATS was the most common first-line treatment for retained hemothorax used in 33.5% of patients. Many of these patients required second interventions, with 20.4% requiring thoracotomy.[13] The most recent Eastern Association for the Surgery of Trauma (EAST) practice management guidelines for retained hemothorax recommend that if an initial chest tube does not result in resolution of the hemothorax early, VATS should be performed rather than placement of a second chest tube. There is some debate in the literature with regard to the optimal timing of early VATS, but the EAST practice management guidelines recommend it be performed in the first 3 to 7 days of admission.[14]

Pneumothorax

Both blunt and penetrating trauma commonly lead to pneumothorax. Most pneumothoraces resolve with chest tube placement. In some patients, however, the air leak persists beyond 72 hours. In such cases, EAST practice management guidelines recommend VATS intervention to decrease the hospital length of stay and complications associated with prolonged chest tube management.[14] Intraoperative injury to lung parenchyma can be treated with staple resection and/or application of tissue sealant. In a retrospective series of blunt chest injuries by Halat et al, four patients had a severe air leak that was managed with VATS stapled wedge resection or stapled pneumorraphy with complete resolution of the air leak. The 50 patients in this study with a minor air leak had resolution with chest tube alone, with most patients resolving their air leak in one day.[15]

Spontaneous pneumothoraces can also be managed with VATS. When blebs are identified either utilizing CT or intraoperatively, they can be resected to prevent recurrent pneumothoraces. Recurrent pneumothoraces can also be treated using mechanical pleurodesis by abrading the parietal pleura during VATS.

Empyema

Empyema can occur after retained hemothorax. In an American Association for the Surgery of Trauma (AAST) multicenter observational study, this was seen in 26.8% of cases.[13] As with retained hemothorax, empyema can be treated with VATS decortication and is more likely to be successful with an early stage, less organized empyema. Compared with the treatment of pneumothorax or retained hemothorax, there is a significantly higher rate of conversion to open associated with empyema.[16] In one series of 125 patients with posttraumatic empyema, all required surgery and 80% were treated with thoracotomy while 12.8% had VATS. Of those with VATS, more than half required conversion to open. Higher stage of empyema was associated with greater likelihood of conversion to open, suggesting earlier intervention may lead to greater success with VATS treatment of posttraumatic empyema.[17]

Intrathoracic Hemorrhage

Hemodynamically stable patients with ongoing hemorrhage requiring operative intervention can have VATS. In one series, 23 patients were managed in the acute setting with VATS and without associated mortality or conversion to thoracotomy.[18] Bleeding from lung parenchyma can be addressed thoracoscopically with stapled resection. Intercostal artery bleeding can frequently be treated with electrocautery. When electrocautery is ineffective, intercostal arteries can be ligated by using a laparoscopic suture passer to pass a suture around both the vessel and adjacent rib and then tying the suture.

Appropriate patient selection is imperative. Hemodynamical compromised patients placed in the lateral decubitus position may experience further deterioration, leading to cardiovascular collapse. In addition, thoracic trauma patients may not tolerate single lung ventilation, which is necessary to perform VATS.

Diaphragmatic Injury

When there is a concern for possible diaphragmatic injury, VATS can be performed to assess the integrity of the diaphragm. In one series of 30 patients, there were no missed diaphragm injuries after VATS.[19] Once found, most injuries require conversion to thoracotomy or an abdominal approach to repair. The VATS approach is of particular benefit in patients with concomitant hemothorax, as it can be evacuated out at the same time as the diaphragmatic assessment is performed.

Thoracic Duct Ligation

Chylothorax infrequently occurs after thoracic trauma or surgery. Trauma to the neck or thorax, and surgical intervention in either of these regions, can result in a lymphatic leak. Milky chest tube output should be evaluated by sending the pleural fluid for analysis. The presence of high triglyceride levels confirms the diagnosis. Nonoperative management is often successful, and surgery is indicated for failure of nonoperative management. Direct ductal ligation via VATS is the preferred operative approach.[20]

Foreign Body Removal

VATS has been performed to remove foreign bodies from the thoracic cavity, including knives and retained surgical sponges.[21] Most thoracic cavity foreign bodies are asymptomatic but when symptomatic, VATS can be used to assist in removal and decrease length of stay.

Diagnosis of Cardiac and Mediastinal Injuries

Cardiac and mediastinal injuries are currently diagnosed utilizing ultrasound, CT, and pericardial window. There are case reports of VATS used to perform evaluation of the pericardium; however, this is not well studied and there is no defined sensitivity to assess for the possibility of missed injuries.[22] The current accepted evaluation and treatment of penetrating mediastinal trauma is well-described by Burack and colleagues.[23] Patients in shock require immediate operation, which carries a substantial mortality. Chest X-ray, CTA, and transthoracic echocardiography (TTE) were performed in stable patients. A negative CTA did not require additional evaluation. Pneumomediastinum on CTA and TTE prompted bronchoscopy, esophagoscopy, and/or esophagram.

7.5 Contraindications and Complications of VATS

While there are many benefits to VATS, it is not without complications and there are several contraindications. VATS should not be performed in hemodynamically unstable patients. Also, as VATS is most effective with single lung ventilation, it is contraindicated in patients with severe pulmonary or cardiac disease. VATS is also relatively contraindicated in patients with prior thoracic surgery due to the potential for significant pulmonary adhesions.[11]

Overall the rate of complications after VATS ranges from 3 to 10%. The most common complications are persistent air leak, bleeding, postoperative pain, and wound infection. Mortality rates after VATS are reported as 2%.[24]

7.6 Open Thoracic Surgery

7.6.1 Operative Exposure

Once the decision is made for operative intervention, the choice of incision is of paramount importance. Whichever incision is chosen, it must provide adequate exposure, be rapidly performed, be versatile, and be one which the surgeon is familiar with. The choice of incision is also influenced if the operation is performed for exploration or definitive repair

For emergent exploration, an anterolateral thoracotomy is preferred. It is the authors' preference to place a bump under the ipsilateral back, extend the ipsilateral arm, and widely prep and drape (▶ Fig. 7.5). The incision is made in the 4th or 5th interspace from sternal border as far posterior as possible, staying in the appropriate interspace. The advantages of the anterolateral thoracotomy are surgeon familiarity, it is rapidly performed, and affords excellent exposure of the pleural space (▶ Fig. 7.6). The main disadvantage is limited exposure of mediastinum and posterior structures.

If mediastinal exploration is necessary, the incision can be extended across the midline as a bilateral anterolateral thoracotomy or a "clamshell." Both pleural cavities and the mediastinum are well-visualized with this approach. When performing a clamshell, it is important to divide the body of the sternum not the xiphoid. Placing the incision too far inferior will limit exposure of the superior mediastinum (▶ Fig. 7.7, ▶ Fig. 7.8).

Median sternotomy is another classic approach to the mediastinum. It is rapid, affords excellent mediastinal exposure, and is versatile. If needed, it can be extended to the neck, clavicle, or abdomen. Among the disadvantages are surgeon experience and the visualization of the posterior mediastinal structures.

In a patient who is not in shock, the mid and distal subclavian vessels may be approached through a periclavicular incision. It can be performed rapidly and affords adequate exposure. The presence of a large hematoma may distort the anatomy and the operative field can be deep and narrow. Transecting the clavicle will improve the exposure but may be time-consuming.

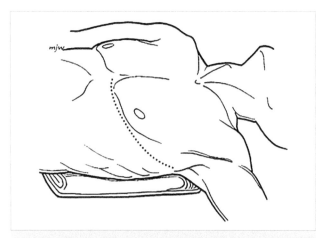

Fig. 7.5 Anterolateral thoracotomy. This versatile incision is preferred for an emergent thoracotomy. If needed, it can be extended as a clamshell or laparotomy. Note the bump under ipsilateral back and extension of the arm, which facilities exposure. (Reproduced with permission of James V. O'Connor. Thoracic Vascular Injuries. In: Thomas M. Scalea. The Shock Trauma Manual of Operative Techniques. New York, NY. Springer-Verlag; 2015; 329–346.)

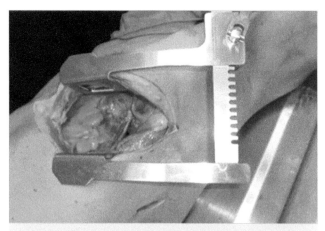

Fig. 7.6 Operative exposure. This cadaveric photograph demonstrates the exposure obtained through a left anterolateral incision. Placing the retractor's handle toward the axilla provides unobstructed access to the sternum and right chest if a clamshell is necessary. (Reproduced with permission of Jay Menaker. Emergency Department Thoracotomy. In: Thomas M. Scalea. The Shock Trauma Manual of Operative Techniques. New York, NY. Springer-Verlag; 2015; 13–35.)

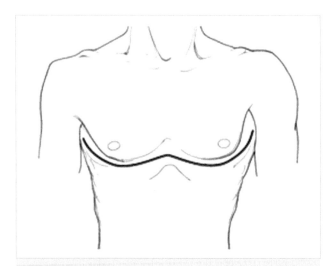

Fig. 7.7 Clamshell thoracotomy. The bilateral anterolateral (clamshell) incision provides excellent exposure to the entire chest. For optimal exposure, the sternal body, not the xiphoid, is divided. (Reproduced with permission of James V. O'Connor. Thoracic Vascular Injuries. In: Thomas M. Scalea. The Shock Trauma Manual of Operative Techniques. New York, NY. Springer-Verlag; 2015; 329–346.)

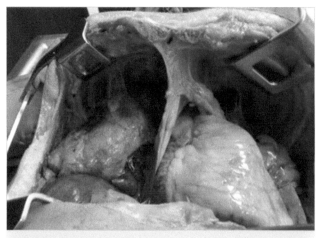

Fig. 7.8 Operative exposure. Excellent exposure of both pleural spaces and the mediastinum is demonstrated in this cadaveric photograph of a clamshell incision. The pericardium has been widely opened and bilateral retractors are placed. (Reproduced with permission of Jay Menaker. Emergency Department Thoracotomy. In: Thomas M. Scalea. The Shock Trauma Manual of Operative Techniques. New York, NY. Springer-Verlag; 2015; 13–35.)

The posterolateral thoracotomy approach is used when a definitive diagnosis has been made, typically an intrathoracic aerodigestive injury. Using a posterolateral incision for exploration, especially in the hemodynamically compromised patient, is fraught with difficulty. Lateral positioning may exacerbate existing compromised hemodynamics and the incision is not at all versatile. Finally, optimal exposure is achieved with single lung ventilation, and placing a double lumen endotracheal tube may not be possible in these patients. The patient's clinical condition, operating for exploration or definite management, nature and location of the injury if known, and surgeon familiarity, will dictate the operative approach. Again, whichever approach is taken, exposure cannot be compromised.

7.6.2 Airway Management

A safe and secure airway is of utmost importance in all trauma patients. Patients who are combative have sustained a traumatic brain injury, have severe facial fractures or a suspected cervical spine injury, pose an additional challenge. Specifically, with thoracic trauma, a tracheobronchial injury needs to be considered. Appropriate equipment including a basic and difficult airway kit, video laryngoscopy, and bronchoscopy are essential. If airway injury is suspected or confirmed, an experienced provider should manage the airway. In this circumstance, video laryngoscopy and

fiberoptic intubation are the authors' preferred approach to secure the airway, since converting a partial to complete airway disruption may have disastrous consequences. A surgical airway is performed if oral or nasal intubation are not possible.

Airway management for an emergent operation is typically accomplished with a single lumen endotracheal tube, since a placing double lumen tube may not be possible. However, there are several options to decrease ventilation to the injured lung if needed. An endobronchial blocker is an attractive option but may dislodge during the operative procedure. Selective mainstem intubation can be utilized if there is sufficient cardiopulmonary reserve, as the maneuver results in considerable shunting. As left mainstem is longer, intubation is straightforward since there is less risk of occluding the upper lobe bronchus. The same cannot be said for the right mainstem. The origin of the right upper lobe bronchus lies closer to the carina and is more easily occluded with mainstem intubation. Mainstem intubation is optimally performed using bronchoscopy. Finally, to facilitate lung repair or resection, ventilation can be briefly interrupted while carefully monitoring carbon dioxide levels and oxygen saturation.

Retrograde intubation, although rarely necessary, is an important adjunct in airway management. It is typically performed in a patient with a proximal tracheal injury and managed with a surgical airway when oral intubation fails. A tube exchanger is passed retrograde from the open trachea into the oral cavity. An endotracheal tube is then passed antegrade, the surgical airway removed, and the endotracheal tube is guided into the distal airway (▶ Fig. 7.9). The airway injury can then be repaired under direct vision (▶ Fig. 7.10).

The surgical approach to an intrathoracic aerodigestive injury is through a posterolateral thoracotomy. In this instance, a double lumen tube, lung isolation, and single long ventilation provides excellent exposure. Lung isolation with a double lumen endotracheal tube is indispensable when performing VATS.

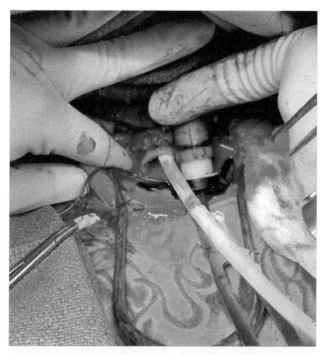

Fig. 7.9 Retrograde intubation. Although rarely necessary, this technique is extremely useful in controlling the airway when oral intubate is not possible. In this intraoperative photograph, a tube exchanger is advanced retrograde through the open trachea. The patient sustained devasting facial injuries and near transection of trachea. The tracheostomy tube was inserted prior to transfer.

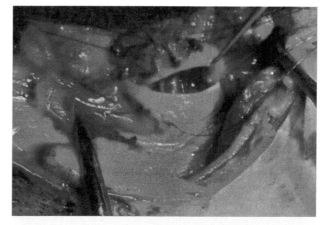

Fig. 7.10 Tracheal repair. This intraoperative photograph is the same patient in ▶ Fig. 7.9. The endotracheal was passed into the distal airway over the tube exchanger. The provided excellent exposure of the tracheal injury, which was repaired in with interrupted absorbable sutures.

7.6.3 Operative Techniques

Lung Injury

Techniques for repair of the injured lung range from suture repair to pneumonectomy. When determining the type of repair required, the surgeon must evaluate the extent of the injury as well as concomitant thoracic injuries. Superficial injuries will be amenable to localized suture repair. If there is an injury tract, not in proximity to the hilum, then a tractotomy can be performed by using a GIA or endostapler.[25,26] Opening the tract will identify bleeding vessels which are then ligated. It is this authors' preference to apply a surgical sealant to raw parenchyma and approximate the staple lines. Although there is a theoretical concern for abscess formation, this has not been observed in practice.

More extensive injuries may be treated with resection. Wedge resection, or a more extensive nonanatomic resection, can be accomplished using a surgical stapler. This is particularly beneficial for injuries located in the lung periphery. If the injury is midlobe or located near the lobar hilum, a formal lobectomy is required. It is optimal to isolate the bronchus from the arterial and venous structures; however, if resection is needed to be quickly performed, the lobe can be taken *en-masse*. Finally, if there is deep parenchymal injury with central hilar hemorrhage, pneumonectomy may be required. Again, it is optimal to take the bronchus separate from the vascular structures. If time and physiology permit, the bronchial stump can be covered with an intercostal muscle flap to decrease the chance of dehiscence. Performing a pneumonectomy is a serious decision and carries a mortality rate as high as 67%.[3] Hemorrhage and acute right heart failure are the most common causes of mortality. Immediately following pneumonectomy, the right heart is subjected to increased pressure and may fail in the postoperative course. Venovenousextracorporeal membrane oxygenation at the time of pneumectomy, and medications to decrease pulmonary vascular resistance and provide right heart inotropic support, should be considered at the time of pneumonectomy.

Vascular Injury

The principles of management of intrathoracic vascular trauma depend on the vessels injured and patient's clinical condition. Much like the tenants of trauma surgery, if the patient is acidotic, hypotensive, hypothermic, and coagulopathic, damage control techniques should be utilized.

Arterial Injuries

With any bleeding vessel, the principles are proximal and distal control. Preoperative planning, adherence to established principles, and precise technical repair are essential. Patients should be widely prepped and draped to allow for adequate exposure of the torso and extremities, and access to veins for harvesting. Proximal control can be obtained at the great vessel origin from the aorta and followed distally. In addition, with the increasing use of endovascular techniques, proximal control of thoracic vessels may be obtained with an endovascular balloon. Once proximal and distal vascular control is achieved, the injured vessel is inspected for any devitalized tissue. It is paramount that in high-velocity injuries such as gunshot wounds, all devitalized tissue should be debrided to ensure proper integrity of the repair. In blunt injuries, arterial stretch can occur over a length of vessel, thus thorough vessel inspection is required to maintain quality tissue and repair integrity.

Prior to repair, antegrade, and retrograde flow must be assessed. If either is inadequate, a thrombectomy should be performed. Most trauma patients are young, thus if inflow if not brisk, the cause is a proximal thrombus rather than preexisting atherosclerotic disease. If thrombectomy fails to improve backbleeding, an intraoperative angiogram may be performed.

Techniques for repair vary in accordance with patient condition, type of injury, and length of vessel damaged. Again, if patients are in a physiologic depleted state, the vessel should be shunted, and definitive repair performed following adequate resuscitation.[5,6] Primary repair may be accomplished with stab wounds, with minimal vessel debridement and a tension-free anastomosis. Partial vessel injuries may be repaired with patch angioplasty, using autologous vein or bovine pericardial patch. With a long segment defect, end-to-end interposition grafting with autologous vein or prosthetic may be necessary. Large caliber great vessels typically require a prosthetic graft rather than vein.

All repairs should be tension-free. After the repair is concluded, vessel patency must be confirmed by the presence of a palpable distal pulse. If there is no palpable pulse, an intraoperative angiogram should be performed, with rapid correction of any problem if encountered. A good rule for repair is to leave the operating room with "a pulse or a picture." Finally, with the advent of endovascular techniques, covered stents and capabilities to bridge arterial occlusions, dissections, and pseudoaneurysms, endovascular repair is an option in select centers.[27]

Vascular repairs should be performed under systemic anticoagulation. In rare circumstance, such as a subdural hematoma or subarachnoid bleeding, local heparization is the alternative. In either case, the heparin is not reversed. It is our practice not to use postoperative systemic anticoagulation but typically prescribe an antiplatelet medication.

Venous Injuries

The same principles exist for venous injury, including exposure and proximal and distal control. Venous injuries may be repaired; however, this is time-consuming and often results in thrombosis and possible embolization of the venous vessel. The exception is the intrathoracic inferior and superior vena cava, which should be repaired without lumen compromise. Ligation of the great veins can be accomplished with little consequence; however, coordination and communication with the anesthesia team is imperative to ensure no central lines are present. Facial edema and limb swelling are the sequela of ligating large veins, which resolves with time and elevation.

Intercostal and Internal Mammary Injuries

Intercostal injuries are commonly injured in penetrating, blunt, and iatrogenic trauma. Intercostal and mammary arteries, while small, are under systemic pressure without substantial surrounding tissue to provide tamponade. These vessels are often difficult to expose and may be tamponaded by the rib retractor. Often overlooked at the initial operation, persistent bleeding will require reoperation. Most chest wall vessels are amenable to proximal and distal ligation by passing a large absorbable suture around the rib. Posterior or inferior vessels, however, are often difficult to control. Posteriorly, the intercostal space is narrow, and the diaphragm may obscure inferior vessel injuries. In this instance, a suture passer may be used to facilitate ligation above and below the rib.[28]

Internal mammary arteries may be injured in penetrating trauma, transected in clamshell thoracotomy, or be injured with a sternotomy. Similar to intercostal arteries, sternal and rib retractors may tamponade the vessel. It is essential to inspect intercostal and internal mammary arteries after retractor removal to ensure there is no injury. These arteries are best controlled with direct ligation.

Pulmonary Vascular Injuries

Unlike their arterial counterpart, the pulmonary vasculature is thin-walled and has limited media and thus will not develop vasospasm. Injures, although rare, may produce impressive bleeding. Due to the low pressure within the pulmonary system, the bleeding encountered in these injuries is like that of a major venous structure. Intestinal Allis clamps may be used to control hemorrhage without occluding the vein. Repair is performed with a running nonabsorbable suture deep to the clamp. Similarly, a side-biting, partial occluding vascular clamp may be used. Widely opening the pericardium will allow the surgeon to gain inflow control to these large venous structures.

Chest Closure

The chest should be closed as expeditiously as possible, when the patient's physiology allows. Typical thoracotomy incisions should be closed in layers, with good approximation of the ribs and appropriate soft tissue coverage. Sternotomy incisions should be closed with the surgeon's system of choice, with care taken to have enough soft tissue coverage over the sternal wires. Importantly, prior to any chest closure, retractors should be slowly removed, and the chest wall examined for any bleeders that have been tamponaded by the retractor.

If the patient's physiology does not allow for definitive closure, there exist varying techniques for temporary closure. Large-bore pleural tubes, pleural packing, and a modified vacuum assist closure device can be placed rapidly if a damage control procedure is performed. Damage control thoracotomy is addressed in another section.

7.7 Complications

Complications in thoracic surgery are related to the specific operation and organs involved. Patients may develop bleeding, atelectasis, respiratory failure, and renal failure due to the initial hypotensive insult and direct lung injury.

Infections are always a risk with thoracic surgery. Due to the robust blood supply of the thoracic wall, thoracotomy wound infections are relatively uncommon and may be managed with local wound care. Sternal wound infection treatment depends on the depth of infection and the presence of sternal dehiscence. With superficial involvement and no dehiscence, this complication may be managed with local wound care and antibiotic therapy. Sternal dehiscence without mediastinitis is managed with operative debridement and closure. The presence of a deep mediastinal infection complicates the management. The principles are adequate drainage, debridement, often multiple, of devitalized bone, cartilage and soft tissue, antibiotics, and definitive closure when the infection is controlled. A vacuum assist closure device may be used until the wound can be closed.[29] Often, a rotational muscle flap is required, and the pectoralis is the ideal choice.[30]

Empyema, although rare, is a serious complication of thoracic surgery. The diagnosis is suspected with persistent leukocytosis, fever, opacity on chest radiograph, and enhancing parietal pleura on chest CT. Diagnosis is confirmed with pleural cultures that guide antibiotic therapy and duration. Direct catheter drainage and antibiotics may resolve a simple empyema. More organized empyema requires decortication with VATs or thoracotomy.[17] Whichever approach is used, the pleural space must be adequately drained and the lung fully expanded.

7.8 Cardiac Injuries

While cardiac injures can result from either blunt or penetrating mechanisms, this section will focus on penetrating injuries. Penetrating cardiac trauma results in substantial mortality, with only slight improvement over decades. One large retrospective study reported cardiac injury in 6% of patients with a penetrating thoracic trauma, with an 80% overall mortality. A prospective study reported an overall mortality of 60%. As expected, gunshot wounds were more lethal than stab wounds. In descending frequency, the chambers involved are the right ventricle, left ventricle, right atrium, and left atrium.[31,32,33]

7.8.1 Presentation and Evaluation

Although penetrating precordial injury has a higher association with cardiac trauma, any thoracic wound can result in myocardial injury, producing hemorrhage or cardiac tamponade. The initial evaluation for penetrating thoracic trauma was discussed in a previous section, but several points need emphasis. The clinical presentation covers the spectrum from normotensive to cardiac arrest, and a seemingly stable compensated patient can rapidly deteriorate to cardiovascular collapse. During the initial evaluation, particular attention should be paid to labile hemodynamics and neck vein distention. Beck's triad, the classic description of tamponade with muffled heart sounds, hypotension and jugular venous distension, is rarely present. Bedside cardiac ultrasound (eFAST) is a crucial modality, with an accuracy of diagnosing hemopericardium approaching 100%. The important limitation is the presence of a hemothorax, since a cardiac injury may decompress into the pleural space, resulting in little or no blood in the pericardium.[34] In this circumstance, or if the image quality is not optimal, a pericardial window is performed in the operating room under general anesthesia. The typical approach is subxiphoid but a transdiaphragmatic technique is used if a concomitant laparotomy is indicated. If the window is positive, a sternotomy is performed. There is no role for a thoracoscopic procedure.[35]

It is imperative that a potential cardiac injury be completely evaluated since a missed injury can be catastrophic.

While the definite treatment of cardiac tamponade is operative, the anesthetic and fluid management are vitally important. Tamponade is highly preload dependent; therefore, adequate preoperative volume resuscitation is essential. Likewise, medications administered during anesthetic induction can result in vasodilation, loss of preload, and cardiovascular collapse. Prepping and draping the patient with tamponade, especially those with compromised hemodynamics prior to induction, facilitates rapid pericardial decompression.

7.8.2 Treatment

Penetrating cardiac injuries require immediate operative repair. The mediastinum can be explored through a median sternotomy or bilateral anterolateral thoracotomy (clamshell), as both provide adequate surgical exposure. The clamshell approach starts as a standard anterolateral thoracotomy, wherein the sternum is divided, and the incision extended to right. The advantages of the clamshell are: general surgeons are familiar with this approach, it can be performed rapidly, and it also provides suitable exposure. Dividing the sternum too inferiorly will limit exposure, particularly to the superior mediastinum, which is the major disadvantage of this approach. The body of the sternum is divided, not the xiphoid. Sternotomy provides exceptional mediastinal exposure and can be expeditiously performed, but may not be as familiar to the general surgeon. Whichever incision is used, the pericardium is widely incised, from the diaphragm to the pericardial reflection superiorly, avoiding the phrenic nerves. A pericardial sling is constructed by tacking the pericardium to the adjacent chest wall. After the pericardium is opened and tamponade relieved by evacuating the hemopericardium, the next priority is hemorrhage control. Direct digital pressure and placement of a Foley catheter and staples are among the options to temporarily control bleeding. The Foley catheter may dislodge, enlarging the cardiac injury, and the staples may be ineffective; therefore, digital control is the authors' favored technique. Once temporary control is achieved, definitive repair is performed.

Although an extensive discussion is beyond the scope of this chapter, there are several salient technical points. Atrial injuries may be amenable to control with a partial occlusion clamp or intestinal Allis clamps. The injury is then closed with a running or horizontal mattress suture, typically 3–0 or 4–0 polypropylene. The posteriorly positioned left atrium is the least frequent injury chamber but can be challenging to repair. Ventricular injuries are generally repaired with 3–0 polypropylene as either a running or interrupted horizontal mattress suture. Using a needle with a larger curve facilitates precise suture placement, which must be coordinated with cardiac contractions. Teflon pledgets can be used for thin or friable ventricular wall.

Following definitive repair and hemostasis, the chest is closed if damage control is not indicated (see section on damage control). Drains are placed in the mediastinum and pleural spaces, if opened. The postoperative care is routine, but a few points are worth mentioning. A postoperative echocardiogram should be obtained. Also, pericarditis (Dressler syndrome) may occur. Diffuse ST changes on electrocardiogram are suggestive, a pericardial friction rub may be heard, and an echocardiogram is performed to evaluate pericardial effusion. The treatment is nonsteroidal, anti-inflammatory medication, or colchicine.

References

[1] Kemmerer WT, Eckert WG, Gathright JB, Reemtsma K, Creech O, Jr. Patterns of thoracic injuries in fatal traffic accidents. J Trauma. 1961; 1:595–599

[2] LoCicero J, III, Mattox KL. Epidemiology of chest trauma. Surg Clin North Am. 1989; 69(1):15–19

[3] O'Connor JV, DuBose JJ, Scalea TM. Damage-control thoracic surgery: Management and outcomes. J Trauma Acute Care Surg. 2014; 77(5):660–665

[4] Johnson JW, Gracias VH, Schwab CW, et al. Evolution in damage control for exsanguinating penetrating abdominal injury. J Trauma. 2001; 51(2):261–269, discussion 269–271

[5] Inaba K, Aksoy H, Seamon MJ, et al. Multicenter Shunt Study Group. Multicenter evaluation of temporary intravascular shunt use in vascular trauma. J Trauma Acute Care Surg. 2016; 80(3):359–364, discussion 364–365

[6] Rasmussen TE, Clouse WD, Jenkins DH, Peck MA, Eliason JL, Smith DL. The use of temporary vascular shunts as a damage control adjunct in the management of wartime vascular injury. J Trauma. 2006; 61(1):8–12, discussion 12–15

[7] Garcia A, Martinez J, Rodriguez J, et al. Damage-control techniques in the management of severe lung trauma. J Trauma Acute Care Surg. 2015; 78(1):45–50, discussion 50–51

[8] Hoksch B, Birken-Bertsch H, Müller JM. Thoracoscopy before Jacobaeus. Ann Thorac Surg. 2002; 74(4):1288–1290

[9] SihoeAlan DL. The Evolution of VATS Lobectomy, Topics in Thoracic Surgery, Prof. Paulo Cardoso (ed) [Internet]. InTech; 2012 [cited 2019 Jun 8]. Available from: https://www.intechopen.com/books/topics-in-thoracic-surgery/the-evolution-of-vats-lobectomy

[10] Ben-Nun A, Orlovsky M, Best LA. Video-assisted thoracoscopic surgery in the treatment of chest trauma: long-term benefit. Ann Thorac Surg. 2007; 83(2):383–387

[11] D. Fullum T. Nembhard C, Williams K, Zafar S, Hwabejire J. The role of laparoscopy/thoracoscopy in acute care surgery. In: Acute Care Surgery [Internet]. 2nd ed. 2018 [cited 2019 Jun 8]. p. 341–64. Available from: https://shop.lww.com/Acute-Care-Surgery/p/9781496370044?promocode=WJ03LCZZ&pid=pe-sitewide-lww-paidsearch-wj03lczz-seer_main_pla_shopping_r&gclid=CjwKEAjwue3nBRCCyrqY0c7bw2wSJACSlmGZeD1xFGAacoJ8M7ZhM_KnkCBveahHv1mEp-Bfukc4ExoCbBDw_wcB

[12] Komatsu T, Neri S, Fuziwara Y, Takahashi Y. Video-assisted thoracoscopic surgery (VATS) for penetrating chest wound: thoracoscopic exploration and removal of a penetrating foreign body. Can J Surg. 2009; 52(6):E301–E302

[13] DuBose J, Inaba K, Okoye O, et al. AAST Retained Hemothorax Study Group. Development of posttraumatic empyema in patients with retained hemothorax: results of a prospective, observational AAST study. J Trauma Acute Care Surg. 2012; 73(3):752–757

[14] Mowery NT, Gunter OL, Collier BR, et al. Practice management guidelines for management of hemothorax and occult pneumothorax. J Trauma. 2011; 70(2):510–518

[15] Halat G, Negrin LL, Chrysou K, Hoksch B, Schmid RA, Kocher GJ. Treatment of air leak in polytrauma patients with blunt chest injury. Injury. 2017; 48(9):1895–1899

[16] Smith JW, Franklin GA, Harbrecht BG, Richardson JD. Early VATS for blunt chest trauma: a management technique underutilized by acute care surgeons. J Trauma. 2011; 71(1):102–105, discussion 105–107

[17] O'Connor JV, Chi A, Joshi M, DuBose J, Scalea TM. Post-traumatic empyema: aetiology, surgery and outcome in 125 consecutive patients. Injury. 2013; 44(9):1153–1158

[18] Goodman M, Lewis J, Guitron J, Reed M, Pritts T, Starnes S. Video-assisted thoracoscopic surgery for acute thoracic trauma. J Emerg Trauma Shock. 2013; 6(2):106–109

[19] Bagheri R, Tavassoli A, Sadrizadeh A, Mashhadi MR, Shahri F, Shojaeian R. The role of thoracoscopy for the diagnosis of hidden diaphragmatic injuries in penetrating thoracoabdominal trauma. Interact Cardiovasc Thorac Surg. 2009; 9(2):195–197, discussion 197–198

[20] Bender B, Murthy V, Chamberlain RS. The changing management of chylothorax in the modern era. Eur J Cardiothorac Surg. 2016; 49(1):18–24

[21] Milanchi S, Makey I, McKenna R, Margulies DR. Video-assisted thoracoscopic surgery in the management of penetrating and blunt thoracic trauma. J Minim Access Surg. 2009; 5(3):63–66

[22] Andrade-Alegre R. Pericardioscopy for diagnosing penetrating cardiac trauma. Ann Thorac Surg. 2015; 99(5):e115–e116

[23] Burack JH, Kandil E, Sawas A, et al. Triage and outcome of patients with mediastinal penetrating trauma. Ann Thorac Surg. 2007; 83(2):377–382, discussion 382

[24] Lochowski MP, Kozak J. Video-assisted thoracic surgery complications. Wideochir Inne Tech Malo Inwazyjne. 2014; 9(4):495–500

[25] Wall MJ, Jr, Hirshberg A, Mattox KL. Pulmonary tractotomy with selective vascular ligation for penetrating injuries to the lung. Am J Surg. 1994; 168(6): 665–669

[26] Asensio JA, Demetriades D, Berne JD, et al. Stapled pulmonary tractotomy: a rapid way to control hemorrhage in penetrating pulmonary injuries. J Am Coll Surg. 1997; 185(5):486–487

[27] Matsagkas M, Kouvelos G, Peroulis M, Xanthopoulos D, Bouris V, Arnaoutoglou E. Endovascular repair of blunt axillo-subclavian arterial injuries as the first line treatment. Injury. 2016; 47(5):1051–1056

[28] Park H, Glaser J, Florecki K, et al. A novel, minimally invasive approach to assure hemostasis for intercostal bleeding after trauma. J Trauma Acute Care Surg. 2018; 84(6):1027–1029

[29] Agarwal JP, Ogilvie M, Wu LC, et al. Vacuum-assisted closure for sternal wounds: a first-line therapeutic management approach. Plast Reconstr Surg. 2005; 116(4):1035–1040, discussion 1041–1043

[30] Jones G, Jurkiewicz MJ, Bostwick J, et al. Management of the infected median sternotomy wound with muscle flaps. The Emory 20-year experience. Ann Surg. 1997; 225(6):766–776, discussion 776–778

[31] Tyburski JG, Astra L, Wilson RF, Dente C, Steffes C. Factors affecting prognosis with penetrating wounds of the heart. J Trauma. 2000; 48(4):587–590, discussion 590–591

[32] Asensio JA, Murray J, Demetriades D, et al. Penetrating cardiac injuries: a prospective study of variables predicting outcomes. J Am Coll Surg. 1998; 186(1):24–34

[33] Mandal AK, Sanusi M. Penetrating chest wounds: 24 years experience. World J Surg. 2001; 25(9):1145–1149

[34] Ball CG, Williams BH, Wyrzykowski AD, Nicholas JM, Rozycki GS, Feliciano DV. A caveat to the performance of pericardial ultrasound in patients with penetrating cardiac wounds. J Trauma. 2009; 67(5):1123–1124

[35] Paci M, Ferrari G, Annessi V, de Franco S, Guasti G, Sgarbi G. The role of diagnostic VATS in penetrating thoracic injuries. World J Emerg Surg. 2006; 1:30

**Expert Commentary on
Thoracic Trauma by**
Gregory J. Jurkovich

Expert Commentary on Thoracic Trauma

Gregory J. Jurkovich

Thoracic trauma, as the authors have pointed out, is a special subset of trauma patients. While I might dispute the statement that 50% of all trauma deaths under the age of 40 are due to thoracic trauma (old data), there is no doubt that breathing and cardiac output are essential to life. The airway, breathing, and circulation (ABC) of trauma care, as promoted by the elegant simplicity of the advanced trauma life support (ATLS) course, emphasize the importance of a patent airway (A) to provide oxygen inflow to the lungs, and adequate mechanics of breathing (B) to allow air–blood oxygen exchange. These essential components of life are often disrupted by thoracic trauma, and the goal of any management strategy should be to correct abnormalities in this system.

Intubation techniques including medications, devices, and adjuncts have rapidly changed in the past decade, along with the more widespread (but unproven) use of airway devices that avoid the technical expertise needed for endotracheal intubation. While there is debate on this topic, the best airway control device remains endotracheal intubation. The authors comment on the use of the extended focused assessment with sonography in trauma (eFAST) to evaluate the sliding of the pleura and the pericardial space in addition to the standard abdominal component of the examination, but this expanded use of FAST is just beginning to be widely adopted, albeit with incomplete data on its accuracy in nonexpert hands. A chest radiograph to supplement a competent physical examination remains the standard of care in chest trauma of any nature.

Immediate indications for operation following thoracic trauma remain unusual, or at least uncommon, as the majority of chest trauma pathology can be managed with airway control and a chest tube. However, massive hemorrhage or ongoing significant bleeding remains an important indication for surgery that should neither be avoided nor should clinicians adopt a "wait and see" attitude. I agree with the authors advise that 1500 mL immediate output, and I would add 500 mL per hour over 3 hours, are clear indications for a thoracotomy; I would also add that a second chest tube during any monitoring of thoracic blood loss might be needed to avoid the pitfall of an occluded tube thoracostomy and unrecognized ongoing thoracic bleeding.[1]

Diagnosing esophageal injury remains a challenge and, in order to be sure, computed tomography (CT) or video-esophagography is an excellent diagnostic technique. Most transmediastinal penetrating wounds, particularly those with a posterior trajectory, mandate esophageal imaging. It is reassuring that CT of the chest as part of the workup of thoracic trauma for a pneumomediastinum is accurate (100% sensitivity and 85% specificity) in identifying patients with major blunt aerodigestive trauma.[2]

It is appropriate for the authors to have some extended comments on less invasive methods of examining the pleural space and repairing some injures. Video-assisted surgical procedures have clear advantages, and the chest cavity, particularly if the lung can be collapsed intentionally, is nicely amendable to inspection, evacuation of retained blood or empyema, and repair of simple lung and diaphragm injuries. Timing and use of video-assisted thoracoscopic surgery (VATS) to evacuate retained fluid collections remain an area in need of better clarity, as does the role of rib-plating.

Every trauma surgeon, indeed every general surgeon, must be competent in gaining access to the thoracic cavity and mediastinum. The lateral thoracotomy and the median sternotomy must remain essential components of training of the acute care surgeon. The authors provide little technical details on these procedures, but I assume that this is because they too feel all trainees in surgery must have mastered these highly technical skills. Managing an injury to the pulmonary hilum is too rare to be an expectation of expertise of all surgeons. However, trauma OR rooms should have readily available, or on the wall, key anatomical illustrations of this anatomy, and surgical expertise in thin-vessel suture ligation is essential. Finally, the control of cardiac wounds is nicely described, but the use of the skinstapler to provide temporary control of ventricular wounds should be emphasized over the use of the Foley catheter and balloon, as the balloon may migrate and may compromise outflow.[3]

References

[1] Karmy-Jones R, Jurkovich GJ, Nathens AB, et al. Timing of urgent thoracotomy for hemorrhage after trauma: a multicenter study. Arch Surg. 2001; 136(5): 513–518

[2] Dissanaike S, Shalhub S, Jurkovich GJ. The evaluation of pneumomediastinum in blunt trauma patients. J Trauma. 2008; 65(6):1340–1345

[3] Shamoun JM, Barraza KR, Jurkovich GJ, Salley RK. In extremis use of staples for cardiorrhaphy in penetrating cardiac trauma: case report. J Trauma. 1989; 29(11):1589–1591

8 Vascular Trauma

Jason Pasley, Megan Brenner, and Raul Coimbra

Summary

Rapid identification and treatment of vascular injuries is of utmost importance in trauma patients. Physical exam, along with adjuncts, such as X-ray and ultrasound, can help identify likely sources. A strong knowledge of anatomic approaches and operative considerations from the neck, torso, to the extremities is needed. In addition to open definitive management of vascular trauma, damage control methods for vascular trauma should be considered for patients in extremis, including tourniquets, pelvic binders, as well as vascular shunts. Depending on the facility and capability of the operative team, endovascular methods can be considered to assist in diagnosis, temporizing hemorrhage (resuscitative endovascular balloon occlusion of the aorta [REBOA]), definitive control or in some cases, a hybrid procedure.

Keywords: Vascular injury, operative exposure, REBOA, angiographic considerations

8.1 Introduction

Vascular injury and associated hemorrhage are significant causes of mortality in trauma. In mature trauma systems with developed prehospital care, interventions such as tourniquet placement and permissive hypotension allow patients with life-threatening hemorrhage to arrive at hospitals alive but in need of emergent management of bleeding. External bleeding can be at times easily identified, however, some cases of vascular trauma may not be immediately life-threatening or apparent. Therefore, in the polytrauma patient, a high index of suspicion is necessary and appropriate workup must ensue.

The common types of arterial injury are: intimal injuries (flaps, disruptions, or subintimal/intramural hematomas); partial or completely transmural defects with pseudoaneurysm or hemorrhage; transection with occlusion and/or hemorrhage; arteriovenous (AV) fistulas and arterial spasm. Blunt trauma usually causes intimal flaps and intramural hematomas, whereas penetrating trauma typically causes partial or complete transections, AV fistulas, and hemorrhage and/or thrombosis.[1]

Patients who present to the trauma bay with hypotension are considered to be in hemorrhagic shock and a bleeding source (s) must be identified. This may include a solid organ injury or a vascular injury. The advanced trauma life support (ATLS) principles should be followed, including external hemorrhage control with direct pressure, tourniquets, or clamps, if available and needed. Mechanism of injury can clue the provider to specific areas to investigate further; for example, a chest X-ray following a head-on collision with steering wheel abrasions on the chest may demonstrate signs of a thoracic aortic injury such as an apical cap or widened mediastinum that would require further imaging and treatment. A pelvic X-ray can be helpful in determining if likely significant bleeding is ongoing and if bedside intervention is needed, such as a binder. It can also help determine from which side of the pelvis hemorrhage is likely occurring.

Peritonitis on physical examination can clue the physician into an intra-abdominal injury which may be solid organ bleeding, vascular injury, perforated viscus, or a combination of perforation and hemorrhage. The focused abdominal sonography for trauma (FAST) may be used to visualize free fluid in the abdominal cavity, although the examination is not adequately sensitive to determine which type of fluid is present.

Hard signs and symptoms of vascular injury in the extremity include active/pulsatile bleeding, expanding or pulsatile hematoma, pulselessness, audible bruit, palpable thrill, shock not explained by other injuries, or evidence of regional ischemia (pain, pallor, paresthesia, paralysis, or pulselessness). Patients with hard signs of vascular injury require emergent proximal control and open or endovascular repair.

Soft signs and symptoms suggestive of vascular trauma include a stable/nonexpanding hematoma, slow bleeding, wounds in the proximity of a major neurovascular tract, peripheral nerve injury, and diminished pulses. Patients with soft signs should undergo diagnostic testing at the very least, if not exploration when other injuries permit.

Long bone fractures or dislocations can alter anatomic relationships after injury. If these are present, reduction should be performed and a complete vascular examination conducted to figure which additional workup is necessary. Documentation of perfusion before and after reduction should be thorough, and objective measures such as the ankle–brachial index can aid in determining when a further workup is required. Posterior knee dislocations are associated with popliteal artery injuries; therefore, further workup should ensue if distal perfusion is not baseline or equal to the contralateral limb.

8.2 Diagnostic Testing

The chest X-ray (CXR) is the primary screening modality for thoracic aortic injury. The aorta is typically injured at fixation points, most commonly the ligamentumarteriosum, just distal to the takeoff of the left subclavian artery. Other areas include the aortic root, near the isthmus, and at the entrance to the diaphragm. Key radiographic signs suggestive of an aortic injury on CXR are a widened mediastinum of 8 cm at the level of T4, obliteration of the aortic knob, rightward tracheal deviation, pleural cap usually on the left but occasionally bilaterally, rightward shift and elevation of the right mainstem bronchus, depression of the left mainstem bronchus, loss of the aorto-pulmonary window, deviation of the nasogastric tube to the right, and left pleural effusion.[2] No single sign reliably confirms or excludes aortic injury, but a widened mediastinum (with a mechanism consistent with possible injury) is the most consistent finding on CXR, prompting further evaluation. Some patients with traumatic aortic injury will have a normal CXR; therefore, liberal use of contrast-enhanced computed tomography (CT) with angiography (CTA) scanning should be performed.[2]

A pelvic X-ray should be performed in the trauma bay, especially in a hypotensive patient. Specific patterns, such as vertical shear fractures, bilateral pubic rami (butterfly) fractures,

fractures with involvement of the posterior elements (sacrum and iliac bone/joint), and fractures leading to increased pelvic volume due to pubic symphysis diastasis of more than 2.5 cm, are associated with a higher likelihood of arterial bleeding.[3,4]

If an open book pelvic fracture is diagnosed, an abdominal binder, sheet, or another method for temporary stabilization should be employed to reduce pelvic volume and decrease hemorrhage. Ligamentous disruption requires a significant force; however, the presence of a major ligamentous disruption does not necessarily lead to hemorrhage, therefore the fracture pattern should not be the sole method to be used for determining the need for angiography. Pelvic injuries can be classified into mild, moderate, and severe. The World Society of Emergency Surgery (WSES) developed a system to group these fractures. Minor pelvic fractures are WSES grade I, including anteroposterior compression (APC) I and lateral compression (LC) I hemodynamically stable pelvic ring injuries. Moderate

pelvic fractures are noted as WSES grade II, including APC II–III and LC II–III hemodynamically stable pelvic ring injuries, as well as WSES grade III, including vertical shear (VS) and combined mechanism (CM) hemodynamically stable pelvic ring injuries. Severe pelvic injuries are WSES grade IV and include any hemodynamically unstable pelvic ring injury.[5]

Physiology, grade, associated injuries, and response to resuscitation should help guide diagnosis and treatment (▶ Fig. 8.1).[5] Further imaging tests can define patients who may benefit from angiography.[6]

Extremity vascular injuries can be complex. Initial suspicion should be high in the presence of hard and soft signs of injury. Pseudoaneurysms, AV fistulas, and intimal tears will not result in diminished pulses or altered acquired brain injuries (ABIs). These injuries can only be identified by CTA, angiography, or arterial duplex exams. The "injured extremity index (IEI)" can reliably determine if further testing is indicated to rule out a

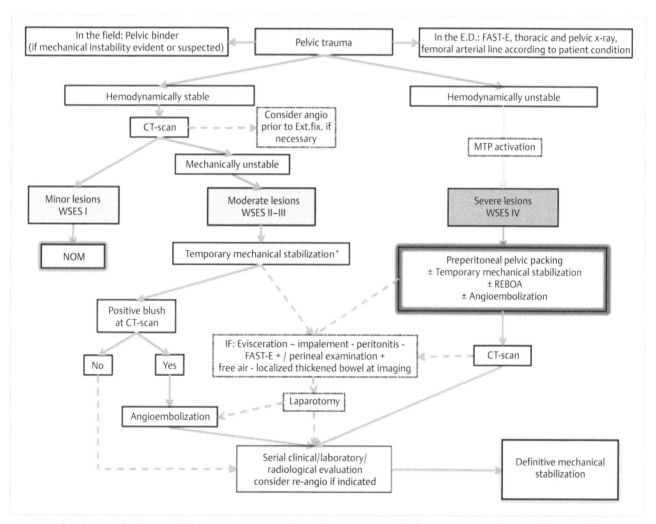

Fig. 8.1 Pelvic trauma algorithm based on World Society of Emergency Surgery (WSES) Classification and Guidelines. Pelvic trauma management algorithm (*: patients hemodynamically stable and mechanically unstable, with no other lesions requiring treatment and negative CT scan, can proceed directly to definitive mechanical stabilization. MTP: massive transfusion protocol, FAST-E: Eco-FAST extended, ED: emergency department, CT: computed tomography, NOM: nonoperative management. Hemodynamic stability is the condition in which the patients achieve a constant or an amelioration of blood pressure after fluids with a blood pressure > 90 mmHg and heart rate < 100 bpm. Hemodynamic instability is the condition in which the patient has an admission systolic blood pressure < 90 mmHg, or > 90 mmHg, but requiring bolus infusions/transfusions and/or vasopressor drugs, admission base deficit [BD] > 6 mmol/l, shock index > 1, or transfusion requirement of at least 4–6 units of packed red blood cells within the first 24 h).

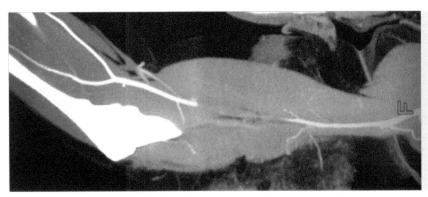

Fig. 8.2 Computed tomography angiography of the upper extremity showing brachial disruption.

vascular injury. A blood pressure cuff is inflated over the injured extremity while using a Doppler to assess the pulse. This systolic pressure is then divided by the systolic arterial pressure of an unaffected limb, resulting in a value. An index above 0.9 excludes injury, while a value of less than 0.9 warrants further investigation including CTA, angiogram, or surgical exploration.[7,8]

CTA has replaced conventional angiography as the initial screening tool for vascular evaluation in the neck, chest, abdomen, pelvis, and extremities. CTA can be performed rapidly with a high-sensitivity for vascular injury[9,10] (▶ Fig. 8.2). If the patient is in the operating room for other more urgent injuries, an angiogram can be performed if the correct equipment is available (OSI table, vascular C-arm, or endovascular supplies). The hybrid operating room is particularly attractive for this purpose, as diagnosis and treatment of these injuries can occur in a single setting.

8.3 Operative Considerations and Approaches

An angiographic compatible operating room (OR) bed is key for assistance in injury identification or additional intraoperative imaging. The affected area, as well as potential sites for vein harvest and distal vascular pulse examinations, should be widely prepped and draped.

Proximal and distal control of the injured artery or vein is the basic tenant of vascular surgery. Once the injury is identified, local control can be obtained with vascular clamps, bulldogs, or vessel loops. Standard teaching recommends obtaining proximal control away from the zone of injury. For example, control of a mid-superficial femoral artery (SFA) injury can occur through a separate incision at the common femoral artery (CFA) or proximal SFA, or the incision can be made directly over the area of injury and extended proximally and distally. If the injury is noted in the neck or upper extremity, the chest should be prepped, in case a sternotomy, thoracotomy or a clavicular incision is needed for proximal control. In a lower extremity injury, the abdomen should be prepped, in case retroperitoneal access is needed to the external iliac arteries. If the injury is to an extremity and it is distal to the groin or axilla, a sterile pneumatic tourniquet can serve as inflow control until the vessel can be properly dissected and controlled. In all vascular cases, bilateral groin and thigh areas should be included, as saphenous vein from the uninjured extremity may be harvested as a potential conduit.

Once the injured vessel is isolated both proximally and distally, vessel loops and/or clamps are used for inflow and outflow control (▶ Fig. 8.3a, b). The injury should be assessed as to whether a simple or complex repair is required (see repair options) (▶ Fig. 8.3c, d). Additional injuries and the patient's hemodynamic status should be considered. In the case of complex injury and/or if the patient is unstable, vessel shunting can be used as a temporizing damage control measure (see shunt section).

In stable patients with an isolated vascular injury, systemic heparinization should be considered. Usually 5000 (50–75 units/kg) units IV should suffice, and a heparin drip at 500 U should be considered through the course of the procedure. If the patient has an associated torso or head injury, systemic heparin should be avoided and local heparinization should be used instead. Proximal and distal injection of heparinized saline of 20 to 25 mL per site (50 U/mL) should be given prior to repair to aid in preventing thrombosis.

Prior to repair and local heparinization, an appropriately sized Fogerty catheter must be passed proximally and distally to clear the vessel of any thrombus. Distally, the catheter should be passed until no clot has returned on two consecutive passes. Appropriately sized Fogerty catheters include a #6 for the common and external iliac arteries, #4 to #5 for the CFA, #4 for the SFA, #3 to #4 for the popliteal artery, and a #3 for the other arteries of the leg. Tissue plasminogen activator (tPA) can be administered locally as well for distal thrombosis. Papaverine or nitroglycerin must be available for injection in cases of vasospasm. Angiography should be used liberally to confirm that no distal thrombus is present both before and after repair. Embolectomy catheters should not be passed in venous injuries as they will disrupt the veins due to valves.[11]

After a vascular repair is complete, a palpable pulse should be noted distally and compared to the contralateral side, if applicable. If there is any doubt about blood distal flow, an angiogram with access proximal to the anastomosis should be performed to assess patency of the repair, run-off, and distal perfusion.

8.3.1 Thoracic Aorta and Great Vessels

If the patient is *in extremis*, the best open surgical approach to the descending aorta is via a left anterolateral thoracotomy and further access to the aortic arch and great vessels via a clamshell thoracotomy. The patient should be in the supine position with the left arm extended above the head. For a left-sided

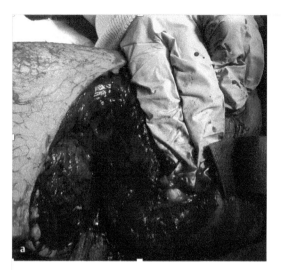
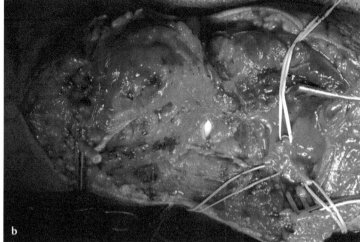
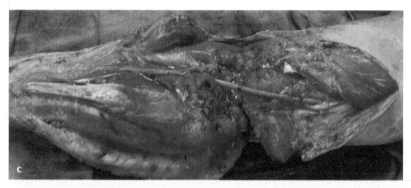
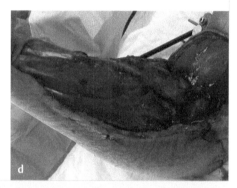

Fig. 8.3 **(a)** Right brachial artery transection with manual compression for proximal control during prepping and draping. **(b)** Brachial artery transection. Proximal control with clamp at brachial artery, vessel loops around interosseus, and radial andulnar arteries. The injury transected the median, ulnar nerves, and cephalic and basilic veins down to the radial head. **(c)** The brachial artery and cephalic veins were repaired with interposition grafts from the left reversed greater saphenous vein. **(d)** The median and ulnar nerves were repaired primarily after external fixation in a semi-flexed position, and muscle flaps were used to cover the vascular repairs.

thoracotomy, the initial incision should start just to the right side of the sternum and continue along the 5th intercostal space toward the left axilla in a curved fashion. Anatomically, this space is delineated just below the nipple line in males and the inframammary crease in females. The incision is started on the right side of the sternum in case sternal division is required for a clamshell thoracotomy. The skin, subcutaneous tissue, and chest wall muscle are divided sharply. Once the intercostal muscle is encountered, this is taken down sharply with either a scalpel or scissors, attempting to stay on the superior portion of the rib to avoid injuring the neurovascular bundle. Once the cavity is entered, a Finochietto retractor can be placed and the ribs spread to facilitate exposure. If further exposure is required, the sternum can be divided with a Lebshe knife and the right-sided chest wall divided in a similar fashion to the left. From there, the pericardium can be opened longitudinally and anteriorly to the phrenic nerve in order to provide access to the heart and the aortic root. Further dissection and division of the innominate vein can provide access to the aortic arch and great vessels. Digital pressure is typically the best initial method for hemorrhage control, until vascular clamps can be positioned appropriately. If a clamshell thoracotomy is performed, both the

left and right internal mammary arteries must be identified and ligated proximally and distally to prevent postoperative hemorrhage and return to the operating room.[12]

In stable patients, a sternotomy is the best approach for visualization of the aortic arch and great vessels. The sternotomy can be extended to the neck if further exposure is needed for the subclavian or carotid arteries. With regard to a median sternotomy, the incision is made from the sternal notch to the xiphoid. The xiphoid is typically excised. Blunt finger dissection is then performed to free any pericardial attachments from both the superior and inferior direction. A sternal saw is then used to divide the sternum in the midline. The sternal retractor is thereafter placed. The pericardium can be entered, and the arch vessels exposed as described above.[12]

The proximal right subclavian and innominate arteries are best approached through a median sternotomy. The proximal left subclavian artery is best approached through a left anterolateral thoracotomy, although the exposure of the proximal left subclavian artery is completely feasible by a median sternotomy incision. A trap-door incision, combining a left anterolateral thoracotomy with partial median sternotomy and left clavicular incision, is rarely needed and is painful and morbid. Clavicular division or resection is sometimes necessary. In rare circumstances, the subclavian artery can be ligated distal to the takeoff of the vertebral artery.[12]

A left posterolateral thoracotomy is the best approach for a descending aortic injury not amenable to endovascular treatment. The patient is placed in a right lateral decubitus position with the left side up and intubated with a double-lumen tube to collapse the left lung during the critical portions of the operation. The incision is made two fingerbreadths below the tip of the scapula, following the rib contour both anteriorly and posteriorly. The muscles can be divided or spared. If further posterior visualization is needed, the latissimus dorsi muscle may be divided or retracted. Once the pleura is entered, the Finnochieto retractor is placed. Occasionally, a rib is transected for further exposure. Proximal control of the aorta is usually obtained between takeoff of the left carotid artery and the left subclavian artery. Blunt aortic injury is rarely treated by the open technique, but when indicated, patients benefit tremendously from a peripheral partial bypass with the Biomedicus pump.

8.3.2 Neck Exposure

The neck can be divided into three zones. Zone I extends from the clavicle to the cricoid cartilage, Zone II extends from the cricoid cartilage to the angle of the mandible, and Zone III from the angle of the mandible to the skull base. The easiest zone to explore is Zone II. With injuries in Zone I and Zone III, additional imaging is typically helpful in surgical planning and repair options. In patients with acute active bleeding, hemodynamic instability, pulsatile hematoma, or signs of aerodigestive injuries, operative intervention should be performed.

8.3.3 Carotid Artery

The carotid artery and the internal jugular vein can be exposed by an anterior sternocleidomastoid (SCM) incision. The head and chest should also be included in the operative field, in case entry into the chest or further cranial dissection is needed. The incision is carried out from the mandible to the clavicular head. If superior extension is necessary, the incision should be curved posteriorly toward the mastoid process to avoid injuring the mandibular branch of the facial nerve. The platysma is divided, exposing the SCM muscle. The SCM is retracted laterally, exposing the neurovascular sheath. The facial vein, which crosses the bifurcation of the common carotid to the internal and external carotid arteries, is usually divided. The carotid sheath can be entered anteriorly, extending the dissection cranially and caudally, and exposing the internal jugular vein, the vagus nerve and the common carotid artery. Near the bifurcation of the common carotid artery, the hypoglossal nerve runs in a perpendicular fashion and care should be taken to not injure it. If additional exposure is required, the omohyoid and digastric muscles can be divided. For high-neck injuries, subluxation or an osteotomy of the mandible may be needed for additional exposure of the internal carotid artery. Assistance from oral and maxillofacial surgery (OMFS) is recommended for these procedures. Alternatively, these high injuries may be best approached by using endovascular techniques.[12]

8.3.4 Vertebral Artery Exposure

A significant portion of the vertebral artery (C6–C2) is covered by the bony canal of the cervical spine. Due to this, most injuries should be addressed by an endovascular approach. If an open approach is required, the SCM incision noted above is performed. With medial retraction of the carotid sheath and lateral retraction of the scalene fat pad, the anterior scalene muscle and inferior thyroid artery are identified. The vertebral artery will be visualized after division of the inferior thyroid artery and lateral retraction of the anterior scalene muscle. Another approach to the origin of the vertebral artery is via a supraclavicular incision and division of the SCM, providing access to the proximal common carotid artery and origin of the vertebral artery from the subclavian artery.[12] Temporization of vertebral artery hemorrhage can be achieved with Foley insertion and balloon inflation until exposure can be obtained. If bleeding does not stop, an osteotomy of the transverse process may provide direct access to the bleeding site, where a Fogarty catheter may be inserted and its balloon inflated for bleeding control.

8.3.5 Axillary Artery Exposure

The axillary artery begins after the subclavian artery crosses beneath the first rib. Overlying this, the pectoralis minor muscle divides the artery into three portions. As the artery courses across the lower border of the Teres Major muscle, it becomes the brachial artery. To access the axillary artery, the initial incision begins at the inferior edge of the center of the clavicle running in the deltopectoral groove. If the patient is hemodynamically stable, the pectoralis major can be retracted or split at the level of its fibers or, if unstable, can be divided 2 cm from its insertion into the humeral head. The pectoralis minor can then be divided using electrocautery. This provides access to the second portion of the axillary artery. The axillary artery is superior to the brachial plexus and the axillary vein usually courses just inferior to the artery.[12]

8.3.6 Brachial Artery

The brachial artery courses in a subcutaneous fashion in the biceps groove between the biceps and triceps on the medial side of the upper extremity. It courses laterally at the antecubital fossa with collaterals arising around the elbow. Two veins accompany the artery, usually on either side. The median nerve runs anterior to the brachial artery and the ulnar nerve posteriorly. Midway down the arm, the median nerve crosses the artery and runs along the posteromedial side of the artery.[12]

The operative incision is carried out over the groove between the triceps and biceps muscle bellies. The incision can be extended obliquely across the antecubital fossa laterally if exposure of the bifurcation to the radial and ulnar arteries is needed. Veins in this area should be preserved. The brachial or basilic vein in this area can sometimes be used as a replacement conduit for an injured brachial artery, so care should be taken not to injure them in dissection. Distally, the bicipital tendon can be divided if the bifurcation of the brachial artery needs to be exposed. The median cubital vein sits on top of the tendon.[12]

8.3.7 Abdominal Aorta and the Inferior Vena Cava (IVC)

All Zone I retroperitoneal hematomas encountered at laparotomy should be explored, whether the injury is penetrating or blunt. Proximal control of the aorta at the diaphragmatic hiatus can be performed by vertically incising the lesser omentum and creating a window between the distal esophagus and liver. The left crus can either be split along its fibers or divided. Blunt dissection is carried out, typically with a finger to clear the aorta from the loose connective tissue. At this point, the aorta can be occluded manually, with a sponge stick, or clamp.[12]

Other options for proximal abdominal aortic control include endovascular balloon occlusion, or distal thoracic aortic cross-clamping through a left anterior lateral thoracotomy. Balloon occlusion and descending thoracic aortic clamping possess the advantage of achieving proximal control away from the area of injury/hematoma.

Proximal Zone I retroperitoneal bleeding injuries are usually approached through the abdomen with a left medial visceral rotation. The white line of Toldt is divided laterally and the colon is mobilized medially. The spleen is mobilized by freeing the lienosplenic ligament, either bluntly, sharply, or with electrocautery. The spleen, stomach, tail of the pancreas, and colon are all rotated medially to expose the aorta. The kidney may be left in its normal anatomic position or mobilized anteriorly, depending on the area of the aorta requiring exposure. Through an extensive medial visceral rotation, the celiac, superior mesenteric, and inferior mesenteric arteries can be identified at their origin.[12]

Distal Zone I retroperitoneal injuries are approached by a right-sided medial visceral rotation. The white line of Toldt is divided lateral to the ascending colon from the cecum to the hepatic flexure. The colon is then rotated medially and upward, dissecting the mesentery of the small bowel to the root of the retroperitoneum. The duodenum can be medialized by a Kocher maneuver, incising the lateral peritoneal attachments. The suprarenal and infrarenal IVC from the inferior liver to the iliac bifurcation can be visualized. Using this maneuver, the IVC and aortic bifurcations, right-sided common, internal and external iliac arteries, veins and the proximal portion of the left common iliac artery, and vein are visible.[12] In certain cases, where the bleeding source is arterial, the infrarenal aorta can be best exposed by mobilizing the small bowel to the right side of the abdomen, as well as the left colon, similar to the surgical approach to ruptured infrarenal abdominal aortic aneurysms. The retroperitoneum is opened at the ligament of Treitz, exposing the aorta. Further dissection can then be carried out distally to expose the necessary area of the aorta or common iliac arteries for the purpose of repair.[12]

Retrohepatic and suprahepatic IVC injuries require division of the hepatic ligaments and mobilization of the right lobe of the liver. Considerations for approaching these injuries include atrial–caval shunting or total hepatic exclusion.[13] Atrial–caval shunting is performed by passing a large-bore chest tube from the right atrium into the vena cava via a thoracotomy or sternotomy. A purse-string suture is placed in the right atrium and the atrium is opened. An additional side hole is cut into the distal part of the chest tube to allow for blood flow to enter the right atrium. The proximal chest tube is fed down the atrium into the juxtarenal IVC, umbilical tapes placed above and below the renal veins will secure the shunt in place, allowing blood flow from the infrarenal IVC as well as from the renal veins to enter the shunt and be delivered into the right atrium. At the right atrium, the distal end of the chest tube is clamped, and the purse- string is tightened.

Total hepatic exclusion is performed by obtaining proximal control of the IVC above the renal veins as well as above the liver by clamping the suprahepatic IVC, either in the abdomen or inside the pericardial sac. To access the intrapericardial portion of the IVC, the central tendon of the diaphragm can be divided, pericardial sac opened, and vascular clamp placed in the IVC, below its entrance in the right atrium. This maneuver is advantageous as it does not require opening the chest. Alternatively, a median sternotomy or a thoracophrenotomy may be performed to expose the suprahepatic IVC. A Pringle maneuver is also performed to complete the total hepatic isolation. Attempts can then be made to repair the injured portion of the IVC. Mortality rates following retrohepatic or suprahepatic IVC injuries vary from 50 to 90%.[14,15] An additional option for total hepatic isolation is a Pringle maneuver and endovascular balloon occlusion of both the IVC and supraceliac aorta.

8.3.8 Celiac Artery

The celiac artery can be approached from the side by exposing it via a left medial visceral rotation or anteriorly, through the lesser sac, by dividing the gastrohepatic and left triangular ligaments.[16,17,18] Atraumatic clamps or vessel loops can be used for vascular control. Injuries in this area can be repaired or even ligated due to significant collaterals from the superior mesenteric artery (SMA). If the celiac artery is ligated, a cholecystectomy should be performed as gallbladder ischemia is common.[19]

8.3.9 Superior Mesenteric Artery (SMA)

Exposure of the proximal SMA can be performed using a left medial visceral rotation or via the lesser sac with or without transection of the pancreatic neck or at the root of the mesentery underneath the pancreas.[20] Distal SMA injuries can be approached from the left side by dividing the ligament of Treitz, or from the right side by mobilizing the duodenum off of the SMA. SMA repair should be performed if possible; however, in the unstable patient, it can be ligated or shunted. SMA ligation was noted to be well-tolerated in two large series;[21] however, bowel ischemia may occur, particularly when additional injuries are present. Therefore, patients should undergo temporary abdominal closure and a second-look exploration within 24 hours.

8.3.10 Inferior Mesenteric Artery (IMA)

IMA injuries can be approached directly through the mesentery and repaired. Ligation can be performed for lesions that are complex or destructive or in the unstable patient, due to extensive collateral circulation.[20] Rarely, ligation may lead to distal colon and rectal ischemia, which is similar to the ischemia noted from covering the IMA in endovascular repair of abdominal aortic aneurysms. Colonic ischemia monitoring is necessary, especially in patients with poor collateral flow, atherosclerotic disease, or prior bowel resection.[18]

8.3.11 Portal Vein (PV) and Superior Mesenteric Vein (SMV)

PV and SMV injuries are rare and usually associated with penetrating trauma.[22,23,24] Injuries to surrounding structures are frequent and mortality is high. A Pringle maneuver should be performed with either a vessel loop or clamp. A direct approach is usually used as the hematoma has often completed much of the dissection of the portal structures. Once the hematoma is evacuated, the injury should be visualized. Formal proximal and distal control can then be obtained. In order to access the proximal PV, duodenal mobilization with a Kocher maneuver can be extended to a right medial visceral rotation. Pancreatic neck division is required at times for full exposure of the distal SMV and splenic vein junction.

PV injuries can be repaired, reconstructed, or ligated. Ligation may be tolerated if the hepatic artery is patent. Studies have shown that if ligation is performed for damage control, it should be performed as early as possible for improved survival, as compared to late ligation.[25] Mesenteric venous congestion may ensue with reduced systemic venous return. SMV injuries can also be repaired, reconstructed, or ligated. Intestinal ischemia and compartment syndrome may occur if the vein is ligated; therefore, temporary abdominal closure and a second look laparotomy is warranted, given the risks of intestinal ischemia from venous outflow obstruction and abdominal compartment syndrome. For patients in extremis, shunts may be considered as opposed to ligation as a damage control strategy for SMV and PV injuries.[23]

8.3.12 Renal Artery and Vein

Zone II retroperitoneal hematomas due to penetrating injury should be explored. Blunt injuries need to be explored if the hematoma is expanding or has pulsatile bleeding. A majority of the injuries will be sustained by the renal parenchyma itself, although injuries to the renal artery and vein can also occur.

For Zone II hemorrhage, the kidney and renal artery and vein are approached from either a lateral to medial fashion, or a medial to lateral fashion. More commonly, a lateral approach is used by performing the previously described medial visceral rotation. Gerota's fascia is then opened laterally and the kidney is elevated to expose the renal hilum for control with manual pressure, clamps, or vessel loops. Otherwise, from a medial technique, the renal aorta is identified by dividing the mesentery next to the ligament of Treitz; then, vessel loops or clamps may be applied to the proximal renal artery/vein before opening Gerota's fascia laterally. The patient's physiologic status as well as the degree of injury will dictate if complex repairs should be performed, or if nephrectomy is indicated.

Zone III retroperitoneal hematomas due to penetrating injury should be routinely explored, while blunt injuries should be explored only if the hematoma is expanding or is pulsatile and a femoral pulse is absent. Hematomas in Zone 3, associated with pelvic fractures, may be best treated by either extraperitoneal pelvic packing through a separate incision or angiography and

embolization. Placement of an intra-aortic balloon in cases of severe hypotension can also be used.

Injuries in Zone 3 include the distal aorta, infrarenal IVC, or the common, internal, and external iliac arteries or veins. The ureter crosses over the common iliac arteries at the level of the bifurcation bilaterally, so care should be taken while dissecting in this area and it should be evaluated for associated injury. A medial visceral rotation, as described above, will give adequate exposure to this area. The common iliac veins are densely adherent to the back wall of the common iliac arteries; therefore, dissection should be done carefully, so as to not injure them with dissection. The right common iliac artery crosses over the distal bifurcation of the IVC and the confluence of iliac veins. Historically, division of the right common iliac has been advocated to visualize and repair venous injuries located at the confluence of the iliac veins.

Iliac vessel repair depends on the extent of the injured vessel, degree of contamination, and the overall disease burden of the patient. For patients in extremis, arterial shunting should be performed. Venous injury can be primarily repaired or ligated. In addition to primary repair, reconstruction options include grafts with saphenous vein or polytetrafluoroethylene (PTFE) in an anatomic or extra-anatomic bypass fashion. Extra-anatomic bypass is considered when there is concern for gross contamination from other injuries. If a significant portion of the external iliac artery is injured, the internal iliac artery can be ligated distally and transposed anteriorly to construct an end-to-end anastomosis with the distal external iliac artery.

The external iliac artery can be exposed via a transperitoneal approach or retroperitoneal approach. Accessing the artery in an extraperitoneal fashion can be performed by using a "hockey stick" incision, carrying out the same from the groin to above the inguinal ligament in an oblique and lateral direction above the iliac crest. The fibers of the external and internal oblique muscles can be bluntly split and the retroperitoneal space entered, which is similar to a kidney transplant approach. Self-retaining retractor and lap pads are helpful in rotating the peritoneum medially to expose the psoas muscle and the vessels. If needed, the inguinal ligament can be divided to access the most distal portion of the external iliac artery, as it transitions to the CFA. Care must be taken not to injure the ureter which can be found at the level of the bifurcation of the common iliac artery.[12]

8.3.13 Common Femoral Artery (CFA) and Vein

The CFA extends from the inguinal ligament until it divides into the SFA and profunda femoral (PFA) arteries. When approaching the CFA, the incision should begin just above the inguinal ligament and brought down longitudinally along the medial border of the sartorius muscle. Dissection to identify the artery should begin laterally, as the vein and lymph channels are on the medial side. Once the femoral sheath is identified, it can be opened and the artery exposed. Bridging veins may occasionally be encountered above the artery and these can be ligated. Careful dissection can then be carried out to the bifurcation using vessel loops to help retract the artery from the surrounding structures while sharp dissection continues.[12] If there is difficulty exposing the proximal CFA, the inguinal ligament can be divided, or a transverse incision made so as to expose and control the external iliac artery.

8.3.14 Proximal SFA and Profunda Femoral Artery (PFA)

The PFA is typically found coursing posterolaterally. Once the bifurcation of the CFA is dissected, the takeoff of the PFA can be seen, as the CFA shows a decrease in its diameter, leading to the SFA. Traction of the CFA and SFA can be performed using vessel loops, and the origin of the PFA can be identified. Proximal control of the PFA can be obtained with a clamp or vessel loop, thereby avoiding damage to the lateral circumflex vein.[12]

8.3.15 Distal SFA

The distal SFA runs under the sartorius muscle until it enters the popliteal (Hunter's) canal. Hunter's canal, the adductor hiatus, is a fascial lined cleft located medially to the vastus muscles and lateral to the adductor muscles in the midthigh. The suprageniculate popliteal artery lies distal to the hiatus. Full exposure of the SFA is achieved through a medial upper leg incision, paralleling the lateral border of the sartorius muscle, which is then retracted medially to expose the roof of the canal to allow entry to the vessels. With large hematomas, anatomy in this region may be distorted and more proximal control may be needed. When operating in this area, the sartorius can be used as an excellent coverage option following vascular repair. Associated venous injury is common with arterial injury, therefore identification of the vein is necessary with repair or ligation as needed.[12]

8.3.16 Popliteal Artery

Between the adductor hiatus and the lower border of the popliteus muscle lies the popliteal artery. The semitendinosus muscle and its confluence with gracilis, sartorius, and semimembranosus muscles run medially, covering the popliteal fossa and its vessels. The associated veins are typically adherent to the artery. The tibial nerve is loosely attached to the vessel sheath within the popliteal fossa. The distal end of the popliteal artery is located at the hiatus by the origin of the soleus muscle. To access this site, the knee should be bent to 30 degrees and laterally rotated. The skin incision is carried out between the vastusmedialisand sartorius muscles. The saphenous vein should be maintained and ideally left with the posterior skin flap, if possible. Distally, the incision is carried out to the knee, one centimeter posteriorly to the tibia. Full exposure is usually needed; therefore, the semimembranosus, semitendinosus, gracilis, and sartoriusmuscles are divided 2 to 3 cm from their bony insertion. These are all tagged, so they can be reapproximated later for knee stability. For the distal portion of the popliteal artery, the medial head of the gastrocnemius muscle needs to be divided.[12]

8.4 Extremity Injuries

With long bone fractures and associated vascular injury, a combined approach with orthopedic surgery should be opted for. Minimizing the interval between injury and reperfusion is critical. Ideally, ischemia time should be less than 6 hours. Restoration of blood flow via vascular shunting should take priority over skeletal stabilization if an unstable fracture or dislocation is present. Once blood flow has been restored, orthopedic stabilization can proceed with either external fixator or open reduction and internal fixation, depending on the patient's hemodynamic stability and associated injuries. In stable patients, definitive reconstruction of the injured vessel should be always attempted.

8.5 Reconstructive Options

Primary repair, when possible, is always the best option to restore blood flow in an artery that has been completely transected. The injured vessel must be adequately debrided to healthy tissue both proximally and distally. Length can be gained by dividing the side branches of the vessel, depending on the location and covering gaps up to 3 cm; however, care must be taken when dividing small collateral branches, as those may be important to maintain collateral flow if the repair fails. For longer defects, an interposition graft is necessary.[11] The choice of conduit depends on the size and location of the injured vessel. Typically, the greater saphenous vein from the uninjured leg is the first choice for conduit.

8.5.1 Saphenous Vein

The contralateral saphenous vein is the ideal conduit for the repair of most extremity vascular injuries. It can be used as a primary conduit (▶ Fig. 8.2c), venous patch, or spiraled venous graft for reconstruction of larger vessels. Small side branches should be ligated with 2–0 or 3–0 silk. The vein is reversed and secured to an olive tip catheter with silk suture in order to inject heparinized saline to dilate the vein and assess for any leaks. Once the conduit is satisfactory, it is placed in a heparinized saline bath. Other venous options for conduits include the lesser saphenous or cephalic or brachial veins.[1]

8.5.2 Polytetrafluoroethylene (PTFE)

PTFE grafts can be used for larger arterial vascular injuries in the thorax, abdomen, or in the upper and lower extremities proximal to the axilla or to the knee. Vein should be used for distal injuries in the extremities because the diameter of the injured vessel is small, and inherently smaller PTFE grafts tends to clot. PTFE has shown improved patency (70–90% short term) and rare infection, even in contaminated wounds[26,27] After PTFE repair, patients should be placed on ASA 162 to 325 mg daily × 3 months postoperatively, with this recommendation extrapolated from data from aortosaphenous bypass for myocardial revascularization as well as from bypass for peripheral vascular disease.[28] PTFE is available in a variety of sizes and can be ringed or nonringed.

8.5.3 Other Conduits

Artergraft, made of bovine carotid artery, or Cryovein can also be used for vascular repair. These tissue conduits may be better options than PTFE if the autologous saphenous vein is of poor quality or there is a significant size mismatch. Some consider using these conduits in infected fields. However, there is little published data on these techniques and none in the trauma literature.

8.6 Venous Injuries

Basic options for management of venous injury include ligation or simple repair. Location of the injury as well as the hemodynamic status dictate optimal management. If the patient is hemodynamically stable and the repair will not significantly delay the treatment of associated injuries, simple or more complex repairs can be undertaken. Patients in extremis or hemodynamically unstable are better served by venous ligation. Lateral venorrhaphies that minimally narrow the lumen of the repaired vein have the highest patency rates. Complex venous repairs can be carried out either with end-to-end or spatulated venous or PTFE grafts. Synthetic and interposition repairs have the lowest reported patency rates. Edema and thrombosis rates are high, regardless of the type of repair.[29] Many veins tolerate ligation due to an abundance of collateral flow. The IVC can be ligated in the infrarenallocation, however, significant limb edema may occur. This requires significant compression wrapping and elevation in the early postoperative stages, and long-term surveillance for signs and symptoms of postthrombotic syndrome. If the IVC is ligated above the renal veins, renal failure will ensue due to outflow obstruction. The portal vein/SMV can also be ligated; however, significant bowel edema and potential bowel ischemia will ensue. Hepatic artery inflow as well as the splenic vein must be intact to aid in redistribution of flow.

8.7 Considerations After Repair of Extremity Injuries

Isolated vascular injuries with prolonged ischemia time as well as combined arterial and skeletal injuries pose a high-risk for compartment syndrome. In these circumstances, fasciotomies should be strongly considered.[29] Similarly, patients with combined arterial and venous injuries, especially those undergoing venous ligation, should be candidates for fasciotomy. In patients with an altered mental status unable to be examined, such as head injured patients or patients on mechanical ventilation, fasciotomies should be considered, as clinical examination alone can be inaccurate when subjective aspects of the diagnosis are lost. Serial measurement of compartment pressures can be performed, but they are time-consuming and some compartments may be missed on evaluation.

8.8 Role of Endovascular Interventions

With technological advancement and skills training, endovascular techniques have moved beyond the elective setting and into the acute setting for vascular trauma. These techniques are useful specifically in areas that are difficult to access through standard open surgical exposure. Endovascular therapy should be a consideration for any type of bleeding, and it can be used as a diagnostic modality, temporizing measure, bridge to definitive control, part of a combined procedure, or definitive therapy. Specific techniques depend on physician skills, institutional resources and, most importantly, the patient's injuries, physiology, and preexisting conditions. For Zones 1 to 3, retroperitoneal hematomas found intraoperatively, angiography is a potentially helpful diagnostic tool, as it can demonstrate endoluminal lesions which may not be appreciated on open inspection of the vessel wall. Furthermore, treatment with endovascular, open, or hybrid procedure can occur. Hemodynamic instability is no longer an absolute contraindication for endovascular therapy. Temporary occlusion of the aorta with a balloon catheter for proximal vascular control can aid in resuscitation and stabilize the patient, bridging them to definitive treatment.

Covered stents are one of the mainstays in endovascular treatment and can be used in traumatic hemorrhage when preservation of flow is required (▶ Fig. 8.4a, b). Key components to a successful stent deployment include a healthy proximal and distal landing zone while not occluding critical branches. If a guidewire can typically be passed through an area of partial transection or occluded vessel, a stent can be deployed, reestablishing flow. Even with complete transection, advanced techniques above and below the area of the injury can be used to successfully pass a wire across the injured segment with a conduit placed to reestablish flow. Specific injuries require advanced techniques and novel methods such as fenestrated, branched, or chimney stents. Placement of these devices are time-consuming and are not useful in an unstable patient. Covered stents are typically either self-expanding nitinol or balloon-expandable. Balloon deployment will allow for accurate placement and appropriate opposition of the stent against the vessel wall. Standard stents are not durable in areas of compression or kinking such as the knee or shoulder joints.

Angioembolization is an important bleeding control technique after trauma in nearly any anatomical location. This method occludes blood flow by placing thrombogenic material in the lumen of the blood vessel and activating the clotting cascade, leading to clot formation in a particular area. Various materials can be used for embolization, including metallic coils and plugs, particles, and liquid agents. Vessel size, patient's anatomy, and experience of the provider all lend to the decision-making of which device to use. Material choice is dependent on the particular scenario, with each device having pros and cons.

Metallic coils are frequently used for vessel occlusion. These coils cause local thrombosis, using the patient's clotting factors for thrombus formation. Coils are made up of metallic wires with various diameters and lengths, which take a "coiled" shape when deployed. Some coils have thrombogenic fibers coating the metal which aid in the activation of the coagulation cascade. Standard coils are 0.035 mm or 0.038 mm in thickness and require 5F catheter for deployment. Standard coils are usually used for occluding larger proximal vascular structures. Smaller coils can be deployed via a microcatheter if more distal/selective embolization is required. Coils are detachable and retrieval can be performed prior to deployment, if needed (▶ Fig. 8.5 a–c).

Plugs can be used for proximal occlusion in a larger diameter vessel, such as the splenic artery. Sheath system delivery allows for a more controlled and precise delivery. They can be recaptured and positioned to the desired location if the original position is not satisfactory. Migration is infrequent. Since the plugs are relatively inflexible, use of this product is limited to certain areas where little torque has built up in the sheath or catheter.

Particle embolization is typically performed with Gelfoam, providing nonselective vessel occlusion. Gelfoam can be used to

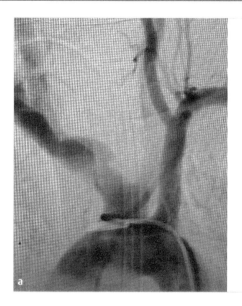
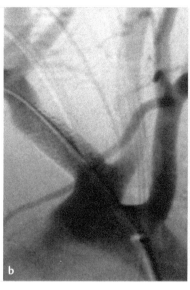

Fig. 8.4 (a) Pseudoaneurysm of the left innominate artery. (b) Covered stent–graft repair of the pseudoaneurysm.

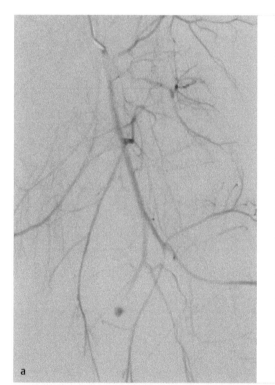
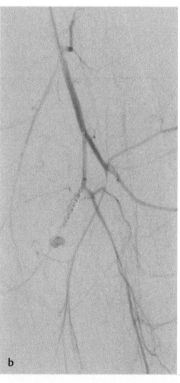
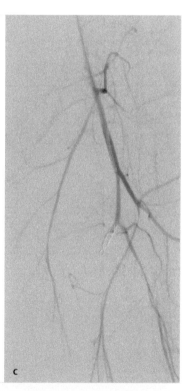

Fig. 8.5 (a) Active extravasation is seen from a branch of the left profunda femoral artery after a stab wound to the thigh with hematoma and compartment syndrome. (b) Coils were used to selectively embolize the injured branch. (c) Completion angiogram demonstrating no flow beyond coil embolization. The patient then underwent a thigh fasciotomy in the hybrid operating room, with minimal blood loss.

control bleeding of multiple branching vessels, such as proximal deployment in the internal iliac artery. Distal ischemia is more common with Gelfoam embolization. Particle size is important, as smaller particles can occlude smaller vessels with less collateral flow; therefore, marked ischemia and necrosis may occur. Gelfoam can be cut into small pieces, leading to more consistent particles. It can also be "slurried" by mixing small pieces back and forth through a syringe system, although this leads to various small size particles. One benefit of the use of

Gelfoam is thrombosis, which is typically not permanent as recanalization usually occurs after 2 weeks.

The hallmark of using stent grafts in vascular trauma lies in the treatment of blunt thoracic aortic injuries (BTAI). Demetriades et al has shown, in two multi-institutional studies of the American Association for the Surgery of Trauma (AAST), that thoracic endovascular repair of the aorta (TEVAR) has resulted in marked improvement in morbidity and mortality rates when compared to open aortic repair.[30] With a blunt mechanism, the thoracic aorta is typically injured distal to the takeoff of the left subclavian artery. Initial CT imaging can be used for specific diameter measurements for graft sizing. Further details can be determined with intra-operative angiogram and intravascular ultrasound (IVUS). Important considerations include the landing zone, aortic diameter, and lesion characteristics. Some injuries have a short proximal landing zone, and the left subclavian artery (LSCA) may need to be covered. With appropriate patient selection, minimal morbidity has been noted by covering this artery. With a patent vertebral artery, collateral flow can limit complications of covering the LSCA. Assessment for postoperative upper extremity ischemia is standard practice and intervention conducted only if clinically warranted. In certain patient populations with insufficient vertebral artery flow or prior coronary artery bypass grafting with left internal mammary artery, a left carotid subclavian bypass is indicated if the LSCA is to be covered by an endovascular graft.

Endovascular management is also useful and indicated in patients sustaining blunt injuries to the carotid or vertebral arteries. Injuries to the internal carotid or vertebral arteries are fairly inaccessible from an open approach. Treatment of these injuries is based on grade and include medical and surgical approaches. When medical therapy is contraindicated or if lesions are worsening with medical therapy, endovascular therapy should be considered. Endovascular treatment can be tailored to the particular injury based on the collateral circulation, location, and grade of injury. Options include stenting certain injuries, occluding vertebral artery injuries, or coil embolizing pseudoaneurysms.[31,32,33] Routine stenting is not recommended and should be reserved for select cases.[34]

Bleeding sources from the liver, spleen, kidney, as well as pelvis can all potentially be controlled with angioembolization. Selective or nonselective embolization can occur in the various vascular beds, depending on the site of injury and desired effect. Experienced interventionalists are capable of embolizing bleeding intercostal arteries. This technique is time- and labor-intensive, since both sides of the intercostal artery may require an intervention to prevent ongoing bleeding; therefore, it should not be performed in an unstable patient.

Pelvic bleeding can be from a variety of sources, depending on the mechanism of injury and the fracture pattern. Pelvic hemorrhage may be arterial, venous, muscular, or from the fractured bones. Deep branches of the internal iliac artery can cause significant bleeding which is difficult and contraindicated to control via an open approach. Angioembolization is recommended in such cases. Pelvic bleeding from venous injuries are usually self-limiting due to the natural tamponade effect of an intact retroperitoneum. Alternatively, venous outflow can be decreased with associated angioembolization of the arterial vasculature in the region. In patients with significant pelvic trauma, a multimodal treatment is usually needed. Therapy is based on the specific injury as well as the patient's hemodynamic status. Temporizing measures may be performed with a pelvic binder or REBOA placement. Preperitoneal packing, exploratory laparotomy, with or without external fixator placement may also be necessary. Angiography may play a role, performed either in a hybrid room or sequentially, after the other methods have been implemented.

Angiographic embolization should be part of the algorithm for management of splenic injuries. Embolization should be considered for patients who either fail nonoperative management (NOM) of splenic trauma (grade I/II/III) or as initial therapy for patients with higher levels of injury (grade III/IV/V) with or without active extravasation (▶ Fig. 8.6a), although widespread use of this technique in high-grade injuries without a blush on CT is controversial. If a patient is hemodynamically unstable or a nonresponder to transfusions, splenectomy should be performed. However, if a patient responds to resuscitation or is stable, embolization of the spleen may be able to control the injury, avoiding an exploratory laparotomy and potentially a splenectomy. Recent data suggests the success rate of angioembolization in grade IV injuries being greater than 95%.[35,36] The higher the grade of the injury, the more likely NOM will fail; therefore, in patients with grade V injuries, aggressive management including splenectomy should be strongly considered in transient responders or those requiring successive blood transfusions. NOM of splenic injuries can be augmented by angioembolization, although some patients will continue to bleed even after embolization. If an injury is managed either nonoperatively or with proximal splenic artery embolization, follow-up imaging should be performed at 48 to 72 hours to search for any evidence of intrasplenic arterial pseudoaneurysm as these can cause late bleeding.[37] If a pseudoaneurysm is noted on follow-up imaging, additional embolization or operative management is indicated. Embolization of splenic artery injury was initially described by Sclafani et al in 1991.[38]

Proximal coil or plug embolization of the main splenic artery is performed, leading to a significant reduction of inflow of the splenic artery, and allowing the injured area to thrombose and remodel (▶ Fig. 8.6b, c). The spleen remains viable, based on collateral flow from the short gastric arteries, retaining some degree of function. Selective embolization can also be used with microcatheter placement and target directed embolization, if there is normal flow to the remainder of the spleen. An issue with this type of embolization is partial splenic infarction and possible abscess formation.

Due to significant differences in the vascular anatomy of the liver, angiographic approaches are different than those used in splenic trauma. Venous hemorrhage is common in liver trauma, and both the hepatic veins and portal venous system must be considered when evaluating liver trauma. Proximal arterial embolization cannot be used in liver trauma due to the lack of collateral flow. Due to the various blood sources to the liver, hepatic ischemia is difficult to predict. Several liver injuries are successfully treated nonoperatively, regardless of injury grade; therefore, angioembolization should be used in rare cases. In unstable patients with liver injury, angioembolization plays a role, usually after the initial damage control laparotomy. Multiple operative techniques are used in attempts to control the liver, including packing, sutures, and other methods. Angioembolization is an important adjunct to treat significant hepatic hemorrhage, as an adjunct to other treatment modalities. Distal embolization should be performed when at all possible. If needed, nonselective embolization can be used; however, this can lead to a significant area of hepatic necrosis in up to 40% of patients, and some of these patients may require significant hepatic resection due to this complication.[39]

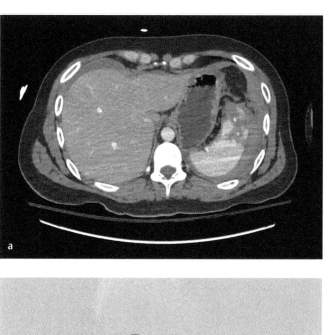
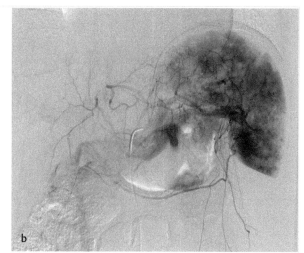
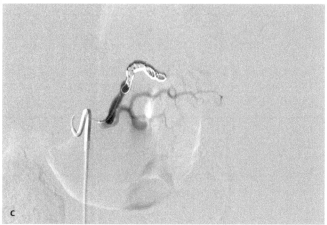

Fig. 8.6 **(a)** CT scan with IV contrast showing Grade 4 splenic injury with active extravasation. **(b)** Angiogram showing corresponding splenic lesion. **(c)** Proximal coiling of splenic artery to decrease inflow.

Proximal mesenteric vascular injuries can be difficult to approach in an open fashion, therefore, endovascular repair can be an attractive option in a stable patient. Several case reports have noted successful control of SMA injuries with no significant procedural complications.[40,41]

Although endovascular techniques have been used in multiple other areas of the body with success, the data is limited in those regions.[42,43,44,45,46] Renal injuries, chest wall injuries, intercostal injuries, lumbar arteries, external carotid artery branches, profundal femoral artery, thyrocervical trunk, axillary artery, and pulmonary artery have all been treated by endovascular means.

8.8.1 Shunts

In damage control situations or if an associated orthopedic injury is noted, a shunt should be used to reestablish vascular flow to the injured extremity.[47] Various commercial shunts are available in many sizes and configurations. Any tubular conduit may be used if commercial shunts are not available and this can range from IV tubing, pediatric feeding tubes, or even chest tubes, depending on the size of the injured vessel. The shunt size chosen

should be the largest diameter that will fit into the injured vessel. Venous shunting may be considered depending on location; however, they typically clot and in true exsanguination, ligation is recommended.

For arterial shunting, after proximal and distal control and clots have been cleared with Fogerty catheters, local heparin should be injected and the shunt placed. The distal end is inserted first, ideally with back-bleeding appreciated. The proximal side is instilled with heparinized saline to prevent air embolism. 2–0 silk suture is used to secure the shunt at both sides, tying the sutures close to the ends of the injured vessel, as this area of the vessel must be resected for the definitive repair later on (▶ Fig. 8.7). Shunt patency should be confirmed with palpation of a pulse or with Doppler wave flow. Muscle should be loosely approximated over the area if possible, or a moist dressing should be placed to avoid desiccation of the native vessel.

8.8.2 Tourniquets

Temporary vascular control can be performed in the field or site of injury with direct pressure or tourniquet placement. Military data showed decreased mortality for patients with

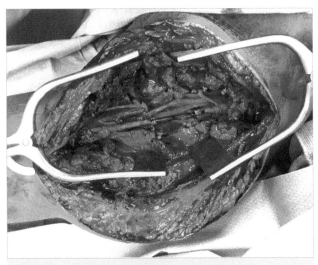

Fig. 8.7 Argyle shunt in brachial artery.

exsanguinating extremity hemorrhage when a tourniquet was applied correctly and rapidly.[48] Increased survival is noted for patients who have tourniquets applied before shock ensues. Civilian tourniquet usage has increased,[49] providing early temporary control of potentially life-threatening bleeding.

Tourniquet placement should be above the site of an injured extremity. This can be performed over clothing if necessary, and joints, such as the knees and elbows, should be avoided as the devices can slip when applied over these anatomic sites. Whichever device is used, it is important to document that bleeding has stopped. This should be monitored in route to the hospital, or in the hospital, to ensure the rebleeding has not occurred when the patient is resuscitated or has elevated blood pressure due to pain. It is important to tighten these devices as much as possible, because if they are not tight enough, they may only act as a venous tourniquet, leading to an increase in bleeding if the artery is not controlled.

If a patient comes to the emergency room or the trauma bay with a tourniquet in place, the remainder of the standard ATLS treatment should begin. If the patient is stable, the tourniquet can be taken down to assess the wound and document if there is significant bleeding requiring operative intervention. If no bleeding is appreciated, a pressure dressing can be placed, while perfusing the rest of the limb. If there is bleeding, suggesting an arterial injury, direct pressure or another tourniquet just proximal to the wound can be placed for control until operative control can be performed. Blind clamping bleeding vessels in the emergency department is discouraged, as this can cause undue injury to surrounding structures.

8.8.3 REBOA

Resuscitative endovascular balloon occlusion of the aorta (REBOA) can be performed in patients with life threatening torso hemorrhage, specifically in patients with abdominal, pelvic or junctional bleeding. After the primary survey has been performed, along with chest/pelvis X-ray and FAST, balloon occlusion should be considered if life-threatening hemorrhage below the diaphragm is noted.

When rapid percutaneous arterial cannulation is achieved, REBOA is noted to be faster than emergency department thoracotomy (EDT).[50] Some trauma centers have moved to initially placing small-bore CFA arterial lines in all hypotensive patients arriving at the trauma center, as the access site rapidly hastens REBOA placement if the decision is made to proceed with aortic occlusion.

REBOA should be considered for transient or nonresponder patients sustaining abdominal or pelvic bleeding. It can be performed in the hypotensive patient, before arrest, offering an attractive alternative to EDT. If the patient falls into one of the above categories, balloon occlusion should be performed at the appropriate level (Zone 1 or Zone 3), in an attempt to stabilize the patient for definitive therapy. Zone 1 is located in the thoracic aorta between an area distal to the takeoff of the left subclavian artery and the diaphragm. Occlusion in this area provides decreased inflow for any bleeding below the level of the diaphragm (▶ Fig. 8.8a). Occlusion times in this location are limited as blood flow to the abdominal viscera is compromised. Zone 3 is located from the renal arteries to the aortic bifurcation. Occlusion in this area provides inflow occlusion to pelvic or junctional bleeding in the groin (▶ Fig. 8.8b). Device placement can be performed in the resuscitation area, ideally with image guidance using X-ray or fluoroscopy. External landmarks are used for approximate distances, measuring the p-tip of the device to the sheath. For Zone 1, the p-tip can be placed at the sternal notch with the end of the catheter at the length of the femoral access sheath. This should result in the balloon landing in Zone 1, which is above the diaphragm. For Zone 3, the p-tip can be placed at the xiphoid process and the catheter measured to the femoral access sheath. This should result in the balloon ending up at the distal aorta above the bifurcation. Once the device is in, an X-ray image should be taken to confirm appropriate placement of the balloon before inflation. Full aortic occlusion can be confirmed by virtue of an improvement in systolic blood pressure upon inflation or by noting the disappearance of the contralateral femoral pulse. Occlusion volumes are different in all patients, so care in inflation is paramount, so balloons do not burst or vessels are not injured. Using a mixture of 1:3 contrast and saline can help visualize the balloon under radiographic imaging.[51]

Sheath placement is either performed via an open surgical approach or percutaneously with or without ultrasound guidance. In a recent study, 50% required surgical cutdown,[40] but current evidence demonstrates increased use of percutaneous cannulation.[52] Main challenges in this procedure stem from access of the CFA,[50] particularly in patients in cardiac arrest without a palpable pulse. In these patients, moving quickly to an open technique is recommended, if percutaneous methods are unsuccessful. Accessing the SFA or cannulating the common femoral vein (CFV) vein instead of the CFA are two complications that can occur at this step.[53] Once balloon occlusion has been performed, patients should be rapidly transported to the operating room, endovascular suite, hybrid room, or location of definitive care, so definitive therapy can commence and ischemia can be limited. A sense of urgency must be kept up with the team, as balloon occlusion is essentially the same as open aortic occlusion. Once hemorrhage control or more distal control can be obtained, the next priority should be deflating the balloon. This should be done

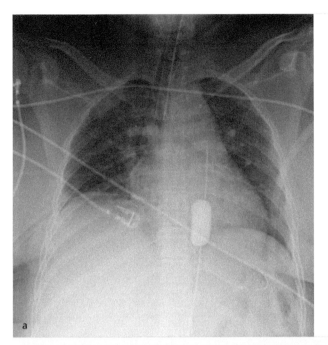 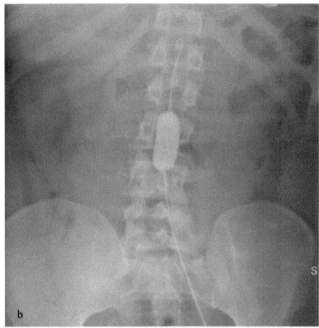

Fig. 8.8 (a) REBOA at Zone 1. **(b)** REBOA at Zone 3. REBOA, resuscitative endovascular balloon occlusion of the aorta.

methodically with good communication with the operating team and anesthesia. Slow deflation should take place as anesthesia continues with resuscitation and other medication to decrease the impact of ischemia and reperfusion. Once the balloon is deflated and flow is reestablished, it is advisable to complete the remainder of the damage control operation. When it is time to completely remove the balloon, care is taken to attach the syringe and hold negative pressure on the balloon to assure all of the air is out. The balloon should come easily out of the sheath. If for some reason it does not, further imaging can aid in determining what the issues are. If the balloon still does not come out, the patient may need a cut down with en bloc removal of the sheath and catheter.[53] Once the balloon is removed, sheath management is key. If the patient needs to go to interventional radiology, the radiologist may use the sheath for angiography or embolization. If this is not the case, the distal circulation of the limb should be interrogated in the OR. An angiogram can be obtained through the sheath to rule out distal ischemia. If none are noted and the device was placed percutaneously, the device can be removed and manual compression held for 30 minutes. If the device was placed in an open fashion or there is persistent hemorrhage after adequate compression, an open repair can be performed. Postprocedure monitoring should be performed with neurovascular checks. If there is any concern for pulse differential or issues with the ipsilateral leg, additional imaging or intervention should be performed. Ultrasound evaluation of the puncture site should be performed at 24 to 48 hours in order to search for a pseudoaneurysm.[53]

8.9 Conclusion

Vascular injury can lead to significant mortality. Significant knowledge of different approaches is critical to obtaining appropriate vascular control for various wounds. Certain wounds lend themselves to endovascular diagnosis and therapy, so a team-based approach to the injured patient is crucial. Tourniquets can aid in decreasing extremity bleeding, both in the prehospital environment and the emergency department. Damage control techniques such as shunting can help salvage severely injured patients, or those with combined orthopedic injuries, to bridge them to definitive care. When patients are in extremis with torso injuries, consideration for REBOA can stabilize patients while they are being resuscitated and moved to the operating room or undergoing interventional radiology for definitive control. It is imperative that the acute care trauma surgeon keeps all of these options in mind when taking care of this patient population.

References

[1] Feliciano DV, Moore FA, Moore EE, et al. Evaluation and management of peripheral vascular injury. Part 1. Western Trauma Association/critical decisions in trauma. J Trauma. 2011; 70(6):1551–1556

[2] Woodring JH, Dillon ML. Radiographic manifestations of mediastinal hemorrhage from blunt chest trauma. Ann ThoracSurg. 1984; 37(2):171–178

[3] Young JW, Burgess AR, Brumback RJ, Poka A. Pelvic fractures: value of plain radiography in early assessment and management. Radiology. 1986; 160(2): 445–451

[4] Eastridge BJ, Starr A, Minei JP, O'Keefe GE, Scalea TM. The importance of fracture pattern in guiding therapeutic decision-making in patients with hemorrhagic shock and pelvic ring disruptions. J Trauma. 2002; 53(3):446–450, discussion 450–451

[5] Coccolini F, Stahel PF, Montori G, et al. Pelvic trauma: WSES classification and guidelines. World J EmergSurg. 2017; 12:5

[6] Sarin EL, Moore JB, Moore EE, et al. Pelvic fracture pattern does not always predict the need for urgent embolization. J Trauma. 2005; 58(5):973–977

[7] Fox N, Rajani RR, Bokhari F, et al. Eastern Association for the Surgery of Trauma. Evaluation and management of penetrating lower extremity arterial trauma: an Eastern Association for the Surgery of Trauma practice management guideline. J Trauma Acute Care Surg. 2012; 73(5) Suppl 4:S315–S320

[8] Johansen K, Lynch K, Paun M, Copass M. Non-invasive vascular tests reliably exclude occult arterial trauma in injured extremities. J Trauma. 1991; 31(4): 515–519, discussion 519–522

[9] Inaba K, Branco BC, Reddy S, et al. Prospective evaluation of multidetector computed tomography for extremity vascular trauma. J Trauma. 2011; 70(4): 808–815

[10] Inaba K, Branco BC, Menaker J, et al. Evaluation of multidetector computed tomography for penetrating neck injury: a prospective multicenter study. J Trauma Acute Care Surg. 2012; 72(3):576–583, discussion 583–584, quiz 803–804

[11] Feliciano DV, Moore EE, West MA, et al. Western Trauma Association critical decisions in trauma: evaluation and management of peripheral vascular injury, part II. J Trauma Acute Care Surg. 2013; 75(3):391–397

[12] Fildes J, Meredith JW, Hoyt DB, et al. Trauma ACoSCo. ASSET (Advanced Surgical Skills for Exposure in Trauma): Exposure Techniques When Time Matters. Chicago, IL: American College of Surgeons. 2010

[13] Schrock T, Blaisdell FW, Mathewson C, Jr. Management of blunt trauma to the liver and hepatic veins. Arch Surg. 1968; 96(5):698–704

[14] David Richardson J, Franklin GA, Lukan JK, et al. Evolution in the management of hepatic trauma: a 25-year perspective. Ann Surg. 2000; 232(3): 324–330

[15] Hansen CJ, Bernadas C, West MA, et al. Abdominal vena caval injuries: outcomes remain dismal. Surgery. 2000; 128(4):572–578

[16] Asensio JA, Forno W, Roldán G, et al. Visceral vascular injuries. SurgClin North Am. 2002; 82(1):1–20, xix

[17] Asensio JA, Soto SN, Forno W, et al. Abdominal vascular injuries: the trauma surgeon's challenge. Surg Today. 2001; 31(11):949–957

[18] Dente C, Feliciano D. Abdominal vascular injury. In: Feliciano DV, Mattox KL, Moore EE, eds. Trauma. New York, NY: McGraw Hill; 2008:737–757

[19] Asensio JA, Petrone P, Kimbrell B, Kuncir E. Lessons learned in the management of thirteen celiac axis injuries. South Med J. 2005; 98(4):462–466

[20] Hoyt DB, Coimbra R, Potenza BM, Rappold JF. Anatomic exposures for vascular injuries. SurgClin North Am. 2001; 81(6):1299–1330, xii

[21] Asensio JA, Britt LD, Borzotta A, et al. Multiinstitutional experience with the management of superior mesenteric artery injuries. J Am CollSurg. 2001; 193 (4):354–365, discussion 365–366

[22] Coimbra R, Filho AR, Nesser RA, Rasslan S. Outcome from traumatic injury of the portal and superior mesenteric veins. Vasc Endovascular Surg. 2004; 38 (3):249–255

[23] Fraga GP, Bansal V, Fortlage D, Coimbra R. A 20-year experience with portal and superior mesenteric venous injuries: has anything changed? Eur J VascEndovascSurg. 2009; 37(1):87–91

[24] Asensio JA, Petrone P, Garcia-Nuñez L, Healy M, Martin M, Kuncir E. Superior mesenteric venous injuries: to ligate or to repair remains the question. J Trauma. 2007; 62(3):668–675, discussion 675

[25] Stone HH, Fabian TC, Turkleson ML. Wounds of the portal venous system. World J Surg. 1982; 6(3):335–341

[26] Feliciano DV, Mattox KL, Graham JM, Bitondo CG. Five-year experience with PTFE grafts in vascular wounds. J Trauma. 1985; 25(1):71–82

[27] Martin LC, McKenney MG, Sosa JL, et al. Management of lower extremity arterial trauma. J Trauma. 1994; 37(4):591–598, discussion 598–599

[28] Feliciano DV. Management of peripheral arterial injury. CurrOpinCrit Care. 2010; 16(6):602–608

[29] Arrillaga A, Bynoe R, Frykberg E, et al. Practice Management Guidelines for Penetrating Trauma to the Lower Extremity: Practice Parameter for Evaluation and Management of Combined Arterial and Skeletal Extremity Injury from Penetrating Trauma. EAST Guidelines 2002

[30] Demetriades D, Velmahos GC, Scalea TM, et al. Diagnosis and treatment of blunt thoracic aortic injuries: changing perspectives. J Trauma. 2008; 64(6): 1415–1418, discussion 1418–1419

[31] DiCocco JM, Fabian TC, Emmett KP, et al. Optimal outcomes for patients with blunt cerebrovascular injury (BCVI): tailoring treatment to the lesion. J Am CollSurg. 2011; 212(4):549–557, discussion 557–559

[32] Desouza RM, Crocker MJ, Haliasos N, Rennie A, Saxena A. Blunt traumatic vertebral artery injury: a clinical review. Eur Spine J. 2011; 20(9):1405–1416

[33] Cohen JE, Gomori JM, Rajz G, et al. Vertebral artery pseudoaneurysms secondary to blunt trauma: Endovascular management by means of neurostents and flow diverters. J ClinNeurosci. 2016; 32:77–82

[34] Burlew CC, Biffl WL, Moore EE, et al. Endovascular stenting is rarely necessary for the management of blunt cerebrovascular injuries. J Am CollSurg. 2014; 218(5):1012–1017

[35] Schurr MJ, Fabian TC, Gavant M, et al. Management of blunt splenic trauma: computed tomographic contrast blush predicts failure of nonoperative management. J Trauma. 1995; 39(3):507–512, discussion 512–513

[36] Miller PR, Chang MC, Hoth JJ, et al. Prospective trial of angiography and embolization for all grade III to V blunt splenic injuries: nonoperative management success rate is significantly improved. J Am CollSurg. 2014; 218(4):644–648

[37] Leeper WR, Leeper TJ, Ouellette D, et al. Delayed hemorrhagic complications in the nonoperative management of blunt splenic trauma: early screening leads to a decrease in failure rate. J Trauma Acute Care Surg. 2014; 76(6): 1349–1353

[38] Sclafani SJ, Weisberg A, Scalea TM, Phillips TF, Duncan AO. Blunt splenic injuries: nonsurgical treatment with CT, arteriography, and transcatheter arterial embolization of the splenic artery. Radiology. 1991; 181(1):189–196

[39] Dabbs DN, Stein DM, Scalea TM. Major hepatic necrosis: a common complication after angioembolization for treatment of high-grade liver injuries. J Trauma. 2009; 66(3):621–627, discussion 627–629

[40] Hagiwara A, Takasu A. Transcatheter arterial embolization is effective for mesenteric arterial hemorrhage in trauma. EmergRadiol. 2009; 16(5):403–406

[41] Asayama Y, Matsumoto S, Isoda T, Kunitake N, Nakashima H. A case of traumatic mesenteric bleeding controlled by only transcatheter arterial embolization. CardiovascInterventRadiol. 2005; 28(2):256–258

[42] DuBose JJ, Rajani R, Gilani R, et al. Endovascular Skills for Trauma and Resuscitative Surgery Working Group. Endovascular management of axillo-subclavian arterial injury: a review of published experience. Injury. 2012; 43(11):1785–1792

[43] Simeone A, Demlow T, Karmy-Jones R. Endovascular repair of a traumatic renal artery injury. J Trauma. 2011; 70(5):1300

[44] Antevil JL, Holmes JF, Lewis D, Battistella F. Successful angiographic embolization of bleeding into the chest wall after blunt thoracic trauma. J Trauma. 2006; 60(5):1117–1118

[45] Nemoto C, Ikegami Y, Suzuki T, et al. Repeated embolization of intercostal arteries after blunt chest injury. Gen ThoracCardiovascSurg. 2014; 62(11): 696–699

[46] Yuan KC, Hsu YP, Wong YC, Fang JF, Lin BC, Chen HW. Management of complicated lumbar artery injury after blunt trauma. Ann Emerg Med. 2011; 58(6):531–535

[47] Inaba K, Aksoy H, Seamon MJ, et al. Multicenter Shunt Study Group. Multicenter evaluation of temporary intravascular shunt use in vascular trauma. J Trauma Acute Care Surg. 2016; 80(3):359–364, discussion 364–365

[48] Kragh JF, Jr, Walters TJ, Baer DG, et al. Survival with emergency tourniquet use to stop bleeding in major limb trauma. Ann Surg. 2009; 249(1):1–7

[49] Teixeira PGR, Brown CVR, Emigh B, et al. Texas Tourniquet Study Group. Civilian prehospital tourniquet use is associated with improved survival in patients with peripheral vascular injury. J Am CollSurg. 2018; 226(5):769–776.e1

[50] Romagnoli A, Teeter W, Pasley J, et al. Time to aortic occlusion: It's all about access. J Trauma Acute Care Surg. 2017; 83(6):1161–1164

[51] DuBose JJ, Scalea TM, Brenner M, et al. AAST AORTA Study Group. The AAST prospective Aortic Occlusion for Resuscitation in Trauma and Acute Care Surgery (AORTA) registry: data on contemporary utilization and outcomes of aortic occlusion and resuscitative balloon occlusion of the aorta (REBOA). J Trauma Acute Care Surg. 2016; 81(3):409–419

[52] Dubose JJ, Morrison J, Brenner M, et al. (2018, September). Comparison of 7 and 11–12 French access for REBOA: results from the AAST Aortic Occlusion for Resuscitation in Trauma and Acute Care Surgery (AORTA Registry). Quickshot presentation at the 77th Annual Meeting of the American Association for the Surgery of Trauma. San Diego, CA

[53] Davidson AJ, Russo RM, Reva VA, et al. BEST Study Group. The pitfalls of reboa: risk factors and mitigation strategies. J Trauma Acute Care Surg. 2017

Expert Commentary on Vascular Trauma by *David V. Feliciano*

Expert Commentary on Vascular Trauma

David V. Feliciano

Incisions/Exposures

An anterolateral thoracotomy performed in a woman is accomplished by manually and vigorously elevating the breast superiorly, so that the skin incision can be placed over the appropriate rib.

Exposure of the distal first portion of the subclavian artery on the right and the second portion bilaterally is improved significantly by division of the clavicle at its midpoint or by a partial claviculectomy of the middle 1/3rd. Either of these maneuvers is quicker than trying to disarticulate the sternoclavicular joint. The divided clavicle or segment removed can later be reapproximated by placing one drilled hole on either end, passing a sternal wire as a "U" from back to front, and tightening the wire anteriorly by twisting.

The first and second portions of the axillary artery are exposed by means of an infraclavicular incision and manually splitting the fibers of the pectoralis major muscle until the tendon of the pectoralis minor is visualized. An incision in the deltopectoral groove can be utilized for injuries of all three portions of the axillary artery, but is most commonly an extension of an infraclavicular incision.

For proximal hematomas in the groin, longitudinal division of 2 cm of the inguinal ligament may allow for control of the distal external iliac artery without the need to perform a formal "transplant" incision. Division of the entire inguinal ligament compromises coverage of an interposition graft in the common femoral artery.

Abdominal Vascular

With blunt trauma, a retroperitoneal hematoma in zone II or III should be opened if it is pulsatile, rapidly expanding, or partially ruptured.

The proximal superior mesenteric artery (Fulton zones I, II, and probably III) and common and external iliac arteries should NEVER be ligated and are always shunted at the first damage control operation.

While the use of atriocaval shunt is rare, the ideal size is a 38 Fr thoracostomy tube with an extra hole cut 20 cm proximal to the most proximal hole in the tube.

Extremity Vascular

"Regional" heparin (2000–2500 units of unfractionated heparin) injected after passage of Fogarty catheters into a peripheral artery is a reasonable option when associated injuries to the brain, a solid organ, or pelvis are present; however, data on its efficacy are lacking.

The two main indications for insertion of a temporary intraluminal vascular shunt are a Gustilo IIIC fracture in an extremity or the need for "damage control" in the presence of a major arterial injury. The most common size of an arterial shunt is 14 Fr, and a thoracostomy tube should be used for the femoral, common femoral, iliac, or axillary veins. If the size of the overlying injury to soft tissue precludes appropriate temporary coverage of the shunt until it is removed, formal reconstruction should be performed in an extra-anatomic fashion.

If the surgeon is not a believer in using compartment pressures to determine the need for a fasciotomy, the following are suggested as indications for "prophylactic" fasciotomy: hypotension in the field, crush injury, disproportionate pain and swelling in distal extremity, delay > 4 hours in reestablishing arterial inflow, need for simultaneous clamping of adjacent major artery and vein, and need for ligation of injured vein.

9 Appendicitis

Edward Lineen, Yee Wong, and Nicholas Namias

Summary

Appendicitis, although common, remains a significant challenge worldwide. Diagnosis and management continue to evolve. In this chapter, we have reviewed the most recent trends.

Keywords: Appendicitis, peritonitis, intraabdominal infection

9.1 Introduction

Appendicitis is an affliction of the masses. It is a disease that affects both toddlers and the elderly, and occurs throughout the world irrespective of ethnic or socioeconomic differences. Although it has a well-recognized classical presentation, it frequently does not follow the standard textbook presentation, leading to diagnostic dilemmas. The evaluation has changed from clinical to primarily radiographic with dramatic increases in cost and risk of radiation-induced malignancy. What was once believed to be a surgical disease has now become the subject of considerable debate between operative and nonoperative management. The advent of minimally invasive surgery has brought on a new series of approaches, which have dramatically changed not only the technique but also the economics of the disease. During the 1983 Southern Surgical Presidential Address, Dr. G. Rainey Williams summarized what was true then and is true to date: "the history of appendicitis includes examples of great resistance to changing concepts, brilliant but unaccepted early observations, the importance of timing, and, finally, the development of highly satisfactory solutions."[1]

For much of recorded history, the appendix was not well-considered. Discussion and debate about the true pathology of the right iliac fossa often neglected the appendix. The appendix was first described in 1552[2] by Berengarius Carpus. Claudius Amyand performed the first appendectomy in 1735, but it was not until the 19th century that the disease appendicitis was recognized and a treatment developed for it. Fortunately, at the same time, the development of ether as an anesthetic and the concept of antisepsis by Lister were beginning. The first great debate concerning appendicitis came about when Francois Melier battled with the more influential Guillaume Dupuytren in his 1827 paper, describing postmortem diagnosis of appendicitis and suggesting treatment with appendectomy, instead of attributing all right-sided maladies as diseases of the cecum.[1,3,4] Finally in 1886, Reginald H Fitz formally described the disease and expressed his desired treatment, which was early surgical removal of the appendix, coining the term appendicitis.[5]

Case reports and series described drainage and stone removal for right lower quadrant (RLQ) infections throughout the mid and late 19th century, but in 1887, Morton performed the first deliberate appendectomy that survived.[6] Through the turn of the century, the technique was developed and refined, including the development of the muscle splitting incision by McBurney[7] and the transverse incision with extension through the lateral border of the rectus by Rocky and Davis[8].

The next 7 decades showed the introduction and evolution of antibiotic use, improvements in the safety of anesthesia, and debates on the types of incisions. However, the disease was still deadly if not treated optimally. The obituary from the New York Times of Harry Houdini from November 1st, 1926, describes his death due to the development of perforated appendicitis, delay in treatment, and subsequent development of peritonitis.

Not until 1980, when Dr. Kurt Stemm performed and reported his first laparoscopic appendectomy, was there a more radical change in the treatment of appendicitis.[9] This led to changes in both surgical procedure and patient management. New variants such as single port, robotic, and natural orifice appendectomy rose to add to the new debate on optimal management. Now, the 21st century has seen the turn toward less operative management, antibiotic-only management, and observational management without antibiotics.[10]

9.2 Epidemiology

The incidence of appendicitis had increased in the United States since its description in 1886, peaking in the 1940 s. In 1948, the peak incidence in the United States was 383 per 100,000 person-years.[11] The rate decreased to 152 in 1970,[12] 110 in 1984,[13] and 94 in 1997.[14] In the 21st century, the rate of appendicitis has remained stable at 100 per 100,000 person-years. However, Ferris and Kaplan studied incidence rates and showed that in economically developing areas such as Asia (206), the Middle East (160) and South America (206), rates are on the rise.[15] Implicated but not proven factors are changes in diet, air quality, rates of smoking, and possible introduction of novel infectious agents by increased air travel. The MAGIC study showed that the presentation, severity of disease, and treatment varied throughout the world based on gross national income per capita.[16] Specifically, patients presenting at a younger age in lower income countries underwent less CT scans and less laparoscopic operations. However, there was no difference in death rates or complications in low-income versus high-income countries.

Addiss examined the National Hospital Inpatient Survey and, using data from 1979 to 1984, described a lifetime risk of appendicitis in males (8.6%) and females (6.7%) with a lifetime rate of appendectomy in males (12%) and females (23.1%).[13] This disparity is accounted for by the 12x higher rate of incidental appendectomy in women, probably due to the broader differential diagnosis. The 21st century, with the increased use of nonoperative management, has witnessed a decrease in the rates of appendectomy.[17] There also has been a decrease of 46% in the age standardized death rate from appendicitis.[18]

Seasonal variation of appendicitis is a well-known entity. Fares reviewed 11 studies from 1970 to 2012 and showed an increased incidence of appendicitis in the summer months except in Nigeria and Turkey.[19] Possible explanations include change to a more constipating diet, exposure to more allergens producing lymphoid hyperplasia, possibility of more enteral infections, and possible increased exposure to air pollution. Two recent studies in Europe and Asia confirmed seasonal variation and proposed allotting increased resources during the summer to deal with this phenomenon.[20,21]

While many centers turned to an acute care surgery model to deal with surgical emergencies including appendicitis, there have been mixed results with regard to a benefit in cost and outcome to this allotment of resources. While Bandy showed increased cost ($28,000 to $30,000), higher complications (odds ratio [OR]1.2), and length of stay (2.92 days to 3.31 days) with ACS managed cases, these outcomes differences vanished after adjustment for insurance and comorbidities.[22] Ladhani showed that acute care-trained surgeons were more efficient with less time to OR, shorter hospital stays, and less emergency department cost.[23]

Racial disparities in the treatment of appendicitis still exist in the 21st century. Black patients are more likely than Whites to experience serious postoperative complications.[24] Other studies have shown that with equal access to care, these racial and economic disparities disappear,[25] except that Blacks and lower income patients still underwent minimally invasive procedures less frequently.[26] While there is a large amount of literature about socioeconomic and ethnic disparities throughout medicine, recent studies continue to show the importance of access to care being one of the most important factors. The 2010 Dependent Coverage Provision provided the ability to young adults to remain on their parent's insurance and thus have early access to care. Reductions in the uninsured rate in 19- to 25-year-old patients led to a significant decrease in perforated appendicitis as compared to 26- to 34-year-old patients.[27] Major improvements in the treatment of appendicitis can be made by increasing access to care. Even in the military, in groups where access to care may be limited, such as marine recruits, increased rates of perforated appendicitis have been found as compared to their active duty counterparts.[28]

Most of the epidemiology studies have been based on administrative data. Since the clinical diagnosis can be questionable, and because of incidental appendectomy or appendectomy carried out for diagnoses other than appendicitis, the validity of this approach has been called into question. Coward et al showed that the use of a pathological based registry gave significantly different results when compared to administrative databases.[29] Specifically, administrative databases overestimated the rate of appendicitis and perforated appendicitis with PPV of 83% and 52%, respectively. This calls into question the use of administrative databases where the coding may not accurately reflect the disease.

9.3 Pathogenesis

Appendicitis, a mix of Greek and Latin, is defined as inflammation of the appendix. Classically, the inciting event involves the obstruction of the lumen of the appendix. This can be due to a fecalith, lymphoid hyperplasia, parasites, or malignancy. The obstruction then leads to increased intraluminal pressure and mucosal ischemia, bacterial translocation, further infection and necrosis, perforation (usually within 24 to 36 hours), consequent localized or generalized peritonitis, and possible abscess formation. This classical teaching may not be accurate. The same

process may not be taking place in uncomplicated and complicated appendicitis. The concept of the appendix as a neuroendocrine organ also points to other possible mechanisms of pathogenesis.

Fecaliths are often described by radiologists as supporting evidence for a radiologic diagnosis of appendicitis. However, in one study, the positive predictive value was only 44.8% for appendicitis. Fecaliths were found more commonly in negative appendectomy specimens (28%) than in appendicitis specimens (18%); however, they were significantly more common in perforated/complicated (39%) than nonperforated/uncomplicated appendicitis specimens (14%).[30] This may point to different etiologies of uncomplicated appendicitis and complicated appendicitis. The fact that there may not be true mechanical obstruction of the lumen in uncomplicated appendicitis may also partially explain the phenomenon of spontaneous resolution of appendicitis seen in uncomplicated appendicitis. Another argument for different pathological bases for uncomplicated and complicated appendicitis is the fact that in-hospital delay in treatment does not lead to increased rates of perforation.[31] Delays in surgery for up to 24 hours did not increase the rate of perforation or complication.[32,33] A 2018 meta-analysis showed that delaying appendectomy by up to 24 hours in uncomplicated appendicitis did not show progression to complicated appendicitis, postoperative surgical site infection, or morbidity.[34]

Genetic factors may predispose to appendicitis. The relative risk for appendicitis is 3.4 in twins, 1.98 in siblings, and 6.7 in 1st degree relatives.[35] This may be related to immunologic factors, as shown by fact that children with an Immunoglobulin E (IgE)-mediated allergy had a significantly lower rate of complicated appendicitis (19 vs. 46%).[36]

The concept of the appendix as a neuroendocrine organ with neural transmitter-mediated appendicitis has been studied, with implicating factors being increased levels of VIP and substance P.[37] The patient with ongoing pain but normal imaging presents a dilemma. Often the appendix appears normal but symptoms are relieved after the surgery. The pathology report is negative for acute inflammation, and the results are often attributed to a placebo effect of the surgery. However, the surgery may have been therapeutic. Bouchard showed that many of these patient's appendices had increased neuroproliferation in the lamina propria mucularis and specifically stained for VIP and substance P. The substance P expression was higher or the same in specimens with acute inflammation.[38]Although schizophrenia clearly is a risk factor for perforation due to delays in seeking treatment, schizophrenia has been shown to be protective for appendicitis with an odds ratio of 0.51.[39] This is been explained by the lower levels of VIP in the brain and peripheral nervous system of schizophrenics.

Factors other than host-related factors play a significant role in the pathogenesis. The most important is the microbiome. Recent studies have shown that alteration of the microbiome can lead to anastomotic leaks and fistula formation. While culturing appendicitis has shown to have little to no clinical value, the recent publication by Subramanian showed prognostic significance with regard to culturing purulent fluid.[40] *Streptococcus anginosus* was present in 26% of appendectomy specimens, and was significantly associated with complicated appendicitis, longer

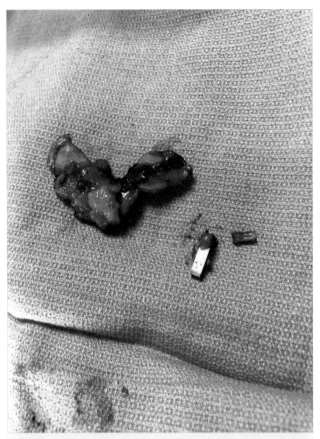

Fig. 9.1 Iatrogenic appendicitis caused by clipping of appendix during tubal ligation.

length of stay, and increased likelihood of developing postoperative complications (OR = 2.4).[41] The treatments for HIV and AIDS have changed dramatically in the last few decades, so that HIV infection alone does not increase the risk of complications, but AIDS still increases postoperative infectious complications (OR 2.12).[42]

Other causes of appendicitis are traumatic and iatrogenic. The incidence of appendicitis is reported at 0.9% of blunt trauma.[43] The mechanism is similar to other hollow viscus injuries, and it has been associated with seat belts signs.[44] The main clinical scenarios are RLQ pain, which is similar to that of nontraumatic appendicitis, presenting 24 or 72 hours after blunt trauma, or vague abdominal pain with small bowel distention and a fluid-like classic blunt hollow viscus injury.[45] Iatrogenic appendicitis is also rare but has been associated with barium procedures and postcolonoscopy, specifically in ulcerative colitis patients.[46] It has also been reported as a complication of surgery to adjacent structures, most commonly observed in urologic and gynecologic procedures. ▶ Fig. 9.1 shows a post tubal ligation appendicitis with clips across the appendix.

9.4 Diagnosis

The diagnosis of appendicitis has classically been clinical in nature. The difficulty in diagnosis can be seen in the historically acceptable negative appendectomy rate of 20 of 25%.[47] The classic history of periumbilical pain which migrates to the RLQ,

and is associated with fever, nausea, vomiting, anorexia, followed by rebound, guarding, Rovsing's sign, psoas sign, and obturator sign is taught in medical school to this day. A survey by Yeh et al showed that 73% of experienced general surgeons would not require further imaging if the patient had the classical presentation and presented within 12 hours from the onset of symptoms.[48]

In 1986, signs, symptoms, and laboratory work were characterized and made part of the Alvarado scoring system that has been validated to varying degrees over the last 30 years.[49] Alvarado described a score of 1 to 4 with 33% chance, 5 to 6 with a 66% chance, and 7 to 10 with a 93% chance of appendicitis (see ▶ Fig. 9.2). In 2011, Ohle performed a meta-analysis of 42 studies, and showed that a cutoff of 5 for ruling out appendicitis had a sensitivity of 96% in men and 99% in women and children.[50] He also performed a calibration analysis of predicted/observed across the three risk strata and three different patient groups (men, women, and children). The Alvarado score was good for ruling out appendicitis with a score less than 5, but for a score over 5, the risk is generally overestimated by the Alvarado score, suggesting the more liberal use of diagnostic imaging.

Coleman and Rozycki,[51] in an attempt to limit the use of CT scan in the emergency room, showed that in males a score of 9 or greater and in women a score of 10 could proceed to the operating room without further diagnostics, with 100% pathology-proven appendicitis. They also showed that 5% of females with a score of less than 2 and 0% of males with a score less than 1 had appendicitis and thus could be safely discharged. Ebell further evaluated the clinical validity by adding a pretest probability to the algorithm,[52] but the clinical significance is of questionable value, as the pretest probability varies between institutions.

Appendicitis is the most common condition in pregnancy requiring abdominal surgery. The incidence in the United States in 2014 was 100 cases in 100,000 births.[53] The rate of sepsis and shock, however, is double that of the general population. Making the diagnosis is important, as appendectomy for negative appendicitis leads to an increased risk of fetal loss, even more so than for uncomplicated appendicitis.[54] A quick and accurate diagnosis is needed in pregnancy. A retrospective review of pregnant and nonpregnant females using the Alvarado score showed equivalent sensitivities in pregnant and nonpregnant women, respectively.[55] Therefore, the Alvarado score can be used as a diagnostic tool in pregnancy.

There is a clear need for imaging modalities to decrease the rates of both missed diagnosis and negative appendectomy. Ultrasound and CT scan have been the default modalities, with MRI generally used only in pregnant patients. A retrospective review of patients from 1992 to 2014 showed that use of CT scan for diagnosing appendicitis significantly increased from 2.8 to 82%.[56] The use of ultrasound in the study period decreased from 4.4 to 2.5% and the use of MRI increased from 0 to 1.7%, neither statistically significant changes. Interestingly, complete omission of imaging decreased from 91 to 2.5%. In a review of the Washington State surgical outcome database, investigators evaluated consecutive appendectomy patients in 15 hospitals from 2006 to 2007. They demonstrated that the use of ultrasound and CT scan significantly decreased the negative

Symptoms		Value
Symptoms	Migration	1
	Anorexia-acetone	1
	Nausea-vomiting	1
Signs	Tenderness in right lower quadrant	2
	Rebound pain	1
	Elevation of temperature	1
Laboratory	Leukocytosis	2
	Shift to the left	1
Total score		10

Fig. 9.2 The Alvarado score for the diagnosis of appendicitis. Scores less than 5 are helpful to rule out appendicitis. Scores grater than 5 may overestimate the risk of appendicitis. (Reproduced with permission of Alvarado A. A practical score for the early diagnosis of acute appendicitis. Ann Emerg Med. 1986;15(5):557–564.)

appendectomy rate.[57] The clinical benefit from additional diagnostic studies is balanced by cost. A 2018 study by D'Souza evaluated whether there was a financial benefit to imaging studies making the diagnosis. After calculating the negative appendectomy rate of 22% at his facility and the financial burden to the hospital of negative appendectomies, he calculated the cost of imaging that would be required to drop the rate of negative appendectomy to 5%. He showed that adding a diagnostic imaging study to the workup would provide significant savings: MRI ($33,866), CT ($105,896) scan and ultrasound ($132,296), respectively.

9.4.1 Ultrasound

Ultrasound is accurate, cost-effective, and bereft of ionizing radiation, but the CT scan remains the default imaging test for most ER patients with abdominal pain. The main drawback of ultrasound is operator dependency. The graded compression ultrasound technique was first used for the diagnosis of appendicitis in 1986,[58] measuring the diameter of the appendix, thickness of the wall, and compressibility. Since then, the technique has not significantly changed. In Europe, the use of contrast-enhanced ultrasound[59] has added to the ability to view vascularity of the appendix and surrounding tissue, but the approach has not been widely used in the United States. The use of ultrasound has been validated using the cutoff of greater than 6 mm for diagnosis of appendicitis. For a diameter of less than 3 mm, between 3 and 6-mm and greater than 6 mm, the rates of appendicitis are 2.6%, 65% and 96%, respectively[60] (▶ Fig. 9.3). Despite these findings, the sensitivity and specificity has been shown to be variable ranging from 44 to 100% and 47 to 99%, respectively.[61] A 2008 meta-analysis showed that CT had better posttest probabilities for both positive and negative examinations.[62]

Factors that may lead to an inconclusive test and the need for further imaging have been evaluated, and include advanced age, BMI, atypical location, and complicated appendicitis.[63] The most common reason for a nondiagnostic ultrasound examination is lack of visualization of the appendix, but is lack of visualization really nondiagnostic? A review of 1383 pediatric patients from 2004 to 2013 showed that lack of visualization of the appendix had an 86% negative predictive value.[64] In 2014, using an algorithm based on clinical suspicion and a nondiagnostic/nonvisualized appendix, 526 out of 968 patients had nonvisualized appendices.[65] Of that group, 59% were discharged, 11% went to the operating room, and 30% were admitted. Only 15% of the 526 had appendicitis, but more importantly, only 0.3% discharged home were ultimately found to have appendicitis. This shows that an algorithm using clinical suspicion and a nonvisualized appendix can be adequate for ruling out appendicitis in the right population. Algorithms have been shown to decrease the amount of CT scans performed.[66]

Newer ideas in ultrasound include the addition of short-interval follow-up ultrasound. Of the 111 children studied with appendicitis, the diagnosis was made without CT in 108.[67] The use of a 5-category scoring system has led to a more accurate diagnosis. The five categories include positive, intermediate, and negative, and nonvisualized with or without secondary findings. In the positive group, the appendicitis rate was 92%; in the intermediate or nonvisualized with findings, the rate was 39%; and in the negative or nonvisualized without secondary findings, the rate was 3.8%.[68] In a period of healthcare emphasizing patient throughput, length of stay and speed of care, and emergency physician point of care, ultrasound has a sensitivity of 84% in adults and 95% in children.[69] The benefits in children are clear, but as age increases, the use of ultrasound alone is probably not sufficient unless the clinical suspicion is strong and the study is positive. That does not mean ultrasound does

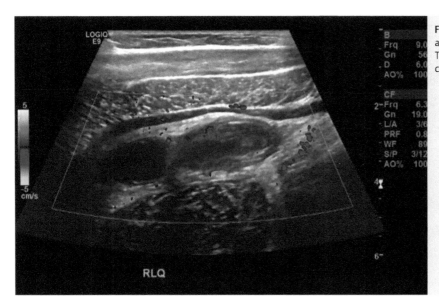

Fig. 9.3 Ultrasound diagnosis of appendicitis. The appendix measures up to 1.3 cm in diameter. There is adjacent increased echogenicity compatible with inflammation.

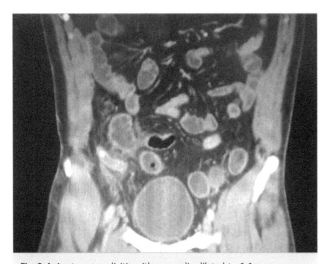

Fig. 9.4 Acute appendicitis with appendix dilated to 1.1 cm, peri-appendiceal fat stranding, no air in appendix, and fecalith.

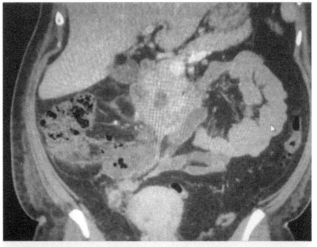

Fig. 9.5 Appendicitis with abscess formation.

not play a role in adults. Using a protocol including ultrasound as the first diagnostic test in patients with a clinical suspicion for appendicitis, CT scan utilization decreased by 50%, with comparable sensitivity but slightly decreased specificity.[70]

9.4.2 Computed Tomography

CT scan (▶ Fig. 9.4, ▶ Fig. 9.5, ▶ Fig. 9.6, ▶ Fig. 9.7) has become the imaging test of choice in adults in the United States. In a 2018 survey of general surgeons from the Eastern Association of the Surgery for Trauma, CT scan was the diagnostic tool of choice in all presentations of RLQ abdominal pain, except for the classic history and physical presentation with less than 12 hours of pain. The rate of preference for CT increased from 26% in the classic presentation, with less than 12 hours of pain, to 65% in a young female and 85% in an older male.[48] The survey also showed that only 38% would use oral contrast, while 81% would use intravenous (IV) contrast.

Various protocols for CT scans have been used, including no contrast, rectal contrast, oral contrast, and IV contrast. All come with their benefits and risks. IV contrast can lead to contrast extravasation which, in turn, could lead to tissue loss, allergic reaction, and contrast-induced nephropathy. Oral contrast can be uncomfortable, carries the risk of aspiration, and, importantly in the modern world of medicine, may lead to increased emergency room times and worsen throughput. Rectal contrast is now rarely used because of its limited benefit and obvious discomfort involved in the technique.

Is there a benefit to oral contrast? Anderson compared the use of oral and IV contrast versus IV contrast alone; a 64 multidetector computed tomography (MDCT) showed no benefit to the addition of oral contrast in sensitivity (100%, 100%) or specificity (97%, 97%).[71] Kepner in 2012 confirmed these findings and also showed that patients who received IV contrast alone had significantly shorter times to emergency

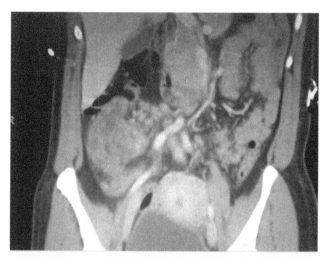

Fig. 9.6 Appendicitis with perforation and phlegmon formation.

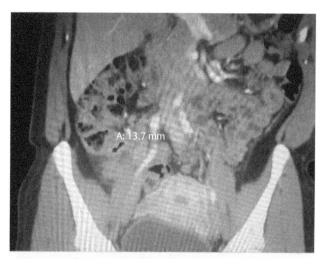

Fig. 9.7 Resolved appendiceal phlegmon with resolution of inflammation and recannalization of the appendix.

department and operating room disposition (1 hour 31 minutes and 1 hour 10 minutes, respectively).[72] Even with CT, there is a risk of nonvisualization of the appendix which can lead to a diagnostic dilemma. The appendix may be nonvisualized in up to 14% of cases; the benefit of oral and IV contrast is that nonvisualization of the appendix reliably excludes appendicitis. Therefore, if not visualized with oral and IV contrast, there is a 98% negative rate for appendicitis.[73] Does nonvisualization rule out appendicitis if oral contrast is not used? Rates of nonvisualization of the appendix improve with the addition of oral contrast, but it does not improve diagnostic accuracy.[74] As fat water content provides contrast between adjacent structures, nonvisualization has been an issue with low body mass index (BMI) patients. However, nonoral contrast CT scan protocols in patients with a BMI of less than 25 do not have diminished accuracy in diagnosing appendicitis.[75] Therefore, we can probably extrapolate that a nonvisualized appendix in an IV only contrast study can exclude appendicitis. The use of oral contrast in the emergency room to rule out appendicitis is unnecessary and inefficient.

The real debate is whether contrast is needed at all. IV contrast entails risks and can introduce delays in centers where renal function laboratory tests are performed prior to scan. A systematic review of the literature revealed the diagnostic accuracy for noncontrast CT scan in adults to be adequate for clinical decision-making, with a sensitivity of 92.7% and a specificity of 96.1%.[76] A meta-analysis in the pediatric population showed similar results in accuracy between noncontrast and IV contrast studies.[77] The need for follow-up with an IV contrast scan for inconclusive results shows that only 5.3% of the time was additional information obtained and only 1.9% of the time was management changed.[78] Therefore, the use of IV contrast is not needed when the suspicion is strong for appendicitis, but the addition of IV contrast may be useful in making the diagnosis of other processes causing RLQ pain when the diagnosis is less clear.

Many studies have now shown the use of low-dose radiation CT scan protocols are as accurate as standard protocols. In the highest risk group for malignancy, low-dose (2mSv) CT was noninferior to conventional (8mSv) CT of the abdomen and pelvis to evaluate for appendicitis in a multicenter randomized trial including 3000 patients. More importantly, it showed that there was no change in outcome, with a similar negative appendectomy rate between the low-dose (3.9%) and conventional dose groups (2.7%).[79] Most recently, the OPTICAP trial showed that a low-dose protocol (3.3mSv) is noninferior to a standard protocol (4.44mSv) in diagnosing appendicitis or differentiating between uncomplicated or complicated appendicitis.[80] Using the lowest dose of radiation and limiting the total number of CT scans should be the goal. An assessment of CT scans from the United States in 2007 showed that an estimated 29,000 future cancers could be related to CT scans performed in 2007, half of those would result in death, and the largest contribution would come from CT scans of the abdomen and pelvis.[81] When performing a diagnostic or therapeutic procedure, we, as physicians, balance risks and benefits. In 2015, Rogers evaluated the possible risk and benefit of universal CT scans. In young adults at the institution studied, 2000 CT scans led to 58 appendectomies. Using the Biological Effects of Ionizing Radiations exposure data, 2000 CT scans should lead to one death. The negative appendectomy rate was 1.7%; thus, the benefit of CT scanning was to avoid 12 negative appendectomies.[82] Is the avoidance of 12 negative appendectomies worth one future cancer death? Limiting the amount of radiation by selectively using CT scanning and changing to low-dose protocols should be the goal.

What is the real impact of CT scanning on clinical outcomes? A 2011 meta-analysis showed that by using CT scans, an institution can decrease its rate of negative appendectomy (16.7 to 8.7%). Time to surgery was increased but this did not increase the rate of perforation.[83] CT scanning has a clear role and can be cost-effective when used in combination with adequate clinical judgement. Long-term malignancy risk is real, so surgical groups need to work with their emergency departments to set-up algorithms such as the one proposed by Coleman and Rozycki to optimize outcomes, costs, and radiation risks.[51]

9.4.3 MRI

MRI has evolved into a viable alternative to CT scanning for appendicitis. The main benefit it has is that it does not expose patients to radiation. This has led to its increased use in pregnancy and children. One of the criticisms of MRI is that except in large volume institutions, experience with reading MRI for appendicitis has been variable. A meta-analysis from 2016 showed that in 30 studies with 2665 patients, the sensitivity and specificity for appendicitis was 96% and 96%, respectively.[84] Subgroup analysis in pregnant patients (94%, 97%) and children (96%, 96%) showed similar results. A 2018 single center study, however, showed that a positive MRI had a positive predictive value of 100% but a sensitivity of only 18%, with two MRIs positive, 29 negative, and 21 inconclusive.[85] Therefore, in this single center study, in contrast to the meta-analysis, a negative or inconclusive MRI could not rule out appendicitis. These two studies highlight the problem of variable accuracy rates with MRI. It has been shown that reader inaccuracy can be improved in attending and resident radiologists with structured training and direct feedback in only 25 cases.[86] MRI does, however, come with a cost. One center's four-year experience from 2012 to 2016 showed that an ultrasound first protocol can reduce the CT scan rate.[87] However, the rate of MRI increased up to 26% and their imaging cost increased as a result.

One of the more interesting and clinically important developments in MRI technology is the development of "Fast MRI.". Different MRI protocols are being developed to make MRI scanning more accessible and limit its cost and time. Ultrafast MRI[88] can be completed in less than 9 minutes, requiring no sedation and no contrast. Clinically, it has a 100% negative predictive value and a 98% positive predictive value in the diagnosis of appendicitis.

9.5 Treatment

From the time of Fitz until 1983, the treatment of appendicitis involved open appendectomy. The first laparoscopic appendectomy in 1983 changed the debate from transverse versus oblique incision to laparoscopic versus open. Up until the 21st century, surgery was the mainstay for treatment, whether it was laparoscopic or open. In the 21st century, the debate changed from laparoscopic versus open surgery to surgery versus antibiotic therapy.

The open appendectomy can be performed with the help of many incisions. A midline laparotomy, the "incision of indecision," is often used when the diagnosis is unclear or when the inflammation is so extreme that partial colectomy may be needed. The two more common incisions are the Rocky–Davis, which is a transverse incision through McBurney's point, (2/3 of the way from the umbilicus to the right anterior superior iliac spine) and the modified McBurney incision, which is an oblique incision along the Langer lines through McBurney's point. This incision is also easier to extend superiorly if more mobilization, or even a colectomy, is needed. Notably, the classic incision is through McBurney's point, but care has to be made to understand the imaging studies preoperatively, as one may need to place the incision higher or more lateral based on the position of the appendix. Placing the incision too low will make it

extremely difficult to mobilize the appendix and cecum into the operative field. The external abdominal oblique fascia is opened along the length of the incision, sometimes extending medially into the rectus sheet if exposure is needed. Then, a muscle-splitting incision is used to carry down to the peritoneum, which is again opened sharply. Appendiceal retractors keep the incision open over the area of interest. Blunt dissection can be used to mobilize the cecum, and the appendix is found at the convergence of the three taenia coli, usually at the base of the cecum. The appendix is then mobilized and its mesentery divided. The base of the appendix is crushed with a clamp and then ligated. Some surgeons will cauterize the mucosa. Some surgeons recommend inverting the appendiceal stump into the cecum and closing the cecum over it with sutures. The peritoneum is then closed and the anterior fascia closed. If the appendix is perforated, management of the skin wound remain a topic of controversy. There are proponents of primary closure, delayed primary closure, closure by secondary intention, and a variety of adjuncts to primary closure (probing, wicks, and negative pressure wound therapy over a closed incision).

The laparoscopic approach classically uses three ports, one at the umbilicus with a 10 to 12 mm trocar, and two other ports of 5 to 10 mm. The risk of placing 10 mm ports is hernia formation, with the rate of hernia increased from 0.5% for 5 mm ports to 5% for 10 mm ports.[89] The two nonumbilical ports can be placed in order to triangulate, but surgeon preference is variable and can be adjusted for adhesions or a gravid uterus. The loop suture technique has been shown to decrease device costs, but these savings were negated by increased operating room time,[90] while others concluded that the loop technique did, in fact, lead to a cost savings over other techniques.[91] More importantly than cost, Beldi showed that in 6486 patients, the rate of intra-abdominal infection was significantly increased by endoloop (1.7%) versus stapled closure (0.7%).[92]

Irrigation after removal of the appendix is another point of contention. There have been a series of contradictory studies. Some studies show copious irrigation (greater than or equal to 2 liters) leads to decreased intra-abdominal abscess rates in patients with complicated appendicitis.[93] Others, using large volumes with short controlled irrigations, showed a significant decrease in intra-abdominal infections with both complicated and uncomplicated patients.[94] Others show a suction-only approach leads to significantly decreased incidence of abscesses,[95] whereas still others show no difference.[96] Recent surveys of pediatric surgeons showed 58% irrigate only if contaminated.[97] The surgical concept of keeping the infection localized and not spreading through uncontrolled lavage of the abdomen, however, follows sound surgical principles.

9.5.1 Laparoscopic Versus Open Appendectomy

Surveys of surgeons reveal that the laparoscopic approach is preferred over the open approach. Pediatric surgeons prefer laparoscopy in the treatment of simple (89%) and perforated appendicitis (81%),[97] with similar findings among adult surgeons.[48]

The most extensive recent study comparing open versus laparoscopic appendectomy was a 2017 meta-analysis study of three randomized controlled trials and 23 case control trials with

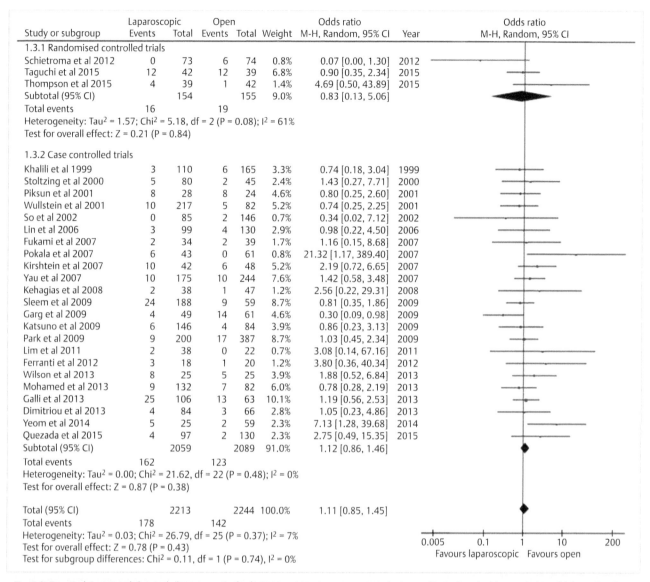

Study or subgroup	Laparoscopic		Open			Odds ratio		Odds ratio
	Events	Total	Events	Total	Weight	M-H, Random, 95% CI	Year	M-H, Random, 95% CI
1.3.1 Randomised controlled trials								
Schietroma et al 2012	0	73	6	74	0.8%	0.07 [0.00, 1.30]	2012	
Taguchi et al 2015	12	42	12	39	6.8%	0.90 [0.35, 2.34]	2015	
Thompson et al 2015	4	39	1	42	1.4%	4.69 [0.50, 43.89]	2015	
Subtotal (95% CI)		154		155	9.0%	0.83 [0.13, 5.06]		
Total events	16		19					
Heterogeneity: Tau^2 = 1.57; Chi^2 = 5.18, df = 2 (P = 0.08); I^2 = 61%								
Test for overall effect: Z = 0.21 (P = 0.84)								
1.3.2 Case controlled trials								
Khalili et al 1999	3	110	6	165	3.3%	0.74 [0.18, 3.04]	1999	
Stoltzing et al 2000	5	80	2	45	2.4%	1.43 [0.27, 7.71]	2000	
Piksun et al 2001	8	28	8	24	4.6%	0.80 [0.25, 2.60]	2001	
Wullstein et al 2001	10	217	5	82	5.2%	0.74 [0.25, 2.25]	2001	
So et al 2002	0	85	2	146	0.7%	0.34 [0.02, 7.12]	2002	
Lin et al 2006	3	99	4	130	2.9%	0.98 [0.22, 4.50]	2006	
Fukami et al 2007	2	34	2	39	1.7%	1.16 [0.15, 8.68]	2007	
Pokala et al 2007	6	43	0	61	0.8%	21.32 [1.17, 389.40]	2007	
Kirshtein et al 2007	10	42	6	48	5.2%	2.19 [0.72, 6.65]	2007	
Yau et al 2007	10	175	10	244	7.6%	1.42 [0.58, 3.48]	2007	
Kehagias et al 2008	2	38	1	47	1.2%	2.56 [0.22, 29.31]	2008	
Sleem et al 2009	24	188	9	59	8.7%	0.81 [0.35, 1.86]	2009	
Garg et al 2009	4	49	14	61	4.6%	0.30 [0.09, 0.98]	2009	
Katsuno et al 2009	6	146	4	84	3.9%	0.86 [0.23, 3.13]	2009	
Park et al 2009	9	200	17	387	8.7%	1.03 [0.45, 2.34]	2009	
Lim et al 2011	2	38	0	22	0.7%	3.08 [0.14, 67.16]	2011	
Ferranti et al 2012	3	18	1	20	1.2%	3.80 [0.36, 40.34]	2012	
Wilson et al 2013	8	25	5	25	3.9%	1.88 [0.52, 6.84]	2013	
Mohamed et al 2013	9	132	7	82	6.0%	0.78 [0.28, 2.19]	2013	
Galli et al 2013	25	106	13	63	10.1%	1.19 [0.56, 2.53]	2013	
Dimitriou et al 2013	4	84	3	66	2.8%	1.05 [0.23, 4.86]	2013	
Yeom et al 2014	5	25	2	59	2.3%	7.13 [1.28, 39.68]	2014	
Quezada et al 2015	4	97	2	130	2.3%	2.75 [0.49, 15.35]	2015	
Subtotal (95% CI)		2059		2089	91.0%	1.12 [0.86, 1.46]		
Total events	162		123					
Heterogeneity: Tau^2 = 0.00; Chi^2 = 21.62, df = 22 (P = 0.48); I^2 = 0%								
Test for overall effect: Z = 0.87 (P = 0.38)								
Total (95% CI)		2213		2244	100.0%	1.11 [0.85, 1.45]		
Total events	178		142					
Heterogeneity: Tau^2 = 0.03; Chi^2 = 26.79, df = 25 (P = 0.37); I^2 = 7%								
Test for overall effect: Z = 0.78 (P = 0.43)								
Test for subgroup differences: Chi^2 = 0.11, df = 1 (P = 0.74); I^2 = 0%								

0.005   0.1   1   10   200
Favours laparoscopic   Favours open

Fig. 9.8 Forest plot– intra-abdominal abscesses rate for laparoscopic versus open appendectomy. (Reproduced with permission of Athanasiou C, Lockwood S, Markides GA. Systematic review and meta-analysis of laparoscopic versus open apendicectomy in adults with complicated appendicitis: an update of the literature. World J Surg. 2017; 41(12):3083–3099.)

a total of 4439 patients. The findings showed clear advantages of laparoscopy with a significant benefit in surgical site infection, time to tolerate oral intake, and length of stay, and no difference in intra-abdominal abscesses[98] (▸ Fig. 9.8, ▸ Fig. 9.9, ▸ Fig. 9.10).

A 2010 Cochrane database review of 67 trials also compared the two techniques.[99] The rate of wound infection decreased by 50% when laparoscopy was compared with the open technique, with extremely low heterogeneity. However, laparoscopic appendectomy led to a 3-fold increase in intra-abdominal abscess, not attributable to the technique of stump closure (loop versus stapler). Laparoscopy was also associated with less pain. There was also a 1.1 day reduction of length of stay, but this was qualified by the authors because the two largest studies showing no difference in length of stay were excluded, as they only reported the mean length of stay, and the remaining studies showed a high-heterogeneity. Laparoscopy yielded an earlier return of bowel function, as well as earlier return to work (2 days) and

daily activities (5 days earlier), but it increased hospital costs. Again, the authors qualified the findings of increased hospital costs, as cost benefits outside the hospital seem to cancel out the increase in hospital costs. The findings in children were similar, with the strongest finding being a decrease in superficial surgical site infection, but no conclusion could be made on the issue of intra-abdominal abscess due to the rarity of the finding in the studies examined. The study concluded that the laparoscopic approach was superior, but that the open approach was acceptable. Finally, single center results from 2011 to 2013 showed that length of stay and morbidity were higher in the open appendectomy group, with the risk of Clavien Dindo 3 or greater complications being 2.6 times more likely with an open procedure.[100]

The evolution of laparoscopic appendectomy and the developing comfort with the procedure among surgeons has led to changes in the overall management of appendicitis. The less

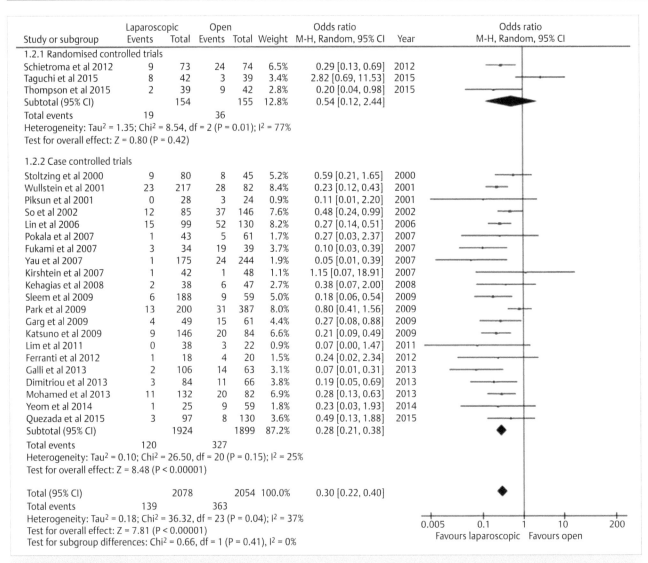

Study or subgroup	Laparoscopic Events	Total	Open Events	Total	Weight	Odds ratio M-H, Random, 95% CI	Year
1.2.1 Randomised controlled trials							
Schietroma et al 2012	9	73	24	74	6.5%	0.29 [0.13, 0.69]	2012
Taguchi et al 2015	8	42	3	39	3.4%	2.82 [0.69, 11.53]	2015
Thompson et al 2015	2	39	9	42	2.8%	0.20 [0.04, 0.98]	2015
Subtotal (95% CI)		154		155	12.8%	0.54 [0.12, 2.44]	
Total events	19		36				
Heterogeneity: Tau^2 = 1.35; Chi^2 = 8.54, df = 2 (P = 0.01); I^2 = 77%							
Test for overall effect: Z = 0.80 (P = 0.42)							
1.2.2 Case controlled trials							
Stoltzing et al 2000	9	80	8	45	5.2%	0.59 [0.21, 1.65]	2000
Wullstein et al 2001	23	217	28	82	8.4%	0.23 [0.12, 0.43]	2001
Piksun et al 2001	0	28	3	24	0.9%	0.11 [0.01, 2.20]	2001
So et al 2002	12	85	37	146	7.6%	0.48 [0.24, 0.99]	2002
Lin et al 2006	15	99	52	130	8.2%	0.27 [0.14, 0.51]	2006
Pokala et al 2007	1	43	5	61	1.7%	0.27 [0.03, 2.37]	2007
Fukami et al 2007	3	34	19	39	3.7%	0.10 [0.03, 0.39]	2007
Yau et al 2007	1	175	24	244	1.9%	0.05 [0.01, 0.39]	2007
Kirshtein et al 2007	1	42	1	48	1.1%	1.15 [0.07, 18.91]	2007
Kehagias et al 2008	2	38	6	47	2.7%	0.38 [0.07, 2.00]	2008
Sleem et al 2009	6	188	9	59	5.0%	0.18 [0.06, 0.54]	2009
Park et al 2009	13	200	31	387	8.0%	0.80 [0.41, 1.56]	2009
Garg et al 2009	4	49	15	61	4.4%	0.27 [0.08, 0.88]	2009
Katsuno et al 2009	9	146	20	84	6.6%	0.21 [0.09, 0.49]	2009
Lim et al 2011	0	38	3	22	0.9%	0.07 [0.00, 1.47]	2011
Ferranti et al 2012	1	18	4	20	1.5%	0.24 [0.02, 2.34]	2012
Galli et al 2013	2	106	14	63	3.1%	0.07 [0.01, 0.31]	2013
Dimitriou et al 2013	3	84	11	66	3.8%	0.19 [0.05, 0.69]	2013
Mohamed et al 2013	11	132	20	82	6.9%	0.28 [0.13, 0.63]	2013
Yeom et al 2014	1	25	9	59	1.8%	0.23 [0.03, 1.93]	2014
Quezada et al 2015	3	97	8	130	3.6%	0.49 [0.13, 1.88]	2015
Subtotal (95% CI)		1924		1899	87.2%	0.28 [0.21, 0.38]	
Total events	120		327				
Heterogeneity: Tau^2 = 0.10; Chi^2 = 26.50, df = 20 (P = 0.15); I^2 = 25%							
Test for overall effect: Z = 8.48 (P < 0.00001)							
Total (95% CI)		2078		2054	100.0%	0.30 [0.22, 0.40]	
Total events	139		363				
Heterogeneity: Tau^2 = 0.18; Chi^2 = 36.32, df = 23 (P = 0.04); I^2 = 37%							
Test for overall effect: Z = 7.81 (P < 0.00001)							
Test for subgroup differences: Chi^2 = 0.66, df = 1 (P = 0.41), I^2 = 0%							

Favours laparoscopic   Favours open

Fig. 9.9 Forest plot– surgical site infection rate for laparoscopic versus open appendectomy. (Reproduced with permission of Athanasiou C, Lockwood S, Markides GA. Systematic review and meta-analysis of laparoscopic versus open apendicectomy in adults with complicated appendicitis: an update of the literature. World J Surg. 2017; 41(12):3083–3099.)

invasive nature led to a decrease in the length of stay, which then led to surgeons decreasing length of stay for the conventional open procedure. In many cases, appendectomy is now an ambulatory procedure. A 1997 randomized trial showed that there was no difference between length of stay or postop pain, but it did show increased operating room time and hospital costs for laparoscopic appendectomy.[101] In 2011, a review of 40337 patients from the University Health System Consortium database looked at mortality, morbidity, readmission rate, length of stay, and hospital cost. It showed improved outcomes for laparoscopy in uncomplicated appendicitis but not improved cost ($7,825 for laparoscopy and $7,841 for open). For complicated appendicitis, surgical outcomes were improved and costs were reduced ($12,125 for laparoscopy and $17,495 for open).[102] Presently, enhanced recovery programs for appendicitis have been developed. These protocols led to similar surgical outcomes and complications, but the average length of stay was significantly improved, with over 90% of patients successfully completing

ambulatory management.[103] Notably, the length of stay in the enhanced recovery group was down to 9 hours and the rate of readmission was no different.

Another benefit to laparoscopy was seen in the statistically nonsignificant decreased rate of negative appendectomy and statistically significant decreased rate of unestablished diagnosis reported in the Cochrane review.[99] Reiertsen, in a randomized controlled trial of open versus laparoscopic appendectomy, showed a significant decrease in negative appendectomy rates with laparoscopy.[104] Laparoscopy allows for a clearer exploration of adnexal processes, inflammatory bowel disease, and malignancy.

Stump appendicitis, which can occur when a residual segment of appendix is left behind, causes significant morbidity, increased cost, and further surgery. The recurrent appendicitis in the stump can lead to perforation and possible fistula if the staple line or loop is distal to an obstruction. A 2018 review of 3000 appendectomies over 10 years showed a rate of stump

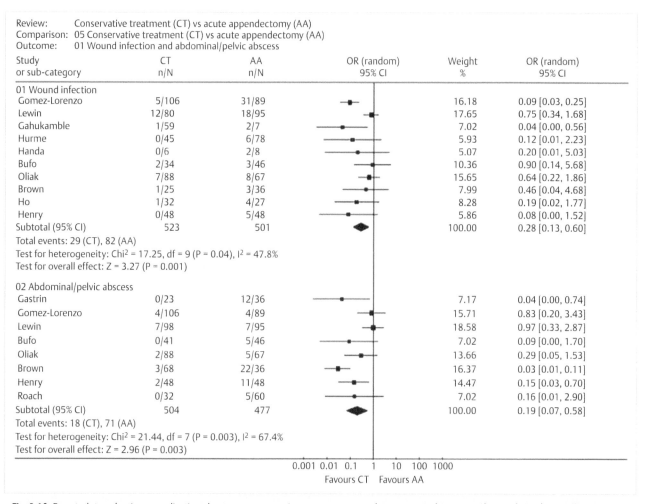

Review: Conservative treatment (CT) vs acute appendectomy (AA)
Comparison: 05 Conservative treatment (CT) vs acute appendectomy (AA)
Outcome: 01 Wound infection and abdominal/pelvic abscess

Study or sub-category	CT n/N	AA n/N	OR (random) 95% CI	Weight %	OR (random) 95% CI
01 Wound infection					
Gomez-Lorenzo	5/106	31/89		16.18	0.09 [0.03, 0.25]
Lewin	12/80	18/95		17.65	0.75 [0.34, 1.68]
Gahukamble	1/59	2/7		7.02	0.04 [0.00, 0.56]
Hurme	0/45	6/78		5.93	0.12 [0.01, 2.23]
Handa	0/6	2/8		5.07	0.20 [0.01, 5.03]
Bufo	2/34	3/46		10.36	0.90 [0.14, 5.68]
Oliak	7/88	8/67		15.65	0.64 [0.22, 1.86]
Brown	1/25	3/36		7.99	0.46 [0.04, 4.68]
Ho	1/32	4/27		8.28	0.19 [0.02, 1.77]
Henry	0/48	5/48		5.86	0.08 [0.00, 1.52]
Subtotal (95% CI)	523	501		100.00	0.28 [0.13, 0.60]

Total events: 29 (CT), 82 (AA)
Test for heterogeneity: Chi² = 17.25, df = 9 (P = 0.04), I² = 47.8%
Test for overall effect: Z = 3.27 (P = 0.001)

02 Abdominal/pelvic abscess					
Gastrin	0/23	12/36		7.17	0.04 [0.00, 0.74]
Gomez-Lorenzo	4/106	4/89		15.71	0.83 [0.20, 3.43]
Lewin	7/98	7/95		18.58	0.97 [0.33, 2.87]
Bufo	0/41	5/46		7.02	0.09 [0.00, 1.70]
Oliak	2/88	5/67		13.66	0.29 [0.05, 1.53]
Brown	3/68	22/36		16.37	0.03 [0.01, 0.11]
Henry	2/48	11/48		14.47	0.15 [0.03, 0.70]
Roach	0/32	5/60		7.02	0.16 [0.01, 2.90]
Subtotal (95% CI)	504	477		100.00	0.19 [0.07, 0.58]

Total events: 18 (CT), 71 (AA)
Test for heterogeneity: Chi² = 21.44, df = 7 (P = 0.003), I² = 67.4%
Test for overall effect: Z = 2.96 (P = 0.003)

0.001 0.01 0.1 1 10 100 1000
Favours CT   Favours AA

Fig. 9.10 Forest plot evaluating complications between conservative management and acute appendectomy with complicated appendicitis. (Reproduced with permission of Similis C, Symeoonides P, Shorthouse AJ, Tekkis PP. A meta-analysis comparing conservative treatment versus acute appendectomy for complicated appendicitis(abscess or phlegmon). Surgery. 2010;147(6):818–829.)

appendicitis of 0.15%.[105] Up to 40% may go on to perforate. Care must be taken to clearly identify the base of the appendix during the initial operation.[106]

9.5.2 Alternative Minimal Invasive Techniques

The age of minimally invasive surgery has spurred surgeons to develop more minimally invasive and more technically advanced approaches. The most common are single incision laparoscopic surgery and robotic surgery. Natural orifice transluminal endoscopic surgery (NOTES) saw a period of interest, but currently has seen no widespread use. The technology has advanced fast and the research into safety, benefits, and costs have not fully caught up. A Cochrane review of single port laparoscopic appendectomy from 2011 stated that no conclusions can be drawn in comparing single port versus conventional multiport laparoscopic surgery[107] because there have been no appropriate randomized controlled trials to appropriately compare these two laparoscopic approaches.

Single port laparoscopic surgery was designed to improve cosmesis and, to some extent, improve pain and time to recovery. However, safety and efficacy have to be noninferior to multiport surgery to fully adopt single port surgery. The steep learning curve for these procedures is well-documented, so experience in the procedure is important, and that may be the reason why there has been such heterogeneity of results in the literature.[108] Most studies have shown little to no benefit in terms of pain improvement and some have even showed worse pain. A 2014 randomized trial showed worsened pain and increased opiate use with single port laparoscopy, while showing no improvement in perceived cosmesis.[109]

Most, if not all, studies showed increased operative time and cost. The most worrisome issue is the intermittent finding of increased trocar hernia rate in single port laparoscopic surgery.[110,111] The normal rate of trocar hernia in multiple port hernia is 1.7 to 1.8% increasing to up to 5.8% in one study in single port surgery. More recent studies have continued to show very little benefit with increased time, later postop functional recovery, length of stay, and cost.[112] At this point in time, it can be concluded that single port laparoscopic appendectomy is a safe and effective form of appendectomy, but there is little, if any, benefit and increased costs.

Robotic and natural orifice appendectomy have been used sparingly. There are no randomized trials and reports on complication rates for appendectomy. The lack of evidence with regard to advantages of robotic appendectomy over other minimally invasive techniques implies that robotic appendectomy should be only conducted under research protocols.[113] NOTES and, more precisely, distant target NOTES (which is the category for natural orifice appendectomy) have not been widely adapted. Atallah, in his review of NOTES, showed that "enthusiasm" with respect to distant target NOTES is decreasing due to well-described NOTES-specific complications.[114] A 2017 report of a prospective observational trial of transgastric appendectomy showed no benefits in relation to transgastric surgery.[115] Both robotic and NOTES have very limited data to support any recommendation regarding their use.

9.5.3 Appendectomy Versus Antibiotics

Since the first description of acute appendicitis was published in the late 19th century, appendectomy has been considered the gold standard therapy of the disease. However, over the past 2 decades, some have been challenging this standard of care in favor of nonoperative management with antimicrobial therapy. In cases of complicated appendicitis with abscess formation, nonoperative treatment with percutaneous drainage of fluid collections and antibiotics is well-accepted as primary therapy. Initial treatment with antimicrobials for acute nonperforated appendicitis has been the center of debate in recent years.

9.5.4 Uncomplicated

Proponents of this alternative treatment argue that treating with antibiotics eliminates the risks of abdominal surgery, such as wound infection, intra-abdominal sepsis, small bowel obstruction from adhesions, and risk of general anesthesia, especially in patients with comorbidities. In 2014, DiSaverio, in the prospective observational NOTA trial, assessed nonoperative management in a large group of patients over a 2-year period.[116] He showed the recurrence rate over the 2-year period was 13.8%. More importantly, the failure rate of nonoperative management in the first week was 11.9%. In addition, the authors observed a rapid rise in the recurrence rate to approximately 10% before reaching 13.8% at 2 years.

A meta-analysis of three randomized controlled trials found that antibiotics were only successful in treating 68% of patients with an initial presentation of uncomplicated appendicitis. Even though there was a trend toward reduced risk of complications in patients treated with antibiotics, there was a high crossover rate of 42% from the antibiotics-only group to surgery, either due to failure of nonoperative therapy or readmission for appendicitis. Therefore, the authors concluded that antibiotics only in the treatment of uncomplicated appendicitis may not be superior to appendectomy. In addition, a major limitation of these studies was that they lacked a systematic assessment for the diagnosis of acute appendicitis. Diagnosis was often made based on clinical presentation alone.[117]

Vons et al performed a randomized controlled trial utilizing CT scan to confirm the diagnosis of uncomplicated appendicitis, and then assigned patients to antibiotics with amoxicillin and clavulanic acid or immediate appendectomy. The group that received antibiotics experienced persistent abdominal pain or peritonitis more often than the appendectomy group within 30 days after treatment. The authors also found that antibiotics alone were successful in treating 68% of patients with the remaining subjects undergoing appendectomy either within 30 days or one-year postintervention. The presence of an appendicolith on CT was associated with a significantly increased rate of complicated appendicitis and failure of antibiotic management. The rate of recurrence after nonoperative management within 1 year of follow-up was 25% in the study, which is significantly higher than 14% reported in other studies. The authors concluded that immediate appendectomy remains the standard of care for acute uncomplicated appendicitis, especially in those with risk factors associated with failure of conservative management.[118]

The 2015 APPAC trial attempted to show noninferiority of antibiotic therapy in CT-proven uncomplicated appendicitis.[119] The antibiotic therapy group received 3 days of IV ertapenem and 7 days of oral levofloxacin and metronidazole. The overwhelming majority (256 out of 257) of patients had one-year follow-up in the antibiotic group, with 72.7% percent not requiring appendectomy. However, the 27% failure rate of antibiotic therapy was greater than the assumed acceptable level of 24%, thereby rejecting noninferiority. The complication rates were lower in the antibiotic group (2.8%), and continued to be lower in the failed antibiotic group (7%), as compared to the surgery-only group (20.5%). The most common complication was surgical wound infection. Since only 15% underwent laparoscopy, the wound infection rate was high, which was not reflective of current laparoscopic experience. Interestingly, there was a 1.5% rate of neoplasm. This highlights the potential for delaying the diagnosis and treatment of malignancy with nonoperative management. In the 2018 update of the APPAC trial, 3-year and 5-year failure rates were 37% and 39%, respectively.[120]

A more recent meta-analysis showed an initial failure rate of 19.4% and a 1-year failure rate of 36.2%.[121] Overall complications were greater in the surgery group (23.6 vs. 7.7%), which is understandable, as surgery has more identifiable complications than antibiotics. Notably, differing from previous studies, the rate of abscess formation was significantly increased in the group that failed antibiotics versus the appendectomy group. Finally, patients who failed antibiotic therapy had a relative risk of 2.83 for the development of wound infection as compared to the appendectomy group, which differed from the APPAC trial.

Surgeons continue to debate the issue of appendectomy versus antibiotics and individual biases seem to let surgeons come to different conclusions from the same data. Maybe if we could predict a group less likely to fail antibiotic treatment, we could better come to a consensus on treating appendicitis. Loftus designed a clinically relevant protocol to help improve outcomes with nonoperative management.[122] Patients were directed into the appendectomy or nonoperative management pathway based on CT scan evidence of appendicitis and a modified Alvarado score greater or less than 6, and compared outcomes to preprotocol treatment. This protocol led to a decrease in total appendectomy and decreased hospital stay. However, there was a very high failure rate of nonoperative management

(33%), so he concluded that his criteria were not adequate. He also showed an increased risk of perforation in the failed nonoperative management group by up to 28%.

Loftus, in a retrospective review, showed that duration of symptoms greater than 25 hours (OR 4.17), lack of fever during the first 6 hours of admission (OR 8.07), modified Alvarado score less than 4 (OR 9.06), and appendiceal diameter of less than 13 mm (OR 17.55)[123] were all related to successful nonoperative management. Although there was a trend toward the presence of a fecalith having an increased risk of failed management, it did not reach statistical significance. In this study no patient had all four criteria, but the successful management rates were 67% for three criteria, 54% for two criteria, and 29% for one criterion. Using these types of predictors, we may be able to improve our selection of nonoperative management in uncomplicated appendicitis.

The debate may have a new twist. Parks shows that patients randomized to either no antibiotics or a 4-day course of antibiotics had no difference in treatment failure rate, with a shorter hospital stay and decreased cost.[124] The failure rate was 23% in the no antibiotics group and 20% in the antibiotic group. This points to the fact that not all cases of appendicitis behave similarly and have the same clinical course; some will resolve without any treatment. As we improve our ability to identify subgroups of patients suited for antibiotics, no antibiotics, and surgery, we will not only improve failure rates but will also optimize cost of therapy. An analysis of the APPAC trial for cost-effectiveness showed operative therapy to be 1.6 times more expensive than antibiotic therapy. This not only considered total hospital charges but also societal costs, including productivity losses. Treatment costs represented a smaller proportion of the overall costs compared to societal costs. Sick leave time was the most expensive component of cost. Therefore, protocols designed to improve postop care and return to activity earlier can help decrease costs. However, the APPAC trial compared antibiotics with open appendectomy. The cost of appendectomy can vary depending on open or laparoscopic and differ based on techniques of laparoscopic appendectomy. Therefore, to truly understand differences in cost, data on surgical technique and postoperative care would need to be included in the analysis.

9.5.5 Complicated Appendicitis

Of the 300,000 appendectomies performed each year in the United States, 25% are associated with complicated appendicitis, generally defined as perforated with phlegmon or abscess. Nonoperative management with IV antibiotics alone or with drainage has been a mainstay of treatment. Nonoperative management is associated with a decreased rate of wound infections (OR 0.24), intra-abdominal abscess (OR 0.19), and ileus/obstruction (OR 0.35)[125] (see ▸ Fig. 9.10). A recent study of complicated appendicitis showed a significant increase in nonoperative management rate with age (greater than 42 years) and delay in presentation. Patients managed initially nonoperatively had significant increased lengths of stay, but no increase in cost and increase in intra-abdominal abscesses.[126] A significant percentage (33%) of patients with complicated appendicitis who managed nonoperatively failed treatment. The rate of partial colectomy was 2/247 for early appendectomy and 2/58 for late

appendectomy. A Cochrane review analyzed early versus delayed appendectomy in complicated appendicitis. There were only two randomized controlled trials with 80 patients. They concluded there was insufficient evidence to determine if early appendectomy prevents complications.[127]

In children, nonoperative therapy for perforated and phlegmonous appendicitis has been dogma. A recent meta-analysis showed decrease rates of complication (OR 0.22) and specifically wound infection (OR 0.40) with conservative management. A survey of European pediatric surgeons showed that the presence of a phlegmon or abscess is the most common contraindication for immediate surgery.[97]

Whether or not to perform an interval appendectomy is influenced by complication rates, costs, and risk of malignancy. The risk of recurrence after nonoperative management of complicated appendicitis is 12 to 17%.[128,129] A meta-analysis of over 1,900 patients showed no difference in morbidity or length of stay between interval appendectomy and recurrent appendicitis managed nonoperatively. Senekjian showed that for likelihood of cost-effectiveness, interval appendectomy is the preferred strategy up until 33 years of age, after which no interval appendectomy becomes more likely to be cost-effective.[130] Wright showed that the rate of neoplasm was 0.5% in uncomplicated and 12% in complicated appendicitis.[131] The need for colonoscopy prior to interval appendectomy or after nonoperative management has not been well-studied. However, patients diagnosed with acute appendicitis and over 40 years of age showed a 7.4% rate of colonic neoplasm, supporting the importance of performing colonoscopy after an episode of uncomplicated or complicated appendicitis managed nonoperatively if age is greater than 40 years.[132]

The debate on antibiotics versus surgery is further clouded by the different antibiotic regimens used. There is not adequate data to recommend any specific antibiotic protocol. It seems clear that when treating complicated appendicitis, and the source is controlled, patients do not need more than 4 days of antibiotics.[133] It is also clear that if a patient is able to tolerate per os (PO), then treatment with enteral antibiotics in the first 3 days after surgery is noninferior to IV antibiotics.[134]

9.6 Appendicitis in the Elderly

Although appendectomy is one of the most commonly performed procedures, the overall mortality rate is between 0.07 to 0.7% for nonperforated and 0.5 to 2.4% for perforated appendicitis. The risk of mortality increases with age: 2.6% for patients over 70 years old, 6.8% over 80, and 16.4% over 90.[135] The elderly pose a challenge due to their comorbidities and variability in presentation.

Classic symptoms are frequently absent in the elderly population. White blood cell count can sometimes be normal or mildly elevated. Less than one-third of older patients present with all four signs and symptoms of fever, anorexia, RLQ pain, and leukocytosis.[136,137] Therefore, the diagnosis of acute appendicitis is often delayed in the elderly because of atypical presentation. By the time they present to the hospital, many of those patients may have experienced 3 to 7 days of symptoms. In fact, half of these patients are found to have a perforated appendix with abscess formation at the time of surgery.[138] When comparing perforated and nonperforated appendicitis in patients over 60 years old, delay in presentation is associated with a higher rate of complicated appendicitis, whereas delay in surgical treatment after admission is not.[137] Early and routine use of CT imaging in elderly patients with abdominal pain reduced the rate of perforated appendicitis from 72 to 51% over a few decades.[136] Perhaps because of the increased use of imaging modalities, the incidence of negative appendectomy is also significantly lower in the elderly group.[139]

Very few studies have evaluated antibiotics for appendicitis in the elderly. Nonetheless, a case-control study by Horn et al explored the incidence, demographics, and outcomes of nonoperative management in the United States, spanning from 1998 to 2014 and found that patients who were older and had more comorbidities were more likely to have acute appendicitis managed nonoperatively. In addition, the study found a positive association between nonoperative management and mortality, leading the authors to conclude that early operative treatment may be more beneficial for elderly patients and for those with multiple comorbidities.[140] Nevertheless, a randomized controlled trial in this patient population may help guide the treatment strategy for acute appendicitis.

While the risk of neoplasm associated with acute appendicitis is low, the risk increases with age, and the consequences of delayed diagnosis of malignancy can be devastating with dissemination of tumor within the peritoneal cavity. As there is no consensus with regard to the practice of interval appendectomy, clinicians should err on the side of caution when treating an elderly patient with acute appendicitis. Interval appendectomy should be considered with a dilated appendix greater than 15 mm on imaging at the initial episode. Repeat ultrasound or CT may be helpful after completion of antibiotics to evaluate for an appendiceal mass.

Since these patients often present with complicated appendicitis, the operative time and the hospital length of stay are both significantly longer than in the younger population. In addition, the rate of conversion from laparoscopy to open is also significantly greater in the elderly compared to younger patients, mostly secondary to increased rate of perforation and severe inflammation.[139] Furthermore, this patient population also has a higher rate of comorbidities, such as ischemic heart disease, diabetes mellitus, pulmonary conditions, and previous abdominal operations, which can all contribute to increased mortality and morbidity rate.[141] One retrospective study did not find a significant difference in postoperative morbidity unrelated to the surgical procedure, but had a higher incidence of cardiac complications in the elderly group.[139] Half of the deaths associated with appendicitis occur in the elderly.[138] Mortality is often associated with intra-abdominal sepsis and comorbidities related to pulmonary and cardiac diseases.[137] In addition, patients over 60 years old are also more likely to be discharged to a rehabilitation facility, skilled nursing home, or long-term care facility after undergoing treatment for appendicitis.[141]

Even though acute appendicitis is one of the most commonly treated diseases in the world, a few obstacles remain before optimizing management of the condition in the elderly. Despite appendicitis being a disease of the young, clinicians must remain cognizant of the diagnosis when a geriatric patient presents with abdominal pain. Delayed and atypical presentation can often confuse the clinical picture. Early utilization of imaging studies such as ultrasound and/or CT can help with the diagnosis and may decrease the rate of perforation. It can also identify complicated appendicitis with abscess and promptly initiate nonoperative treatment with percutaneous drainage and antibiotics. Primary therapy with antimicrobials can be considered in selected low-risk patients in order to minimize risks of surgery and anesthesia, as some studies have shown efficacy in acute, nonperforated, appendicitis in the adult population, but treating physicians must be aware that conservative management in this setting has not been well-studied in the elderly. Because the risk of appendiceal neoplasm increases for patients over 40 years, clinicians must be vigilant when an elderly patient presents with appendicitis. Interval appendectomy should be performed when there is a suspicion of malignancy to prevent progression of disease. Appendicitis-associated mortality remains higher in the elderly compared to the younger population, but this may be due to more comorbid conditions that contribute to complications. However, mortality rate may be improved by reducing delay to presentation, earlier use of imaging modalities, recognition of complications related to comorbidities, and aggressive treatment of sepsis.

9.7 Pregnancy

Appendicitis is the most common surgical abdominal emergency during pregnancy with 101 cases of appendicitis per 100,000 live births.[53] In 2017, Won evaluated over 62,000 appendectomies in women from 2005 to 2011. Pregnancy was associated with higher negative appendectomy rates and pregnant patients were less likely to undergo laparoscopic appendectomy. Appendectomy increased preterm birth but over time the risk normalized.[142] The diagnosis of appendicitis is important because negative appendectomy increases fetal loss. Both perforated appendicitis and negative appendectomy increase risks of fetal loss with OR of 2.68 and 1.88, respectively.[54]

The need for a clear and accurate diagnosis is very important. If MRI is not available, a protocol using low-dose CT scan can lead to a sensitivity of 100% and specificity of 92%.[143] At the radiation dose used, there exists no real risk of teratogenicity, but probably still a doubling in the rate of childhood cancer.[144]

Laparoscopy is safe in pregnancy in all three trimesters. In a retrospective cohort study of over 6000 pregnant patients undergoing laparotomy or laparoscopy for benign conditions, a significantly lower rate of fetal adverse events and preterm labor (0.41 to 1.8%, respectively) were observed following laparoscopy.[145] Previously, laparoscopy was considered to be risky and ineffective in late pregnancy. Recently it has been shown that there is no increased risk of complications in the late second and third trimesters.[146] Open appendectomy in pregnancy may be needed based on patient factors and surgeon comfort, but the technique should not change, not even the incision. It has been shown that the appendix does not migrate with increasing gestational age.[147,148]

In conclusion, appendicitis is a common disease. Uncomplicated appendicitis can be self-resolving and does not progress aggressively to complicated appendicitis, probably due to different pathology. Laparoscopic appendectomy is the gold standard, safe and effective, but the benefits of antibiotics may be proven in subgroups of patients with uncomplicated appendicitis. Complicated appendicitis is more safely treated with antibiotics, but the true need for interval appendectomy is not clear, especially with the risk of malignancy being a real problem. Due to its high incidence and cost to the healthcare system, continued research to define optimal management strategies of different forms of acute appendicitis is warranted.

References

[1] Williams GR. Presidential address: a history of appendicitis. With anecdotes illustrating its importance. Ann Surg. 1983; 197(5):495–506

[2] Deaver JB. Appendicitis. 3rd ed. Philadelphia: P Blakiston's Son and Co;1905

[3] de Moulin D. Historical notes on appendicitis. Arch Chir Neerl. 1975; 27(2):97–102

[4] Meade RH. The evolution of surgery for appendicitis. Surgery. 1964; 55:741–752

[5] Fitz RH. Perforating inflammation of the vermiform appendix: with special reference to its early diagnosis and treatment. Am J Med Sci. 1886; 92:321–346

[6] Streck CJ, Jr, Maxwell PJ, IV. A brief history of appendicitis: familiar names and interesting people. Am Surg. 2014; 80(2):105–8

[7] McBurney C. The incision made in the abdominal wall in cases of appendicitis, with a description of a new way of operating. Ann Surg. 1894; 20(1):38–43

[8] Davis GG. A transverse incision for the removal of the appendix. Ann Surg. 1906; 43(1):106–110

[9] Semm K. Endoscopic appendectomy. Endoscopy. 1983; 15(2):59–64

[10] Andersson RE. The natural history and traditional management of appendicitis revisited: spontaneous resolution and predominance of prehospital perforations imply that a correct diagnosis is more important than an early diagnosis. World J Surg. 2007; 31(1):86–92

[11] Lembcke PA. Measuring the quality of medical care through vital statistics based on hospital service areas; I. Comparative study of appendectomy rates. Am J Public Health Nations Health. 1952; 42(3):276–286

[12] Rutkow IM, Zuidema GD. Surgical rates in the United States: 1966 to 1978. Surgery. 1981; 89(2):151–162

[13] Addiss DG, Shaffer N, Fowler BS, Tauxe RV. The epidemiology of appendicitis and appendectomy in the United States. Am J Epidemiol. 1990; 132(5):910–925

[14] Davies GM, Dasbach EJ, Teutsch S. The burden of appendicitis-related hospitalizations in the United States in 1997. Surg Infect (Larchmt). 2004; 5(2):160–165

[15] Ferris M, Quan S, Kaplan BS, et al. The global incidence of appendicitis: A systemic review of population based studies. Ann Surg. 2017; 266(2):237–241

[16] Gomes CA, Abu-Zidan FM, Sartelli M, et al. Management of Appendicitis Globally Based on Income of Countries (MAGIC) Study. World J Surg. 2018; 42(12):3903–3910

[17] Sahm M, Pross M, Otto R, Koch A, Gastinger I, Lippert H. Clinical health service research on the surgical therapy of acute appendicitis: comparison of outcomes based on 3 German multicenter quality assurance studies over 21 years. Ann Surg. 2015; 262(2):338–346

[18] D'Inca R, Neri L, Daperno M, et al. Poor adherence is associated with impaired quality of life and increased illness intrusiveness in patients with ulcerative colitis and Crohn disease. Dig Liver Dis. 2015; 47:e183

[19] Fares A. Summer appendicitis. Ann Med Health Sci Res. 2014; 4(1):18–21

[20] Ahmed W, Akhtar MS, Khan S. Seasonal variation of acute appendicitis. Pak J Med Sci. 2018; 34(3):564–567

[21] Eisenberg N, Gockel J, von Dercks N. Seasonal variation in surgical diseases: Is an economic resource management necessary? Chiurg. 2018; 90(3):202–210

[22] Bandy NL, DeShields SC, Cunningham TD, Britt RC. Statewide assessment of surgical outcomes and the acute care surgery model. J Surg Res. 2017; 220:25–29

[23] Ladhani HA, Posillico SE, Zosa BM, Verbus EA, Brandt CP, Claridge JA. Efficiency of care and cost for common emergency general surgery conditions: Comparison by surgeon training and practice. Surgery. 2018; 164(4):651–656

[24] Scarborough JE, Bennett KM, Pappas TN. Racial disparities in outcomes after appendectomy for acute appendicitis. Am J Surg. 2012; 204(1):11–17

[25] Lee SL, Shekherdimian S, Chiu VY. Effect of race and socioeconomic status in the treatment of appendicitis in patients with equal health care access. Arch Surg. 2011; 146(2):156–161

[26] Lee SL, Yaghoubian A, Stark R, Shekherdimian S. Equal access to healthcare does not eliminate disparities in the management of adults with appendicitis. J Surg Res. 2011; 170(2):209–213

[27] Scott JW, Rose JA, Tsai TC, et al. Impact of ACA insurance expansion on perforated appendix rates among young adults. Med Care. 2016; 54(9):818–826

[28] Prieto JM, Thompson KA, Wessels L, et al. Healthcare disparity among marine recruits treated for acute appendicitis. Mil Med. 2018; 184(1–2):e186–e189

[29] Coward S, Kareemi H, Clement F, et al. Incidence of appendicitis over time: a comparative analysis of an administrative healthcare database and pathology proven appendicitis registry. PLoS One. 2016; 11(11):e0165161

[30] Singh JP, Mariadason JG. Role of the faecolith in modern-day appendicitis. Ann R Coll Surg Engl. 2013; 95(1):48–51

[31] Almström M, Svensson JF, Patkova B, Svenningsson A, Wester T. In-hospital surgical delay dose not increase risk of perforated appendicitis in children: a single center retrospective cohort study. Ann Surg. 2017; 265(3):616–621

[32] Kim SH, Park SJ, Park YY, Choi SI. Delayed appendectomy is safe in patients with acute nonperforated appendicitis. Int Surg. 2015; 100(6):1004–1010

[33] Drake FT, Mottey NE, Farrokhi ET, et al. Time to appendectomy and risk of perforation in acute appendicitis. JAMA Surg. 2014; 149(8):837–844

[34] van Dijk ST, van Dijk AH, Dijkgraaf MG, Boermeester MA. Meta-analysis of in-hospital delay before surgery as a risk factor for complications in patients with acute appendicitis. Br J Surg. 2018; 105(8):933–945

[35] Li HM, Yeh LR, Huang YK, Hsieh MY, Yu KH, Kuo CF. Familial risk of appendicitis: a nationwide population survey. J Pediatr. 2018; 203:330–335.e3

[36] Salö M, Gudjonsdottir J, Omling E, Hagander L, Stenström P. Association of IGE mediated allergy with risk of complicated appendicitis in a pediatric population. JAMA Pediatr. 2018; 172(10):943–948

[37] Di Sebastiano P, Fink T, di Mola FF, et al. Neuroimmune appendicitis. Lancet. 1999; 354(9177):461–466

[38] Bouchard S, Russo P, Radu AP, Adzick NS. Expression of neuropeptides in normal and abnormal appendices. J Pediatr Surg. 2001; 36(8):1222–1226

[39] Lauerma H, Lehtinen V, Joukamaa M, Järvelin M-R, Helenius H, Isohanni M. Schizophrenia among patients treated for rheumatoid arthritis and appendicitis. Schizophr Res. 1998; 29(3):255–261

[40] Akingboye AA, Davies B, Tien T. Pus samples in complicated appendicitis: an important investigation or a waste of resources: a prospective cohort study. Scand J Surg. 2019; 108(1):55–60

[41] Subramanian T, Jerome E, Jones I, Jester I. Streptococcus anginosus is associated with postoperative intraabdominal collections in appendicitis. J Pediatr Surg. 2018; 53(2):237–240

[42] Smith MC, Chung PJ, Constable YC, Boylan MR, Alfonso AE, Sugiyama G. Appendectomy in patients with human immunodeficiency virus: Not as bad as we once thought. Surgery. 2017; 161(4):1076–1082

[43] Ciftci AO, Tanyel FC, Büyükpamukçu N, Hiçsönmez A. Appendicitis after blunt abdominal trauma: cause or coincidence? Eur J Pediatr Surg. 1996; 6(6):350–353

[44] Takagi Y, Yasuda K, Abe T. Seat belt compression appendicitis. J Clin Gastroenterol. 2000; 31(2):184

[45] Toumi Z, Chan A, Hadfield MB, Hulton NR. Systematic review of blunt abdominal trauma as a cause of acute appendicitis. Ann R Coll Surg Engl. 2010; 92(6):477–482

[46] Bachir NM, Feagins LA. Postcolonoscopy appendicitis in a patient with active ulcerative colitis. World J Gastrointest Endosc. 2010; 2(6):232–234

[47] Tan WJ, Acharyya S, Goh YC, et al. Prospective comparison of the Alvarado score and CT scan in the evaluation of suspected appendicitis: a proposed algorithm to guide CT use. J Am Coll Surg. 2015; 220(2):218–224

[48] Yeh DD, Sakran JV, Rattan R, et al. A survey of the practice and attitudes of surgeons regarding the treatment of appendicitis. Am J Surq. 1986; 218(1):106–112

[49] Alvarado A. A practical score for the early diagnosis of acute appendicitis. Ann Emerg Med. 1986; 15(5):557–564

[50] Ohle R, O'Reilly F, O'Brien KK. Fahey Tom, Dimitrov BD, The Alvarado score for predicting acute appendicitis: a systemic review. BMC Med. 2011; 9:139

[51] Coleman JJ, Carr BW, Rogers T, et al. The Alvarado score should be used to reduce emergency department length of stay and radiation exposure in select patients with abdominal pain. J Trauma Acute Care Surg. 2018; 84(6):946–950

[52] Ebell MH, Shinholser J. What are the most clinically useful cutoffs for the Alvarado and Pediatric Appendicitis Scores? A systematic review. Ann Emerg Med. 2014; 64(4):365–372.e2

[53] Abbasi N, Patenaude V, Abenhaim HA. Management and outcomes of acute appendicitis in pregnancy-population-based study of over 7000 cases. BJOG. 2014; 121(12):1509–1514

[54] McGory ML, Zingmond DS, Tillou A, Hiatt JR, Ko CY, Cryer HM. Negative appendectomy in pregnant women is associated with a substantial risk of fetal loss. J Am Coll Surg. 2007; 205(4):534–540

[55] Tatli F, Yucel Y, Gozeneli O, et al. The Alvarado Score is accurate in pregnancy: a retrospective case-control study. Eur J Trauma Emerg Surg. 2019; 45(3):411–416

[56] Repplinger MD, Weber AC, Pickhardt PJ, et al. Trends in the use of medical imaging to diagnose appendicitis at an academic center. J Am Coll Radiol. 2016; 13(9):1050–1056

[57] D'Souza N, Marsden M, Bottomley S, Nagarajah N, Scutt F, Toh S. Cost-effectiveness of routine imaging of suspected appendicitis. Ann R Coll Surg Engl. 2018; 100(1):47–51

[58] Puyleart JB. Acute appendicitis: Ultrasound evaluation using graded compression. Radiology. 1986; 161:691–695

[59] Incesu L, Yazicioglu AK, Selcuk MB, Ozen N. Contrast-enhanced power Doppler US in the diagnosis of acute appendicitis. Eur J Radiol. 2004; 50(2):201–209

[60] Trout AT, Towbin AJ, Fierke SR, Zhang B, Larson DB. Appendiceal diameter as a predictor of appendicitis in children: improved diagnosis with three diagnostic categories derived from a logistic predictive model. Eur Radiol. 2015; 25(8):2231–2238

[61] Pinto F, Pinto A, Russo A, et al. Accuracy of ultrasonography in the diagnosis of acute appendicitis in adult patients: review of the literature. Crit Ultrasound J. 2013; 5 Suppl 1:S2

[62] van Randen A, Bipat S, Zwinderman AH, Ubbink DT, Stoker J, Boermeester MA. Acute appendicitis: meta-analysis of diagnostic performance of CT and graded compression US related to prevalence of disease. Radiology. 2008; 249(1):97–106

[63] Pelin M, Paquette B, Revel L, Landecy M, Bouveresse S, Delabrousse E. Acute appendicitis: factors associated with inconclusive ultrasound study and the need for additional computed tomography. Diagn Interv Imaging. 2018; 99 (12):809–814

[64] Cohen B, Bowling J, Midulla P, et al. The non diagnostic ultrasound in the pediatric population. A non visualized appendix the same as a negative study? J Pediatis Surg. 2015; 50(6):923–927

[65] Ross MJ, Liu H, Netherton SJ, et al. Outcomes of children with suspected appendicitis and incompletely visualized appendix on ultrasound. Acad Emerg Med. 2014; 21(5):538–542

[66] Wagenaar AE, Tashiro J, Wang B, et al. Protocol for suspected pediatric appendicitis limits computed tomography utilization. J Surg Res. 2015; 199 (1):153–158

[67] Schuh S, Chan K, Langer JC, et al. Properties of serial ultrasound clinical diagnostic pathway in suspected appendicitis and related computed tomography use. Acad Emerg Med. 2015; 22(4):406–414

[68] Larsen DB, Trout AT, Fierke SR, Towbin AJ. Improvement on diagnostic accuracy of ultrasound of the pediatric appendix through the use of equivicable interpretative categories. AJR Am J Roentgenol. 2015; 294: 849–856

[69] Lee SH, Yun SJ. Diagnostic performance of emergency physician-performed point-of-care ultrasonography for acute appendicitis: A meta-analysis. Am J Emerg Med. 2019; 37(4):696–705

[70] Atema JJ, Gans SL, Van Randen A, et al. Comparison of imaging strategies with conditional versus immediate contrast enhanced computed tomography in patients with clinical suspicion of acute appendicitis. Eur Radiol. 2015; 25(8):2445–2452

[71] Anderson SW, Soto JA, Lucey BC, et al. Abdominal 64-MDCT for suspected appendicitis: the use of oral and IV contrast material versus IV contrast material only. AJR Am J Roentgenol. 2009; 193(5):1282–1288

[72] Kepner AM, Bacasnot JV, Stahlman BA. Intravenous contrast alone vs intravenous and oral contrast computed tomography for the diagnosis of appendicitis in adult ED patients. Am J Emerg Med. 2012; 30(9):1765–1773

[73] Ganguli S, Raptopoulos V, Komlos F, Siewert B, Kruskal JB. Right lower quadrant pain: value of the nonvisualized appendix in patients at multidetector CT. Radiology. 2006; 241(1):175–180

[74] Wadhwani A, Guo L, Saude E, et al. Intravenous and oral contrast vs intravenous contrast alone computed tomography for the visualization of appendix and diagnosis of appendicitis in emergency department patients. Can Assoc Radiol J. 2016; 67(3):234–241

[75] Ramalingam V, Bates DD, Buch K, et al. Diagnosing acute appendicitis using a nonoral contrast CT protocol in patients with a BMI of less than 25. Emerg Radiol. 2016; 23(5):455–462

[76] Hlibczuk V, Dattaro JA, Jin Z, Falzon L, Brown MD. Diagnostic accuracy of noncontrast computed tomography for appendicitis in adults: a systematic review. Ann Emerg Med. 2010; 55(1):51–59.e1

[77] Kim DW, Yoon HM, Lee JY, et al. Diagnostic performance of CT for pediatric patients with suspected appendicitis in various clinical settings: a systematic review and meta-analysis. Emerg Radiol. 2018; 25 (6):627–637

[78] Agarwal MD, Levenson RB, Siewert B, Camacho MA, Raptopoulos V. Limited added utility of performing follow-up contrast-enhanced CT in patients undergoing initial non-enhanced CT for evaluation of flank pain in the emergency department. Emerg Radiol. 2015; 22(2):109–115

[79] LOCAT Group. Low-dose CT for the diagnosis of appendicitis in adolescents and young adults (LOCAT): a pragmatic, multicentre, randomised controlled non-inferiority trial. Lancet Gastroenterol Hepatol. 2017; 2(11):793–804

[80] Sippola S, Virtanen J, Tammilehto V, et al. The accuracy of low dose computed tomography protocol in patients with suspected appendicitis: the OPTICAP trial. Ann Surg. 2018; 271(2):332–338

[81] Berrington de González A, Mahesh M, Kim KP, et al. Projected cancer risks from computed tomographic scans performed in the United States in 2007. Arch Intern Med. 2009; 169(22):2071–2077

[82] Rogers W, Hoffman J, Noori N. Harms of CT scanning prior to surgery for suspected appendicitis. Evid Based Med. 2015; 20(1):3–4

[83] Krajewski S, Brown J, Phang PT, Raval M, Brown CJ. Impact of computed tomography of the abdomen on clinical outcomes in patients with acute right lower quadrant pain: a meta-analysis. Can J Surg. 2011; 54(1):43–53

[84] Duke E, Kalb B, Arif-Tiwari H, et al. A systematic review and meta-analysis of diagnostic performance of MRI for evaluation of acute appendicitis. AJR Am J Roentgenol. 2016; 206(3):508–517

[85] Aguilera F, Gilchrist BF, Farkas DT. Accuracy of MRI in diagnosing appendicitis during pregnancy. Am Surg. 2018; 84(8):1326–1328

[86] Leeuwenburgh MM, Wiarda BM, Bipat S, et al. Acute appendicitis on abdominal MR images: training readers to improve diagnostic accuracy. Radiology. 2012; 264(2):455–463

[87] Anderson KT, Bartz-Kurycki M, Austin MT, et al. Approaching zero: implications of a computed tomography reduction program for pediatric appendicitis evaluation. J Pediatr Surg. 2017; 52(12):1909–1915

[88] Johnson AK, Filippi CG, Andrews T, et al. Ultrafast 3-T MRI in the evaluation of children with acute lower abdominal pain for the detection of appendicitis. AJR Am J Roentgenol. 2012; 198(6):1424–1430

[89] Holihan JL, Chen JS, Greenberg J, et al. Incidence of port site hernias: a survey and literature review. Surg Laparosc Endosc Percutan Tech. 2016; 26(6): 425–430

[90] Mehdorn M, Schürmann O, Mehdorn HM, Gockel I. Intended cost reduction in laparoscopic appendectomy by introducing the endoloop: a single center experience. BMC Surg. 2017; 17(1):80

[91] Kim S, Weireter L. Cost effectiveness of different methods of appendiceal stump closure during laparoscopic appendectomy. Am Surg. 2018; 84(8): 1329–1332

[92] Beldi G, Vorburger SA, Bruegger LE, Kocher T, Inderbitzin D, Candinas D. Analysis of stapling versus endoloops in appendiceal stump closure. Br J Surg. 2006; 93(11):1390–1393

[93] Sun F, Wang H, Zhang F, et al. Copious irrigation versus suction alone during laparoscopic appendectomy for complicated appendicitis in adults. J Invest Surg. 2018; 31(4):342–346

[94] LaPlant MB, Saltzman DA, Rosen JL, Acton RD, Segura BJ, Hess Dj. Standardized irrigation technique reduces intraabdominal abscess after appendectomy. J Pediatr Surg. 2018; 54(4):728–732

[95] Hartwich JE, Carter RF, Wolfe L, et al. The effects of irrigation on outcomes in cases of perforated appendicitis in children. J Surg Res. 2013; 180(2):222–225

[96] St Peter SD, Adibe OO, Iqbal CW, et al. Irrigation versus suction alone during laparoscopic appendectomy for perforated appendicitis: a prospective randomized trial. Ann Surg. 2012; 256(4):581–585

[97] Zani A, Hall NJ, Rahman A, et al. European Paediatric Surgeons Association Survey on the Management of Pediatric Appendicitis. Eur J Pediatr Surg. 2018

[98] Athanasiou C, Lockwood S, Markides GA. Systematic review and meta-analysis of laparoscopic versus open apendicectomy in adults with complicated appendicitis: an update of the literature. World J Surg. 2017; 41(12):3083–3099

[99] Sauerland S, Jaschinski T, Neugebauer EA. Laparoscopic versus open surgery for suspected appendicitis. Cochrane Database Syst Rev. 2010(10):CD001546

[100] Dumas RP, Subramanian M, Hodgman E, et al. Laparoscopic appendectomy: a report of 1164 operations at single institution, safety net hospital. Am Surg. 2018; 84(6):1110–1116

[101] Minné L, Varner D, Burnell A, Ratzer E, Clark J, Haun W. Laparoscopic vs open appendectomy. Prospective randomized study of outcomes. Arch Surg. 1997; 132(7):708–711, discussion 712

[102] Tiwari MM, Reynoso JF, Tsang AW, Oleynikov D. Comparison of outcomes of laparoscopic and open appendectomy in management of uncomplicated and complicated appendicitis. Ann Surg. 2011; 254(6):927–932

[103] Trejo-Ávila ME, Romero-Loera S, Cárdenas-Lailson E, et al. Enhanced recovery after surgery protocol allows ambulatory laparoscopic appendectomy in uncomplicated acute appendicitis: a prospective, randomized trial. Surg Endosc. 2019; 33(2):429–436

[104] Reiertsen O, Larsen S, Trondsen E, Edwin B, Faerden AE, Rosseland AR. Randomized controlled trial with sequential design of laparoscopic versus conventional appendicectomy. Br J Surg. 1997; 84(6):842–847

[105] Dikicier E, Altintoprak F, Ozdemir K, et al. Stump appendicitis: a retrospective review of 3130 consecutive appendectomy cases. World J Emerg Surg. 2018; 13:22

[106] Leff DR, Sait MR, Hanief M, Salakianathan S, Darzi AW, Vashisht R. Inflammation of the residual appendix stump: a systematic review. Colorectal Dis. 2012; 14(3):282–293

[107] Rehman H, Rao AM, Ahmed I, Cochrane Review Library, July 11, 2011

[108] Farach SM, Danielson PD, Chandler NM. Impact of experience on quality outcomes in single-incision laparoscopy for simple and complex appendicitis in children. J Pediatr Surg. 2015; 50(8):1364–1367

[109] Carter JT, Kaplan JA, Nguyen JN, Lin MY, Rogers SJ, Harris HW. A prospective, randomized controlled trial of single-incision laparoscopic vs conventional 3-port laparoscopic appendectomy for treatment of acute appendicitis. J Am Coll Surg. 2014; 218(5):950–959

[110] Agaba EA, Rainville H, Ikedilo O, Vemulapali P. Incidence of port-site incisional hernia after single-incision laparoscopic surgery. JSLS. 2014; 18 (2):204–210

[111] Alptekin H, Yilmaz H, Acar F, Kafali ME, Sahin M. Incisional hernia rate may increase after single-port cholecystectomy. J Laparoendosc Adv Surg Tech A. 2012; 22(8):731–737

[112] Kang BM, Choi SI, Kim BS, Lee SH. Single-port laparoscopic surgery in uncomplicated acute appendicitis: a randomized controlled trial. Surg Endosc. 2018; 32(7):3131–3137

[113] Akl MN, Magrina JF, Kho RM, Magtibay PM. Robotic appendectomy in gynaecological surgery: technique and pathological findings. Int J Med Robot. 2008; 4(3):210–213

[114] Atallah S, Martin-Perez B, Keller D, Burke J, Hunter L. Natural-orifice transluminal endoscopic surgery. Br J Surg. 2015; 102(2):e73–e92

[115] Schoenberg MB, Magdeburg R, Kienle P, Post S, Eisser PP, Kähler G. Hybrid transgastric appendectomy is feasible but does not offer advantages compared with laparoscopic appendectomy: results from the transgastric appendectomy study. Surgery. 2017; 162(2):295–302

[116] Di Saverio S, Sibilio A, Giorgini E, et al. The NOTA Study (Non Operative Treatment for Acute Appendicitis): prospective study on the efficacy and safety of antibiotics (amoxicillin and clavulanic acid) for treating patients with right lower quadrant abdominal pain and long-term follow-up of conservatively treated suspected appendicitis. Ann Surg. 2014; 260(1):109–117

[117] Varadhan KK, Humes DJ, Neal KR, Lobo DN. Antibiotic therapy versus appendectomy for acute appendicitis: a meta-analysis. World J Surg. 2010; 34(2):199–209

[118] Vons C, Barry C, Maitre S, et al. Amoxicillin plus clavulanic acid versus appendicectomy for treatment of acute uncomplicated appendicitis: an open-label, non-inferiority, randomised controlled trial. Lancet. 2011; 377(9777):1573–1579

[119] Salminen P, Paajanen H, Rautio T, et al. Antibiotic therapy versus appendectomy for treatment of uncomplicated acute appendicitis. The APPAC randomized clinical trial. JAMA. 2015; 313(23):2340–2348

[120] Salminen P, Tuominen R, Paajanen H, et al. Five year follow-up of antibiotic therapy for uncomplicated acute appendicitis in the APPAC randomized clinical trial. JAMA. 2018; 320(12):1259–1265

[121] Sakran JV, Mylonas KS, Gryparis A, et al. Operation versus antibiotics—The "appendicitis conundrum" continues: a meta-analysis. J Trauma Acute Care Surg. 2017; 82(6):1129–1137

[122] Loftus TJ, Dessaigne CG, Croft CA, et al. A protocol for non-operative management of uncomplicated appendicitis. J Trauma Acute Care Surg. 2018; 84(2):358–364

[123] Loftus TJ, Brakenridge SC, Croft CA, et al. Successful nonoperative management of uncomplicated appendicitis: predictors and outcomes. J Surg Res. 2018; 222:212–218.e2

[124] Park HC, Kim MJ, Lee BH. Randomized clinical trial of antibiotic therapy for uncomplicated appendicitis. Br J Surg. 2017; 104(13):1785–1790

[125] Simillis C, Symeonides P, Shorthouse AJ, Tekkis PP. A meta-analysis comparing conservative treatment versus acute appendectomy for complicated appendicitis (abscess or phlegmon). Surgery. 2010; 147(6):818–829

[126] Helling TS, Soltys DF, Seals S. Operative versus non-operative management in the care of patients with complicated appendicitis. Am J Surg. 2017; 214 (6):1195–1200

[127] Cheng Y, Xiong X, Lu J, Wu S, Cheng N. Early versus delayed appendicectomy for appendiceal phlegmon or abscess. Cochrane Datebase Syst Rev. 2017; 6: CD011670

[128] Darwazeh G, Cunningham SC, Kowdley GC. A systematic review of perforated appendicitis and phlegmon: Interval appendectomy or wait and see? Am Surg. 2016; 82(1):11–15

[129] Samdani T, Fancher TT, Pieracci FM, Eachempati S, Rashidi L, Nash GM. Is interval appendectomy indicated after non-operative management of acute appendicitis in patients with cancer? A retrospective review from a single institution. Am Surg. 2015; 81(5):532–536

[130] Senekjian L, Nirula R, Bellows B, Nelson R. Interval appendectomy: finding the breaking point for cost effectiveness. J Am Coll Surg. 2016; 223(4):632–643

[131] Wright GP, Mater ME, Carroll JT, Choy JS, Chung MH. Is there truly an oncologic indication for interval appendectomy? Am J Surg. 2015; 209(3):442–446

[132] Sylthe Pedersen E, Stornes T, Rekstad LC, Martinsen TC. Is there a role for routine colonoscopy in the follow-up after acute appendicitis? Scand J Gastroenterol. 2018; 53(8):1008–1012

[133] Sawyer RG, Claridge JA, Nathens AB, et al. STOP-IT Trial Investigators. Trial of short-course antimicrobial therapy for intraabdominal infection. N Engl J Med. 2015; 372(21):1996–2005

[134] Kleif J, Rasmussen L, Fonnes S, et al. Enteral antibiotics are non inferior to intravenous antibiotics after complicated appendicitis in adults: A retrospective multicenter non-inferiority study. World J Surg. 2017; 41(11):2706–2714

[135] Sakorafas GH, Sabanis D, Lappas C, et al. Interval routine appendectomy following conservative treatment of acute appendicitis: is it really needed. World J Gastrointest Surg. 2012; 4(4):83–86

[136] Storm-Dickerson TL, Horattas MC. What have we learned over the past 20 years about appendicitis in the elderly? Am J Surg. 2003; 185(3):198–201

[137] Omari AH, Khammash MR, Qasaimeh GR, Shammari AK, Yaseen MK, Hammori SK. Acute appendicitis in the elderly: risk factors for perforation. World J Emerg Surg. 2014; 9(1):6

[138] Spangler R, Van Pham T, Khoujah D, Martinez JP. Abdominal emergencies in the geriatric patient. Int J Emerg Med. 2014; 7:43

[139] Kirshtein B, Perry ZH, Mizrahi S, Lantsberg L. Value of laparoscopic appendectomy in the elderly patient. World J Surg. 2009; 33(5):918–922

[140] Horn CB, Tian D, Bochicchio GV, Turnbull IR. Incidence, demographics, and outcomes of nonoperative management of appendicitis in the United States. J Surg Res. 2018; 223:251–258

[141] Bhullar JS, Chaudhary S, Cozacov Y, Lopez P, Mittal VK. Acute appendicitis in the elderly: diagnosis and management still a challenge. Am Surg. 2014; 80 (11):E295–E297

[142] Won RP, Friedlander S, Lee SL. Management and outcomes of appendectomy during pregnancy. Am Surg. 2017; 83(10):1103–1107

[143] Poletti PA, Platon A. Suspicion of appendicitis in pregnant women: emergency evaluation by sonography and low-dose CT with oral contrast. Eur Radiol. 2019; 29(1):345–352

[144] Hurwitz LM, Yoshizumi T, Reiman RE, et al. Radiation dose to the fetus from body MDCT during early gestation. AJR Am J Roentgenol. 2006; 186 (3):871–876

[145] Shigemi D, Yasunaga H, et al. Safety of laparoscopic surgery for benign diseases during pregnancy: a nationwide retrospective cohort study. J Minim Invasive Gynecol. 2019; 26(3):501–506

[146] Kwon H, Lee M, Park HS, Yoon SH, Lee CH, Roh JW. Laparoscopic management is feasible for nonobstetric surgical disease in all trimesters of pregnancy. Surg Endosc. 2018; 32(6):2643–2649

[147] Ishaq A, Khan MJH, Pishori T, Soomro R, Khan S. Location of appendix in pregnancy: does it change? Clin Exp Gastroenterol. 2018; 11:281–287

[148] Popkin CA, Lopez PP, Cohn SM, Brown M, Lynn M. The incision of choice for pregnant women with appendicitis is through McBurney's point. Am J Surg. 2002; 183(1):20–22

Expert Commentary on
Appendicitis by
Purvi P. Patel, Brendan Ringhouse,
Christian Renz, and Fred A. Luchette

Expert Commentary on Appendicitis

Purvi P. Patel, Brendan Ringhouse, Christian Renz, and Fred A. Luchette

Appendicitis remains the most common disease process encountered by general surgeons and its diagnosis and management continues to evolve. Lineen et al provides a comprehensive review of the pathophysiology, diagnosis, and treatment of acute appendicitis. Although historically appendicitis was thought to be a result of obstructive pathology at the appendiceal orifice, current data suggests there may be different etiologies with varying clinical presentations. Many patients present with uncomplicated appendicitis who may successfully be managed nonoperatively with antibiotics. In contrast, others experience a much more complicated course at presentation,that is, perforation with or without abscess. As in the pediatric population, the majority of these patients will respond to nonoperative management with antibiotics and/or percutaneous drainage.

Prior to settling on a treatment plan, one must confirm the diagnosis of appendicitis, uncomplicated or complicated. This article does an exceptional job reviewing the paradigm shift from clinical examination to computed tomography (CT) imaging being used to confirm a majority of cases. It also calls into question the need for oral or IV contrast which can prolong time taken to diagnose and treat. The group also highlights the use of alternative imaging modalities, including ultrasound and magnetic resonance imaging. Both eliminate the exposure to ionizing radiation. Of the two, sensitivity and specificity of ultrasound is comparable to CT scan. Thus, it is easy to understand why bedside ultrasound evaluation of the right lower quadrant for signs of appendicitis is the preferred modality in pediatric patients. Its use in the adult population is increasing annually.

Now, we address the controversy regarding operative versus nonoperative management. The treatment of appendicitis has transitioned from open appendectomy to laparoscopic appendectomy with the most recent studies investigating the efficacy of nonoperative management. As noted by the authors, it is no surprise that nonoperative management with antibiotics will reduce morbidity, cost, and time to resume normal activities associated with appendectomy. However, the recurrence (failure) rate is not insignificant. The Appendicitis Acuta (APPAC) randomized control trial and its five-year follow-up emphasize antibiotics only as an alternative to immediate surgery; however, this study did demonstrate that 27% of patients initially allocated to antibiotics underwent an operation in the first year, with that number rising to 39% at the end of five years. This was higher than the recurrence (failure) threshold set for noninferiority at 24%, suggesting an early operation is still the best option in the treatment of acute appendicitis. Also, this study excluded the pediatric and elderly populations, limiting its applicability, as these are the ages with the highest incidence of appendicitis. An additional area that requires further investigation with the increased use of antibiotics is the need for an interval appendectomy. Especially in the setting of complicated appendicitis or concern for an appendiceal mass, many advocate interval appendectomy due to the fear of recurrent appendicitis and to rule out malignancy. An alternative approach is to screen all adult patients who were managed nonoperatively with a screening colonoscopy. Regardless, close clinical follow-up remains essential, as there remains no consensus on how to best manage this growing cohort of patients.

Lineen et al provides a comprehensive assessment of the current literature regarding diagnosis and treatment of appendicitis. However, additional studies are needed to define the optimal management of patients presenting with acute or complicated appendicitis.

10 Acute Cholecystitis

Giana H. Davidson and Eileen M. Bulger

Summary

Biliary disease is one of the most common and costly gastrointestinal illnesses in the United States and cholecystectomy is one of the most common general surgical procedures. While asymptomatic cholelithiasis is common, symptomatic biliary disease has a significant impact on quality of life and health care utilization.

This chapter will review the epidemiology and clinical manifestations of biliary disease, diagnostic work up, complications of biliary disease, considerations for intervention including laparoscopy, open surgery, and percutaneous drainage, management of surgical complications, and consideration for special populations including pregnant people, those with cirrhosis, and older adults.

Keywords: Cholelithiasis, cholecystitis, choledocholithiaiss, gallstone pancreatitis

10.1 Introduction

Biliary disease affects 10 to 15% of Americans, including approximately 6.3 million men and 14.2 million women with a broad range of morbidity.[1,2,3,4,5,6,7,8,9,10] Among people with asymptomatic gallstones, 1 to 4% of people per year and up to 15 to 25% within 10 years will require treatment,[5,11,12,13,14] a majority for biliary colic rather than complications of cholelithiasis, such as acute cholecystitis, obstructive jaundice, or gallstone pancreatitis. Acute cholecystitis typically originates from gallstones although additional rare cases can include ischemia, infections, motility disorders, protozoa or parasites, collagen disease, and adverse drug reactions.[1,15] Acalculous cholecystitis is typically associated with systemic insult, including critical illness, trauma, burns, recent operation, or parental nutrition. This chapter will include an overview of the workup, data to support surgical recommendations, operative decision-making, and the management of surgical complications related to biliary disease.

10.2 Diagnostic Evaluation

The workup of a patient with biliary disease includes physical examination, and laboratory and radiographic evaluation. The majority of patients with symptomatic biliary diseases present with right upper quadrant or epigastric abdominal pain. The pain classically radiates to the right upper back, right shoulder, or subscapular area. It is constant and usually lasts for more than 30 minutes. Patients often have associated nausea and vomiting. In patients with uncomplicated biliary disease, physical examination shows moderate right upper quadrant or epigastric abdominal tenderness and lack of systematic signs of an inflammatory process. Among patients with complicated biliary disease, severe tenderness and fever are noted. Generalized peritonitis may be present in patients with free perforation although this is a rare complication of gallbladder necrosis. Murphy's sign, which refers to the patient abruptly halting inspiration due to the pain elicited upon touching the gallbladder by the examiner's hand that is pressed into the right subcostal margin, is frequently present with a sensitivity and specificity of 97% and 48%, respectively, and a positive predictive value of 70%.[16,17] However, it may be less accurate in patients over the age of 60 years.[18]

When gallbladder disease is suspected, complete blood count (CBC) and liver function tests should be completed. The clinical presentation is typically accompanied by an elevated white blood cell count. If associated with elevated bilirubin, alkaline phosphatase, alanine aminotransferase, and aspartate aminotransferase, then cholangitis should be suspected. Cholestasis is characterized by elevation of conjugated bilirubin and a rise in alkaline phosphatase. Serum alanine aminotransferase and aspartate aminotransferase may be normal or mildly elevated. Chronic cholecystitis patients often have normal laboratory values even during periods of symptomatic disease.

Transabdominal ultrasonography is the initial imaging modality of choice to evaluate for biliary disease, given the high sensitivity and accuracy (>95%) for biliary disease, lack of ionizing radiation, and potential for evaluation of solid organs.[1] It is highly dependent on the operator's skills and experience, as it is dynamic, and may be limited in subpopulations including those with an elevated body mass index, those with ascites, and those with distended bowel. Biliary cholescintigraphy and biliary radionuclide scanning (HIDA scan) has a sensitivity and specificity approaching 95% and 90%, respectively.[19,20,21,22,23,24,25] However, limitations include false positive results in subpopulations, including patients on total parenteral nutrition, with severe hepatocellular dysfunction, hyperbilirubinemia, pancreatitis, inadequate (<2 hours) or prolonged (>24 hours) fasting, alcohol and opiate abuse, biliary sphincterotomy, and cystic duct obstruction in the absence of acute cholecystitis.[23,26] Computed tomography (CT) may be helpful for abdominal pain when biliary disease is lower on the differential diagnosis, and evaluation of cholecystenteric fistula, porcelain gallbladder, and suspected malignancy. Magnetic resonance cholangiopancreatography (MRCP) is frequently used for evaluation of choledocholithiasis, with a sensitivity of 95% and a specificity of 89%, as well as evaluation of malignancy. There is variability in the use of MRCP for the first-line diagnostic workup of suspected common bile duct stones versus endoscopic retrograde cholangiopancreatography (ERCP) which can be also used for therapeutic purposes. Clinical protocols for workup may be driven, in part, by local hospital resource availability and cost.

10.3 Indications and Timing for Operative Intervention

Laparoscopic cholecystectomy is the definitive treatment of acute cholecystitis. There has been controversy regarding the optional timing of surgery with historical support for operative intervention within 72 hours of presentation of symptoms. This is due to observations in pathology proposing progression from edematous cholecystitis to necrotizing and finally suppurative cholecystitis[15] and retrospective studies, with a conversion from laparoscopic to open rate that increases with increased time with symptoms.[15]

Laparoscopic cholecystectomy during the initial period of presentation with symptoms of acute cholecystitis has been shown to be safe when compared with delayed laparoscopic cholecystectomy, and early intervention may be associated with shorter overall hospital stay.[12,27,28,29,30,31,32,33,34,35,36,37]

10.4 Symptomatic Gallbladder Disease

10.4.1 Acute Cholecystitis

Approximately 120,000 cholecystectomies are performed for acute cholecystitis annually in the United States but this rate is decreasing, likely due to an increase in laparoscopic cholecystectomy for symptomatic gallstone disease (biliary cholic).[38,39] Acute cholecystitis not only affects 20% of the people who are admitted to the hospital for biliary disease[40,41,42] but is also the cause of 3 to 11% of hospital admissions.[43,44,45,46] It is more common in women[47] and has a mortality rate of 0 to 10%,[48,49,50,51,52] largely dependent on severity of disease and patient comorbid conditions. Acute cholecystitis is the most common complication of cholelithiasis due to inflammation of the gallbladder which is frequently associated with obstruction of the cystic duct, most often due to gallstones.[15,53,54] Classic presentation includes acute onset of right upper quadrant abdominal or epigastric pain lasting for more than four to six hours, fever, nausea, vomiting, and anorexia.[55,56] While classically described as pain associated with ingestion of fatty food an hour before its onset, in practice, association with food or specifically fatty food is variable. Murphy's sign is prevalent in more than 95% of patients with acute cholecystitis,[17] with a sensitivity and specificity of 97% and 48%, respectively, and a positive predictive value of 70%.[16] Laboratory abnormalities commonly include a leukocytosis ($12,000–15,000$ cells/mm^3) with a left shift.

Patients typically require admission to the hospital with supportive care, including intravenous fluid hydration, correction of electrolyte abnormalities, pain control, and intravenous antibiotics. Adequate pain control should be achieved with a combination (when possible) of nonsteroidal anti-inflammatory drugs (NSAIDs) and, if needed opioids. Although the sphincter of Oddi prevents enteric bacteria from entering the biliary system, infection of the gallbladder can occur as a result of cystic duct obstruction and bile stasis which allows bacterial proliferation and infection. Empiric antibiotic therapy should cover common pathogens of the biliary tree including anaerobes and enteric Gram-negative organisms including *Escherichia coli, Enterococcus, Klebsiella,* and *Enterobacter.*[38,57] Regimens like third-generation cephalosporin with appropriate anaerobic coverage, or second-generation cephalosporin combined with metronidazole, are used. An aminoglycoside with metronidazole should be used in patients allergic to cephalosporins.[57]

Cholecystectomy is the definitive treatment for acute cholecystitis[58] as 2% of patients with nonsevere cholecystitis experience a recurrence within 8 to 10 weeks[15] and 11% of

cholelithiasis patients within the following 1.5 to 4 years.[59] Cholecystectomy during the initial presentation has been advocated for, as it offers definitive treatment during index admission, reduced length of stay, and decreased hospital costs.[12,29,30,31,33,34,60,61] There is not a homogenous definition of early cholecystectomy but a meta-analysis concluded there was no significant difference between rates of conversion to open cholecystectomy and rates of complications between patients operated on within 4 days or 7 days from the onset of symptoms.[61]

10.4.2 Percutaneous Cholecystostomy

Percutaneous cholecystostomy can be performed under local analgesia for those who are unfit for surgery. This is typically performed by interventional radiology but may be done laparoscopically or, rarely, in an open surgical operation. If the patient doesn't improve, which is usually due to gangrene or perforation of the gallbladder, surgery may be needed during the index admission. A cholecystostomy tube can be removed once cholangiography through it shows a patent cystic duct, and cholecystectomy can be scheduled once the patient is medically optimized for surgery.[62] For the small subgroup of patients who cannot tolerate surgery, stone retrieval can be attempted via the cholecystostomy tube before its removal.[63]

10.4.3 Chronic Cholecystitis

About two-thirds of patients with gallstones disease present with chronic cholecystitis. This is manifested as right upper quadrant pain, often radiating to the right upper back, right shoulder, or subscapular area, and is often triggered following fatty meals. Despite the common use of the term "biliary colic" to describe uncomplicated gallstone disease, in chronic cholecystitis, the pain is not colicky but rather constant. Nausea without vomiting is often described.

Atypical symptoms of chronic cholecystitis may include left upper back pain, lower right quadrant pain, regurgitation, abdominal distension/bloating, fullness after meals/early satiety, chest pain, and belching. Ultrasound should be used to confirm the presence of gallstones. Laboratory tests are usually normal in patients with uncomplicated gallstones both during asymptomatic periods and pain attacks.

10.5 Complicated Biliary Disease

10.5.1 Choledocholithiasis

The incidence of common bile duct (CBD) stones in patients with cholelithiasis is not known, but it is estimated to be between 5 to 21% at the time of cholecystectomy,[64,65,66,67,68,69,70] and they are found in 6% of asymptomatic patients getting routine intraoperative cholangiography[71] with increasing incidence with advancing age.[64] CBD stones are classified into primary and secondary stones. Primary stones are cholesterol stones that are formed in the bile ducts and are formed in the setting of bile stasis (e.g., cystic fibrosis patients, biliary stricture, papillary stenosis, or tumors) and infection.[64] Secondary stones, which constitute the vast majority of CBD stones in

Western countries, are formed within the gallbladder and migrate down the cystic duct to the CBD.[64]

Choledocholithiasis may cause complete or incomplete obstruction, jaundice, gallstone pancreatitis, or cholangitis. Thus, prompt intervention is indicated once identified. The pain associated with choledocholithiasis is similar to that of biliary colic caused by impaction of a stone in the cystic duct. Choledocholithiasis should be suspected in those with laboratory findings of direct hyperbilirubinemia, imaging with intrahepatic biliary dilatation, and dilated CBD. Early in the course of CBD obstruction, there is an elevation of both serum alanine aminotransferase (ALT) and aspartate aminotransferase (AST); later on, there is an increase in serum bilirubin, alkaline phosphatase and gamma-glutamyl transpeptidase (GGT), exceeding the elevation of serum AST and ALT.

In patients suspected to have CBD stones, either preoperative MRCP, ERCP, or intraoperative cholangiogram may confirm choledocholithiasis.[72] Preoperative ERCP is both diagnostic and therapeutic. If ERCP confirms stones, sphincterotomy and ductal clearance of the stones is typically completed, followed soon by laparoscopic cholecystectomy. If a preoperative ERCP is unsuccessful, alternative methods of stone extraction are used including laparoscopic CBD exploration by a trained surgeon at the same time as laparoscopic cholecystectomy. The transcystic approach for stone extraction is completed by exposing 2 to 3 cm of the cystic duct and placing a clip on the gallbladder side of the cystic duct proximally. The duct is incised with scissors and a cholangiogram catheter is introduced. Contrast is injected under fluoroscopy to confirm anatomy and presence of stones in the CBD. The CBD can be flushed with 30 mL of saline via the catheter which is often successful in flushing small stones. If stones remain, 1 mg of glucagon is given intravenously to allow relaxation of the sphincter of Oddi and flushing is repeated. If flushing attempts fail, fluoroscopic-guided basket retrieval may be completed using a 4 Fr Fogarty balloon inserted through the cystic ductotomy, passed distally, inflated, and withdrawn to pull stones retrograde through the ductotomy. In experienced hands, choledochoscopy may be performed. A guidewire is passed via the cystic ductotomy into the common duct (confirmed by fluoroscopy) and an 8 Fr angioplasty balloon used to dilate the orifice. A 12 Fr introducer catheter is used to facilitate passage of the choledochoscope. A retrieval basket can be inserted under direct visualization through the choledochoscope.[73,74,75]

A choledoctotomy may be also be required if ERCP is unavailable or fails. The CBD is exposed and a vertical 5 mm ductotomy is completed on the anterior surface of the duct, distal to the cystic–CBD junction. The techniques for stone clearance include the use of a Fogarty catheter (described above). The choledochotomy site is managed with a T-tube sutured in place, with absorbable suture closed over a stent which can later be removed by ERCP. T-tube removal should be completed 4 to 6 weeks postoperatively, following cholangiogram, to assure clearance of stones from the biliary ductal system. Retained stones can be extracted either endoscopically or via the T-tube once it has matured (2 to 4 weeks). An endoscopic sphincterotomy may be completed to allow stone retrieval and spontaneous passage of retained and recurrent stones.

Sensitivity and specificity of choledocholithiasis via intraoperative cholangiogram is highly surgeon dependent and will demonstrate CBD stones with a sensitivity of 59 to 100% and a specificity of 93 to 100%.[76,77,78,79] If laparoscopic exploration of CBD is not completed (due to feasibility or surgeon experience), consideration should be given to a drain placement adjacent to the cystic duct, and an ERCP with endoscopic sphincterotomy may be scheduled the following day.[80]

10.5.2 Cholangitis

The first known report of acute biliary fever was made by Charcot in 1877, "The symptoms of hepatic fever";[81] from this work, "Charcot's triad" was used to describe intermittent fever, right upper quadrant pain, and jaundice. In 1969, obstructive cholangitis was defined by Charcot's triad, in addition to lethargy or confusion and shock, and called Reynold's Pentad.[82] The lifetime incidence in patients with gallstones is 0.3 to 1.6%[83,84] with an associated 2.7 to 10% mortality rate which is primarily driven by sepsis and multisystem organ failure.[84]

The development of acute cholangitis requires biliary obstruction and bacterial overgrowth in the biliary system and its causes are multifactorial.[85,86] Common bacteria isolated included *Escherichia coli*, *Klebsiella spp.*, *Pseudomonas spp.*, and *Enterobacter* and less commonly *Acinetobacter spp.*, *Citrobacter spp.*, *Streptococcus spp.*, *Staphylococcus*, and anaerobes,[84] with a high proportion of polymicrobial, Gram-negative, and anaerobic infections.[87]

In 2013, the Tokyo Guidelines helped in establishing diagnostic criteria for acute cholangitis. Diagnosis is based on the following: 1. Systemic inflammation (fever, shaking chills, white blood cells [WBC] <4 cells/McL or >10 cells/McL or C-reactive protein >1 mg/dL) 2. Cholestasis (jaundice and liver function tests >1.5x normal) and 3. Imaging findings supporting biliary ductal obstruction (e.g., ductal dilation).[88]

10.5.3 Gallstone Pancreatitis

Gallstone pancreatitis is one of the most common complications of biliary disease with severe pancreatitis occurring in 10 to 25% of patients with gallstone pancreatitis. Presentation includes epigastric pain, fever, nausea, and vomiting, with laboratory values revealing elevated liver function tests including bilirubin, alkaline phosphatase, ALT, and AST.

Mild gallstone pancreatitis should be treated with cholecystectomy during the initial hospitalization to prevent recurrence[89] and decrease hospital length of stay[90] Recurrence rates without operative intervention are high, with estimates ranging from 25 to 63%.[91] In cases of severe pancreatitis, cholecystectomy should be delayed several weeks as it is associated with higher morbidity and mortality rates if performed during the initial hospitalization. There may be a higher conversion from laparoscopic to open cholecystectomy in this population. ERCP may be performed in surgically unfit patients with either mild or severe gallstone pancreatitis, aiming at clearing the duct.[90,91,92] Abdominal ultrasound is the preferred imaging technique to detect gallstone pancreatitis.

10.5.4 Gangrenous Cholecystitis

Gangrenous cholecystitis occurs often due to cystic artery thrombosis by infection and inflammation, leading to ischemia, gangrene of the gallbladder wall, liquefaction necrosis, and may progress to perforation of the gallbladder. Gangrenous cholecystitis accounts for 2 to 36% of patients with acute cholecystitis,[93,94,95,96,97,98,99,100,101] with a higher proportion among older patients and those with underlying small vessel diseases such as diabetes.[102] Perforation of the gallbladder may cause a pericholecystic abscess. Free perforation may result in bile-stained ascites, generalized peritonitis, and is associated with highmortality rates. Gangrenous cholecystitis is difficult to diagnose preoperatively because patients present with clinical findings indistinguishable from patients with nongangrenous acute cholecystitis.[103] Although there are some suggestive factors of gangrenous cholecystitis like advanced age, significant comorbidities, and a palpable gallbladder on physical examination, they have a low predictive value.[93,97,98,104] It is associated with a higher conversion rate to open surgery. In cases of confirmed or suspected gangrenous cholecystitis, laparoscopic cholecystectomy should be performed as soon as possible, with preparation of conversion to an open procedure if needed.[93]

10.5.5 Acalculous Cholecystitis

Acalculous cholecystitis is inflammation of the gallbladder due to stasis and ischemia, without the presence of gallstones primarily affecting critically ill patients with severe comorbidities, including sepsis, immunosuppression, and/or those receiving parenteral nutrition[105] It constitutes 10% of all cases of acute cholecystitis and is associated with highmorbidity and mortality rates.[105] In a patient who is able to provide a reliable history, symptoms mimic those of acute calculous cholecystitis, with fever, right upper quadrant tenderness to palpation, and positive Murphy's sign. In sedated or unconscious patients, clinical features are obscure, but patients frequently have fever, leukocytosis, elevated alkaline phosphatase, and elevated conjugated bilirubin.

For clinically suspected cases, abdominal sonography is the diagnostic test of choice which often reveals distended gallbladder with a thickened wall, pericholecystic fluid, biliary sludge and possible evidence of abscess. CT, which has the same accuracy of ultrasonography, could be used to visualize the abdominal and thoracic cavities in order to exclude other causes of infection. Cholescintigraphy may fail to opacify the gallbladder at one hour. It is associated with a higher false positive rates in patients who are fasting, on total parenteral nutrition, or afflicted with liver disease. In addition, the test often take multiple hours limiting feasibility in critically ill patients.[106] Once the diagnosis is made, prompt intervention is indicated with percutaneous ultrasound or CT-guided cholecystostomy. For the small percentage of patients who do not improve with percutaneous cholecystostomy, open cholecystostomy or cholecystectomy may be indicated, depending on the ability to tolerate surgery and general anesthesia.

10.5.6 External Compression of the Common Bile Duct: Mirizzi's and Lemmel Syndrome

Mirizzi's syndrome is rare, ranging from 0.05 to 4% in patients with gallstone disease,[107]but most common among the female sex and those who have reached an advanced age.[108] It is defined as obstructive jaundice caused by external compression of the CBD due to impacted stones in the cystic duct or gallbladder infundibulum. Two types of Mirizzi's syndrome have been described: Type 1 involves bile duct compression from the left by stones in the gallbladder neck and cystic ducts with pericholecystic inflammatory change. Type II is secondary to biliobiliary fistulization which is caused by pressure necrosis of the bile duct due to cholecystolithiasis. Presentation includes fever, jaundice, and right upper quadrant pain. Serum concentrations of alkaline phosphatase and direct bilirubin are elevated in 90% of the patients with Mirizzi's syndrome.[109] Lemmel syndrome comes about due to a duodenal parapapillary diverticulum compression on the bile duct or pancreatic duct opening, effectively obstructing the passage of bile and resulting in cholestasis, jaundice, cholangitis, and pancreatitis.[110]

10.5.7 Hydrops

Long-standing impaction of stones in the cystic duct leads to a distended gallbladder, often filled with clear mucoid "white bile" due to the absence of bile entry to the gallbladder and absorption of bilirubin. Other causes of gallbladder hydrops include cystic fibrosis, tumors, and mechanical obstruction of the cystic duct including external compression by inflammatory or neoplastic masses. In children, gallbladder hydrops is relatively common during acute phases of inflammatory and infectious diseases including typhoid, streptococcal infections, mesenteric adenitis, viral hepatitis, leptospirosis, familial Mediterranean fever, and Kawasaki disease.[111]

Abdominal pain, nausea, vomiting, and right upper quadrant pain are often presenting symptoms with right upper quadrant tenderness and/or right upper abdominal mass. Symptoms usually resolve by treating the underlying disease, for example, cholecystectomy if cholelithiasis is the underlying cause. If surgery is contraindicated, external drainage can be completed to treat persistent gallbladder hydrops.[112]

10.5.8 Cholecystenteric Fistula (Gallstone Ileus)

Fistula formation may be due to pressure necrosis from cholelithiasis, leading to gangrene and perforation. Perforation can be localized, leading to the formation of pericholecystic abscess; into the peritoneum, resulting in peritonitis; or into the small or large intestine, developing a cholecystenteric fistula.[113] A stone that passed through a cholecystenteric fistula can lead to gallstone ileus which is a cause of mechanical bowel obstruction.[114,115] Presentation may include episodic or subacute obstruction and occasional hematemesis due to hemorrhage at the site of the cholecystenteric fistula. When gallstone is impacted, it causes symptoms of pain and vomiting due to bowel obstruction. Gallbladder wall thickening, pneumobilia, intestinal obstruction, and obstructing gallstones may be seen on CT scan.[116] CT scan may be used to evaluate for evidence of ischemia, necrosis, or bowel perforation. Surgical candidates should be treated with enterolithotomy to relieve the intestinal obstruction and cholecystectomy with cholecystenteric fistula closure. Surgically unfit patients may be managed with enterolithotomy and observation.[113,115,117,118,119]

10.5.9 Porcelain Gallbladder

Porcelain gallbladder is defined as gallbladder wall calcification. There is an incidence of 0.2% in patients who undergo a cholecystectomy.[120,121,122,123,124,125,126] It is five times more common in females than males, typically presenting in the sixth decade of life. Approximately one in five patients are asymptomatic or report nonspecific symptoms.[127] Diagnosis is typically made via abdominal CT, identifying calcified wall of the gallbladder, and classified depending on the extent of calcification to complete intramural calcification. Porcelain gallbladder is weakly associated with gallbladder carcinoma.[124,125,127] Incidental gallbladder carcinoma is identified in 0.8% of patients who underwent cholecystectomies; of those cases, 15% had an association with porcelain gallbladder.[120,121,122,123,124,125,126] Cholecystectomy is recommended in patients with porcelain gallbladder, symptomatic disease, but not for radiographic findings alone.[124,125,127]

10.6 Special Populations

10.6.1 Cholecystitis in Pregnancy

Biliary diseases in pregnancy may be, in part, due to the physiological actions of estrogen and progesterone promoting cholesterol secretions and biliary stasis, leading to biliary sludge and stone formation.[128,129] Approximately 3.5% of pregnant patients are found to have cholelithiasis and 0.05 to 0.8% develop symptomatic gallstone disease during pregnancy. It is the second most common urgent surgical operation in pregnant women following appendectomy.[130] Pregnant patients present with symptoms similar to that of nonpregnant patients. White blood cells are normally elevated in pregnancy, but the presence of a left shift suggests infection. Diagnosis is made using abdominal ultrasound as in the nonpregnant patient.

Laparoscopic cholecystectomy is a safe option in all three trimesters of pregnancy.[130,131,132,133] Surgery during the initial hospitalization is the preferred treatment for acute cholecystitis in pregnant people due to the recurrence of symptoms in the same pregnancy in patients who only had medical management,[130,134,135] shorter hospital stays,[130,132,134,136] lower rates of preterm labor, preterm delivery, and fewer hospital admissions.[134] For pregnant patients at high-risk for surgery, percutaneous or open gallbladder decompression can be considered.

10.6.2 Cirrhosis

Gallstones occur frequently in cirrhotic patients and contributes to mortality in cirrhotic patients.[137,138,139,140,141,142] Historically, open cholecystectomy in patients with cirrhosis has been associated with a mortality rate of 7 to 20% with primary cause of morbidity and mortality related to blood loss (intraoperative and associated gastrointestinal bleeding), infections, or uncontrolled ascites.[138,143,144,145,146,147,148] Laparoscopic cholecystectomy should be considered if technically possible, taking care on entry to the abdomen for collateral venous drainage.

Patients with severe symptomatic biliary cholic or cholecystitis, Child-Pugh C cirrhotic patients, are generally offered medical treatment directed to improve their liver function, control ascites, improve nutrition and coagulation parameters, and when possible, portal vein pressure reduction to allow for safer elective operation. When medical management fails, percutaneous cholecystostomy tube can be considered.

Operative planning for patients with Child-Pugh A or B cirrhosis should include preoperative coagulation correction. Given hypertrophy of liver tissue and nodularity from cirrhotic changes, surgeons should anticipate the potential for difficulty in exposure of the cholecystohepatic triangle. Increased portal venous hypertension, thrombocytopenia, and friability of the liver tissue increases the risk of intraoperative bleeding and may limit the ability to provide adequate retraction on the gallbladder. Surgeons may consider placing extra ports for retraction of the liver, having an additional qualified assistant in the case, and/or using intraoperative packing (such as a vaginal pack) to optimize exposure in laparoscopic cases. Subtotal cholecystectomy may be considered though there is a high rate of postoperative biliary leakage and prophylactic drains should be considered.[149]

10.6.3 Older Population with Cholecystitis

While typical management of acute cholecystitis is laparoscopic cholecystectomy, operative morbidity in the elderly is higher compared to the general population. In patients aged 69 years or older, acute cholecystitis complications occurred in 23.2% compared to 12.0% of those in the younger cohort. Comorbidities were higher in the elderly cohort with a higher proportion also requiring emergency surgery, higher rate of conversion to an open procedure, prolonged LOS in the hospital, and higher proportion with CBD stones.[150,151,152,153,154] Among patients who are unable to receive general anesthesia, percutaneous cholecystostomy or intravenous antibiotics may prove to be definitive management.[155,156] Surgery remains the recommended treatment for cholelithiasis; however, in subpopulations with high perioperative risk factors, consideration should be given to preoperative optimization when possible and/or treatment consideration for cholecystostomy tube and antibiotic management. In a retrospective study of patients over the age of 65 and admitted to two institutions with acute cholecystitis, it was found that 97.6% of patients who initially managed without surgery did not have recurrence over a mean follow-up of 2.5 years.[157]

10.7 The Role of Minimally Invasive Surgery

In the United States, nearly 300,000 cholecystectomies are performed annually.[158] Laparoscopic cholecystectomy was introduced in the mid 1980s[159] and is the standard of care for patients unless there is a contraindication to laparoscopic approach. The critical view of safety (CVS) is the view of a "window" crossed by the cystic duct and artery which is ideally seen in all laparoscopic cholecystectomy. This is achieved following clearance of fibrous and fatty tissue from Calot's triangle and separating the gallbladder of the lower third of its attachment to the liver visualizing the cystic plate.

Two tubular structures, cystic duct and artery, entering into the base of the gallbladder can be visualized (▶ Fig. 10.1). This should be achieved before any clipping or dividing of tubular structures is implemented to secure the correct identification of those structures and avoid common bile duct injury.[158,160] In practice, CVS technique is used variably by surgeons[161] Cholangiogram, intraoperative ultrasound, and indocyanine green (ICG) should be considered if there is any question regarding biliary anatomy to ensure there is no injury to the CBD.

In cases with significant inflammation or dense fibrotic tissue in the cystic triangleobscuring clear biliary anatomy, consideration should be given to damage control maneuvers in order to decrease complication risk including: subtotal cholecystectomy, laparoscopic top-down ("fundus-first") cholecystectomy, biliary drainage via placement of a laparoscopic cholecystostomy tube and, ultimately, conversion to open procedure.[160,161,162,163,164] As resident training in the past 15 years has largely favored laparoscopic experience for cholecystectomy, there is concern that experience with open cholecystectomy is limited, laparoscopic damage control may be attempted first, depending on the surgeon skill set,[165,166] and there has been a paradigm shift in that difficult laparoscopic cholecystectomy should be directly converted to an open procedure.

Subtotal cholecystectomies may be performed laparoscopically and are divided into "reconstituting" (leaving a remnant

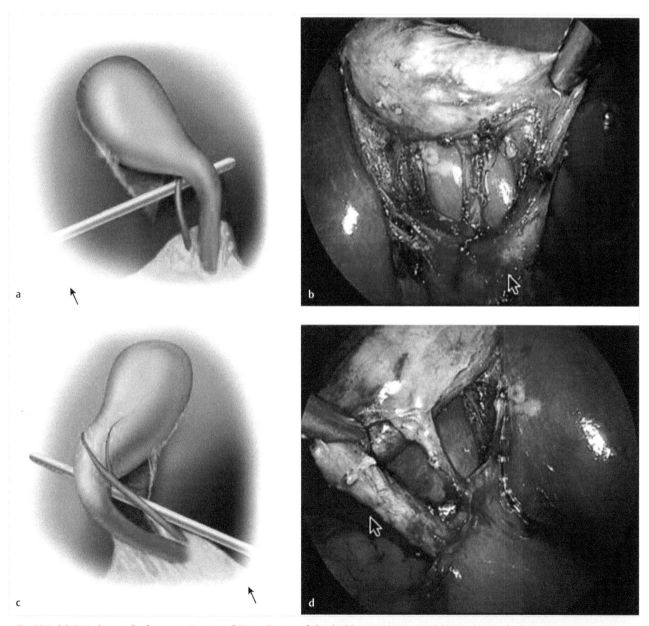

Fig. 10.1 (a) Critical view of safety posterior view. (b) Visualization of the doublet view (posterior) (c) Critical view of safety anterior view. (d) Visualization of the doublet (anterior view). (Reproduced with permission of Sages. The Sages safe cholecystectomy program: strategies for minimizing bile duct injuries: adopting a universal culture of safety in cholecystectomy. Available at: https://www.sages.org/safe-cholecystectomy-program/).

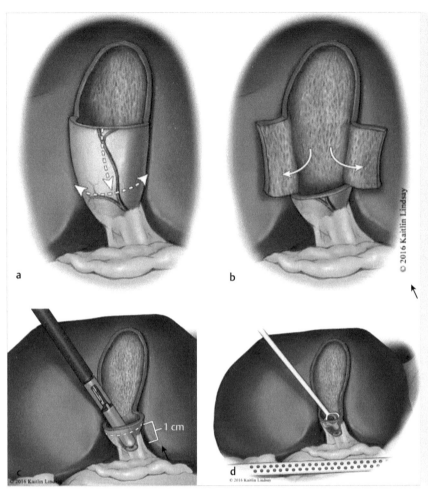

Fig. 10.2 (a–d) Laparoscopic subtotal cholecystectomy. (Reproduced with permissions of Sharmila D. A step-by-step guide to laparoscopic subtotal fenestrating cholecystectomy: a damage control approach to the difficult gallbladder. Journal of the American College of Surgeons 2016; 223(2): e15–e18.)

gallbladder) and "fenestrating"[167,168]. Subtotal reconstituting cholecystectomy decreases the incidence of postoperative fistula, and increases the risk of recurrent biliary symptoms and need for a higher morbid operation for future remnant cholecystectomy.[162] Subtotal fenestrating cholecystectomy leaves the lower end of the gallbladder open, making it more susceptible for postoperative fistula and prolonged leakage but decreases the risk of recurrent cholelithiasis symptoms as a remnant gallbladder is not created.[169] Laparoscopic subtotal cholecystectomy (▶ Fig. 10.2) is a damage control maneuver intended to decrease the risk of major bile duct injury. Biliary leak typically resolves in the first 2 weeks postoperatively.[149,168,170,171,172,173,174,175,176,177,178,179,180,181] ERCP and stenting may be performed following subtotal cholecystectomy[162,173,174,175,177,182,183] and due to retained stones, persistent bile leaks, and CBD strictures or Mirizzi's syndrome.

A "top-down," "retrograde," or "fundus-first" laparoscopic cholecystectomy refers to the traditional approach that starts with gallbladder fundus dissection and proceeds toward the portal triad and Calot's triangle. This approach is performed to facilitate the identification of the cystic duct and artery, as they are the only remaining structures attached to the gallbladder.[159,184] Risks associated with the top-down laparoscopic cholecystectomy include vascular and biliary injury due to the significant inflammation from underlying disease.[184,185,186] In all cases of damage

control laparoscopic cholecystectomy, conversion to an open cholecystectomy should be considered.

10.7.1 Role of Intraoperative Cholangiogram (IOC), Intraoperative Ultrasound, and Indocyanine Green (ICG)

Bile duct injury rates during laparoscopic cholecystectomies occur at a rate of approximately 0.3 to 0.7%[187] with significant associated morbidity and cost.[188,189,190,191,192,193] Intraoperative cholangiogram is used to delineate anatomy, and confirm vascular and biliary anatomy, ensuring there is no injury to the CBD, common hepatic duct or branches, and there are no retained stones in the CB. The primary cause of biliary duct injury is misinterpretation of biliary anatomy.[194]

IOC is associated with lower risk of common bile duct injury;[195,196] however, evidence that CBD injuries are preventable with routine use of IOC is lacking.[189] IOC may increase operative time,[197] but it has been cost-effective in considering the cost of a delayed CBD injury.[189,198] Routine cholangiography, especially in resident training settings or in the early surgical career, allows for development of critical surgeon experience in cannula insertion and interpretation and identification of intraoperative injury.

Intraoperative ultrasound may be used to evaluate the biliary and vascular anatomy. Appropriate training of use and interpretation of results may prevent bile duct injury.[199] It can be equivalent to intraoperative cholangiogram in detecting stones, performed 50% faster, does not include the use of radiation or dye exposure, and has superior cost-effectiveness.[200] Limitations include appropriate training in intraoperative biliary ultrasound, adequate evaluation of intrahepatic anatomy, and ability to detect anatomic anomalies with the same level of IOC.[199,200]

Fluorescent cholangiography is based on the principle that ICG is excreted into bile and protein-bound ICG emits light when illuminated with near-infrared light. Preoperatively, one milliliter (2.5 mg/mL) of ICG is injected approximately two hours prior to surgery and lasts for up to 125 minutes. Advantages include the lack of radiation and no dissection of the triangle of Calot, and in a retrospective study of 43 patients comparing IOC and ICG, potential saving in in cost and operative time.[201] Limitations include frequency of visualization decreasing with increasing body mass index.[202]

10.8 Contraindications to an MIS Approach

Absolute contraindications for laparoscopic cholecystectomy include inability to tolerate pneumoperitoneum or general anesthesia and is most often due to a systemic illness, uncontrolled coagulopathy, end-stage liver disease, and metastatic disease.[158]

10.8.1 Open Cholecystectomy

The conversion rate from laparoscopic cholecystectomy to open cholecystectomy in the US is 5 to 10%.[203] Risk factors include choledocholithiasis or severe inflammation near Calot's triangle, male sex, age > 50, obesity, and previous abdominal surgery.[203,204,205,206] Conversion rate to an open procedure is higher early in a surgeon's career and decreases as overall operative experience increases.[203] Indications for conversation from a laparoscopic to an open procedure have complications including hemorrhage from a vascular injury, suspected aberrant anatomy unable to be identified laparoscopically, bowel or bile duct injury, or inability to safely progress during a laparoscopic cholecystectomy due to fibrosis tissue or inflammation.

10.9 The Role for Nonoperative Management

Nonoperative management should be considered in cases in which the patient declines surgery or has significant comorbid conditions, raising their operative risk to unacceptable levels for an elective procedure. Optimal medical management may include collaboration with gastroenterology and/or the primary care team to ensure symptom management. Ursodeoxycholic acid (UDCA) may reduce the risk of biliary tract pain, surgery, and acute cholecystitis in symptomatic patients.[207] Treatment with extracorporeal shock wave lithotripsy (ESWL) with dissolution therapy achieved complete elimination of gallstones in 87% of patients with uncomplicated, symptomatic biliary disease[208] and may be an effective method in selected patients with favorable stones. Therefore, it appears that this method of treatment makes it possible to achieve a high-rate of elimination in a select group of patients (including those with smaller, radiolucent stones).[209,210,211] Patient should be aware of the recurrence risk.[212] UDCA has not been shown to be effective in cholelithiasis prevention in high-risk populations (e.g., those with rapid weight loss).[213,214]

10.9.1 Percutaneous Cholecystostomy

A percutaneous ultrasound-or CT-guided cholecystostomy is the insertion of a pigtail catheter over a guidewire passed into the gallbladder through the abdominal wall and the liver. It may be both diagnostic and therapeutic. It is used to drain the distended, inflamed, hydropic, or purulent gallbladder in surgically unfit patients, for cholecystectomy, and patients with acalculous cholecystitis. The catheter is removed after inflammation has been resolved, the patient's condition has improved, and cholangiography reveals a patent cystic duct. If the patient is fit for surgery, laparoscopic cholecystectomy is performed after 6 weeks of placement.

10.9.2 Perforated Cholecystitis with Hepatic Abscess

Guidelines for moderate to severe acute cholecystitis with local complications such as biliary peritonitis and pericholecystic abscess include emergency cholecystectomy and abdominal cavity drainage,[215] if the patient is able to undergo general anesthesia. In high-risk surgical patients, emergency gallbladder drainage via percutaneous cholecystostomy and abscess drainage, antibiotic therapy, and intensive care support may be initially recommended with interval cholecystectomy.

10.10 The Management of Complications

Intraoperative complications for laparoscopic cholecystectomy in 452,936 patients with cholelithiasis between 1990 and 2013 included bile duct injury (0.63%), conversation to open procedure (3.6%), conversation to open procedure for bleeding typically due to the cystic artery of liver bed (0.51%), and organ injuries (0.26%).[216] Prevention of bile duct injuries is critical and most major injuries are due to misidentification of biliary structures.[217] A critical view of safety should be used to identify the cystic duct and cystic artery during laparoscopic cholecystectomy.[218] A critical view should include the following: 1) The hepatocystic triangle is identified by the cystic duct, common hepatic duct, and inferior edge of the liver. 2) The lower portion of the gallbladder is dissected to expose the liver bed and 3) Only two structures should be seen entering the gallbladder.

Postoperative bile leak is often related to late perforation due to heat damage, bile outflow obstruction (secondary to a clip), or patent duct of Luschka.[216] Appropriate radiographic evaluation to determine etiology is necessary. Drainage of biloma should be performed and ERCP with placement of a biliary or nasobiliary drain is recommended[219] as biliary leaks typically close with appropriate drainage. Intraoperative bleeding is often secondary to 1) vascular injury 2) misplaced or failed clip on the cystic artery, and 3) liver bed bleeding. Vascular bleeding is frequently the most devastating and is usually encountered while establishing pneumoperitoneum or during dissection within Calot's triangle.[220] Operating room management for unexpected major bleeding should always include the following: immediately alerting anesthesia, ensuring adequate vascular access and blood product availability, considering urgently calling an experienced surgical colleague for assistance, and keeping in mind to call for additional instruments in order to optimize exposure and rapidly convert an open procedure if indicated.

Up to 41% of patients report some postoperative persistence of abdominal pain[221,222,223,224] and usually in the initial period postoperatively. "Post-cholecystectomy syndrome" was defined for the first time by Womack and Crider in 1947 as "the presence of symptoms after cholecystectomy." It contains a group of abdominal symptoms that recur and/or persist after cholecystectomy. Those symptoms, which can be biliary or extra biliary, include biliary or nonbiliary-like abdominal pain, dyspepsia, vomiting, with or without jaundice, fever, and cholangitis.[162,225,226,227,228]

References

[1] Shaffer EA. Gallstone disease: Epidemiology of gallbladder stone disease. Best Pract Res Clin Gastroenterol. 2006; 20(6):981–996

[2] Ansaloni L, Pisano M, Coccolini F, et al. "2016 WSES guidelines on acute calculous cholecystitis". World Journal of Emergency Surgery. 2016; 11:25

[3] Everhart JE, Khare M, Hill M, Maurer KR. Prevalence and ethnic differences in gallbladder disease in the United States. Gastroenterology. 1999; 117(3): 632–639

[4] Aerts R, Penninckx F. The burden of gallstone disease in Europe. Aliment Pharmacol Ther. 2003; 18 Suppl 3:49–53

[5] Gracie WA, Ransohoff DF. The natural history of silent gallstones: the innocent gallstone is not a myth. N Engl J Med. 1982; 307(13):798–800

[6] Shaffer EA, S.E.A. Epidemiology and risk factors for gallstone disease: has the paradigm changed in the 21st century? Curr Gastroenterol Rep. 2005; 7(2): 132–140

[7] Kratzer W, Mason RA, Kächele V. Prevalence of gallstones in sonographic surveys worldwide. J Clin Ultrasound. 1999; 27(1):1–7

[8] Pedersen G, Hoem D, Andrén-Sandberg A. Influence of laparoscopic cholecystectomy on the prevalence of operations for gallstones in Norway. The European Journal of Surgery. 2011; 168(8)(9):464–469

[9] Attili AF, Carulli N, Roda E, et al. Epidemiology of gallstone disease in Italy: prevalence data of the Multicenter Italian Study on Cholelithiasis (M.I.COL.). Am J Epidemiol. 1995; 141(2):158–165

[10] Beckingham IJ. Gallstones. Surgery. 2017; 35(12):682–691

[11] Halldestam I, Enell EL, Kullman E, Borch K. Development of symptoms and complications in individuals with asymptomatic gallstones. Br J Surg. 2004; 91(6):734–738

[12] Gurusamy KS, Davidson C, Gluud C, Davidson BR. Early versus delayed laparoscopic cholecystectomy for people with acute cholecystitis. Cochrane Database Syst Rev. 2013; 6(6):CD005440

[13] CapocacciaL, the GREPCO group. Clinical symptoms and gallstone disease: Lessons from a population study. In: Epidemiology and Prevention of Gallstone Disease. Dordrecht: Springer Netherlands;1984:153

[14] Barbara L, Sama C, Morselli Labate AM, et al. A population study on the prevalence of gallstone disease: the Sirmione study. Hepatology. 1987; 7(5): 913–917

[15] Kimura Y, Takada T, Kawarada Y, et al. Definitions, pathophysiology, and epidemiology of acute cholangitis and cholecystitis: Tokyo Guidelines. J Hepatobiliary Pancreat Surg. 2007; 14(1):15–26

[16] Singer AJ, McCracken G, Henry MC, Thode HC, Jr, Cabahug CJ. Correlation among clinical, laboratory, and hepatobiliary scanning findings in patients with suspected acute cholecystitis. Ann Emerg Med. 1996; 28(3):267–272

[17] Simeone JF, Brink JA, Mueller PR, et al. The sonographic diagnosis of acute gangrenous cholecystitis: importance of the Murphy sign. AJR Am J Roentgenol. 1989; 152(2):289–290

[18] Adedeji OA, McAdam WA. Murphy's sign, acute cholecystitis and elderly people. J R Coll Surg Edinb. 1996; 41(2):88–89

[19] Shea JA, Berlin JA, Escarce JJ, et al. Revised estimates of diagnostic test sensitivity and specificity in suspected biliary tract disease. Arch Intern Med. 1994; 154(22):2573–2581

[20] Chatziioannou SN, Moore WH, Ford PV, Dhekne RD. Hepatobiliary scintigraphy is superior to abdominal ultrasonography in suspected acute cholecystitis. Surgery. 2000; 127(6):609–613

[21] Freitas JE, Mirkes SH, Fink-Bennett DM, Bree RL. Suspected acute cholecystitis. Comparison of hepatobiliary scintigraphy versus ultrasonography. Clin Nucl Med. 1982; 7(8):364–367

[22] Jamieson NV, Friend PJ, Wraight EP. A two year experience with 99mTC HIDA cholescintigraphy in teaching hospital practice. Surg Gynecol Obstet. 1986; 163(1):29–32

[23] Kalimi R, Gecelter GR, Caplin D, et al. Diagnosis of acute cholecystitis: sensitivity of sonography, cholescintigraphy, and combined sonography-cholescintigraphy. J Am Coll Surg. 2001; 193(6):609–613

[24] Kiewiet JJS, Leeuwenburgh MMN, Bipat S, Bossuyt PMM, Stoker J, Boermeester MA. A systematic review and meta-analysis of diagnostic performance of imaging in acute cholecystitis. Radiology. 2012; 264(3): 708–720

[25] Lauritsen KB, Wied U, Henriksen JH. [Cholescintigraphy in suspected cholecystitis. Further experience with a diagnostic test]. Ugeskr Laeger. 1985; 147(8):698–700

[26] Lambie H, Cook AM, Scarsbrook AF, Lodge JPA, Robinson PJ, Chowdhury FU. Tc99m-hepatobiliary iminodiacetic acid (HIDA) scintigraphy in clinical practice. Clinical Radiology. 2011; 66(11):1094–1105. W.B. Saunders

[27] Wu XD, Tian X, Liu MM, Wu L, Zhao S, Zhao L. Meta-analysis comparing early versus delayed laparoscopic cholecystectomy for acute cholecystitis. British Journal of Surgery. 2015; 102(11):1302–1313. John Wiley & Sons, Ltd

[28] Saber A, Hokkam EN. Operative outcome and patient satisfaction in early and delayed laparoscopic cholecystectomy for acute cholecystitis. Minim Invasive Surg. 2014; 2014:162643

[29] Gutt CN, Encke J, Köninger J, et al. Acute cholecystitis: early versus delayed cholecystectomy, a multicenter randomized trial (ACDC study, NCT00447304). Ann Surg. 2013; 258(3):385–393

[30] Roulin D, Saadi A, Di Mare L, Demartines N, Halkic N. Early versus delayed cholecystectomy for acute cholecystitis, are the 72 hours still the rule? A randomized trial. Ann Surg. 2016; 264(5):717–722

[31] Lo CM, Liu CL, Fan ST, Lai EC, Wong J. Prospective randomized study of early versus delayed laparoscopic cholecystectomy for acute cholecystitis. Ann Surg. 1998; 227(4):461–467

[32] Lai PB, Kwong KH, Leung KL, et al. Randomized trial of early versus delayed laparoscopic cholecystectomy for acute cholecystitis. Br J Surg. 1998; 85(6): 764–767

[33] Johansson M, Thune A, Blomqvist A, Nelvin L, Lundell L. Management of acute cholecystitis in the laparoscopic era: results of a prospective, randomized clinical trial. J Gastrointest Surg. 2003; 7(5):642–645

[34] Kolla SB, Aggarwal S, Kumar A, et al. Early versus delayed laparoscopic cholecystectomy for acute cholecystitis: a prospective randomized trial. Surg Endosc. 2004; 18(9):1323–1327

[35] Macafee DAL, Humes DJ, Bouliotis G, Beckingham IJ, Whynes DK, Lobo DN. Prospective randomized trial using cost-utility analysis of early versus delayed laparoscopic cholecystectomy for acute gallbladder disease. Br J Surg. 2009; 96(9):1031–1040

[36] Yadav RP, Adhikary S, Agrawal CS, Bhattarai B, Gupta RK, Ghimire A. "A comparative study of early vs. delayed laparoscopic cholecystectomy in acute cholecystitis. Kathmandu Univ Med J. 2009; 7(25):16–20

[37] Gul R, Dar RA, Sheikh RA, Salroo NA, Matoo AR, Wani SH. Comparison of early and delayed laparoscopic cholecystectomy for acute cholecystitis: experience from a single center. N Am J Med Sci. 2013; 5(7):414–418

[38] Strasberg SM. Clinical practice. Acute calculous cholecystitis. N Engl J Med. 2008; 358(26):2804–2811

[39] Urbach DR, Stukel TA. Rate of elective cholecystectomy and the incidence of severe gallstone disease. CMAJ. 2005; 172(8):1015–1019

[40] Halpin V. "Acute cholecystitis." BMJ Clin Evid. 2014:2014

[41] Fialkowski E, Halpin V, Whinney RR. "Acute cholecystitis." BMJ Clin Evid. 2008:2008

[42] Halpin V, Gupta A. "Acute cholecystitis." BMJ Clin Evid. 2011:2011

[43] Hilsden R, Leeper R, Kolchupulos J, et al. Point-of-care biliary ultrasound in the emergency department (BUSED): implications for surgical referral and emergency department wait times. Trauma Surg Acute Care Open. 2018; 3 (1):e000164

[44] Hastings RS, Powers RD. Abdominal pain in the ED: a 35 year retrospective. Am J Emerg Med. 2011; 29(7):711–716

[45] Miettinen P, Pasanen P, Lahtinen J, Alhava E. Acute abdominal pain in adults. Ann Chir Gynaecol. 1996; 85(1):5–9

[46] Irvin TT. Abdominal pain: a surgical audit of 1190 emergency admissions. Br J Surg. 1989; 76(11):1121–1125

[47] Blaivas M, Adhikari S. Diagnostic utility of cholescintigraphy in emergency department patients with suspected acute cholecystitis: comparison with bedside RUQ ultrasonography. J Emerg Med. 2007; 33(1):47–52

[48] Ransohoff DF, Miller GL, Forsythe SB, Hermann RE. Outcome of acute cholecystitis in patients with diabetes mellitus. Ann Intern Med. 1987; 106(6): 829–832

[49] Meyer KA, Capos NJ, Mittelpunkt AI. Personal experiences with 1,261 cases of acute and chronic cholecystitis and cholelithiasis. Surgery. 1967; 61(5): 661–668

[50] Bedirli A, Sakrak O, Sözüer EM, Kerek M, Güler I. Factors effecting the complications in the natural history of acute cholecystitis. Hepatogastroenterology. 2001; 48(41):1275–1278

[51] Addison NV, Finan PJ. Urgent and early cholecystectomy for acute gallbladder disease. Br J Surg. 1988; 75(2):141–143

[52] Girard RM, Morin M. Open cholecystectomy: its morbidity and mortality as a reference standard. Can J Surg. 1993; 36(1):75–80

[53] Roslyn JJ, DenBesten L, Thompson JE, Jr, Silverman BF. Roles of lithogenic bile and cystic duct occlusion in the pathogenesis of acute cholecystitis. Am J Surg. 1980; 140(1):126–130

[54] Morris CR, Hohf RP, Ivy AC. An experimental study of the role of stasis in the etiology of cholecystitis. Surgery. 1952; 32(4):673–685

[55] Diehl AK, Sugarek NJ, Todd KH. Clinical evaluation for gallstone disease: usefulness of symptoms and signs in diagnosis. Am J Med. 1990; 89(1): 29–33

[56] Indar AA, Beckingham IJ. Acute cholecystitis. BMJ. 2002; 325(7365): 639–643

[57] Solomkin JS, Mazuski JE, Bradley JS, et al. Diagnosis and management of complicated intra-abdominal infection in adults and children: guidelines by the Surgical Infection Society and the Infectious Diseases Society of America. Clin Infect Dis. 2010; 50(2):133–164

[58] Acar T, Kamer E, Acar N, et al. Laparoscopic cholecystectomy in the treatment of acute cholecystitis: comparison of results between early and late cholecystectomy. Pan Afr Med J. 2017; 26:49

[59] Vetrhus M, Søreide O, Eide GE, Solhaug JH, Nesvik I, Søndenaa K. Pain and quality of life in patients with symptomatic, non-complicated gallbladder stones: results of a randomized controlled trial. Scand J Gastroenterol. 2004; 39(3):270–276

[60] Papi C, Catarci M, D'Ambrosio L, et al. Timing of cholecystectomy for acute calculous cholecystitis: a meta-analysis. Am J Gastroenterol. 2004; 99(1): 147–155

[61] Zhou MW, Gu XD, Xiang JB, Chen ZY. Comparison of clinical safety and outcomes of early versus delayed laparoscopic cholecystectomy for acute cholecystitis: a meta-analysis. ScientificWorldJournal. 2014; 2014:274516

[62] Chikamori F, Kuniyoshi N, Shibuya S, Takase Y. Early scheduled laparoscopic cholecystectomy following percutaneous transhepatic gallbladder drainage for patients with acute cholecystitis. Surg Endosc. 2002; 16(12):1704–1707

[63] Patel M, Miedema BW, James MA, Marshall JB. Percutaneous cholecystostomy is an effective treatment for high-risk patients with acute cholecystitis. Am Surg. 2000; 66(1):33–37

[64] Ko CW, Lee SP. "Epidemiology and natural history of common bile duct stones and prediction of disease". Gastrointestinal Endoscopy. 2002; 56 Suppl. 6:S165–9

[65] Almadi MA, Barkun JS, Barkun AN. Management of suspected stones in the common bile duct. CMAJ. 2012; 184(8):884–892

[66] de Sousa S, Tobler O, Iranmanesh P, Frossard JL, Morel P, Toso C. Management of suspected common bile duct stones on cholangiogram during same-stay cholecystectomy for acute gallstone-related disease. BMC Surg. 2017; 17(1):39

[67] Kharbutli B, Velanovich V. Management of preoperatively suspected choledocholithiasis: a decision analysis. J Gastrointest Surg. 2008; 12(11): 1973–1980

[68] Ebner S, Rechner J, Beller S, Erhart K, Riegler FM, Szinicz G. Laparoscopic management of common bile duct stones. Surg Endosc. 2004; 18(5): 762–765

[69] Costi R, Gnocchi A, Di Mario F, Sarli L. Diagnosis and management of choledocholithiasis in the golden age of imaging, endoscopy and laparoscopy. World J Gastroenterol. 2014; 20(37):13382–13401

[70] Martin DJ, Vernon D, Toouli J. Surgical versus endoscopic treatment of bile duct stones. Cochrane Database Syst. Rev. 2006; CD003327:1–52

[71] Majeed AW, Ross B, Johnson AG, Reed MWR. Common duct diameter as an independent predictor of choledocholithiasis: is it useful? Clin Radiol. 1999; 54(3):170–172

[72] Tranter SE, Thompson MH. Comparison of endoscopic sphincterotomy and laparoscopic exploration of the common bile duct. Br J Surg. 2002; 89(12): 1495–1504

[73] Lyass S, Phillips EH. "Laparoscopic transcystic duct common bile duct exploration." Surg Endosc. 2006; 20(Suppl 2):S441–5

[74] Topal B, Aerts R, Penninckx F. Laparoscopic common bile duct stone clearance with flexible choledochoscopy. Surg Endosc. 2007; 21(12):2317–2321

[75] Martin IJ, Bailey IS, Rhodes M, O'Rourke N, Nathanson L, Fielding G. Towards T-tube free laparoscopic bile duct exploration: a methodologic evolution during 300 consecutive procedures. Ann Surg. 1998; 228(1):29–34

[76] Gurusamy SK, Giljaca V, Takwoingi Y, et al. "Endoscopic retrograde cholangiopancreatography versus intraoperative cholangiography for diagnosis of common bile duct stones." Cochrane Database Syst Rev. 2015(2): CD010339

[77] Machi J, Tateishi T, Oishi AJ, et al. Laparoscopic ultrasonography versus operative cholangiography during laparoscopic cholecystectomy: review of the literature and a comparison with open intraoperative ultrasonography. J Am Coll Surg. 1999; 188(4):360–367

[78] Videhult P, Sandblom G, Rasmussen IC. How reliable is intraoperative cholangiography as a method for detecting common bile duct stones?: A prospective population-based study on 1171 patients. Surg Endosc. 2009; 23 (2):304–312

[79] Hamy A, Hennekinne S, Pessaux P, et al. Endoscopic sphincterotomy prior to laparoscopic cholecystectomy for the treatment of cholelithiasis. Surg Endosc. 2003; 17(6):872–875

[80] Lilly MC, Arregui ME. A balanced approach to choledocholithiasis. Surg Endosc. 2001; 15(5):467–472

[81] Charcot M. De la fievre hepatique symptomatique. Comparison avec la fievre uroseptique. Lecons sur les maladies du foie des voies biliares et des reins. Paris: Bourneville et Sevestre; 1877:176–185

[82] Reynolds BM, Dargan EL. Acute obstructive cholangitis; a distinct clinical syndrome. Ann Surg. 1959; 150(2):299–303

[83] Lamberts MP. Indications of cholecystectomy in gallstone disease. Curr Opin Gastroenterol. 2018; 34(2):97–102

[84] Kimura Y, Takada T, Strasberg SM, et al. TG13 current terminology, etiology, and epidemiology of acute cholangitis and cholecystitis. J Hepatobiliary Pancreat Sci. 2013; 20(1):8–23

[85] Gigot JF, Leese T, Dereme T, Coutinho J, Castaing D, Bismuth H. Acute cholangitis. Multivariate analysis of risk factors. Ann Surg. 1989; 209(4): 435–438

[86] Lipsett PA, Pitt HA. Acute cholangitis. Surg Clin North Am. 1990; 70(6): 1297–1312

[87] Lee CC, Chang IJ, Lai YC, Chen SY, Chen SC. Epidemiology and prognostic determinants of patients with bacteremic cholecystitis or cholangitis. Am J Gastroenterol. 2007; 102(3):563–569

[88] Kiriyama S, Takada T, Strasberg SM, et al. Tokyo Guidelines Revision Committee. TG13 guidelines for diagnosis and severity grading of acute cholangitis (with videos). J Hepatobiliary Pancreat Sci. 2013; 20(1):24–34

[89] Aboulian A, Chan T, Yaghoubian A, et al. Early cholecystectomy safely decreases hospital stay in patients with mild gallstone pancreatitis: a randomized prospective study. Ann Surg. 2010; 251(4):615–619

[90] Jee SL, Jarmin R, Lim KF, Raman K. Outcomes of early versus delayed cholecystectomy in patients with mild to moderate acute biliary pancreatitis: a randomized prospective study. Asian J Surg. 2018; 41(1):47–54

[91] Duncan CB, Riall TS. Evidence-based current surgical practice: calculous gallbladder disease. J Gastrointest Surg. 2012; 16(11):2011–2025

[92] da Costa DW, Bouwense SA, Schepers NJ, et al. Dutch Pancreatitis Study Group. Same-admission versus interval cholecystectomy for mild gallstone pancreatitis (PONCHO): a multicentre randomised controlled trial. Lancet. 2015; 386(10000):1261–1268

[93] Wu B, Buddensick TJ, Ferdosi H, et al. Predicting gangrenous cholecystitis. HPB (Oxford). 2014; 16(9):801–806

[94] Kanaan SA, Murayama KM, Merriam LT, et al. Risk factors for conversion of laparoscopic to open cholecystectomy. J Surg Res. 2002; 106(1):20–24

[95] Aydin C, Altaca G, Berber I, Tekin K, Kara M, Titiz I. Prognostic parameters for the prediction of acute gangrenous cholecystitis. J Hepatobiliary Pancreat Surg. 2006; 13(2):155–159

[96] Nikfarjam M, Niumsawatt V, Sethu A, et al. Outcomes of contemporary management of gangrenous and non-gangrenous acute cholecystitis. HPB (Oxford). 2011; 13(8):551–558

[97] Merriam LT, Kanaan SA, Dawes LG, et al. Gangrenous cholecystitis: analysis of risk factors and experience with laparoscopic cholecystectomy. Surgery. 1999; 126(4):680–685, discussion 685–686

[98] Wilson AK, Kozol RA, Salwen WA, Manov LJ, Tennenberg SD. Gangrenous cholecystitis in an urban VA hospital. J Surg Res. 1994; 56(5):402–404

[99] Morfin E, Ponka JL, Brush BE. Gangrenous cholecystitis. Arch Surg. 1968; 96 (4):567–573

[100] Kiviluoto T, Sirén J, Luukkonen P, Kivilaakso E, Hanks J, Jones R. Randomised trial of laparoscopic versus open cholecystectomy for acute and gangrenous cholecystitis. Lancet. 1998; 351(9099):321–325

[101] Landman M, Papanicolaou GC, Sulem C, Sulem PL, Wang XP. Stability of isotropic self-similar dynamics for scalar-wave collapse. Phys Rev A. 1992; 46(12):7869–7876

[102] Reiss R, Nudelman I, Gutman C, Deutsch AA. Changing trends in surgery for acute cholecystitis. World J Surg. 1990; 14(5):567–570, discussion 570–571

[103] Revel L, Lubrano J, Badet N, Manzoni P, Degano SV, Delabrousse E. Preoperative diagnosis of gangrenous acute cholecystitis: usefulness of CEUS. Abdom Imaging. 2014; 39(6):1175–1181

[104] Ahmad MM, Macon WL, IV. Gangrene of the gallbladder. Am Surg. 1983; 49 (3):155–158

[105] Ganpathi IS, Diddapur RK, Eugene H, Karim M. Acute acalculous cholecystitis: challenging the myths. HPB (Oxford). 2007; 9(2):131–134

[106] Yasuda H, Takada T, Kawarada Y, et al. Unusual cases of acute cholecystitis and cholangitis: Tokyo guidelines. J Hepatobiliary Pancreat Surg. 2007; 14 (1):98–113

[107] Acquafresca P, Palermo M, Blanco L, García R, Tarsitano F. [Mirizzi Syndrome: Prevalence, diagnosis and treatment]. Acta Gastroenterol Latinoam. 2014; 44(4):323–328

[108] Lacerda PS, Ruiz MR, Melo A, et al. "Mirizzi syndrome: a surgical challenge." ABCD. Arq Bras Cir Dig (São Paulo). 2014; 27(3):226–227

[109] McSherry CK, Ferstenberg H, Virshup M. "The Mirizzi syndrome: suggested classification and surgical therapy. Surg Gastroenterol. 1982; 1:219–225

[110] Lemmel G. Die kliniscle bedeutung der duodenal divertikel. Arch Venduungskrht. 1934; 46:59–70

[111] Khothsymuong RR, Kaminski J. Gallbladder hydrops. J Diagn Med Sonogr. 2004; 20(4):256–259

[112] Irani S, Baron TH, Grimm IS, Khashab MA. EUS-guided gallbladder drainage with a lumen-apposing metal stent (with video). Gastrointest Endosc. 2015; 82(6):1110–1115

[113] Radu C, MeszarosM, CrisanD, et al. Gallstone ileus four months after cholecystectomy. 2015; 7(1):38:41

[114] Ravikumar R, Williams JG. The operative management of gallstone ileus. Ann R Coll Surg Engl. 2010; 92(4):279–281

[115] Nuño-Guzmán CM, Marín-Contreras ME, Figueroa-Sánchez M, Corona JL. Gallstone ileus, clinical presentation, diagnostic and treatment approach. World J Gastrointest Surg. 2016; 8(1):65–76

[116] Walton J. Acute cholecystitis. Practitioner. 1947; 158(943):11–16

[117] Rodríguez Hermosa JI, Codina Cazador A, Gironès Vilà J, Roig García J, Figa Francesch M, Acero Fernández D. [Gallstone Ileus: results of analysis of a series of 40 patients]. Gastroenterol Hepatol. 2001; 24(10): 489–494

[118] Rodríguez-Sanjuán JC, Casado F, Fernández MJ, Morales DJ, Naranjo A. Cholecystectomy and fistula closure versus enterolithotomy alone in gallstone ileus. Br J Surg. 1997; 84(5):634–637

[119] Shiwani MH, Ullah Q. Laparoscopic enterolithotomy is a valid option to treat gallstone ileus. JSLS. 2010; 14(2):282–285

[120] Cornell CM, Clarke R. "Vicarious calcification involving the gallbladder." 1959; 149(2):267–72

[121] Towfigh S, McFadden DW, Cortina GR, et al. Porcelain gallbladder is not associated with gallbladder carcinoma. Am Surg. 2001; 67(1):7–10

[122] Stephen AE, Berger DL. Carcinoma in the porcelain gallbladder: a relationship revisited. Surgery. 2001; 129(6):699–703

[123] Puia ICVladLIancuC, et al. "[Laparoscopic cholecystectomy for porcelain gallbladder]." Chir. (Bucharest, Rom. 1990). 2005; 100(2):187–189

[124] Kim JHH, Kim WH, Yoo BM, Kim JHH, Kim MW. Should we perform surgical management in all patients with suspected porcelain gallbladder? Hepatogastroenterology. 2009; 56(93):943–945

[125] Khan ZS, Livingston EH, Huerta S. Reassessing the need for prophylactic surgery in patients with porcelain gallbladder: case series and systematic review of the literature. Arch Surg. 2011; 146(10):1143–1147

[126] Kwon AH, Inui H, Imamura A, Uetsuji S, Kamiyama Y. Preoperative assessment for laparoscopic cholecystectomy: feasibility of using spiral computed tomography. Ann Surg. 1998; 227(3):351–356

[127] Machado NO. Porcelain gallbladder: decoding the malignant truth. Sultan Qaboos Univ Med J. 2016; 16(4):e416–e421

[128] Ibiebele I, Schnitzler M, Nippita T, Ford JB. Outcomes of gallstone disease during pregnancy: a population-based data linkage study. Paediatr Perinat Epidemiol. 2017; 31(6):522–530

[129] Sharp HT. The acute abdomen during pregnancy. Clin Obstet Gynecol. 2002; 45(2):405–413

[130] Date RS, Kaushal M, Ramesh A. "A review of the management of gallstone disease and its complications in pregnancy." American Journal of Surgery. 2008; 196(4):599–608.– Elsevier

[131] Othman MO, Stone E, Hashimi M, Parasher G. Conservative management of cholelithiasis and its complications in pregnancy is associated with recurrent symptoms and more emergency department visits. Gastrointest Endosc. 2012; 76(3):564–569

[132] Athwal R, Bhogal RH, Hodson J, Ramcharan S. Surgery for gallstone disease during pregnancy does not increase fetal or maternal mortality: a metaanalysis. Hepatobiliary Surg Nutr. 2016; 5(1):53–57

[133] Barone JE, Bears S, Chen S, Tsai J, Russell JC. Outcome study of cholecystectomy during pregnancy. Am J Surg. 1999; 177(3):232–236

[134] Pearl J, Price R, Richardson W, Fanelli R, Society of American Gastrointestinal Endoscopic Surgeons. Guidelines for diagnosis, treatment, and use of laparoscopy for surgical problems during pregnancy. Surg Endosc. 2011; 25(11): 3479–3492

[135] Swisher SG, Schmit PJ, Hunt KK, et al. Biliary disease during pregnancy. Am J Surg. 1994; 168(6):576–579, discussion 580–581

[136] Lu EJ, Curet MJ, El-Sayed YY, Kirkwood KS. Medical versus surgical management of biliary tract disease in pregnancy. Am J Surg. 2004; 188(6):755–759

[137] Aranha GV, Sontag SJ, Greenlee HB. Cholecystectomy in cirrhotic patients: a formidable operation. Am J Surg. 1982; 143(1):55–60

[138] Nicholas P, Rinaudo PA, Conn HO. Increased incidence of cholelithiasis in Laënnec's cirrhosis. A postmortem evaluation of pathogenesis. Gastroenterology. 1972; 63(1):112–121

[139] Bouchier IA. Postmortem study of the frequency of gallstones in patients with cirrhosis of the liver. Gut. 1969; 10(9):705–710

[140] Davidson JF. Alcohol and cholelithiasis: a necropsy survey of cirrhotics. Am J Med Sci. 1962; 244:703–705

[141] McSherry CK, Glenn F. The incidence and causes of death following surgery for nonmalignant biliary tract disease. Ann Surg. 1980; 191(3):271–275

[142] Bloch RS, Allaben RD, Walt AJ. Cholecystectomy in patients with cirrhosis. A surgical challenge. Arch Surg. 1985; 120(6):669–672

[143] Bornman PC, Terblanche J. Subtotal cholecystectomy: for the difficult gallbladder in portal hypertension and cholecystitis. Surgery. 1985; 98(1):1–6

[144] Castaing D, Houssin D, Lemoine J, Bismuth H. Surgical management of gallstones in cirrhotic patients. Am J Surg. 1983; 146(3):310–313

[145] Garrison RN, Cryer HM, Howard DA, Polk HC, Jr. Clarification of risk factors for abdominal operations in patients with hepatic cirrhosis. Ann Surg. 1984; 199(6):648–655

[146] Kogut K, Aragoni T, Ackerman NB. Cholecystectomy in patients with mild cirrhosis. a more favorable situation. Arch Surg. 1985; 120(11): 1310–1311

[147] Sirinek KR, Burk RR, Brown M, Levine BA. Improving survival in patients with cirrhosis undergoing major abdominal operations. Arch Surg. 1987; 122(3):271–273

[148] Brunicardi FC, Andersen DK, Billiar TR, et al. Schwartz's Principles of Surgery, 10e | AccessMedicine | McGraw-Hill Medical. 1981

[149] Palanivelu C, Rajan PS, Jani K, et al. Laparoscopic cholecystectomy in cirrhotic patients: the role of subtotal cholecystectomy and its variants. J Am Coll Surg. 2006; 203(2):145–151

[150] Moyson J, Thill V, Simoens Ch, Smets D, Debergh N, Mendes da Costa P. Laparoscopic cholecystectomy for acute cholecystitis in the elderly: a retrospective study of 100 patients. Hepatogastroenterology. 2008; 55 (88):1975–1980

[151] do Amaral PCG, Azaro Filho EdeM, Galvão TD, et al. Laparoscopic cholecystectomy for acute cholecystitis in elderly patients. JSLS. 2006; 10(4): 479–483

[152] Dubecz A, Langer M, Stadlhuber RJ, et al. Cholecystectomy in the very elderly: is 90 the new 70? J Gastrointest Surg. 2012; 16(2):282–285

[153] Kirshtein D, Bayme M, Bolotin A, Mizrahi S, Lantsberg L. Laparoscopic cholecystectomy for acute cholecystitis in the elderly: is it safe? Surg Laparosc Endosc Percutan Tech. 2008; 18(4):334–339

[154] Coenye KE, Jourdain S, Mendes da Costa P. Laparoscopic cholecystectomy for acute cholecystitis in the elderly: a retrospective study. Hepatogastroenterology. 2005; 52(61):17–21

[155] Ito K, Fujita N, Noda Y, et al. Percutaneous cholecystostomy versus gallbladder aspiration for acute cholecystitis: a prospective randomized controlled trial. AJR Am J Roentgenol. 2004; 183(1):193–196

[156] Morse BC, Smith JB, Lawdahl RB. "Management of acute cholecystitis in critically ill patients: comtemporanry role for cohocyststomy and subsequent cholecystectomy." Am Surg. 2008; 20:708–712

[157] McGillicuddy EA, Schuster KM, Barre K, et al. Non-operative management of acute cholecystitis in the elderly. Br J Surg. 2012; 99(9):1254–1261

[158] Hassler KR, Jones MW. Gallbladder, Cholecystectomy, Laparoscopic. StatPearls Publishing; 2018

[159] Martin IG, Dexter SP, Marton J, et al. Fundus-first laparoscopic cholecystectomy. Surg Endosc. 1995; 9(2):203–206

[160] Avgerinos C, Kelgiorgi D, Touloumis Z, Baltatzi L, Dervenis C. One thousand laparoscopic cholecystectomies in a single surgical unit using the "critical view of safety" technique. J Gastrointest Surg. 2009; 13(3):498–503

[161] Strasberg SM, Brunt LM. The critical view of safety. Annals of Surgery. 2017; 265(3):464–465

[162] Henneman D.W., Da Costa B.C., Vrouenraets B.A., Van Wagensveld S.M., Lagarde. Laparoscopic partial cholecystectomy for the difficult gallbladder: A systematic review. Surgical Endoscopy and Other Interventional Techniques. 2013; 27(2):351–358. Springer-Verlag

[163] Chen CB, Palazzo F, Doane SM, et al. Increasing resident utilization and recognition of the critical view of safety during laparoscopic cholecystectomy: a pilot study from an academic medical center. Surg Endosc. 2017; 31(4):1627–1635

[164] Kimura Y, et al. [Conversion has to be learned: bile duct injury following conversion to open cholecystectomy]. J Hepatobiliary Pancreat Surg. 2007; 153(1):15–26

[165] McCoy AC, Gasevic E, Szlabick RE, Sahmoun AE, Sticca RP. Are open abdominal procedures a thing of the past? An analysis of graduating general surgery residents' case logs from 2000 to 2011. J Surg Educ. 2013; 70(6):683–689

[166] Booij KAC, de Reuver PR, Nijsse B, Busch ORC, van Gulik TM, Gouma DJ. Insufficient safety measures reported in operation notes of complicated laparoscopic cholecystectomies. Surgery. 2014; 155(3):384–389

[167] Strasberg SM, Pucci MJ, Brunt LM, Deziel DJ. Subtotal cholecystectomy-"fenestrating" vs "reconstituting" subtypes and the prevention of bile duct injury: definition of the optimal procedure in difficult operative conditions. J Am Coll Surg. 2016; 222(1):89–96

[168] Dissanaike S. A step-by-step guide to laparoscopic subtotal fenestrating cholecystectomy: a damage control approach to the difficult gallbladder. J Am Coll Surg. 2016; 223(2):e15–e18

[169] Elshaer M, Gravante G, Thomas K, Sorge R, Al-Hamali S, Ebdewi H. Subtotal cholecystectomy for "difficult gallbladders": systematic review and meta-analysis. JAMA Surg. 2015; 150(2):159–168

[170] Davis B, Castaneda G, Lopez J. Subtotal cholecystectomy versus total cholecystectomy in complicated cholecystitis. Am Surg. 2012; 78(7):814–817

[171] Di Carlo I, Pulvirenti E, Toro A, Corsale G. Modified subtotal cholecystectomy: results of a laparotomy procedure during the laparoscopic era. World J Surg. 2009; 33(3):520–525

[172] Douglas PR, Ham JM. Partial cholecystectomy. Aust N Z J Surg. 1990; 60(8):595–597

[173] Hubert C, Annet L, van Beers BE, Gigot JF. The "inside approach of the gallbladder" is an alternative to the classic Calot's triangle dissection for a safe operation in severe cholecystitis. Surg Endosc. 2010; 24(10):2626–2632

[174] Chowbey PK, Sharma A, Khullar R, Mann V, Baijal M, Vashistha A. Laparoscopic subtotal cholecystectomy: a review of 56 procedures. J Laparoendosc Adv Surg Tech A. 2000; 10(1):31–34

[175] Horiuchi A, Watanabe Y, Doi T, et al. Delayed laparoscopic subtotal cholecystectomy in acute cholecystitis with severe fibrotic adhesions. Surg Endosc. 2008; 22(12):2720–2723

[176] Shin M, Choi N, Yoo Y, Kim Y, Kim S, Mun S. Clinical outcomes of subtotal cholecystectomy performed for difficult cholecystectomy. Ann Surg Treat Res. 2016; 91(5):226–232

[177] Beldi G, Glättli A. Laparoscopic subtotal cholecystectomy for severe cholecystitis. Surg Endosc. 2003; 17(9):1437–1439

[178] Memon MR, Bozdar AG, Mirani SH, Arshad S, Shah SQA. Laparoscopic subtotal cholecystectomy without cystic duct clipping. Med Channel. 2012; 19(2):103–106

[179] Soleimani M, Mehrabi A, Mood ZA, et al. Partial cholecystectomy as a safe and viable option in the emergency treatment of complex acute cholecystitis: a case series and review of the literature. Am Surg. 2007; 73(5):498–507

[180] Cakmak A, Genç V, Orozakunov E, Kepenekçi I, Cetinkaya OA, Hazinedaroğlu MS. Partial cholecystectomy is a safe and efficient method. Chirurgia (Bucur). 2009; 104(6):701–704

[181] Cottier DJ, McKay C, Anderson JR. Subtotal cholecystectomy. Br J Surg. 1991; 78(11):1326–1328

[182] Philips JAE, Lawes DA, Cook AJ, et al. The use of laparoscopic subtotal cholecystectomy for complicated cholelithiasis. Surg Endosc. 2008; 22(7):1697–1700

[183] Bonavina L. Laparoscopic subtotal cholecystectomy. J Am Coll Surg. 2007; 204(2):337

[184] Conrad C, Wakabayashi G, Asbun HJ, et al. IRCAD recommendation on safe laparoscopic cholecystectomy. J Hepatobiliary Pancreat Sci. 2017; 24(11):603–615

[185] Strasberg SM, Gouma DJ. 'Extreme' vasculobiliary injuries: association with fundus-down cholecystectomy in severely inflamed gallbladders. HPB (Oxford). 2012; 14(1):1–8

[186] Harilingam MR, Shrestha AK, Basu S. Laparoscopic modified subtotal cholecystectomy for difficult gall bladders: a single-centre experience. J Minim Access Surg. 2016; 12(4):325–329

[187] Buddingh KT, Weersma RK, Savenije RAJ, van Dam GM, Nieuwenhuijs VB. Lower rate of major bile duct injury and increased intraoperative management of common bile duct stones after implementation of routine intraoperative cholangiography. J Am Coll Surg. 2011; 213(2):267–274

[188] Kern KA. Malpractice litigation involving laparoscopic cholecystectomy. Cost, cause, and consequences. Arch Surg. 1997; 132(4):392–397, discussion 397–398

[189] Flum DR, Flowers C, Veenstra DL. A cost-effectiveness analysis of intraoperative cholangiography in the prevention of bile duct injury during laparoscopic cholecystectomy. J Am Coll Surg. 2003; 196(3):385–393

[190] Z'graggen K, Wehrli H, Metzger A, Buehler M, Frei E, Klaiber C, Swiss Association of Laparoscopic and Thoracoscopic Surgery. Complications of laparoscopic cholecystectomy in Switzerland. A prospective 3-year study of 10,174 patients. Surg Endosc. 1998; 12(11):1303–1310

[191] Fletcher DR, Hobbs MS, Tan P, et al. Complications of cholecystectomy: risks of the laparoscopic approach and protective effects of operative cholangiography: a population-based study. Ann Surg. 1999; 229(4):449–457

[192] Waage A, Nilsson M. Iatrogenic bile duct injury: a population-based study of 152 776 cholecystectomies in the Swedish Inpatient Registry. Arch Surg. 2006; 141(12):1207–1213

[193] Nuzzo G, Giuliante F, Giovannini I, et al. Bile duct injury during laparoscopic cholecystectomy: results of an Italian national survey on 56 591 cholecystectomies. Arch Surg. 2005; 140(10):986–992

[194] Way LW, Stewart L, Gantert W, et al. Causes and prevention of laparoscopic bile duct injuries: analysis of 252 cases from a human factors and cognitive psychology perspective. Ann Surg. 2003; 237(4):460–469

[195] Livingston EH, Flum DR, Dellinger EP, Chan L. Intraoperative cholangiography and risk of common bile duct injury. JAMA. 2003; 290(4):459–460, author reply 459–460

[196] Traverso LW. Intraoperative cholangiography lowers the risk of bile duct injury during cholecystectomy. Surg Endosc. 2006; 20(11):1659–1661

[197] Mohandas S, John AK. Role of intra operative cholangiogram in current day practice. Int J Surg. 2010; 8(8):602–605

[198] Massarweh NN, Devlin A, Elrod JAB, Symons RG, Flum DR. Surgeon knowledge, behavior, and opinions regarding intraoperative cholangiography. J Am Coll Surg. 2008; 207(6):821–830

[199] Machi J, Johnson JO, Deziel DJ, et al. The routine use of laparoscopic ultrasound decreases bile duct injury: a multicenter study. Surg Endosc. 2009; 23(2):384–388

[200] Teitelbaum EN, Soper NJ. Intraoperative Ultrasound During Laparoscopic Cholecystectomy. In: Abdominal Ultrasound for Surgeons, New York, NY: Springer New York; 2014:177–185

[201] Dip FD, Asbun D, Rosales-Velderrain A, et al. Cost analysis and effectiveness comparing the routine use of intraoperative fluorescent cholangiography with fluoroscopic cholangiogram in patients undergoing laparoscopic cholecystectomy. Surg Endosc. 2014; 28(6):1838–1843

[202] Pesce A, Piccolo G, La Greca G, Puleo S. Utility of fluorescent cholangiography during laparoscopic cholecystectomy: a systematic review. World J Gastroenterol. 2015; 21(25):7877–7883

[203] Sakpal SV, Bindra SS, Chamberlain RS. Laparoscopic cholecystectomy conversion rates two decades later. JSLS. 2010; 14(4):476–483

[204] Livingston EH, Rege RV. A nationwide study of conversion from laparoscopic to open cholecystectomy. Am J Surg. 2004; 188(3):205–211

[205] Ghazanfar R, Tariq M, Ghazanfar H, Malik S, Changez M, Khan J. Role of different factors as preoperative predictors of conversion of laparoscopic cholecystectomy to open cholecystectomy. Arch. Med. Heal. Sci. 2017; 5(2):157

[206] Simopoulos C, Botaitis S, Polychronidis A, Tripsianis G, Karayiannakis AJ. "Risk factors for conversion of laparoscopic cholecystectomy to open cholecystectomy". Surg Endosc Other Interv Tech. 2005; 19(7):905–9

[207] Tomida S, Abei M, Yamaguchi T, et al. Long-term ursodeoxycholic acid therapy is associated with reduced risk of biliary pain and acute cholecystitis in patients with gallbladder stones: a cohort analysis. Hepatology. 1999; 30(1):6–13

[208] Tsuchiya Y, Takanashi H, Haniya K, et al. An early gallstone clearance following repeat piezoelectric lithotripsy. J Gastroenterol Hepatol. 1994; 9(6):597–603

[209] May GR, Sutherland LR, Shaffer EA. Efficacy of bile acid therapy for gallstone dissolution: a meta-analysis of randomized trials. Aliment Pharmacol Ther. 1993; 7(2):139–148

[210] Sakakibara N, Hiramatu K, Okamoto H, et al. ESWL for cholecystolithiasis using spark shock waves. J Jpn Biliary Assoc. 1990; 4:168–175

[211] Yamaguchi A, Tazuma S, Nishioka S, et al. The modality of nonsurgical treatments for gallstones: factors affecting gallstone recurrence after extracorporeal shock wave lithotripsy (ESWL) and posttherapeutic symptoms. J Jpn Biliary Assoc. 2004; 13:18–108

[212] Villanova N, Bazzoli F, Taroni F, et al. Gallstone recurrence after successful oral bile acid treatment. A 12-year follow-up study and evaluation of long-term postdissolution treatment. Gastroenterology. 1989; 97(3):726–731

[213] Marks JW, Stein T, Schoenfield LJ. Natural history and treatment with ursodiol of gallstones formed during rapid loss of weight in man. Dig Dis Sci. 1994; 39(9):1981–1984

[214] Tsai S, Strouse PJ, Drongowski RA, Islam S, Teitelbaum DH. Failure of cholecystokinin-octapeptide to prevent TPN-associated gallstone disease. J Pediatr Surg. 2005; 40(1):263–267

[215] Miura F, Takada T, Strasberg SM, et al. Tokyo Guidelines Revision Comittee. TG13 flowchart for the management of acute cholangitis and cholecystitis. J Hepatobiliary Pancreat Sci. 2013; 20(1):47–54

[216] Zha Y, Chen XR, Luo D, Jin Y. The prevention of major bile duct injures in laparoscopic cholecystectomy: the experience with 13,000 patients in a single center. Surg Laparosc Endosc Percutan Tech. 2010; 20(6):378–383

[217] A prospective analysis of 1518 laparoscopic cholecystectomies. The Southern Surgeons Club. N Engl J Med. 1991; 324(16):1073–1078

[218] Strasberg SM, Brunt LM. Rationale and use of the critical view of safety in laparoscopic cholecystectomy. J Am Coll Surg. 2010; 211(1):132–138

[219] Pinkas H, Brady PG. Biliary leaks after laparoscopic cholecystectomy: time to stent or time to drain. Hepatobiliary Pancreat Dis Int. 2008; 7 (6):628–632

[220] Kaushik R. Bleeding complications in laparoscopic cholecystectomy: incidence, mechanisms, prevention and management. J Minim Access Surg. 2010; 6(3):59–65

[221] Wennmacker S, Lamberts M, Gerritsen J, et al. Consistency of patient-reported outcomes after cholecystectomy and their implications on current surgical practice: a prospective multicenter cohort study. Surg Endosc. 2017; 31(1):215–224

[222] Wennmacker SZ, Dijkgraaf MGW, Westert GP, Drenth JPH, van Laarhoven CJHM, de Reuver PR. Persistent abdominal pain after laparoscopic cholecystectomy is associated with increased healthcare consumption and sick leave. Surgery. 2018; 163(4):661–666

[223] Lamberts MP, Den Oudsten BL, Gerritsen JJ, et al. Prospective multicentre cohort study of patient-reported outcomes after cholecystectomy for uncomplicated symptomatic cholecystolithiasis. Br J Surg. 2015; 102(11): 1402–1409

[224] Finan KR, Leeth RR, Whitley BM, Klapow JC, Hawn MT. Improvement in gastrointestinal symptoms and quality of life after cholecystectomy. Am J Surg. 2006; 192(2):196–202

[225] Jaunoo SS, Mohandas S, Almond LM. Postcholecystectomy syndrome (PCS). Int J Surg. 2010; 8(1):15–17

[226] Girometti R, Brondani G, Cereser L, et al. Postcholecystectomy syndrome: spectrum of biliary findings at magnetic resonance cholangiopancreatography. Br J Radiol. 2010; 83(988):351–361

[227] Arima N, Uchiya T, Hishikawa R, et al. [Clinical characteristics of impacted bile duct stone in the elderly]. Nippon Ronen Igakkai Zasshi. 1993; 30(11): 964–968

[228] Arora D, Kaushik R, Kaur R, Sachdev A. Postcholecystectomy syndrome: a new look at an old problem. J Minim Access Surg. 2018; 14(3):202–207

Expert Commentary on Acute Cholecystitis by
Ronald Stewart

Expert Commentary on Acute Cholecystitis

Ronald Stewart

Dr. Davidson and Dr. Bulger masterfully crafteda comprehensive overview of the diagnosis and management of cholecystitis and the spectrum of complications from gallstone disease. This chapter provides an overview with ample references and links for the safe management of the spectrum of gallstone-related pathologic conditions.

The authors describe a wide variety of strategies to address difficult situations in the management of complex gallstone disease. J. Bradley Aust, MD, commonly used an aphorism appropriate for these strategies: "The patient needs a life preserver, not a swimming lesson." I provide personal commentary, expanding on how I believe it is best to safely deal with the situation when there is significant inflammation and/or dense fibrotic tissue in the cystic triangle obscuring clear biliary anatomy.

Dr. Davidson and Dr. Bulger describe a variety of approaches in dealing with this situation: "...subtotal cholecystectomy, laparoscopic top-down ("fundus-first") cholecystectomy, biliary drainage via placement of a laparoscopic cholecystostomy tube, and ultimately, conversion to open procedure." The authors discuss the decision to open or continue laparoscopically and describe a tailored approach based on the surgeon's expertise and comfort. In the setting of extensive fibrosis in the cystic triangle and the inability to identify clear anatomy, without hesitation, I recommend conversion from laparoscopy to open. Although it is true that most surgeons trained in the modern era do not have a large experience with open cholecystectomy, the principles and techniques of damage control partial cholecystectomy are not difficult, and, I believe, can be performed safely by all well-trained general surgeons.

The specific type of subtotal cholecystectomy depends on the anatomy and circumstances, but I believe the original description framed 65 years ago by W.A. McElmoyle, a surgeon from the Royal Jubilee Hospital in Victoria, B.C, Canada, provides a solid foundation for this damage control approach. McElmoyle's operative strategy is elegantly and succinctly described in a letter to the editor from Lemuel Pran and colleagues where they write: "The concept of the Shield of McElmoyle, described in 1954, is one of great importance...In a case in which Calot's triangle cannot be safely dissected, this shield, which comprises the cystic duct, part of the body, neck, and infundibulum, is left in situ and untouched. There should be no attempt to dissect structures lying cephalad and medially." When this technique is used, it should be accompanied by a closed-suction fluted drain in the hepatorenal recess. Although this is an admittedly rare situation (when dissection is very difficult or impossible), this approach is safe and leads to resolution of the problem. This fenestrated partial cholecystectomy is often followed by a temporary bile leak which frequently stops and spontaneously with observation. When the bile leak continues, it is usually easily managed by an endoscopically placed biliary stent. This technique of leaving the back wall is also helpful in the face of cirrhosis and coagulopathy as it avoids the hepatic bed dissection, although in this setting, the cystic duct can usually be ligated.

I commend Dr. Davidson and Dr. Bulger for a terrific overview of the complications related to gallstones.

11 Acute Diverticulitis

Maryanne L. Pickett, Joseph P. Minei, and Michael W. Cripps

Summary

The management spectrum of diverticulitis ranges from outpatient supportive care to emergent surgery, depending on the disease severity and patient clinical status. There is a growing trend for nonoperative management of diverticulitis; however, for those who need emergent surgery, worse outcomes occur in patients who have a delay in care. Improvements in clinical and surgical care have significantly decreased adverse outcomes in patients undergoing surgical management of diverticulitis.

Keywords: Hinchey stages, Mannheim peritonitis index, Hartmann's procedure, primary anastomosis, diverting loop ileostomy (DLI)

11.1 Introduction

Complications of diverticular disease remains a significant clinical problem, as 70 to 80% of Americans are afflicted with diverticulosis and 10 to 25% will develop acute diverticulitis. Furthermore, 1 to 2% will require hospitalization, and surgical intervention will be required in up to 12% of those admitted.[1,2,3] Acute care surgeons often serve as the sole surgeon for these patients and should understand the changing management strategies, including indications for surgery and options for surgical approaches. Options for both laparoscopic and open techniques will be reviewed along with timing of stoma reversal and management of postoperative complications.

11.2 Indications for Operative Intervention

The initial priority for acute care surgeons should be to determine if operative or nonoperative intervention is indicated. The American Society of Colorectal Surgeons (ASCRS) 2014 guidelines recommend preoperative workup to include history and physical, laboratories, urine analysis, abdominal X-ray, and abdomen/pelvis computed tomography (CT).[4] The overall clinical presentation of disease severity ultimately guides the management in diverticulitis. There are, however, multiple grading systems, for example, the classic Hinchey scoring system (▶ Table 11.1) that can guide categorization of disease and delineate complications, morbidity, and mortality for each class.

The diverticular stages as described by Sheth et al is based on clinical presentation. Stage 1 patients are asymptomatic but with an incidental finding of diverticula. Uncomplicated, symptomatic disease is classified as stage 2 or acute diverticulitis. Stage 3 encompasses recurrent diverticulitis with symptoms like irritable bowel syndrome. It is critical to discern between these diagnoses, as the treatment options are significantly different. Complicated diverticulitis with abscess, stricture, or peritonitis is classified as stage 4 disease.[1]

Table 11.1 Hinchey scoring system for diverticulitis with suggested management strategies and surgical indications with incidence[1,2,5,6,7,8,9,10]

Hinchey score	Radiologic abscess characteristics	Management	Surgery indications operation (incidence)
I	Small (<2 cm area of distant free air or <4 cm abscess) pericolic abscess, phlegmon, or localized pericolic inflammation	Antibiotics Percutaneous drainage (if abscess location and size amenable)	Depends on abscess size Urgent operation (required in 2.2% of patients) Elective 1-stage operation (undergone by 60% of patients) Elective 2-stage operation (undergone by 9% of patients)
II	Pelvic, distant intra-abdominal or retroperitoneal abscess	Antibiotics Percutaneous drainage (if abscess location and size amenable)	
IIa	Distant abscess amenable to percutaneous drainage		
IIb	Complex, small (<5 cm) pericolic abscess with fistula		
III	Diffuse purulent peritonitis Usually >2 cm foci of distant air or >4 cm abscess	Surgical Slight delay in surgical intervention for those with severe comorbidities that require monitored resuscitation prior to operation	Failed medical management, development of peritonitis Urgent operation (required in 6% of patients) Elective 1-stage operation (50%) Elective 2-stage operation (9%)
IV	Generalized feculent peritonitis, pneumoperitoneum from free perforation, nonloculated free fluid in peritoneal cavity	Surgical Percutaneous abscess drainage or nonoperative intervention is rarely indicated	Failed medical management, development of peritonitis Urgent operation (required in 33–83% of patients) Hartmann's procedure (54–72%) Elective 1-stage operation (17)

Generally, hemodynamically normal patients afflicted with Stage 1 to 2 disease should undergo nonoperative management (NOM). Stage 1 diverticulitis often does not require medication, admission, or intervention. As disease severity increases to stage 2, inpatient admission may be required for serial abdominal examinations, pain control, or percutaneous drainage procedures as a temporizing measure. Inpatient management should be considered for patients that are hypovolemic, have poor oral intake tolerance, are frail, or have minimal home support. Outpatient NOM is approximately 95% successful in uncomplicated stage 2 diverticulitis.[5,6,7]

Radiologic imaging is often obtained prior to surgical consultation and while not always necessary in surgical decision-making, CT imaging is 91% sensitive and 77% specific for diagnosing diverticulitis.[8] While these images are not completely necessary in surgical decision-making, CT imaging is used to classify the severity of acute diverticulitis in the well-known Hinchey classification grading scale. ▶ Table 11.1 describes imaging characteristics, management, and surgical indications for this classification.

11.3 Nonoperative Management

Historically, admission for NOM was intravenous broad-spectrum antibiotics, bowel rest, and discharge home with oral antibiotics.[5,9] However, this standard of care for **uncomplicated diverticulitis** has been challenged in recent randomized control trials. The classic hypothesis that the pathology of uncomplicated diverticulitis is caused by perforations and bacterial infection is replaced by one that suggests the symptoms of uncomplicated diverticulitis are from an inflammatory response only. This would obviate the need for antibiotics altogether. In 2012, the Antibiotika Vid Okomplicerad Divertikulit (AVOD), translated to antibiotics in uncomplicated diverticulitis trial suggested acute, uncomplicated diverticulitis can be managed without antibiotics in outpatient settings. In this trial, patients were randomized into two groups—one group receiving 7 days of antibiotics and the other group received none. No significant difference was found between the two groups in pain, complication rates, length of stay, treatment failure, or progression to complicated disease. There was also no significant difference in rate of emergency and elective resection at 12 months, readmission rates, recurrence, or quality of life between groups. Unfortunately, this study was limited by low accrual volumes and a large constituent with recurrent disease. Similar findings were shown in 2014, when the DIVER (outpatient versus hospitalization management for uncomplicated diverticulitis) study compared treatment of uncomplicated diverticulitis with antibiotics administered in inpatient versus outpatient settings. No difference in quality of life and improved cost savings were also observed in the outpatient antibiotic group.[4,8,11,12] Similarly, the DIABLO (DIverticulitis: AntiBiotics Or cLose Observation) trial in 2017 compared antibiotics to observation for management of initial episodes of acute, uncomplicated diverticulitis. A small cohort of patients with Hinchey IB disease had similar outcomes to Hinchey IA patients, as no differences in complication rates, recurrence, need for surgery, or readmission were shown. Further, a similar proportion of patients had episodes of recurrent acute diverticulitis and complicated diverticulitis when followed for 24 months.[12] These trials show promising data that suggest uncomplicated

diverticulitis in patients without physiologic derangements may be able to be treated without antibiotics. However, until there is more definitive evidence, the American Society of Colon and Rectal Surgeons (ASCRS) practice parameters still recommend at least outpatient antibiotics for uncomplicated diverticulitis.[13] Antibiotics should cover anaerobes and Gram negatives (IV 3rd generation cephalosporin, carbapenem, or piperacillin-tazobactam; PO fluoroquinolone and metronidazole) until symptoms resolve.

11.4 Emergent Operation

The range of indications for emergent surgical treatment of diverticulitis is narrow. Patients with diffuse peritonitis and those who have a worsening clinical picture, despite optimal resuscitation and medical therapy, need immediate operative intervention. When presented with a complex patient afflicted with peritonitis, a scoring system for emergency surgery estimating the morbidity and mortality can be used. The Mannheim peritonitis index (MPI) is one such risk calculator that determines a score based on age, gender, organ failure, malignancy, duration peritonitis, noncolonic source of sepsis, diffuse peritonitis, exudate quality, and guide goals of care discussions with patients and families[14,15] (▶ Table 11.2).

Those who fail NOM also require surgical intervention, but the decision on timing is not as straightforward and the acute care surgeon must determine if surgery should be emergent or nonemergent. In an analysis of the American College of Surgeons National Surgical Quality Improvement Program (ACS-NSQIP) database from 2005 to 2012, Mozer et al found that 57.2% of 2119 patients with preoperative sepsis, who underwent emergent surgical intervention for acute diverticulitis, had surgery within 24 hours of presentation. Further, most patients underwent surgery earlier rather than later, with 26.3% having surgery within 1 to 3 days, 12.9% between 3 to 7 days, while 3.6% underwent emergent operative intervention after 7 days from admission.[16] Worse outcomes are seen in patients who have a delay in emergent surgery, especially in patients who are older, have more comorbidities and higher American Society of Anesthesiologists (ASA) grades, and underwent Hartmann's procedure (HP). However, in patients with ASA level greater than three (who have an inherently higher predicted mortality), aggressive resuscitative efforts should be taken to mitigate operative risks. Being conscientious of a patient's systemic morbidities may mean a delay in operative intervention while their physiologic derangements are addressed. If this option is considered, admission to the surgical intensive care unit (ICU) with close monitoring of resuscitative conduct is required.[16]

11.5 Nonemergent Surgery

Nonemergent operative intervention should be considered for hemodynamically normal patients with mild disease who fail to resolve, pelvic abscesses that are not amenable to interventional drainage, and complications such as fistulizing disease, strictures, or recurrent diverticular bleeding.[2] Repeat imaging should be considered if patient remains inpatient on hospital day five, or sooner if no clinical improvement is seen as operative intervention may be needed. Elective outpatient surgery may be planned for those who show clinical improvement, and repeat imaging shows that free air has resolved and there exists no residual

Table 11.2 Mannheim peritonitis index

Characteristic	Point value
Age > 50 years	5
Female sex	5
Malignancy	4
Organ failure	7
• Creatinine > 177 μmol/L; Urea > 167 mmol/L; Oliguria (urine output < 30 mL/hours)	
• PO_2 < 50 mmHg; PCO_2 > 50 mmHg	
• Shock	
• Intestinal obstruction > 24 hours; complete mechanical ileus	
Organ of sepsis not colonic	6
Preoperative duration of peritonitis > 24 hours	4
Diffuse, generalized peritonitis	6
Intraperitoneal exudates	
• Clear	0
• Cloudy, purulent	6
• Feculent	12

	Total score	
Morbidity	Mortality	MPI score
0%	0%	< 14
15.9%	2.2%	14–21
50%	27.2%	22–29
36.3%	50%	> 29

Adapted from Pattanaik et al.[15]

abscess. These patients should be discharged on oral antibiotics and have scheduled follow-up.[5,7]

The debate regarding use of oral antibiotic bowel prep with (OBP) and/or mechanical bowel prep (MBP) is ongoing, and currently left to the surgeon's discretion and preoperative time allowance. However, based on Level II evidence, the American Society of Colon and Rectal Surgeons Enhanced Recovery Pathway guidelines in 2017 recommend MBP and OBP before colorectal surgery to reduce surgical site infections.[17]

Decisions on bowel continuity need to be tailored to each patient, but generally, bowel is resected in Hinchey III/IV disease.[13] Resection of diseased segments can be accomplished with laparoscopic or open surgical techniques, and should include all sigmoid colon plus a healthy margin, as it is no longer mandated to resect all diverticular disease. In all cases of anastomosis, leak tests should be performed prior to case completion. In elective resections, ASCRS recommends that every effort be made to spare superior hemorrhoidal artery in order to enhance blood flow to the rectal stump.[4,13]

Patients with recurring flares of diverticulitis may eventually need an operation. About 10% of patients with chronic diverticulitis presenting with obstruction will need elective resection of the culpable sigmoid stricture. Historically, the decision for surgery in diverticular disease were based on age (younger patients were thought to have increased risk of recurrence based on total lifetime risk of flares) and the total number of flares (with 2–4 flares being an indication for resection). However, the ASCRS practice parameters for diverticulitis state the decision to perform elective surgery after recovery from a bout of acute diverticulitis should be individualized to the patient. The routine recommendation of elective colectomy after recovery from a bout of uncomplicated diverticulitis to prevent the possibility of needing emergency surgery with ostomy formation in the future should be discouraged. Janes and colleagues calculated the risk of subsequently needing emergency surgery with stoma formation after an episode of diverticulitis at 1 in 2000 patientyears follow-up.[18] Another study found that only 5.5% of all patients who had successful nonoperatively managed diverticulitis went on to need an emergency HP in the future.[19] A full discussion with the patient regarding their overall medical status and how potential future flares may affect the patient both personally and professionally should be weighed against the risks of surgery.[13] Those patients in whom carcinoma cannot be completely excluded should be considered for early resection as should patients with immunosuppression, chronic steroids, chronic renal failure, and collagen vascular disease, due to a high risk of perforation in subsequent acute attacks, high-rate of complicated disease, and high mortality associated with emergent surgery.[3]

Colonoscopy should be performed 6 to 8 weeks after resolution of the acute episode. These routine colonoscopies were initially performed to rule out malignancy. Improvements in CT imaging aid in this specific regard and have questioned whether colonoscopies are antiquated in uncomplicated diverticulitis. Colonoscopies still have a role in management of diverticular disease, especially after complicated episodes, uncertain diagnoses, or if the patient experiences rectal bleeding or change in bowel habits, as they can rule out colonic strictures, inflamed or ischemic bowel, and incidental right- sided lesions.[4]

11.6 Role of Minimally Invasive Surgery

Although open colon resection was regarded as the standard of care, minimally invasive surgery (MIS) is becoming more prevalent in treating acute and chronic diverticulitis. The laparoscopic technique is now preferred for uncomplicated, elective colonic resection due to improved postoperative pain along with faster return to liquid diet and bowel function. This approach allows for a decrease in morbidity, blood loss, anesthesia, length of stay, surgical site infection rate, and rate of ventral hernias.[3]

There are several minimally invasive techniques that can be employed including traditional laparoscopy, laparoscopic-assisted, and robotic-assisted techniques. Each of these techniques can then be combined with the standard open technique of primary anastomosis (PA), PA with fecal diversion via diverting loop ileostomy (DLI), or HP if necessary. During laparoscopic surgery, adjuncts such as preoperatively placed ureteral stents and intraoperative placement of a hand port to convert into a hybrid, open surgical technique may be helpful in prevention of conversion to a full open operation. Use of hand-assisted laparoscopic surgery may be particularly helpful in the disruption of phlegmon or scar tissue that can significantly lengthen procedure time. There are those who argue that MIS should not be used because of increased surgery duration. While this increased duration is a known factor of laparoscopic surgery, it does not result in increased rates of disease recurrence or complications.[3]

Conversion from laparoscopic to open approach occurs in 4.8 to 13% of uncomplicated and 12 to 18.2% of complicated diverticulitis surgeries. Risk factors for conversion include inflammation, failure to identify ureters, chronic abscess cavity, enterotomy, patient body mass index (BMI), adhesions, stricture, and fistula.[4,20]

Despite these conversion rates, the benefits of MIS have been shown in many trials. The findings of these trials similarly show no difference in mortality between open and laparoscopic surgeries, but a clear decrease in morbidity in the MIS groups. Most notably, the SIGMA trial compared laparoscopic (LSR) to open sigmoid resection and found LSR was associated with 15.4% rate reduction in major complications, less pain, and shorter hospital stay.[21] These differences were prominent during the first 6 weeks postoperatively but decreased at 6 months. In addition, the authors noted that despite the expense of longer operating times, there was no significant difference in total healthcare costs when combining operative and hospital costs. In a systematic review and meta-analysis, Siddiqui et al also found that there was no difference in mortality but significantly lower morbidity in LSR groups and decreased incidence of postoperative complications including ileus, anastomotic leaks, wound infection, and bowel obstruction.[22] Some have proposed that the lower morbidity in LSR approach is explained by a younger patient group with lower ASA scores and less cardiopulmonary comorbidities; however, these differences remain when matching for age and ASA score.[2,3,23] Further, it has been noted by Levack and colleagues that despite fewer intra-abdominal leaks with LSR surgery (2.4% compared to 8.2% in open group), there were similar reexploration rates.[24]

Minimally invasive benefits are not limited to elective cases, as the use of laparoscopy is becoming more prevalent in the emergent settings, and it has been shown to decrease wound dehiscence, incisional hernias, and wound infections.[25] Initially, the European Association for Endoscopic Surgery (EAES) guidelines did not recommend LSR surgery for emergent, acute diverticulitis, and ASCRS guidelines only recommended LSR

techniques in an elective setting and in selected patients with complicated disease.[4] This however changed, and after the SIGMA trial was published, an updated EAES guideline followed in 2012 where laparoscopic lavage (LL) and drainage was recommended in Hinchey I/IIa, which failed NOM, Hinchey IIb/III, or perforated diverticulitis.[26,27] At that time, the ASCRS guidelines also recommended using LL with or without drainage to convert purulent peritonitis to localized diverticulitis that could be treated with antibiotics. These recommendations were based on early reports that suggested colonic resection and ostomy may be avoided because of 96% success rate and 10% morbidity with LL.[3,8]

However, use of LL became controversial after subsequent case series showed higher failure rates (34%) and significantly higher morbidity (56%). The Ladies (Laparoscopic peritoneal lavage or resection for generalized peritonitis for perforated diverticulitis) study was designed after these original LL results were irreproducible. Patients were randomized after diagnostic laparoscopy into two arms, LOLA (Laparoscopic lavage and drainage) and DIVA (perforated diverticulitis: sigmoid resection with or without anastomosis), and followed for 12 months. The LOLA arm evaluated patients with purulent peritonitis who were treated with LL and drainage, HP, or sigmoidectomy with primary anastomosis (PA). The DIVA arm evaluated patients with feculent peritonitis who were treated with HP or resection with PA. However, the LOLA arm was stopped early because of increased event rates of in-hospital major morbidity and mortality (35% lavage vs. 18% sigmoidectomy) and reintervention (18 vs. 2 cases) in lavage group. Another critical factor found was that LL fails to account for underlying colorectal cancer, thereby contributing to the increased mortality.[8,27]

After the Ladies trial, Schultz et al performed a randomized controlled trial of 199 patients from 21 hospitals across Norway and Sweden that compared treatment of acute perforated diverticulitis with LL versus sigmoid resection. One-year outcomes confirmed the short-term results of Ladies trial, with a higher risk of early reoperation and abscess drainage after LL compared to primary resection. However, no significant difference in severe complications nor disease-related mortality was noted. One-year quality of life measurements failed to show significant difference in pain, sexual, or social function.[28] The combination of the results in these large trials has significantly called into question the practical utility of LL in patients with acute, complicated diverticulitis.

11.7 Contraindications to MIS

Hemodynamic instability and inability of a patient to tolerate pneumoperitoneum remain absolute contraindications for minimally invasive techniques. Due to difficulty of laparoscopic colorectal surgery for diverticular disease processes, the appropriateness of this technique will depend on surgeon experience and comfort level.[29] Previous contraindications to MIS of peritonitis and small bowel dilation over 4 cm are considered antiquated. Caution should be exercised when performing a LSR resection after three or more episodes of acute diverticulitis, as there may be significant inflammatory scar. Severe diverticulitis may result in a buttressing effect around the affected colon, offering some degree of protection from subsequent attacks, but the inflammation and adhesions extending beyond the sigmoid colon increase technical difficulty, risk of conversion, and postoperative complications. The risk of conversion from LSR to open resection depends on surgeon experience, patient BMI, abdominal surgical history, presence of fistula, and degree of inflammation/adhesions beyond sigmoid colon. As previously discussed, use of LL has not shown reproducible improved results and should be discouraged until further data can better define its indications.[3]

11.8 Open Management Strategies

The traditional approach to emergent operation for complicated diverticulitis was the laparotomy with HP. Now there are multiple surgical techniques that can be employed, and this is typically left up to the surgeon's discretion and patient hemodynamic stability. Interestingly, data has shown that experience and availability of surgical subspecialties will also impact operative procedures. For instance, it appears that colorectal surgeons are more likely to perform PA after emergency resection (68.4%) compared to general surgeons (41.6%).[1] This likely stems from long-held beliefs that anastomoses in emergent surgical settings have untoward effects. Contrary to these beliefs, several studies comparing resection and PA to HP show significantly lower 30-day mortality in PA patients. Overall morbidity rates were comparable, but HP had a higher risk of intra-abdominal sepsis, significantly higher rate of postop complications, and increased hospital and ICU stay. Before shunning HP for PA, be mindful that there may be some intrinsic bias in these data, as more unstable patients are likely to receive an HP, as shown by a 33% mortality rate, compared to 1.2% in PA.[1,14,30]

11.8.1 Hartmann's Procedure

Historically, open colon resection with HP was regarded as the "gold standard" for the management of colonic diverticulitis. HP was used in severe disease, patients with multiple comorbidities, high CRP, and MPI > 10 due to concern for high-risk failure of NOM. Rectosigmoid resection with formation of end colostomy was thought to avoid intra-abdominal sepsis secondary to anastomotic dehiscence by providing fecal diversion.[3,31] Now, HP is more likely to occur in urgent or emergent settings and in patients with BMI > 30 or with higher Hinchey score disease.[4]

When performing an HP, the inferior mesenteric artery (IMA) should be preserved and colostomy created with a small length of normal sigmoid. Lateral to medial dissection allows reflection of the perforated colon segment but a medial to lateral approach facilitates separation of colonic mesentery from retroperitoneum if significant fibrosis is encountered.

11.8.2 Primary Anastomosis (PA), With or Without, Diverting Loop Ileostomy (DLI)

Historical resistance to PA was due to concern for anastomotic dehiscence, subsequent pelvic sepsis, and death. However, in animal models, colonic fecal load was the only factor impacting anastomotic dehiscence. Current evidence supports resection and PA as a safe treatment for acute perforated diverticulitis, even if peritonitis is present.[4] When performing PA, mobilization of the splenic flexure can facilitate a tension-free anastomosis, and transection of the distal rectosigmoid junction should ensure no residual sigmoid colon remains. Further, the rectum should not be significantly inflamed, as this can lead to an increased risk of anastomotic leak.

There are no hardline indications for when to perform fecal diversion after PA. The purpose of DLI is to mitigate the serious complications of anastomotic dehiscence and possibly prevent pelvic sepsis. Therefore, DLI should be given great consideration in those patients who are at greatest risk of leak such as diabetics, obese patients, or those who are on concurrent immunosuppression.[4] Although current evidence supports PA in acute diverticulitis, in emergent colectomies, concomitant fecal diversion with ileostomy is often performed.[31]

A systematic review noted PA with DLI had a mortality of 15%, morbidity of 50%, but no reported anastomotic dehiscence. PA with stoma, with or without lavage, has more favorable outcomes with significantly lower morbidity and mortality than HP and avoids the need for additional Hartmann's reversal surgery.[30,32] In performing DLI, an ileal segment of 30 to 40 cm should be selected that can be exteriorized without tension and held in place with a rubber catheter to prevent twisting until DLI is matured.

11.9 Damage Control

The use of damage control (DC) surgery is a life-saving bailout procedure that can obtain source control, potentially remove the diseased segment, and should be reserved for those patients in severe shock from any source (septic, cardiac, or hemorrhagic). Surgery is performed in a staged approach. The first stage entails a limited resection of diseased segment and placement of negative pressure/wound vacuum therapy until the patient is resuscitated and can return to operating room. Stage two requires a decision of PA versus HP depending on intraoperative findings and patient stability. This stage may require several trips to the operating room, as up to 55% patients will have ongoing peritonitis with visible fibrinous, purulent, or fecal peritoneal fluid in the first take back. When compared to patients without ongoing peritonitis, these patients had a higher rate of organ failure, significantly higher Mannheim peritonitis index (MPI) score, increased operative times (105 vs. 84 min), and were less likely to have an anastomosis created. Attention should be given to those patients with ongoing peritonitis, as it is associated with 35% overall postoperative morbidity and 7% mortality.[1,14] The process of washing out the abdomen and replacing the wound vacuum therapy should continue until the patient can have definitive HP or PA. Caution should be noted that after a few days, the abdominal wall musculature and fascia will retract laterally, potentially leading to a ventral hernia that may require skin grafting and delayed repair. Prolonged periods with an open abdomen markedly increase the risk for entero-atmospheric fistulas and their associated complications. As such, in the postop phase of DC, every effort should be made to perform a definitive procedure and close the abdominal fascia as soon as possible.

11.9.1 Timing of Stoma Reversal

The ideal timing of stoma reversal remains controversial. The general consideration is to delay stoma reversal until the risk from intra-abdominal adhesions is minimal. Unfortunately, there are no high-quality data for when to reverse the ostomy; furthermore, several papers are contradictory to each other. Some have shown decreased colostomy reversal complications when done within 4 months, while others found increased risk of postoperative complications, including anastomotic leak and death, when closure was performed within 6 to 9 months.[33] Ultimately, the decision of stoma reversal timing will be individualized based on patient health and recovery to baseline, comorbidities, and quality of life.

Reversal is advocated due to stoma complications of retraction, obstruction, hernia, ischemia, and high output. However, operative risk of surgical site infections, enterotomy, site hernias, need for reoperation, and anastomotic leaks must be considered.[33] Perioperative planning should include consideration of precipitating incident (peritonitis, bowel ischemia, or infection) that may result in difficult adhesions and distorted surgical anatomy. Oncologic status must be considered before assessing for stoma closure. While not mandatory before an ostomy reversal, preoperative evaluation of the distal rectal stump with endoscopy or contrast studies can be done to evaluate for leak, stricture, inflammation, and masses.[34]

Minimally invasive techniques can also be used during ostomy reversals. Reduced overall 30-day morbidity, wound infection, and postoperative ileus have been found when LSR reversal was compared to open technique. When compared to LSR reversal, open reversal is associated with higher complication rates (31% open vs. 14% laparoscopic), significantly longer hospital stays (10.8 vs. 6.7 days), and longer operative times (187.5 vs. 164 min). From 2005 to 2014, LSR colostomy reversal has 2.9% increased annual incidence, as many have recommended the LSR approach.[33,35] Interestingly, there is some disparity, as LSR reversals are not universally utilized. Some studies have shown that LSR colostomy reversals are more likely to occur in Caucasian patients with lower BMIs who are not currently smoking and have fewer comorbidities. Despite the improved outcomes and increasing use, LSR reversal is considered one of the most demanding procedures in colorectal surgery, attributing to a less than 20% rate of LSR reversals and a rate of conversion to open technique in up to half of patients.[4,36]

Patient anatomy and surgeon capabilities will determine appropriate surgical technique for stoma reversal. Prior splenic flexure mobilization, retained sigmoid colon, anastomosis type, and anatomical configuration should be considered. Multiple studies have failed to prove a significant benefit of hand-sewn or stapled anastomosis. Similarly, no significant difference in postoperative complications has been reported when considering anatomical configuration of anastomosis.[33] The ostomy should be sutured closed, taken down, adhesions lysed, and the rectal stump identified. End-to-end anastomosis is done with transanal circular stapler or hand-sewn anastomosis. Ostomy site skin closure with a purse-string technique decreases wound infections and increases patient satisfaction.[37]

When deciding between a PA with DLI versus an HP, the acute care surgeon should also consider that the morbidity rates after stoma reversal are significantly decreased in patients undergoing ileostomy versus colostomy reversal (13.75 vs. 25.6–33%).[32] One study found patients with DLI (13% were created for diverticulitis and 55% for malignancy) were reversed after a median of 5.6 months, significantly sooner in diverticulitis than for malignancy, and had 80% reversal rate. Presence of an end ileostomy and intra-abdominal abscess independently delayed reversal. Not all stomas are reversed; permanent stomas occur for several reasons. Patient age, high-risk status, and patient refusal all contribute to a 30 to 90% nonreversal rate.[30,38] Other independent risk factors for nonreversal were age over 70 years, end ileostomy, high BMI, and preoperative radiation.[39]

11.9.2 Management of Postoperative Complications

In a systematic review and meta-analysis, overall postoperative complication rate for diverticulitis was 32.6% and was divided into surgical and medical categories. Medical complications included pneumonia (3.7% of patients), urinary tract infection (3.1%), myocardial infarction (1.4%), and pulmonary embolism (0.8%). Surgical complications included incisional hernia (15.1–17% of patients), prolonged ileus (12.8–32.6%), wound infection (6.8%), anastomotic leak (4%), intra-abdominal abscess (3.6%), wound dehiscence (2.2%), and bleeding (2.1%).[2,10,40,41,42] Minor and major postoperative morbidities occurred in 23.3% and 26.9%, respectively, of patients who underwent surgical intervention within 24 hours. There was a significant increase in these complications if there was delay in operative intervention.[16] Exact postoperative mortality and morbidity rates vary according to surgery technique and Hinchey class. See ▶ Table 11.3 for summary of postoperative morbidity and mortality rates.[1,3,4,5,10,27,30,32]

Medical complications should be managed by the surgeon's preferred standard of care. Pneumonia and urinary tract infections should be treated based on presumed etiology and antibiotics compliant with the hospital's antimicrobial stewardship antibiogram. A patient suspected of having a myocardial infarct should have electrocardiogram and troponins checked, followed by prompt cardiology consultation as indicated. Pulmonary embolism (PE) should be treated with resuscitation, oxygenation, pulmonary CT angiography (if stable), and anticoagulation. If a PE causing hemodynamic instability occurs in the early postoperative period, serious consideration should be given to thrombolytic therapy, keeping in mind there may be an associated bleeding risk.

Early surgical complications of anastomotic leak and bleeding should be managed with a return to the operating room. Intra-abdominal abscesses and remote, contained anastomotic leaks can be managed with percutaneous drainage. NOM is usually appropriate for prolonged ileus, wound infection, and wound dehiscence; incisional hernias are best managed with elective repair.

Diverticulitis is not considered a progressive disease and the initial attack is usually the most severe. After the first attack, recurrent diverticulitis occurs in 25 to 33%. Complicated recurrence affects 4 to 10% and 30% will go on to have a third episode.[8,10] The recurrence rate is 6% after NOM, 6.7% in patients with colorectal anastomosis, and in 12% of patients with colocolostomy.[3,4] Complicated recurrent disease usually

Table 11.3 Diverticulitis postoperative morbidity, mortality, and complications[1,3,4,5,11,27,30,32,38,43,44,45,46,47,48,49]

Hinchey score	Morbidity	Mortality	Complications (rate)
Hinchey I–II	4.5–33%	1.9–13.4%	Postoperative leak (2.3%)
Hinchey III–IV	30–43%	3.5–35.3%	Postoperative leak (1.4%) Failure of IR drainage (15–30%) Abscess recurrence (40–50%)
Surgical intervention			
Emergent resection			
–Open approach	40–80%	2.6–35%	Postoperative leak (8.1%)
–Laparoscopic approach	43.6%	0.7–4.1%	Conversion to open (3–8.4%) Postoperative leak (3.3–4.3%) Surgical reintervention (5.1%) Percutaneous reintervention (7.7%) Wound infection (3%)
Elective resection			
–Open approach	15–80%	0.5–4.7%	Postoperative leak (3.2–8.2%)
–Laparoscopic approach	11.2–16.8%	0.1–1.1%	Postoperative leak (2–2.3%)
Laparoscopic Hartmann's procedure	21%	3%	Conversion to open (5.1–29.4%)
Open resection with primary anastomosis	29–41.1%	2–19%	Stoma failure (13.6%) Postoperative leak (3.3–4%)
Open Hartmann's procedure	33.4–48.8%	10–22.6%	Stump leak (3–15%) Stoma failure (31.8%) Reversal failure (30–90%)
Hartmann's reversal	25.6–33%	3.6–10%	Postoperative leak (3.6–8%)

presents with peritoneal contamination, large abscess, inflammatory rind, mesenteric stiffness, and friable tissue with distorted planes, small bowel distention, foreshortened mesentery, or bleeding.[4]

Hospital admission is required in 11.5% of recurrent acute diverticulitis and 3.2% will require multiple admissions. Among readmissions, 17% are readmitted within 30 days. In those readmitted, two-year mortality is 22% for elective surgery and 42% for emergency surgery. Most readmissions for recurrent diverticulitis occur in females younger than 30 years. Increased risk of recurrence is noted if patients were female, smokers, older, obese, had comorbid score > 20, and afflicted with dyslipidemia or complicated diverticular disease. Among patients with recurrent diverticulitis, requiring admission, the most common cause of death is cardiovascular disease and male gender.[50]

In summary, management of diverticulitis for the acute care surgeon should focus on individual case evaluation to determine if a patient needs immediate or delayed intervention. Benign examinations in a hemodynamic normal patient may warrant NOM or even omission of imaging, admission, or antibiotic therapy. While there may be a trend toward NOM for diverticulitis, procedural and surgical advancements are reflected in decreased adverse outcomes in these patients. When emergent surgical intervention is indicated, sound surgical skills with a solid understanding of surgical options and prudent decision-making allows for optimal disease treatment while mitigating potential morbidities.

References

[1] Floch MH, Longo WE. United States guidelines for diverticulitis treatment. J Clin Gastroenterol. 2016; 50 Suppl 1:S53–S56

[2] Masoomi H, Buchberg BS, Magno C, Mills SD, Stamos MJ. Trends in diverticulitis management in the United States from 2002 to 2007. Arch Surg. 2011; 146(4):400–406

[3] Gralista P, Moris D, Vailas M, et al. Laparoscopic approach in colonic diverticulitis: dispelling myths and misperceptions. Surg Laparosc Endosc Percutan Tech. 2017; 27(2):73–82

[4] Mahmoud NN, Riddle EW. Minimally invasive surgery for complicated diverticulitis. J Gastrointest Surg. 2017; 21(4):731–738

[5] Dharmarajan S, Hunt SR, Birnbaum EH, Fleshman JW, Mutch MG. The efficacy of nonoperative management of acute complicated diverticulitis. Dis Colon Rectum. 2011; 54(6):663–671

[6] Hong MK, Tomlin AM, Hayes IP, Skandarajah AR. Operative intervention rates for acute diverticulitis: a multicentre state-wide study. ANZ J Surg. 2015; 85 (10):734–738

[7] Fung AK, Ahmeidat H, McAteer D, Aly EH. Validation of a grading system for complicated diverticulitis in the prediction of need for operative or percutaneous intervention. Ann R Coll Surg Engl. 2015; 97(3):208–214

[8] McDermott FD, Collins D, Heeney A, Winter DC. Minimally invasive and surgical management strategies tailored to the severity of acute diverticulitis. Br J Surg. 2014; 101(1):e90–e99

[9] Siewert B, Tye G, Kruskal J, et al. Impact of CT-guided drainage in the treatment of diverticular abscesses: size matters. AJR Am J Roentgenol. 2006; 186 (3):680–686

[10] Haas JM, Singh M, Vakil N. Mortality and complications following surgery for diverticulitis: systematic review and meta-analysis. United European Gastroenterol J. 2016; 4(5):706–713

[11] Sirany AE, Gaertner WB, Madoff RD, Kwaan MR. Diverticulitis diagnosed in the emergency room: is it safe to discharge home? J Am Coll Surg. 2017; 225 (1):21–25

[12] van Dijk ST, Daniels L, Ünlü Ç, et al. Dutch Diverticular Disease (3D) Collaborative Study Group. Long-term effects of omitting antibiotics in uncomplicated acute diverticulitis. Am J Gastroenterol. 2018; 113(7):1045–1052

[13] Feingold D, Steele SR, Lee S, et al. Practice parameters for the treatment of sigmoid diverticulitis. Dis Colon Rectum. 2014; 57(3):284–294

[14] Sohn MA, Agha A, Steiner P, et al. Damage control surgery in perforated diverticulitis: ongoing peritonitis at second surgery predicts a worse outcome. Int J Colorectal Dis. 2018; 33(7):871–878

[15] Pattanaik SK, John A, Kumar VA. Comparison of Mannheim peritonitis index and revised multiple organ failure score in predicting mortality and

morbidity of patients with secondary peritonitis. International Surgery Journal. 2017; 4(10):3499–3503

[16] Mozer AB, Spaniolas K, Sippey ME, Celio A, Manwaring ML, Kasten KR. Postoperative morbidity, but not mortality, is worsened by operative delay in septic diverticulitis. Int J Colorectal Dis. 2017; 32(2):193–199

[17] Carmichael JC, Keller DS, Baldini G, et al. Clinical practice guidelines for enhanced recovery after colon and rectal surgery from the American Society of Colon and Rectal Surgeons and Society of American Gastrointestinal and Endoscopic Surgeons. Dis Colon Rectum. 2017; 60(8):761–784

[18] Janes S, Meagher A, Frizelle FA. Elective surgery after acute diverticulitis. Br J Surg. 2005; 92(2):133–142

[19] Anaya DA, Flum DR. Risk of emergency colectomy and colostomy in patients with diverticular disease. Arch Surg. 2005; 140(7):681–685

[20] Köckerling F, Schneider C, Reymond MA, et al. Laparoscopic Colorectal Surgery Study Group. Laparoscopic resection of sigmoid diverticulitis. Results of a multicenter study. Surg Endosc. 1999; 13(6):567–571

[21] Klarenbeek BR, de Korte N, van der Peet DL, Cuesta MA. Review of current classifications for diverticular disease and a translation into clinical practice. Int J Colorectal Dis. 2012; 27(2):207–214

[22] Siddiqui MR, Sajid MS, Khatri K, Cheek E, Baig MK. Elective open versus laparoscopic sigmoid colectomy for diverticular disease: a meta-analysis with the Sigma trial. World J Surg. 2010; 34(12):2883–2901

[23] Klarenbeek BR, Bergamaschi R, Veenhof AA, et al. Laparoscopic versus open sigmoid resection for diverticular disease: follow-up assessment of the randomized control Sigma trial. Surg Endosc. 2011; 25(4):1121–1126

[24] Levack M, Berger D, Sylla P, Rattner D, Bordeianou L. Laparoscopy decreases anastomotic leak rate in sigmoid colectomy for diverticulitis. Arch Surg. 2011; 146(2):207–210

[25] Vennix S, Boersema GS, Buskens CJ, et al. Emergency laparoscopic sigmoidectomy for perforated diverticulitis with generalised peritonitis: a systematic review. Dig Surg. 2016; 33(1):1–7

[26] Sher ME, Agachan F, Bortul M, Nogueras JJ, Weiss EG, Wexner SD. Laparoscopic surgery for diverticulitis. Surg Endosc. 1997; 11(3):264–267

[27] Vennix S, Musters GD, Mulder IM, et al. Ladies trial collaborators. Laparoscopic peritoneal lavage or sigmoidectomy for perforated diverticulitis with purulent peritonitis: a multicentre, parallel-group, randomised, open-label trial. Lancet. 2015; 386(10000):1269–1277

[28] Schultz JK, Wallon C, Blecic L, et al. SCANDIV Study Group. One-year results of the SCANDIV randomized clinical trial of laparoscopic lavage versus primary resection for acute perforated diverticulitis. Br J Surg. 2017; 104(10):1382–1392

[29] Naguib N, Masoud AG. Laparoscopic colorectal surgery for diverticular disease is not suitable for the early part of the learning curve. A retrospective cohort study. Int J Surg. 2013; 11(10):1092–1096

[30] Abbas S. Resection and primary anastomosis in acute complicated diverticulitis, a systematic review of the literature. Int J Colorectal Dis. 2007; 22(4):351–357

[31] Cauley CE, Patel R, Bordeianou L. Use of primary anastomosis with diverting ileostomy in patients with acute diverticulitis requiring urgent operative intervention. Dis Colon Rectum. 2018; 61(5):586–592

[32] Gachabayov M, Oberkofler CE, Tuech JJ, Hahnloser D, Bergamaschi R. Resection with primary anastomosis vs nonrestorative resection for perforated diverticulitis with peritonitis: a systematic review and meta-analysis. Colorectal Dis. 2018; 20(9):753–770

[33] Horesh N, Rudnicki Y, Dreznik Y, et al. Reversal of Hartmann's procedure: still a complicated operation. Tech Coloproctol. 2018; 22(2):81–87

[34] Ballian N, Zarebczan B, Munoz A, et al. Routine evaluation of the distal colon remnant before Hartmann's reversal is not necessary in asymptomatic patients. J Gastrointest Surg. 2009; 13(12):2260–2267

[35] Pei KY, Davis KA, Zhang Y. Assessing trends in laparoscopic colostomy reversal and evaluating outcomes when compared to open procedures. Surg Endosc. 2018; 32(2):695–701

[36] Celentano V, Giglio MC, Bucci L. Laparoscopic versus open Hartmann's reversal: a systematic review and meta-analysis. Int J Colorectal Dis. 2015; 30(12):1603–1615

[37] Hendren S, Hammond K, Glasgow SC, et al. Clinical practice guidelines for ostomy surgery. Dis Colon Rectum. 2015; 58(4):375–387

[38] Fleming FJ, Gillen P. Reversal of Hartmann's procedure following acute diverticulitis: is timing everything? Int J Colorectal Dis. 2009; 24(10):1219–1225

[39] Sier MF, van Gelder L, Ubbink DT, Bemelman WA, Oostenbroek RJ. Factors affecting timing of closure and non-reversal of temporary ileostomies. Int J Colorectal Dis. 2015; 30(9):1185–1192

[40] Letarte F, Hallet J, Drolet S, et al. Laparoscopic versus open colonic resection for complicated diverticular disease in the emergency setting: a safe choice? A retrospective comparative cohort study. Am J Surg. 2015; 209(6):992–998

[41] Pogacnik JS, Messaris E, Deiling SM, et al. Increased risk of incisional hernia after sigmoid colectomy for diverticulitis compared with colon cancer. J Am Coll Surg. 2014; 218(5):920–928

[42] Connelly TM, Tappouni R, Mathew P, Salgado J, Messaris E. Risk factors for the development of an incisional hernia after sigmoid resection for diverticulitis: an analysis of 33 patients, operative and disease-associated factors. Am Surg. 2015; 81(5):492–497

[43] Bauer VP. Emergency management of diverticulitis. Clin Colon Rectal Surg. 2009; 22(3):161–168

[44] Antolovic D, Reissfelder C, Koch M, et al. Surgical treatment of sigmoid diverticulitis–analysis of predictive risk factors for postoperative infections, surgical complications, and mortality. Int J Colorectal Dis. 2009; 24(5):577–584

[45] Oomen JL, Engel AF, Cuesta MA. Mortality after acute surgery for complications of diverticular disease of the sigmoid colon is almost exclusively due to patient related factors. Colorectal Dis. 2006; 8(2):112–119

[46] Chapman J, Davies M, Wolff B, et al. Complicated diverticulitis: is it time to rethink the rules? Ann Surg. 2005; 242(4):576–581, discussion 581–583

[47] Schwesinger WH, Page CP, Gaskill HV, III, et al. Operative management of diverticular emergencies: strategies and outcomes. Arch Surg. 2000; 135(5):558–562, discussion 562–563

[48] Schmelzer TM, Mostafa G, Norton HJ, et al. Reversal of Hartmann's procedure: a high-risk operation? Surgery. 2007; 142(4):598–606, discussion 606–607

[49] van Dijk ST, Bos K, de Boer MGJ, et al. A systematic review and meta-analysis of outpatient treatment for acute diverticulitis. Int J Colorectal Dis. 2018; 33(5):505–512

[50] El-Sayed C, Radley S, Mytton J, Evison F, Ward ST. Risk of recurrent disease and surgery following an admission for acute diverticulitis. Dis Colon Rectum. 2018; 61(3):382–389

Expert Commentary on Acute Diverticulitis by *Frederick A. Moore*

Expert Commentary on Acute Diverticulitis

Frederick A. Moore

Over the 20th century, the surgical management of acute diverticulitis evolved considerably, mostly based on expert opinion supported by small retrospective case series. This chapter provides a 21st century expert opinion based on some more recent higher quality information. In the late 1990s, there was a strong consensus among general surgeons that: (1) uncomplicated diverticulitis requires antibiotics and after two episodes, an elective sigmoid resection with anastomosis is warranted, and (2) complicated diverticulitis with significant sepsis was best treated by a "2-staged" Hartmann's procedure followed by delayed colostomy reversal. These dogmas were largely driven by the belief that diverticulitis was a progressive disease and the next episodes would be more severe and morbid. This proved not to be true. With regard to the first issue, it now appears that uncomplicated diverticulitis may not even require antibiotics and an elective resection should be reserved for patients with recurrent bouts, that are limiting their lifestyle, or those associated with immunosuppressive comorbidities. Elective resections are best accomplished by laparoscopic primary resection with anastomosis (PRA). With respect to the second issue, it has been shown that: (1) the initial Hartmann's procedure carries high-morbidity and mortality rates, (2) 50% of colostomies are never reversed, and (3) colostomy reversal is associated with significant complications and prolonged hospital stays. Consequently, two very different alternatives (i.e., minimally invasive laparoscopic lavage and drainage [LLD] versus PRA) were utilized in selected patients and shown to be better options than the traditional Hartmann's procedure.

This evolving literature has caused a lot of confusion. For the acute care surgeon, decision-making is driven by the severity of sepsis and stage of disease at presentation. The modified Hinchey classification provided a good structure for these decisions. In general, grade I disease is associated with mild sepsis that will resolve with IV antibiotics, and elective resection maybe warranted in the future. In grade II disease, one will have more severe sepsis, and abscesses > 4 centimeters should undergo percutaneous drainage. Again, most cases will improve over several days. Postdischarge, these patients warrant delayed colonoscopy to rule out cancer and elective resection. Grade II disease that does not improve with drainage and antibiotics require operative intervention. Depending on the degree of inflammation, patients may require either a resection with PRA, with or without a diverting loop ileostomy, or an open Hartmann's procedure. Hinchey Grade III and IV are difficult to differentiate on presentation and both can be very morbid (IV > III). Those in septic shock should undergo preoperative optimization and proceed to the operating room for damage control resection of the perforated segment of colon and temporary abdominal closure. The controversy at the second laparotomy is about whether a colostomy or anastomosis should be performed. Hinchey III/IV patients who do not present with septic shock have been the focus of three recent prospective randomized trials. These were designed to show that LLD is superior to Hartmann's procedure or PRA with Hinchey III disease, but unfortunately the studies did not show that. Rather, the combined data shows that at 1 year, the outcomes of total hospital days, major morbidity, and mortality are roughly the same. The major issue with LLD is some Hinchey IV perforations were missed and these patients do very poorly without a resection. In addition, roughly 20% of Hinchey III will not respond and require a second operation. However, the remaining 80% of patients recovered uneventfully and avoided a colostomy. While the authors discourage the use of LLD until further data become available, I believe LLD is still a viable option in otherwise healthy patients who can tolerate a failed attempt at LLD.

12 A Modern Approach to Complicated Pancreatitis

Chris Javadi, Monica Dua, and Brendan Visser

Summary

The modern treatment of peripancreatic collections is a multidisciplinary effort involving surgeons, intensivists, interventional endoscopists (gastroenterology), and interventional radiologists. This chapter provides an overview of the various strategies used to manage peripancreatic collections and the evolution of our modern approach to necrosectomy.

Keywords: Pancreatitis, necrosectomy, MIRP, VARD, PANTER, cyst gastrostomy

12.1 Terminology Matters

Is it a "pseudocyst," "walled-off necrosis (WON)," or a "collection"? Words matter: the name we use for a peripancreatic fluid collection can invoke the strategy of its treatment—sometimes incorrectly. When a collection is called a pseudocyst on computed tomography (CT) when it is, in fact, an area of WON that is semisolid, it can lead an inexperienced clinician down an incorrect path, placing a drain into a cavity that will not drain.

The 2012 revision of the Atlanta classification of acute pancreatitis provides four definitions based on the presence or absence of necrosis and the time from pancreatitis onset. These terms are acute peripancreatic fluid collection, pancreatic pseudocyst, acute necrotic collection, and WON.[1] This framework provides a common language to use among multidisciplinary teams; however, these four categories do not capture the complexity of individual patient presentations, and we caution against overly restricting a case into one category or another.

Peripancreatic fluid that develops in the early phase (< 4 weeks) of edematous pancreatitis without necrosis constitutes an acute peripancreatic fluid collection. On CT, acute peripancreatic collections are homogenous with no definable wall. They are adjacent to the pancreas and confined by normal fascial planes. Many will remain sterile and resolve spontaneously without intervention. When an acute collection persists beyond 4 weeks, it becomes a pancreatic pseudocyst, which is a homogenous collection surrounded by a well-defined wall containing predominantly liquid.

During the early phase of necrotizing pancreatitis, a collection with varying amounts of fluid and solid necrotic debris is an acute necrotic collection. Acute necrotic collections are heterogeneous, with no definable wall encapsulating the collection. A mature collection (4 weeks after the onset of necrotizing pancreatitis) of peripancreatic necrosis with a well-defined inflammatory wall is WON. On CT, WON is heterogeneous with liquid and solid components and varying degrees of loculations. WON can be both intrapancreatic and extrapancreatic.

12.2 Necrosis and Infection Exist in a Continuum

We make the mistake of thinking of peripancreatic collections in boxes—"sterile pseudocyst," "infected pseudocyst," "sterile necrosis," or "infected necrosis"—but in reality, collections exist as a continuum (▶ Fig. 12.1).

The texture of a collection is in most cases a mixture of liquid and solid. And while some patients have completely sterilized necrosis and others have grossly infected collections with rip-roaring sepsis, there are many patients who hide an infection of a lesser degree. These patients can hide a low-grade infection for a prolonged period, as the contaminated necrosis is being walled-off.[2]

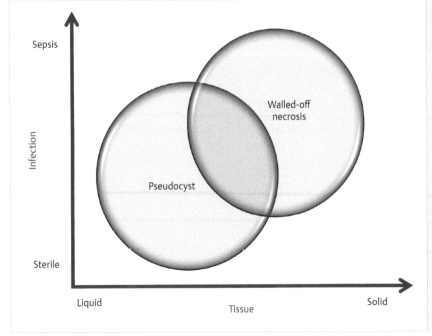

Fig. 12.1 Postpancreatitis collections exist on a continuum from sterile to infected and from liquid to solid.

12.3 Indications for Intervention

The indications for intervention in complicated pancreatitis include unstable anatomy, infected necrosis, deterioration of the patient, and persistent unwellness. Unstable anatomy occurs when there is a disconnected pancreatic duct and living islands of pancreas tissue that have no way to drain. The most common unstable anatomy is a necrotic neck with an intact body/tail, leading to a disconnected left duct.[3,4]

Necrosis is the most frequent indication for intervention and is the focus of this chapter. The most important question with regard to pancreatic necrosis is when to intervene. Acute necrotic collections almost never require intervention early in the course of disease. Asymptomatic WON does not mandate intervention regardless of size, and will often resolve slowly given time.[5,6] Intervention is warranted if the necrosis becomes infected or when WON causes intractable pain or obstruction.[7]

In general, a precipitous decline in the clinical status of the patient implies infected necrosis. Infection of acute necrotic collections may occur at any time during the clinical course of necrotizing pancreatitis, but infections often occur early, as in 3 to 4 weeks after presentation.[7,8,9] Infection is strongly suspected when there is gas evident on CT, clinical development of sepsis, or organ failure in a previously stable patient.

Some patients with WON are afflicted with what Warshaw described as "persistent unwellness." They have residual pain, difficulty eating, and "a general lack of well-being that prevents them from returning to work and other normal activities for many months."[2] Persistent unwellness denotes a patient who is not sick but is not getting better; this can occur with a low-grade, walled-off infection, or with organized sterile necrosis causing disabling symptoms or mechanical obstruction of the stomach or bile ducts.

12.4 What is Our Goal?

The successful management of necrotizing pancreatitis is *not* defined by avoiding surgery. *The goal is to return the patient to prepancreatitis health as quickly as possible.* Avoiding surgery in and of itself should not be the goal, although in published reports, surgical intervention has been reported as an outcome of its own. Many times, the appropriate minimally invasive operation can return the patient to health more quickly than percutaneous drainage or endoscopy alone.

12.5 Evolution of Strategies

Techniques for necrosectomy have evolved over the last 3 decades to reduce the invasiveness of surgery and decrease the morbidity and mortality of open necrosectomy. We will review each strategy and comment on their strengths and weaknesses. Defenders of each technique see every case as a nail for their hammer. There is not one universal approach that is applicable to all patients with necrosis. The treatment strategy should be tailored to the clinical status of the patient, timing of intervention, characteristics of necrosis (on the continuum from pseudocyst to solid necrosum), and anatomic considerations (location and accessibility).

12.5.1 Open Necrosectomy

Traditional open necrosectomy is now required infrequently but is still sometimes unavoidable. The most common situation is in patients who need to undergo another operation in addition to a necrosectomy (except cholecystectomy). For example, a patient with necrotizing pancreatitis who develops perforation of the colon due to thrombosis of the middle colic vessels. Additional clinical scenarios that occasionally accompany severe necrotizing pancreatitis include gastric necrosis causing perforation, and hemorrhage not controlled by angioembolization. These situations demand laparotomy, and open necrosectomy can be performed at the same time.

The drawback to open necrosectomy is, of course, its high morbidity and mortality. Even in institutions with experience, with appropriate delay and good techniques, open necrosectomy continues to be associated with significant early and late morbidity and a mortality of 11 to 16%.[10,11] Even with the good exposure of an open necrosectomy and repeated trips to the operating room, debridement may not always be complete. If there is solid necrosis left behind, the patient may continue to be unwell and will require drains until the solid tissue liquifies.

12.5.2 Laparoscopic Debridement

Given the morbidity of the open operation, less invasive laparoscopic debridements were attempted to decrease physiological stress and improve survival.[12,13,14] Unfortunately, laparoscopic debridement has not been shown to be an improvement over open necrosectomy and has a limited role today. Laparoscopic debridements face several drawbacks: the instrumentation for debridement is limited to 10 mm spoon forceps; it is difficult to remove all of the necrosis in a single operation; repeat laparoscopy is often impossible, unlike open necrosectomy, due to loss of domain; there is poor control if hemorrhage is encountered; and, most importantly, it does not free the patient of the need for drains.[12,15,16]

However, there are occasional patients in whom conventional laparoscopic debridement can be useful, for example, in patients with limited anterior necrosis, necrosis along the paracolic gutters, or necrosis distant from the pancreas (▸ Fig. 12.2).

12.5.3 Retroperitoneal Debridement

In the 2000s, two minimally invasive approaches were developed to access collections in the retroperitoneum: minimally invasive retroperitoneal pancreatectomy (MIRP) and video-assisted retroperitoneal debridement (VARD). Our preferred approach is a two-trocar technique originally described by Horvath, which is a variation on these strategies.[17,18] All of these strategies target retroperitoneal collections via two principle routes: on the left, in a window between the kidney and spleen (the more common location), and on the right, behind the head of the pancreas and adjacent to the duodenum.

Minimally Invasive Retroperitoneal Pancreatectomy

Minimally invasive retroperitoneal pancreatectomy (MIRP) was initially published in 2000 by authors in the UK. MIRP begins with

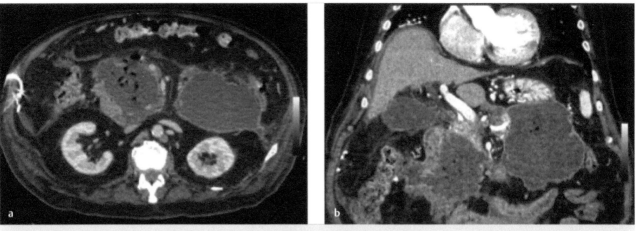

Fig. 12.2 (a, b) Two areas of walled-off necrosis is best approached with laparoscopic necrosectomy. The collections do not abut the abdominal wall, do not abut the stomach, and are not in communication with each other. Laparoscopic necrosectomy with drain placement is the least invasive option that provides adequate debridement.

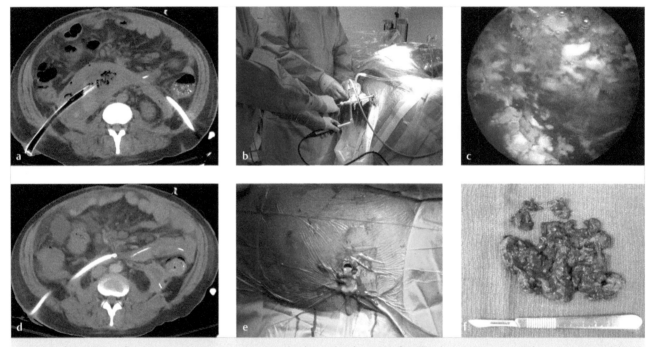

Fig. 12.3 This patient underwent an open necrosectomy at another hospital and was transferred with ongoing sepsis. His late presentation did not allow reopening of his laparotomy, and his collection did not abut the stomach. We performed MIRP. (a) CT showing placement of a 30 Fr sheath into the walled-off necrosis. (b) A nephroscope placed into the sheath for debridement. (c) Intraoperative view through the nephroscope under water irrigation. (d) CT one week after debridement. (e, f) Infected necrosis removed with the nephroscope. CT, computed tomography; MIRP, minimally invasive retroperitoneal pancreatectomy.

placement of a percutaneous drain into the collection. The drain tract is serially dilated to 30 Fr with graduated dilators and radiologic guidance. A 30 Fr Amplatz sheath is then inserted to allow the use of an operating nephroscope. The nephroscope has two channels that allow dissection with small grasping forceps under water irrigation[19] (▶ Fig. 12.3).

However, debridement with the nephroscope is very tedious, and most patients undergoing MIRP require multiple visits to the operating room to achieve an adequate necrosectomy.[19,20]

Video-assisted Retroperitoneal Debridement

Video-assisted retroperitoneal debridement (VARD) was first described in 2001 by a group from the Netherlands. As above, the operation begins with percutaneous drain placement with CT guidance. The drain is upsized to 18 Fr, and a 3 to 5 cm incision is made over the drain. Using a renal vein or lateral retractor, the dissection is performed down the drainage tract until the necrosis cavity is entered. Debridement is performed with sponge forceps

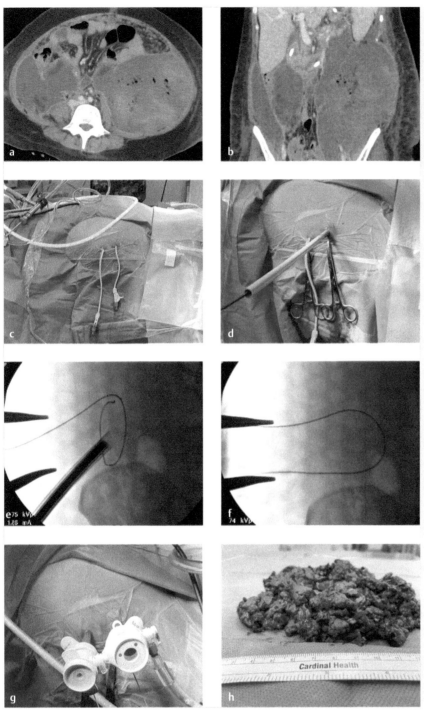

Fig. 12.4 Two trocar technique for retroperitoneal debridement. **(a, b)** Preoperative CT showing large retroperitoneal collections away from the stomach. **(c)** Two percutaneous drains placed by an interventional radiologist. **(d, e)** One tract is serially dilated to 30 Fr, aiming towards the other drain's wire and guided by the nephroscope and fluoroscopy. **(f)** The wire is used to connect the two tracts. **(g, h)** Radially dilating trocars are placed, the cavity is insufflated, and laparoscopic debridement is performed with laparoscopic spoon forceps. CT, computed tomography.

and a Yankauer suction. The technique is video-assisted, although the laparoscope often acts merely as a source of light down the tract.[21,22]

12.5.4 Two Trocar Technique

Our preferred approach is a variation on MIRP and VARD.[18] The goal is to place two laparoscopic trocars to convert the operation to a laparoscopic retroperitoneal approach. An interventional radiologist places two percutaneous drains about 3 to 4 finger-breadths apart (▶ Fig. 12.4). One drain is serially dilated to allow

initial debridement via the nephroscope (in the style of a MIRP). A wire is then placed through the other drain. With a combination of fluoroscopy and direct vision with the nephroscope, the collection is debrided under water irrigation in the direction of the other drain's wire. When this wire is reached, the two drain tracts are now connected. The two drains are then replaced with radially dilating Versastep trocars, which are inserted along the tract of the wire under the vision of the nephroscope. Placing the laparoscopic trocars in this way ensures that they enter the collection and not into the nearby colon, or other structures. A working space can be created with carbon dioxide insufflation (converting the operation from nephroscopic to laparoscopic), and debridement proceeds with 10 mm stone forceps (▶ Fig. 12.4).

Between 2000 to 2010, the retroperitoneal strategy was the best way forward. An important paper from the Dutch group, "A Step-up Approach or Open Necrosectomy for Necrotizing Pancreatitis (the PANTER trial)," was published in 2010.[11] This was the first trial comparing open necrosectomy with VARD. In the study, 88 patients were randomly assigned to open necrosectomy or the minimally invasive step-up approach. Their strategy is called "step-up" because they started with a percutaneous drain and scaled up as needed. Only if patients had not improved with percutaneous drainage, would they perform a retroperitoneal debridement. They did not use VARD to accelerate a patient's course.

The study found that percutaneous drainage alone was sufficient for 35% of patients. Compared to open necrosectomy, VARD caused less surgical trauma, but the overall mortality was the same between the two groups. VARD patients also developed diabetes less often compared with open necrosectomy, presumably because less healthy pancreas was taken along with the necrotic tissue.

Retroperitoneal debridement allows most patients to avoid the ICU postoperatively. The piecemeal debridement of MIRP and VARD, however, often requires repeated trips to the operating room; in the PANTER study, 26% of patients required more than one trip to the OR. Therefore, the total length of stay was not significantly changed, with a median of 50 days in the step-up group. Patients persist for a long time with drains, as the drains must remain until all the necrosis has been liquefied, which can take weeks or months.

12.5.5 Primary Percutaneous Drainage

The PANTER trial demonstrated that percutaneous drainage as a primary strategy can play a role in certain cases. In patients with liquid necrosis, percutaneous drainage alone can be sufficient in 30 to 50% of patients.[11,23] Drains also can be used in the initial control of a septic patient, buying time before a more definitive strategy is undertaken.

As an isolated strategy, though, drains have several drawbacks. While drains effectively temporize sick patients, they contaminate collections that may have otherwise remained sterile. They have a high failure rate as an independent strategy when some degree of solid necrosis is present. Even when drains work well, patients generally require so many drain exchange procedures and persist with drains for so long that an operative approach may be less morbid overall.

12.5.6 Transgastric Debridement

From the 2010s onward, transgastric debridement has become the preferred approach when anatomically feasible. Why does transgastric debridement work so well? Unlike all other approaches, a cyst gastrostomy allows continuous internal debridement. After the initial access and debridement, the persistent connection between the stomach and the collection leads to ongoing auto-debridement. In *in vitro* studies, gastric juice has been shown to accelerate liquefaction of pancreatic necrosis more effectively than saline lavage, enzyme solutions (trypsin, collagenase, or tPA), or even hydrogen peroxide.[24] A cyst gastrostomy avoids the necessity to reoperate, and it is the only strategy that does not require percutaneous drains.

A prerequisite for transgastric techniques is a large enough area where the necrosis is in contact with the gastric wall. If transgastric debridement is anticipated, placement of percutaneous drains should be avoided whenever possible. While placement of percutaneous drains can be life-saving in septic patients, drains disrupt containment of the necrosis and create an external pancreatic fistula, complicating the internal drainage of transgastric approaches.

12.5.7 Endoscopic Transgastric Debridement

The majority of the data on transgastric debridement comes from the endoscopic route. In 2018, the Dutch group published a trial comparing an endoscopic step-up method with the previous surgical step-up strategy, that is, percutaneous drainage and VARD when necessary.[23] Ninety-eight patients were randomized either to endoscopic (51) or surgical (47) step-up. With endoscopic step-up, patients underwent endoscopic, ultrasound-guided transgastric or transduodenal drainage with placement of two 7 Fr double pigtail stents and one 8.5 Fr nasocystic catheter. If drainage alone did not lead to considerable clinical improvement, endoscopic transluminal necrosectomy was performed.

To find 98 patients with necrotizing pancreatitis suitable for either strategy, 418 patients were screened, which is more than four times as many. This matches our clinical experience that patients are often appropriate for one strategy but not another. The median number of interventions was high in both groups, but more or less the same (three endoscopic interventions vs. four surgical). In other publications of endoscopic management, the number of endoscopic reinterventions is even higher, typically four and as high as 15.[23,25]

In those who underwent surgical step-up, 51% were successfully treated with catheter drainage only. This relatively high percentage should be considered with the caveat that their overall strategy is to perform VARD only if the patient is deteriorating with a drain, and not to hasten the patient's recovery. In the endoscopy group, 27% later needed an additional percutaneous drain, mostly for necrosis extending down into the pelvis. The major complication rate was the same (43% endoscopic vs. 45% surgical), and so was the mortality rate (18% endoscopic vs. 13% surgical), but very high in both groups. As expected, patients with percutaneous drains developed many more pancreatic fistulas (5% endoscopic vs. 32% surgical). It should be noted that the patients spent a prolonged time in the hospital after the first procedure– 35 median days in the endoscopic group and 69 in the surgical group.[23] This long postoperative length of stay is the Achilles heel of step-up approaches.

The step-up trials relied on small plastic pigtail stents which were not originally intended for draining thick or partially solid

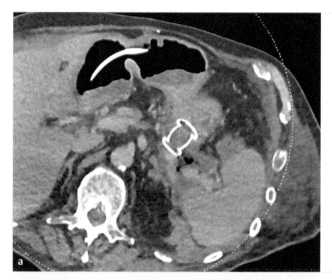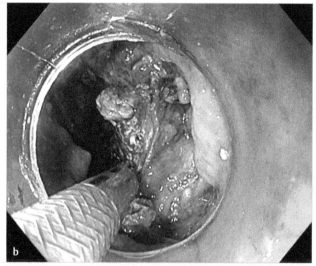

Fig. 12.5 Endoscopic necrosectomy. **(a)** CT after placement of a lumenal apposing Axios stent. **(b)** Endoscopic debridement using the Endorotor resection tool. CT, computed tomography.

collections. Endoscopic debridement has changed dramatically with the introduction of lumenal apposing metal stents (LAMS). At the time of publication, the Axios stent (Boston Scientific) is the only LAMS approved for transgastric endoscopic drainage of pancreatic pseudocysts and WON in the United States.[26,27]

Under combined endoscopic and endoscopic-ultrasound guidance, the LAMS catheter is advanced through the gastric wall and into the target collection using the catheter's cautery tip. The stent is then deployed. Three sizes are available, with the largest containing a 20 mm lumen for drainage. These large-diameter LAMS also allow passage of the endoscope through the stent for irrigation and debridement. The debridement is limited to the tools that fit through the working channel of the endoscope–typically, small deployable nets or endoscopic graspers, although a suction catheter with a rotating blade (Endorotor and Interscope Medical) has recently become available[28] (▶ Fig. 12.5).

Surgical Transgastric Necrosectomy

The alternative to endoscopic approaches is a surgical transgastric necrosectomy. With surgical instruments, a much larger cyst gastrostomy (i.e., to 6 to 10 cm) can be created, and the debridement is more efficient. A surgical approach also allows one to perform a simultaneous cholecystectomy, if indicated.

Pearls

The fundamental principles of surgical transgastric necrosectomy are as follows:[29]

- Ensure a large enough area where the necrosis is in contact with the gastric wall on preoperative imaging.
- Delay intervention by at least 4 weeks to allow a mature wall to form around the necrosis.
- Debride the bulk of necrosum in a single procedure.

- Minimize intraoperative and postoperative hemorrhage through precise tissue handling.
- Ensure durable internal drainage with a large cyst gastrostomy (6 to 10 cm).

Laparoscopic Transgastric Necrosectomy

Laparoscopic transgastric necrosectomy, described previously,[30,31,32] involves endoscopic stomach insufflation for the placement of transgastric trocars. At the beginning of the case, an endoscope is inserted into the stomach. Laparoscopic access is then obtained through the umbilicus, and the potential sites for trocar entry into the stomach are identified. The endoscope is used to maximally distend the stomach, while intra-abdominal insufflation is modestly reduced to allow the anterior abdominal wall and stomach to come together (while maintaining a limited laparoscopic view).

Versastep (Medtronic) radially dilating trocars are used to access the stomach under both laparoscopic and endoscopic vision. Depending on the case, 2 to 3 trocars are used (often two 5 mm and one 12 mm), which are placed in relatively close proximity because the available working area is limited. The laparoscope is then inserted through a transgastric trocar. Insufflation of the abdomen is released and the gastric lumen is insufflated to 15 mm Hg. A laparoscopic aspiration needle and/or laparoscopic ultrasound probe are used to localize the WON. After creating a small gastrotomy with electrocautery, this is extended with a vessel sealer or laparoscopic stapler to allow wide access (10 cm or more) into the WON. Debridement is conducted with standard laparoscopic instruments, leaving the necrosum in the stomach or pushing it through the pylorus. After debridement, the trocar sites on the gastric wall are sutured closed, the endoscope is withdrawn, and the abdominal wall port sites are closed (▶ Fig. 12.6).

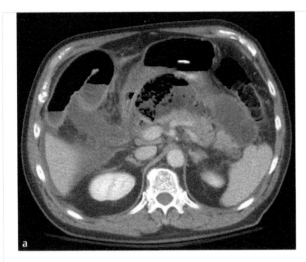

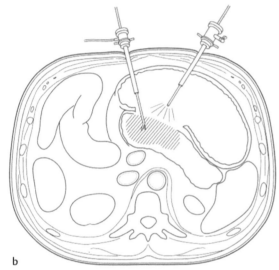

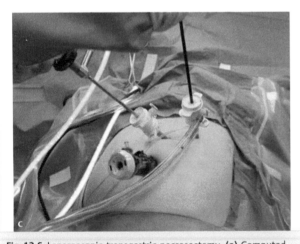

Fig. 12.6 Laparoscopic transgastric necrosectomy. **(a)** Computed tomography is used to guide port placement. **(b)** Schematic showing port placement and approach to the necrosum. **(c)** Final port placement including a 12 mm umbilical port used for initial entry. (Reproduced with permission of Worhunsky, DJ et al. Laparoscopic transgastric necrosectomy for the management of pancreatic necrosis. J Am Coll Surg. 2014;219(4):735–743.)

Surgical necrosectomy remains more effective than endoscopic necrosectomy in patients with significant amounts of solid necrosis. Even the largest LAMS can be obstructed by solid necrosis, and the great majority of patients undergoing endoscopic necrosectomy will require repeated debridements. Suboptimal debridement often prolongs the overall course of unwellness, avoiding frank sepsis from the infected necrosis but leaving a patient who only makes slow incremental progress with each endoscopic debridement (▶ Fig. 12.7).

Open Transgastric Necrosectomy

The same transgastric necrosectomy conducted via an open approach is equally effective and may be more accessible for surgeons wary of placing transgastric trocars. This operation requires a small upper midline laparotomy and anterior gastrostomy. Similar to the laparoscopic approach, a large cyst gastrostomy is performed to allow adequate surgical and then continuous internal debridement.

A multicenter retrospective review of open and laparoscopic transgastric necrosectomies conducted at Stanford University, University of Calgary, and Indiana University was recently published.[29] Among the three centers, 178 patients with WON underwent surgical transgastric necrosectomy. Thirty-nine percent had infected necrosis, and 25% required preoperative stay in the intensive care unit. The median delay between pancreatitis onset and surgery was 60 days. Morbidity and mortality were 38% and 2%, respectively. The median hospital stay was 8 postoperative days, which is significantly shorter than the 35 median days with endoscopic step-up.[23] The majority of patients were discharged home, and 91% had complete resolution of symptoms at a median of 6 weeks follow-up. Readmission or repeat interventions were required in just one-fifth of the patients. This data suggests that surgical transgastric necrosectomy in appropriately selected patients resolves the patient's WON faster and returns the patient to their prepancreatitis health sooner than percutaneous or endoscopic approaches.

12.6 Conclusion

The successful management of complicated pancreatitis requires knowledge of the advantages and limitations of surgical and nonsurgical strategies. The goals of any strategy for debridement and drainage are to minimize procedural morbidity and mortality, avoid multiple procedures and lengthy hospital stays, and expedite recovery to the patient's prepancreatitis health. No one approach to necrosectomy is optimal for all patients. The overall strategy must be tailored to the clinical status of the patient, the timing of intervention, the character of the necrosis on the continuum from pseudocyst to solid necrosum, and anatomic accessibility. When the patient's anatomy allows it, surgical transgastric necrosectomy achieves effective debridement with a single definitive operation and offers significant benefits in postoperative recovery.

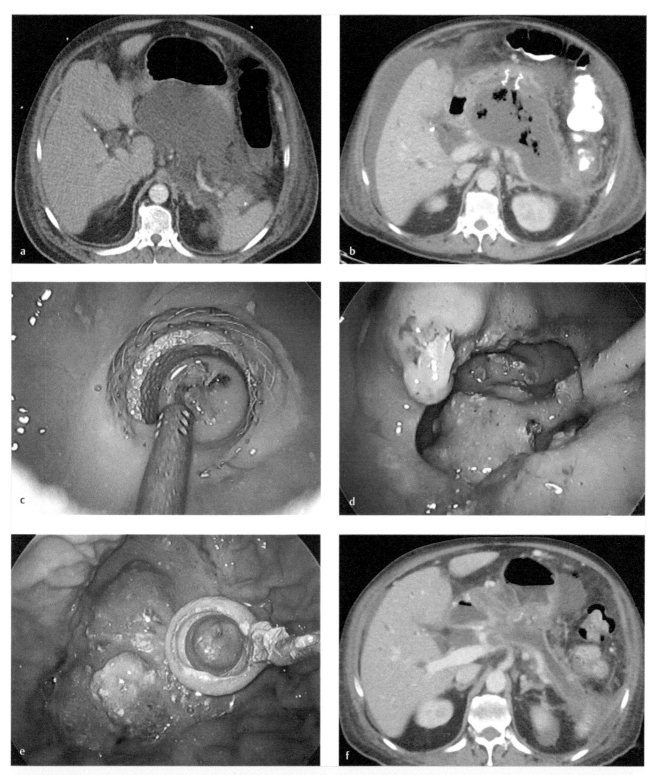

Fig. 12.7 A 56 -year-old man with alcoholic pancreatitis. **(a)** A necrotic collection abuts the stomach, but at this point, it is too immature to intervene, and there is no evidence of infection. Nonetheless, a gastroenterologist placed a LAMS into the collection and performed four serial endoscopic debridements, removing a little of the necrosis each time. The patient returned to the hospital with sepsis. **(b)** The patient's CT after 4 endoscopic debridements. Only modest progress was made removing the necrosis. **(c)** Laparoscopic transgastric view. Note that even the largest LAMS used here is occluded with solid necrotic tissue. **(d)** The stent was removed and the cyst gastrostomy widened to allow laparoscopic debridement. **(e)** Solid necrosum collected in the antrum. Note the large size of the tissue relative to the LAMS. **(f)** CT one week after laparoscopic transgastric necrosectomy. After a single operation, most of the necrosis has resolved. CT, computed tomography; LAMS, lumenal-apposing metal stent.

References

[1] Banks PA, Bollen TL, Dervenis C, et al. Acute Pancreatitis Classification Working Group. Classification of acute pancreatitis–2012: revision of the Atlanta classification and definitions by international consensus. Gut. 2013; 62(1): 102–111

[2] Warshaw AL. Pancreatic necrosis: to debride or not to debride-that is the question. Ann Surg. 2000; 232(5):627–629

[3] Fischer TD, Gutman DS, Hughes SJ, Trevino JG, Behrns KE. Disconnected pancreatic duct syndrome: disease classification and management strategies. J Am Coll Surg. 2014; 219(4):704–712

[4] Murage KP, Ball CG, Zyromski NJ, et al. Clinical framework to guide operative decision making in disconnected left pancreatic remnant (DLPR) following acute or chronic pancreatitis. Surgery. 2010; 148(4):847–856, discussion 856–857

[5] Rau B, Pralle U, Uhl W, Schoenberg MH, Beger HG. Management of sterile necrosis in instances of severe acute pancreatitis. J Am Coll Surg. 1995; 181(4): 279–288

[6] Bradley EL, III. Indications for debridement of necrotizing pancreatitis. Pancreas. 1996; 13(3):219–223

[7] Freeman ML, Werner J, van Santvoort HC, et al. Interventions for necrotizing pancreatitis: summary of a multidisciplinary consensus conference. Pancreas. 2012; 41(8):1176–1194

[8] Runzi M, Niebel W, Goebell H, Gerken G, Layer P. Severe acute pancreatitis: nonsurgical treatment of infected necroses. Pancreas. 2005; 30(3):195–199

[9] Besselink MG, van Santvoort HC, Boermeester MA, et al. Dutch Acute Pancreatitis Study Group. Timing and impact of infections in acute pancreatitis. Br J Surg. 2009; 96(3):267–273

[10] Ashley SW, Perez A, Pierce EA, et al. Necrotizing pancreatitis: contemporary analysis of 99 consecutive cases. Ann Surg. 2001; 234(4):572–579, discussion 579–580

[11] van Santvoort HC, Besselink MG, Bakker OJ, et al. Dutch Pancreatitis Study Group. A step-up approach or open necrosectomy for necrotizing pancreatitis. N Engl J Med. 2010; 362(16):1491–1502

[12] Gagner M. Laparoscopic Treatment of Acute Necrotizing Pancreatitis. Semin Laparosc Surg. 1996; 3(1):21–28

[13] Cuschieri SA, Jakimowicz JJ, Stultiens G. Laparoscopic infracolic approach for complications of acute pancreatitis. Semin Laparosc Surg. 1998; 5(3): 189–194

[14] Pamoukian VN, Gagner M. Laparoscopic necrosectomy for acute necrotizing pancreatitis. J Hepatobiliary Pancreat Surg. 2001; 8(3):221–223

[15] Zhu JF, Fan XH, Zhang XH. Laparoscopic treatment of severe acute pancreatitis. Surg Endosc. 2001; 15(2):146–148

[16] Parekh D. Laparoscopic-assisted pancreatic necrosectomy: a new surgical option for treatment of severe necrotizing pancreatitis. Arch Surg. 2006; 141 (9):895–902, discussion 902–903

[17] Horvath KD, Kao LS, Ali A, Wherry KL, Pellegrini CA, Sinanan MN. Laparoscopic assisted percutaneous drainage of infected pancreatic necrosis. Surg Endosc. 2001; 15(7):677–682

[18] Horvath KD, Kao LS, Wherry KL, Pellegrini CA, Sinanan MN. A technique for laparoscopic-assisted percutaneous drainage of infected pancreatic necrosis and pancreatic abscess. Surg Endosc. 2001; 15(10):1221–1225

[19] Carter CR, McKay CJ, Imrie CW. Percutaneous necrosectomy and sinus tract endoscopy in the management of infected pancreatic necrosis: an initial experience. Ann Surg. 2000; 232(2):175–180

[20] Logue JA, Carter CR. Minimally invasive necrosectomy techniques in severe acute pancreatitis: role of percutaneous necrosectomy and video-assisted retroperitoneal debridement. Gastroenterol Res Pract. 2015; 2015(8656): 693040–693046

[21] van Santvoort HC, Besselink MG, Bollen TL, Buskens E, van Ramshorst B, Gooszen HG, Dutch Acute Pancreatitis Study Group. Case-matched comparison of the retroperitoneal approach with laparotomy for necrotizing pancreatitis. World J Surg. 2007; 31(8):1635–1642

[22] van Brunschot S, van Grinsven J, Voermans RP, et al. Dutch Pancreatitis Study Group. Transluminal endoscopic step-up approach versus minimally invasive surgical step-up approach in patients with infected necrotising pancreatitis (TENSION trial): design and rationale of a randomised controlled multicenter trial [ISRCTN09186711]. BMC Gastroenterol. 2013; 13(1):161

[23] van Brunschot S, van Grinsven J, van Santvoort HC, et al. Dutch Pancreatitis Study Group. Endoscopic or surgical step-up approach for infected necrotising pancreatitis: a multicentre randomised trial. Lancet. 2018; 391 (10115):51–58

[24] Brown L, Hong J, Zyromski N, Connor S, Phillips A, Windsor J. Improving the efficacy of drainage for infected pancreatic necrosis by enzymatic accelerated liquefaction. HPB. 2018; 20 Supplement 2:S524

[25] van Brunschot S, Fockens P, Bakker OJ, et al. Endoscopic transluminal necrosectomy in necrotising pancreatitis: a systematic review. Surg Endosc. 2014; 28(5):1425–1438

[26] Siddiqui AA, Kowalski TE, Loren DE, et al. Fully covered self-expanding metal stents versus lumen-apposing fully covered self-expanding metal stent versus plastic stents for endoscopic drainage of pancreatic walled-off necrosis: clinical outcomes and success. Gastrointest Endosc. 2017; 85(4):758–765

[27] Chen Y-I, Yang J, Friedland S, et al. Lumen apposing metal stents are superior to plastic stents in pancreatic walled-off necrosis: a large international multicenter study. Endosc Int Open. 2019; 7(3):E347–E354

[28] van der Wiel SE, Poley J-W, Grubben MJAL, Bruno MJ, Koch AD. The EndoRotor, a novel tool for the endoscopic management of pancreatic necrosis. Endoscopy. 2018; 50(9):E240–E241

[29] Driedger M, Zyromski NJ, Visser BC, et al. Surgical Transgastric Necrosectomy for Necrotizing Pancreatitis. Ann Surg. 2018(September):1–6

[30] Mori T, Abe N, Sugiyama M, Atomi Y, Way LW. Laparoscopic pancreatic cystgastrostomy. J Hepatobiliary Pancreat Surg. 2000; 7(1):28–34

[31] Gibson SC, Robertson BF, Dickson EJ, McKay CJ, Carter CR. 'Step-port' laparoscopic cystgastrostomy for the management of organized solid predominant post-acute fluid collections after severe acute pancreatitis. HPB (Oxford). 2014; 16(2):170–176

[32] Worhunsky DJ, Qadan M, Dua MM, et al. Laparoscopic transgastric necrosectomy for the management of pancreatic necrosis. J Am Coll Surg. 2014; 219(4):735–743

Expert Commentary on A Modern Approach to Complicated Pancreatitis by
Peter Fagenholz and George C. Velmahos

Expert Commentary on A Modern Approach to Complicated Pancreatitis

Peter Fagenholz and George C. Velmahos

The authors provide a comprehensive review of techniques currently available for the management of pancreatic necrosis. There is no single superior technique of necrosectomy, and the challenge in managing these patients involves matching each patient to the best interventional approach based on their anatomy and clinical status. It follows that provision of optimal care requires these patients to be managed in a multidisciplinary fashion with surgeons, interventional radiologists, and gastroenterologists, who are familiar with the disease and the techniques described here.

Regarding the different techniques, the greatest advantage of transgastricnecrosectomy—surgical or endoscopic—is the lack of external drains. The total drain-related morbidity and resource use due to patient discomfort, nursing services, and repeat radiologic interventions is significant. The endoscopic transgastric approach is the most commonly utilized transgastric technique, but, in selected patients, a surgical approach has the advantages of allowing complete debridement in a single procedure and performance of simultaneous cholecystectomy. This is, however, probably the most technically challenging debridement technique. For those reticent to undertake transgastric port placement, transgastric necrosectomy can also be performed laparoscopically through a wide anterior gastrotomy. If this anterior gastrotomy technique is used, it is important to avoid contamination of the peritoneal cavity.

Retroperitoneal debridement techniques are all preceded by percutaneous drainage. While reasonable rates of successful treatment are achievable with percutaneous drainage alone, this often requires long periods of external drainage and multiple procedures. The purpose of a step-up approach is not to avoid surgery but, to borrow from the authors, "*to return the patient to pre-pancreatitis health as quickly as possible.*" As experience with minimally invasive debridement has grown, there has been a tendency to "step-up" earlier, resulting in a lower rate of purely percutaneous treatment, faster overall recovery, and shorter duration of external drainage. The type of retroperitoneal debridement technique is chosen based on the size and anatomy of the necrosis.

We would differ slightly with the authors on a few points. First, we have not found that percutaneous drainage, if needed to control sepsis, is a major barrier to subsequent transgastric intervention. Any of the retroperitoneal debridement techniques described are compatible with endoscopic transgastric drainage, and we increasingly use combinations of retroperitoneal and transgastric techniques. This approach—termed dual modality therapy—combines the main advantage of the retroperitoneal techniques (rapid necrosectomy) with the main advantage of the transgastric approaches (fistula control) and allows early removal of external drains.

Although the term minimally invasive retroperitoneal pancreatectomy (MIRP) has been attached to dilational necrosectomy with a nephroscope, this technique does not require retroperitoneal access. Transperitoneal tracts can be dilated and used for debridement, and this frequently provides optimal access to collections. While repeat necrosectomy is often needed with MIRP, our median number of interventions with this technique remains one; repeat procedures are often spaced at 48 to 72 hours and may not extend hospital stay.

This excellent chapter focuses largely on technique. Surgeons caring for these patients will also need to be comfortable with initial resuscitation, nutrition, and recognition and management of complications such as arterial pseudoaneurysm and enteric fistulae. For those willing to take on the challenge, a robust and evolving field awaits.

13 Inflammatory/Infectious Bowel Disease

Cigdem Benlice, Ipek Sapci, and Scott R. Steele

Summary

Inflammatory bowel disease, including Crohn's disease and ulcerative colitis, and infectious colitides like *Clostridium difficile* colitis encompass a wide range of presentations and symptoms. While the full spectrum of disease remains not completely understood, there have been a number of advances in evaluation and management in these complex diseases, and this chapter will cover these important topics.

Keywords: Inflammatory bowel disease, Crohn's, ulcerative colitis, pouch, *Clostridium difficile* colitis

13.1 Crohn's Disease

13.1.1 Introduction

Crohn's disease (CD) is an incurable, complex chronic inflammatory bowel disease that may affect any portion of the entire length of the gastrointestinal tract. The exact etiology of this disease remains to be elucidated; therefore, management focuses on treating the complications and not curing the disease. Surgery remains to be a vital component in the management of CD, and up to one third of the patients require at least one bowel resection during their lifetime.[1]

Medical therapy options include corticosteroids, antibiotics, 5-aminosalicylic acid, immunomodulator and biologic agents. Medical management alone is typically ineffective due to the inherent recurrent nature of the disease, and in most cases, surgical intervention is inevitable. Benefits of medical therapy have been described but it also poses certain risks and side effects. Immunosuppressant therapy is given earlier in the disease course; however, this does not decrease the need for surgery or intestinal complications.[2] Surgery can be considered the final option after trialing multiple medications, which could

potentially affect the results of the operation. An important step in the management involves balancing medical therapy and accurately deciding the time of surgery, as surgery in the earlier course of disease has benefits.[3] Surgery at an early stage is considered a valid alternative to medical therapy.[4] Long-term effects of biologic agents are yet to be evaluated; therefore, surgery should not be viewed as a last resort in CD and only when medical alternatives are exhausted.

CD is categorized according to the location (terminal ileum, colon, ileocolon, and upper gastrointestinal tract) and disease behavior (stricturing, penetrating, nonstricturing, and nonpenetrating with an addition of perianal modifier). The most commonly involved part of the gastrointestinal tract is the ileum followed by colon and proximal small bowel (▶ Fig. 13.1 and ▶ Fig. 13.2).[5] Operative/nonoperative methods are selected based on these characteristics. It is common for different behaviors to manifest concurrently and this can make their management more challenging.

As most of the patients with CD undergo multiple surgeries due to recurrences or complications related to the index surgery, and the microscopic margins were not shown to have an effect on recurrence, it is preferred to resect minimal amount of bowel and be adamant about leaving as much healthy bowel as possible.[6] Stricturoplasties are commonly performed to evade bowel removal in stricturing disease and is considered a good option for bowel preservation. Therefore, having a strong understanding of the general principles and technical specifics is important for surgeons.

13.1.2 Indications for Operative Intervention

Operative inventions in CD are reserved for either failed medical treatment or complications arising in the disease. Disease refractory to medical treatment remains the most

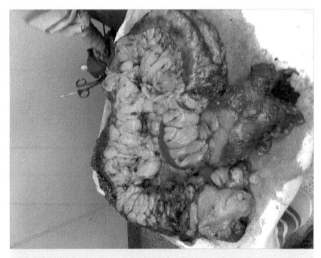

Fig. 13.1 Crohn's colitis with the colon demonstrating fat wrapping and diffuse colitis.

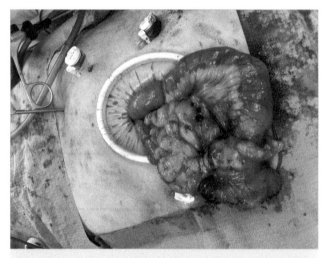

Fig. 13.2 Laparoscopic resection of ileocolic specimen in a patient with Crohn's disease.

common indication for surgery, and complications can be listed as acute perforation in penetrating disease, toxic colitis, abscess, hemorrhage, obstruction, fistula, and neoplasia.

Key technical considerations should be applied toall patients. Before resection, thorough exploration of the abdomen should be performed to identify any additional areas involved in the disease. Normal bowel will present a clearly palpable mesentery, while involved bowel can be distinguished by thickened mesentery and an inflamed appearance.

Abscesses are a common indication for surgery in CD and are most commonly found in ileocecal area with a significant percentage (40%) associated with a fistula.[3] Percutaneous drainage is a valid treatment option, yet majority of the patients will require surgery eventually due to the close relation shared with a fistula. For small abscesses (< 3 cm) that are not feasible for percutaneous drainage, a course of antibiotics can be administered. Percutaneous drainage leads to favorable results and can improve the patients' condition and clinical picture within 24 to 48 hours.[7] The success rate with this technique is over 90% but surgical treatment was found to be more successful in preventing disease recurrence.[8] For postoperative abscesses, percutaneous drainage should be preferred to a reoperation.

Perforation is a rare complication of CD and is associated with obstruction or toxic colitis. Patients may present with sepsis and their status should be optimized prior to surgery. Depending on the underlying reason and location, perforations are treated with either resection and anastomosis or total/subtotal abdominal colectomy with end ileostomy.

Bleeding is another infrequent indication for surgery. After stabilizing the patient, algorithms for gastrointestinal bleeding are followed to investigate the cause of hemorrhage with bleeding scans, angiography, or endoscopy/colonoscopy. The goal is to identify the cause of bleeding in a timely manner and refrain from resecting large bowel segments.

Dysplasia and cancer are topics of concern in inflammatory bowel diseases. CD increases the risk of developing cancer, and the risk for colorectal cancer was shown to increase two to three-fold. Patients who develop cancer on the base of CD also tend to be younger compared to the general population.[9] Stricturing disease pattern is in particular associated with increased incidence of colorectal cancer; therefore, for strictures treated without resections, close observation is advised. Colorectal cancer or high-grade dysplasia can require proctocolectomy in patients who are fit for surgery. Low-grade dysplasia should also be closely monitored or a segmental resection should be performed.[4]

CD can affect any part of the gastrointestinal tract which can behave differently. In order to provide a detailed overview, main indications and operative options based on the disease location and character are provided separately as subtitles.

Stricturing/Obstructing Disease

Fibrostenotic patterns can be observed in any location in CD, especially in the small bowel, and can be of inflammatory, fibrotic or anastomotic origin.[10] Up to 35% of patients can develop stricturing affliction during the course of the disease, which can present with abdominal pain, fever, weight loss, or change in bowel movements.[10] In cases with inflammatory

strictures, initial therapy with steroids can provide symptom resolution, help avoid emergency surgery, which is why it is recommended as the first-line treatment.[11,12]

On the other hand, fibrotic and anastomotic strictures oftentimes require more advanced treatment with endoscopic-balloon dilation or stricturoplasty. Success rates up to 90% have been reported for endoscopic-balloon dilation for treating strictures.[13,14] Recent literature suggests that resection of ileocolic anastomotic strictures result in lower risk of subsequent surgery compared with endoscopic-balloon dilation. In addition, endoscopic-balloon dilation results in increased time interval between the subsequent surgeries. Attempting dilation with endoscopic methods may be beneficial in selected low-risk patients.[14]

If medical and/or endoscopic dilation does not provide symptom relief, surgical treatment should be preferred. Choices of treatment are stricturoplasty, resection, primary anastomosis, and, if necessary, proximal diversion. As the purpose of surgical treatment is not to attain definitive cure, but instead provide symptom relief and avoid extensive bowel resections, stricturoplasties are considered safe options in stricturing jejunoileal disease. Before proceeding with surgery, comprehensive evaluation of the bowel should be completed. Finding additional stricturing segments or fistulas can change the type and approach of surgery, and in these cases, extended resections may be performed instead of localized stricturoplasty.

Since their first description in the 1980s, a variety of stricturoplasty techniques have been described.[4,15] Stricturoplasty relieves the obstruction while preserving maximum length of bowel with low-complication rates.[16] Indications are previous bowel resection of > 100 cm, stricturing disease of small bowel, short-bowel syndrome, recurrent strictures at ileocolic anastomosis, and recurrent strictures within a year of the previous surgery.[4] Conventional stricturoplasties are Heineke–Mikulicz and Finney.[4,11] When there are long or multiple stenotic segments, nonconventional stricturoplasties such as Michelassi stricturoplasty can be preferred.[4] Primary resection with anastomosis should be reserved for patients undergoing their first surgery, those who did not have significant bowel resected in the past, and those who have concomitant symptomatic disease in other bowel segments with multiple strictures. Stricturoplasty is not recommended for colonic strictures,which should be treated with balloon dilation or segmental colon resection.

Heineke-Mikulicz method entails making a longitudinal incision along the antimesenteric border of the bowel with a transverse closure. For the Finney stricturoplasty, a longitudinal U-shaped incision is made along the length of stricture and the segment is folded on itself.[11] In nonconventional methods, an isoperistaltic strictureplasty is constructed in a way that allows anastomosis of narrowed disease segment to the adjacent loop in a side-to-side manner.

Fistulizing/Penetrating Disease

Fistulas related to CD are not uncommon as the inflammation involves all layers of the bowel wall. Longer disease duration is associated with cumulative increase in fistula incidence, and this behavior represents more aggressive disease.[17] Fistulizing/penetrating disease requires evaluation of the disease extent and involvement of a number of organs. If fistulizing disease is suspected, complete evaluation with imaging is necessary. Even with preoperative imaging, incidental discovery intraoperatively is common.[18]

The aim of surgery in fistulizing disease is to alleviate the symptoms and provide relief to the patient. It is imperative to clearly define and separate borders of the diseased bowel from the healthy loops and preserve the healthy tissue. Extent and number of fistulas will determine the surgical approach. If multiple fistulas are present, including multiple organs, then proceeding with minimally invasive surgery (MIS) may not be the optimal choice. Surgeon expertise also affects this choice, as these cases can be unpredictably complicated. Surgical treatment is not essential for all fistulas and if the fistula is enteroenteric between loops in close proximity and is not associated with any symptoms, surgery is not necessary.

Internal fistulas are formed between bowel loops or between bowel and other organs, and external fistulas follow a cutaneous path. The most common type of fistula in CD is enteroenteric, and the terminal ileum is often the origin. Enterocutaneous fistulas can also occur during the course of the disease or as a postoperative complication. Managing enterocutaneous fistulas can be debilitating, as they frequently cause dehydration, electrolyte, and metabolic imbalances. For these, initial treatment involves conservative methods with total parenteral nutrition and electrolyte replacement.[19] In cases where the fistula is not a complication of previous surgery, surgical closure should be attempted almost always.

Ileosigmoid fistulas consist of the majority of internal fistulas in CD, and surgery is considered the initial approach. Protective stoma can be used during repair, and either sigmoid resection or primary sigmoid repair can be performed with comparable results.[18,20]

Fistulas can form between the diseased bowel and the healthy bowel as well as between other organs such as vagina or bladder. When treating the fistulas, the affected bowel should be resected, and the healthy bowel should be preserved with minimal resection or primary closure. During anastomosis construction, stapled side-to-side anastomosis should be favored which was shown to result in fewer overall postoperative complication rates.[21]

Toxic Colitis

Toxic colitis is an acute and life-threatening presentation of colonic involvement in CD. Acute severe colitis is defined as more than six bloody bowel movements per day with at least one sign of systemic toxicity (fever > 37.5 °C, tachycardia, anemia of < 10.5 g/dL, and erythrocyte sedimentation rate >30 mm/h). Diagnosis of toxic megacolon is made when there is total or segmental dilation without obstruction along with the above-mentioned signs of systemic toxicity.[11,12]

Initial evaluation is crucial in toxic colitis as it determines the course of action. Multidisciplinary approach should be preferred and patients' clinical status should be assessed accordingly. Patients presenting with free perforation, unstable condition, or severe hemorrhage need to be adequately resuscitated before emergency surgery.

Conservative management with medical therapy is preferred in patients without these symptoms, and the suggested agent is

corticosteroids with a daily dose of 300 mg.[22] Hydration status should be optimized and any electrolyte imbalances should be corrected. Patients may be put on bowel rest, particularly if an urgent surgery is expected.[11,23]

Emergent surgery should be performed in patients without satisfactory response to medical therapy or if their clinical status deteriorates within 24 to 72 hours. Open total/subtotal abdominal colectomy with end ileostomy is the primary choice of surgery. Emergency proctectomy should be avoided, if possible, unless indicated due to rectal hemorrhage or perforation.[24]

13.1.3 Special Considerations

Upper Gastrointestinal Tract and Duodenal Disease

Disease proximal to the terminal ileum can be extensive and has a worse prognosis. Number, length, and proximity of the diseased bowel segments affect the surgical decision. Primary presentation of the disease in stomach or duodenum is rarely seen, and disease presenting with stricturing characteristics and associated symptoms requires surgery. Stricturoplasty is favored when it comes to treating duodenal strictures, and jejunal disease can be treated with resection, strictureplasty or a combined technique.[4,25] As these sites are prone to development of enteroenteric fistulas, electrolyte and nutrition optimization is important in such cases.

Ileocolic Disease

Ileocolic resection is the most common operation in Crohn's patients since terminal ileum is the most frequently affected location. The abdomen should be explored to assess disease severity. Mobilization of the cecum and terminal ileum are necessary. The colon should be divided proximal to the ileocecal valve and the aim is maximal bowel preservation. The decision to continue with anastomosis or diversion is based on patients' condition, current medications, nutrition status, and presence of contamination with possible perforation. If the conditions are optimal, making an anastomosis is preferred, and wide lumen stapled ileocolic side-to-side anastomosis is favored.[4] Notably, terminal ileitis can resemble CD during laparotomy for appendicitis; however, this should not undergo routine resections.

Colon and Rectum

In instances when surgery is necessary for limited disease in the colon, segmental resections are favored. Segmental resections are equally effective compared with subtotal/total colectomy with similar rates of postoperative complications.[26]

Decision is made based on location of disease, presence of malignancy, and prior resections. Segmental resections are commonly employed with ileocolonic, colo-colonic, and rectal anastomoses. Patients who have pancolitis can undergo a total/subtotal colectomy with ileorectal anastomosis or, alternatively, total proctocolectomy with end ileostomy.

Restorative proctocolectomy with ileal pouch–anal anastomosis (IPAA) can be offered to selected patients who do not have any history of perianal or small bowel disease.[4] After pouch construction, patients with CD are more likely to develop fistula and pouch failure.[27,28] After IPAA construction, CD patients should be actively followed-up in a multidisciplinary manner.

In surgical planning, due to the nature of the disease, certain tips may be helpful. During proctectomy, probability of a nonhealing perineal wound should be kept in mind. An intersphincteric dissection, which maximizes the amount of healthy muscle/tissue remaining, can be performed to avoid this complication. Finally, when appropriate, diversion can be used to alleviate active disease or avoid negative effects of medical therapy on tissue healing.

Perianal Disease

Perianal disease in CD can show a wide range of symptoms which can be the primary presentation of disease. These include skin tags, hemorrhoids, perianal fistulae, and abscesses. It is associated with increased extraintestinal manifestations and steroid resistance.[29,30] In patients without an established diagnosis of CD, waxy perianal edema, painless fissures, edematous tags, and spontaneous ulcerations should raise suspicion of CD, and they should be evaluated thoroughly as these characteristics are associated with granulomas on biopsy.[31]

Most commonly perianal disease manifests as fistula and associated abscess and these require surgical intervention. Abscesses present with increased temperature, swelling, and fluctuance. They can occupy any perirectal space; therefore, a detailed examination is advised. Incision and drainage are part of the standard procedure, preferably from the rectal site. If the infection extends deep into the perirectal space, a mushroom drain can be placed.

Fistulas can be categorized as simple or complex in relation to the tract and association with any abscess. Simple fistulas usually have a single opening and are superficial. Location above the dentate line, transversing the sphincter complex, and connection with an abscess are features of complex fistulas. Examination under anesthesia is considered the gold standard to detect and evaluate the fistula.[4] Medical therapy is also beneficial for perianal fistula in CD, especially with tumor necrosis factor (TNF) antagonists and the recommendation involves combining this with surgical treatment.[32]

Surgical therapy can include seton drainage, fistulotomy, fistula plugs, advancement, and diversion. Symptomatic simple fistulas should be managed with a loose seton which aids in drainage along with antibiotic administration. The objective of surgery is the definitive closure of the fistula tract. Fistulotomy with debridement of tissue is favored for superficial fistulas. Endorectal advancement flaps are advantageous, especially for complex fistulas such as rectovaginal fistulas. This method uses a rectal flap for definitive closure after the internal opening is incised and debrided. If fistulotomy is not feasible, this option can be considered, with success rates varying according to the surgeon expertise, drainage or excision, perioperative antibiotics, and bowel preparation.[32]

Recurrent Disease

CD is known for its recurring nature which may not always be symptomatic. The overall risk of subsequent surgery due to recurrent disease was found to be 28% in a recent series.[33] Risk factors for disease recurrence was also evaluated and it was found that smoking strongly predicts disease recurrence with a two-fold increase in clinical recurrence.[34,35] Disease with penetrating/perforating phenotype is also associated with higher recurrence rates. Recent studies show that biologic agents, especially infliximab can be effective in decreasing recurrence rates.[36]

13.1.4 Minimally Invasive Approaches in Crohn's Disease

Minimally invasive approaches for surgery in Crohn's disease (CD) has been used since the 1990s.[37] Inherent benefits of laparoscopic surgery such as shorter operative time, improved cosmesis, decreased postoperative pain, earlier return of bowel function, and shorter length of hospital stay are well-documented.[38,39,40] Regardless of its common application in CD, use of laparoscopy for complex fistulizing or perforating as well as recurrent disease is debatable and it is recommended based on surgeon expertise.[12]

Laparoscopy can be used for diagnostic purposes in Crohn's patients. Patients presenting with unexplained symptoms can undergo diagnostic laparoscopy to reveal the underlying cause. It can also assist in evaluating existing adhesions and determining practicality of a laparoscopic approach.

Laparoscopic approach is recommended if suitable expertise is available for ileocolic resections in CD and efficacy has been shown in randomized controlled trials.[38,41] Laparoscopy can result in longer operative times but recovery of bowel function, major complications, and length of stay were found to be comparable to open surgery in previous literature.[42] When deciding between open versus laparoscopic approaches, expertise of the surgeon and other patient characteristics should also be considered. As majority of CD patients undergo at least one surgery during their lifetime, starting this process with a minimally invasive method is preferred.

Use of minimally invasive approaches for colonic CD is also common; however, the broad and thick mesentery makes the resections and maneuvering challenging.[43]

Laparoscopic colectomy for CD showed similar results with open surgery in terms of postoperative complications with shorter hospital stay.[44,45] Another known benefit of laparoscopy is prevention of incisional hernia when intracorporeal anastomoses are performed with small transverse incisions for extraction.[46] Possibility of multiple surgeries should always be kept in mind in this population, and laparoscopy should be favored for noncomplex disease when available.

Complex CD with recurrence, perforation, fistulas, and application of minimally invasive approaches is another aspect. CD is progressive and extensive adhesions, multiple affected areas and complications such as fistulas and abscess can make resection more difficult. Laparoscopy can be applied in fistulous, complex, and penetrating CD as the literature reports similar outcomes and supports use of laparoscopy in this subset of patients (▶ Fig. 13.3).[12] It has also been shown to be comparable with the open approach in complex disease involving ileo-sigmoid fistulas.[18] Complexity of the disease does not exclusively guide the decision regarding approach. Surgical decision-making should be based on patients' condition, status

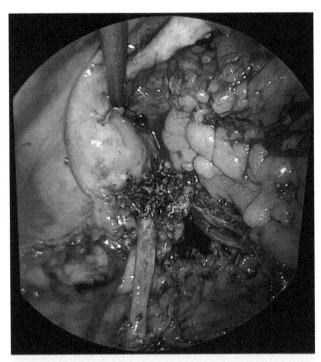

Fig. 13.3 Laparoscopic view of a patient with a colo-ovarian fistula in Crohn's disease.

of adhesions, and knowledge and technical skills of the surgeon. Patients' condition should be stabilized before proceeding with laparoscopy and open approach is preferred in unstable and emergent operations.

Patients who have complex diseases are likely to have recurrences and multiple operations. It is a topic of discussion whether to continue with laparoscopic approach in patients who underwent previous open surgeries. When open and laparoscopy groups were compared in patients with previous midline incisions, two approaches were found to be comparable in terms of operative time, overall morbidity, hospital stay, and reoperation and readmission rates with laparoscopy group having lower rates of wound infection.[47] Therefore, performing the subsequent surgeries with laparoscopy can be beneficial for the patient. Detailed literature reporting the use of minimally invasive approaches in recurrent CD is given in ▶ Table 13.1.

Single incision laparoscopic surgery (SILS) is a subset of laparoscopic surgery that consists of performing the entire procedure and tissue extraction through a single incision[55]. Reports show that SILS has benefits such as decreased pain medication requirement and shorter operative times in complex CD and is considered safe and feasible.[55,56] It must be noted that this is a technically challenging procedure and it should be performed when technical expertise is available. Hand-assisted laparoscopic surgery can also be used as an alternative to conventional laparoscopy which allows manual retraction and tactile feedback. It can be safely applied in complex CD and can decrease the operative time.[57]

The robotic platform is the most recent addition to minimally invasive approaches which enables the surgeon to have enhanced control over the surgical field, dexterity, and improved visualization, especially in the narrow pelvis.[58] It is

not commonly applied in complex CD but it can be useful when completion proctectomy is indicated in selected patients.

When considering the best surgical approach for CD, many factors should be considered such as the location of the disease, extent of the disease, size of the specimen to be extracted, past surgical history of the patient, possibility of adhesions, and expertise of the surgeon.

13.1.5 Conclusion

CD has a progressive course and majority of patients require surgery during their lifetime. Key points in management are timely surgical intervention and maximal bowel preservation. Best surgical treatment and approach is affected by a variety of factors and these should be considered and discussed with the patient.

13.2 Ulcerative Colitis

Ulcerative colitis (UC) is a potentially complex and crippling disease process, which is challenging for both the provider and patient. While many patients are successfully managed with minimal medical intervention, a significant number will progress to severe, debilitating, and intractable disease, ultimately necessitating a high-risk surgery. Multidisciplinary discussion and formation of a solid therapeutic alliance are critical parts of the treatment process, particularly in refractory cases. It should be kept in mind that chronic UC patients often possess an innate understanding of their own disease process that far outweighs clinical data. Individualized medical and surgical care should therefore be the standard. In practice, this principle is not easy to follow, as it necessitates thorough and often lengthy counseling. However, the ability to provide a potentially curative surgery to a patient who has been experiencing the pain and humiliation of UC is a privilege worthy of additional effort. This part of the chapter discusses the indications, role of MIS with contraindications, open management strategies, and postoperative complications of patients afflicted with UC.

13.3 Clinical Manifestations

Signs and symptoms of a UC flare depend largely on the severity and location of disease. The most common findings are blood and mucus in the stool. Tenesmus, urgency, increased stool frequency, fecal incontinence, and pain with defecation are common, as the majority of the disease burden is generally in the rectum. Fecal incontinence is certainly the most distressing and anxiety-producing element of the disease and, as with tenesmus and urgency, is due to noncompliance of the rectum and loss of receptive relaxation. While diarrhea is common, up to 25% of patients may complain of constipation with a sense of incomplete evacuation.[59]

The severity of pain generally signifies severity of inflammation, and as the colonic lumen narrows with edema, the intensity of peristaltic pain increases. Nausea is extremely common, and likely reflects either downstream effects of circulating inflammatory mediators or inflammation of the stomach secondary to direct apposition with inflamed colon as opposed to frank obstruction.

Table 13.1 Literature summary of use of minimally invasive approaches in recurrent disease

Study Year	Authors	Patient number	Study design	Results
1997	Wu et al[48]	116 (46 lap with 24 complex vs. 70 open)	Prospective	Operative time longer in open (p < 0.05), higher blood loss in open (p < 0.05). Shorter LOS in lap (p < 0.01)
2003	Hasegawa et al[49]	52 (61 lap operations, 45 primary vs.16 recurrent [subgroup 7 lap vs. 9 open])	Retrospective	Open and primary groups had shorter operative time in open group (p = 0.042, p = 0.012)
2004	Uchikoshi et al[49]	43 for recurrent disease (17 lap vs. 6 HALS vs. 20 open)	Retrospective	Earliest flatus and shortest LOS in HALS (p < 0.05, p < 0.01)
2004	Moorthy et al[49]	48 (57 lap procedures, 26 recurrent vs. 31 primary)	Retrospective	Conversion higher in recurrent (p = 0.02) Days to soft diet shorter in primary (p = 0.03)
2010	Holubar et al[50]	40 recurrent ileocolic (30 lap-completed vs. 10 lap-converted)	Retrospective	Shorter LOS and days to soft diet in lap (p = 0.002, p = 0.03)
2010	Brouquet et al[51]	57 (62 reoperations– 29 lap vs 33 open)	Retrospective	Need for associated procedures more often in open (p = 0.003) Intraoperative intestinal injuries more in lap (p = 0.01)
2011	Chaudhary et al[52]	59 lap (30 recurrent vs. 29 primary)	Retrospective	Operative time longer in recurrent (p < 0.01)
2011	Pinto et al[53]	130 lap (80 primary resection vs. 50 for recurrent disease)	Retrospective	LOS, complications comparable
2012	Huang et al[54]	130 lap (48 with prior surgery vs. 82 without prior surgery)	Retrospective	Conversion rate, complications comparable

Abbreviations: HALS, hand-assisted laparoscopic surgery; LOS: length of stay.

Weight loss is also common with chronic UC, which is likely a multifactorial phenomenon dependent on protein loss via the inflamed mucosa, avoidance of per os (PO) intake, and metabolic demand of constant inflammation.

13.3.1 Indications for Operative Intervention

Emergent Indications

Colectomy most often follows failure of medical treatment for severe and extensive colitis. Toxic dilatation (colon > 6 cm), perforation, and hemorrhage are less common indications. The decision to operate is taken jointly and involves daily communication between gastroenterology and surgical teams. Patients receiving high-dose intravenous steroids who have a stool frequency of > 8 per day on the third treatment day are likely to require colectomy.[60,61] Similarly those with a stool frequency of 3 to 8 stools per day, and who have a CRP > 45 mg/L, are unlikely to settle. Failure to respond after 5 to 7 days or any significant deterioration during this period is an indication for colectomy. Patients who initially respond but promptly relapse with the reintroduction of diet are also likely to require colectomy. Pouch surgery should be avoided in the acute setting. It is customary to instead perform subtotal colectomy with end ileostomy. The colon is mobilized and vessels taken relatively close to the bowel wall. The sigmoid stump is stapled and left long, allowing it to be secured with sutures in the subcutaneous space at the lower pole of the wound. Any stump dehiscence will then result in an easily manageable fistula rather than a pelvic abscess and the sigmoid will be easy to locate at reoperation. A Foley catheter is used to decompress the rectum for a period of 3 or 4 days.

Life-threatening Severe Colitis

Life-threatening ulcerative colitis, often referred to as fulminant colitis (FC), presents with rapid onset abdominal pain, abdominal distention, persistent bloody diarrhea, and signs of toxicity such as fevers and tachycardia. Many will have anemia and/or a profound leukocytosis as well. These patients must be treated aggressively with fluid resuscitation, electrolyte replacement, and high-dose intravenous steroids. It is important to rule out infectious etiologies before starting corticosteroids. A nasogastric tube may be placed; although, this is unlikely to decompress a colon with a competent ileocecal valve. If the etiology is in question, as it is in the 10% of patients presenting for the first time with FC,[22] the diagnosis should be confirmed with flexible sigmoidoscopy. If the patient remains stable but without substantial improvement over the next 24 to 48 hours, rescue therapy with a calcineurin inhibitor or an anti-TNFα agent may be considered. Short-term results of rescue therapy in this population are encouraging, with 76 to 85% of patients avoiding colectomy on that admission. Long-term patient expectations should be tempered however, as follow-up data suggest that between 58% and 88% of patients who required cyclosporine rescue underwent a colectomy within 7 years.[62,63] "Toxic megacolon" is an extreme variant of FC in which all or a segment of the transverse or left colon is dilated to more than 5.5 cm. It occurs in up to 2.5% of those with UC, and as with FC, may be the initial presentation.[64] Early surgical consultation is an absolute necessity, as a delay in operative management risks perforation and 30% mortality. A lack of response within 24 to 48 hours necessitates either operative intervention or rescue therapy. Rescue therapy, even when successful in the short-term, should be viewed as a bridge to a more "elective" surgery, as at least 35% of these patients will require a proctocolectomy within a year and up to 88% by 7 years.[62]

Massive Hemorrhage

Hemorrhage to the point of hemodynamic instability is a rare occurrence in UC (approximately 1%), although it does account for approximately 10% of urgent colectomies for UC.[65] These cases should be initially managed as any other gastrointestinal bleed with resuscitation, localization, and hemorrhage control. Upper gastrointestinal sources should be ruled out and high-dose intravenous steroids should be administered. A stable patient may be monitored for 24 to 72 hours for improvement on steroids; however, the majority of patients will require surgery. The bleeding is usually from a diffuse mucosal injury and is therefore not amenable to colonoscopic or endovascular hemorrhage control techniques. Massive hemorrhage from both the colon and rectum is likely the one and only indication for an emergent proctocolectomy. If possible, it is preferred to leave rectum in situ in the acute setting to facilitate a staged completion proctectomy with an ileal pouch anastomosis. In approximately 12% of cases, the rectal stump will continue to bleed despite steroids and diversion; however, it is usually relatively minor bleeding that can be managed conservatively.

Perforation

Colonic perforation is related to extent and severity of disease, occurring in as many as 20% of UC patients presenting with fulminant pancolitis. The patients are acutely ill upon presentation, and mortality rate is approximately 50%.[66] Observation with immune suppression therefore plays no role in any patient with a full-thickness perforation. Abdominal colectomy with ileostomy and Hartmann closure of the rectum is the procedure of choice.

Obstruction

Strictures are present in 3 to 17% of patients with UC, with approximately 30% located in the rectum.[67,68] Stricturing disease may ultimately result in a large bowel obstruction, which necessitates surgical excision due to both the risk of perforation and the potential for malignant cells within the stricture.[69] It has been suggested that approximately 40% of resected strictures will have carcinoma in the resected specimen and an additional 33% will have high-grade dysplasia.[70]

Nonemergent Indications

Intractable Disease

Intractable colorectal inflammation is the most common indication for nonemergent surgery in UC.[65] These patients are either unable to tolerate a steroid taper without recurrence of symptoms, intolerant of medical therapy due to severe sideeffects, or have persistent symptoms despite maximal medical therapy.[67] The goldstandard surgery is total proctocolectomy with or without pouch reconstruction. Excision of the entire colon and rectum, regardless of the extent of the disease at the time of surgery, will remove the entirety of the primary disease process and correct several extra-intestinal manifestations. The difficulty in these cases is that maximal medical therapy is a fluid definition, depending on available medications and the person prescribing them. With new biologic therapies in the pipeline, recent studies reporting some success with trialing a third

sequential TNFα-inhibitor, and some clinicians supporting the off-label use of unproven biologics in UC, it is easy to imagine a situation where a smoldering patient is eternally strung along in hopes of a medical "cure." The lack of a clear-cut line in the sand is one of the more frustrating aspects of UC for both patients and surgeons alike, and highlights the necessity for multidisciplinary collaboration.

Dysplasia, Malignancy of the Colon or Rectum, or Cancer Prophylaxis

UC is associated with a 0.5 to 1% increased risk per year after 10 years, regardless of severity of disease activity. This equates to a 20% risk at 20 years and a > 30% risk at 35 years.[71] It stands to reason that patients who are younger at diagnosis are at higher risk of subsequent development of colorectal cancer. Cancer risk is also correlated with extent of disease, as an increase in inflamed surface area imposes a higher mathematical probability of developing inflammation-related cancer. Furthermore, the mere presence of low-grade dysplasia in one portion of the colon suggests that the entirety of the diseased colon and rectum are at risk of synchronous malignancy. Therefore, patients with colorectal malignancy, high-grade dysplasia, dysplasia-associated lesion or mass (DALM), or low-grade dysplasia are candidates for colectomy or proctocolectomy.[72,73] IPAA is not contraindicated in the setting of malignancy, and the decision to proceed with pouch reconstruction is based on tumor location and patient preference rather than a specific algorithm.[65] Caution should be exercised, however, in the setting of more advanced (T3) lesions, as these may represent an aggressive phenotype predisposing to metastases. A conservative approach consisting of abdominal colectomy and end ileostomy,followed by IPAA after an observation period of at least 12 months is recommended in these patients. Patients with low or middle rectal cancer should be advised against IPAA, as they are at increased risk of subsequent radiation therapy (close margins and local recurrence) which renders a pouch poorly functional at best.

13.3.2 The Role of Minimally Invasive Surgery

Since 1951, colectomy with an ileostomy has been the treatment of choice for patients with fulminant (toxic) UC.[74] Nowadays, this procedure is performed laparoscopically more frequently; at a later stage after patient recovery, restorative proctectomy with IPAA is performed. There are no published prospective randomized trials comparing laparoscopic and open total abdominal colectomy for UC. However, several comparative reports have indicated that laparoscopic surgery is safe and feasible in cases of acute severe colitis. Reported conversion rates after laparoscopic total abdominal colectomy have been very acceptable, ranging from 0 to 8%.[75,76,77,78] In addition, most series have reported reduced length of hospital stay after laparoscopic procedures when compared with open counterparts. The great majority of patients who undergo laparoscopic total abdominal colectomy can undergo subsequent proctectomy and IPAA,[74,79] performed either laparoscopically or via a small lower abdominal midline or Pfannenstiel incision, which is an approach that has been described as "minimal access."[80] In this respect, a laparoscopic

Hartmann stump with minimal adhesions could be the ideal setting to initiate a completion proctectomy rather than a longer rectosigmoid stump into the subcutaneous tissue. There is still insufficient data to assess whether a truly laparoscopic restorative proctectomy or a minimal access restorative proctectomy is preferable. In general, a laparoscopic total abdominal colectomy is an effective operation that results in accelerated recovery for patients with acute colitis while retaining comparable morbidity when compared with the open technique. Some of the possible benefits of laparoscopic surgery, such as reduction of pain and cosmesis, have not been formally assessed after total abdominal colectomy, which is generally not considered the definitive operation for patients with UC. A total abdominal colectomy using a laparoscopic approach may prove to be advantageous in appropriate patients. However, the natural history of acute UC makes patient selection for laparoscopic surgery paramount to minimize potentially fatal complications in this often very morbid patient population.[81] SILS for total proctocolectomy with IPAA, as an alternative to the traditional laparoscopic technique, has first been reported in 2010.[82] SILS is expected to have benefits in the early postoperative course with respect to enhanced recovery, length of hospital stay, and cosmesis. So far, the literature is limited to a few caseseries demonstrating the feasibility and safety of both two- and three-stage procedures with complication rates comparable to conventional laparoscopy.[83,84] Additional studies are needed to compare SILS with respect to operative times, convalescence, and (functional) outcomes.[81]

Robotic surgery has also been introduced as a promising technique, especially in technically demanding operations like IPAA.[85] However, so far, all studies demonstrate increased operative time and cost, with no difference in postoperative complications and length of hospital stay when compared to standard laparoscopic colonic surgery.[58,86]

13.3.3 Contraindications to an MIS Approach

In general, the indications for laparoscopic total abdominal colectomy without proctectomy are similar to the established indications for open surgery. In fact, most patients who require an initial total abdominal colectomy are candidates for a laparoscopic approach. However, a subset of patients are not good candidates for laparoscopic total abdominal colectomy, for example, in the case of acute colitis complicated by either colonic perforation or toxic megacolon. Moreover, the patient who is acutely ill with FC might still receive better treatment with a more expeditious open abdominal colectomy than laparoscopic abdominal colectomy.[81] In particular, if the surgeon feels that the tissues are very friable and are at increased risk of intra-abdominal colonic injury during surgical manipulation, he or she might prefer to perform the operation with open technique. In addition, in those rare cases where a Turnbull–Blowhole procedure is considered, such as in pregnant patients,[87] the open technique remains necessary.

13.3.4 Open Management Strategies

The ultimate goal of surgical therapy for UC is removal of the entire intestinal disease burden. Total proctocolectomy is therefore the procedure of choice, and offers the possibility of a surgical "cure." Nevertheless, there are alternative strategies that may play roles in select situations. In all, there are six available surgical options for the UC patient, depending on the clinical scenario. These include subtotal colectomy with end ileostomy, transverse loop ("blowhole") colostomy of Turnbull, total proctocolectomy with end (Brooke) ileostomy, total proctocolectomy with continent (Koch) ileostomy, abdominal colectomy with ileorectal anastomosis, and total proctocolectomy with IPAA.

Subtotal Colectomy with End Ileostomy

In 1951, Crile and Thomas advocated for total abdominal colectomy with end ileostomy to control severe colitis. Adoption of this management strategy reduced the mortality rate of toxic megacolon from 63% (with ileostomy alone) to only 14%.[88] More recent series suggest a mortality rate <10%, with pelvic sepsis rates of approximately 10%, and overall morbidity rates of >30%.[89] The procedure is not definitive. Rather, it is a temporizing measure to control the bulk of the disease burden and ensure colonic decompression while allowing the patient time to wean from steroids and optimize nutrition prior to endeavoring upon a high-risk IPAA. The hidden benefit in this strategy is that it allows for a more accurate pathologic diagnosis, thereby minimizing the risk of a Crohn's "recurrence" in the pouch. There is no urgency to definitive surgery after subtotal colectomy with end ileostomy, as long as the rectal stump is appropriately surveyed for malignancy.

Turnbull-Blowhole Colostomy

Despite improvements in severe UC outcomes with the use of abdominal colectomy and end ileostomy, Turnbull proposed a skin level loop colostomy in addition to loop ileostomy in cases of toxic megacolon. The rationale for this maneuver was twofold: first, it avoided iatrogenic injury secondary to handling of the friable, diseased colon. Second, it avoided the problems associated with management of the difficult rectal stump.[90] The procedure is largely of historical interest, as most do not find that it imparts a benefit over abdominal colectomy in the era of modern medicine. Nevertheless, it continues to play a role in the most unstable patients and in pregnant women in whom colonic dissection around the gravid uterus is undesirable. Another benefit of Turnbull's procedure in pregnant women is that it avoids the need for bringing the rectosigmoid stump out as mucus fistula, which may not be feasible in the presence of a gravid uterus.[87]

Total Proctocolectomy and End Ileostomy

Total proctocolectomy and Brooke ileostomy was the gold-standard for UC surgery prior to the refinement of pouch reconstruction in 1978.[91] The procedure provides outstanding disease control and eliminates any future chance of colorectal cancer. It is also less technically demanding than reconstructive procedures and is routinely performed in a single stage in the nonemergent setting. Reluctance on the patient's behalf to undergo this procedure, as opposed to restorative proctocolectomy,

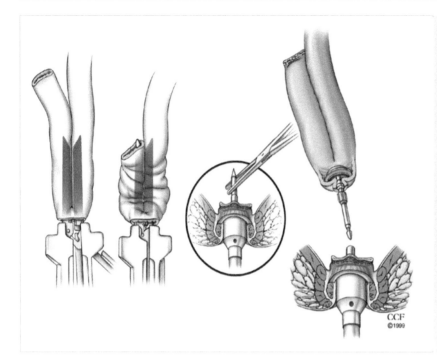

Fig. 13.4 Various stages of construction of the ileal–anal pouch. An enterotomy is made in the curved part of the J. It takes 2 to 3 firings of the GIA 100 to complete the pouch. The tip of the J area should not be long. The spike is brought out the rectal staple line. Finally, the anastomosis constructed. (Reproduced with permission of Cleveland Clinic Center for Medical Art and Photography © 2020. All rights reserved.)

is the presence of a permanent abdominal stoma. While some individual quality of life studies report that ileostomies have a life quality similar to an age-matched cohort of the general population, almost 25% of these patients are restricted in their social and recreational activities, and 15% would consider conversion to pouch reconstruction.[92] In addition, the idea of an uncontrollable fecal stream necessitating the continuous wear of a containment device is unappealing to many.

Total Abdominal Colectomy and Ileorectal Anastomosis

Removal of the diseased colon with ileoproctostomy has been used in various forms since 1943. The benefits of this procedure include preservation of gastrointestinal continuity in addition to avoidance of pelvic dissection, thereby mitigating the risk of impotence, bladder dysfunction, and infertility. Of equal importance is the fact that it leaves other options available should the primary surgery fail. While controversial, it remains an option in UC for select patients with a pliable, distensible rectum and no perianal disease. In the modern era, it is primarily reserved for patients with indeterminate colitis or high-risk patients who are not good candidates for IPAA. It also warrants consideration in teenagers for whom an expeditious return to school is desirable and young women who would like to preserve fertility, but not at the cost of an ileostomy.[93] Clearly, these discussions must be taken on a case-by-case basis, and must include extensive counseling as to the risks and benefits of leaving rectal disease behind. Functional results depend on the level of the anastomosis, state of the rectum, and natural history of the individual patient's UC phenotype (which cannot be accurately predicted). Contraindications to ileorectal anastomosis include a severely diseased and nondistensible rectum, rectal dysplasia or cancer, perianal disease, or a poorly functioning anal sphincter complex.[94]

Total Proctocolectomy and Ileal Pouch–Anal Anastomosis (IPAA)

The earliest ileoanal anastomoses were described by Vignolo in 1912, when he used the distal ileum as an interposition graft between the sigmoid colon and anus to avoid mandatory colostomy after proctectomy.[95] This maneuver, when coupled with his previous description of mucosal proctectomy, set the stage for the anal ileostomy refined by Ravitch and Sabiston in 1947.[95] These concepts mark the foundations of the modern-day restorative proctocolectomy described by Parks in 1978, which has become the gold standard surgical procedure for UC (▶ Fig. 13.4).[91] The allure of a well-functioning IPAA seems obvious in that it avoids a permanent abdominal stoma without compromising quality of life. Nevertheless, the decision between proctocolectomy with Brooke ileostomy and IPAA must not be taken lightly, as complications associated with IPAA can be substantial. At a minimum, the decision to proceed with IPAA subjects the patient to a longer recovery with greater uncertainty. Therefore, IPAA should not be a foregone conclusion in all candidate patients, as some will elect a permanent ileostomy when appropriately counseled.

All UC patients with preserved anal sphincter function, no evidence of small bowel or perineal Crohn's, and without the need for pelvic radiation are technically candidates for restorative proctocolectomy. Relative contraindications include advanced age, desired future pregnancy, history of perianal suppurative disease, obesity, and presence of isolated Crohn's colitis. Each of these findings warrants some concern and should prompt careful consideration prior to proceeding with pouch reconstruction.

13.3.5 The Management of Postoperative Complications

Specific Complications

Pelvic Sepsis

Pelvic abscess is one of the most feared complications after IPAA, as the largest series to date found a significant association between pelvic sepsis and pouch failure (hazard ratio [HR] 3.3, 95% confidence interval (CI) 2.2–4.8; $p < 0.001$).[96] Sepsis is generally due to anastomotic dehiscence or infected pelvic hematoma. Early leaks occur in approximately 5% of patients and account for the majority of cases, although late leaks (seen in 2% of patients) may contribute as well. Acute manifestations include fevers, tenesmus, frequency, or bleeding and purulence from the pouch. Subacute or smoldering abscesses may present later as a perineal fistula. Regardless of the timing of symptoms, CT or MRI should be obtained for diagnosis. Intravenous broad-spectrum antibiotics should be started and fluid collections should be drained. Percutaneous drainage is preferred, although endoanal drainage is a good option, particularly if percutaneous access does not adequately clear the septic source. If the endoanal approach is utilized, it is important to establish wide drainage into the pouch and curette the cavity. Open drainage via laparotomy may be entertained, although this should be considered a last resort after multiple attempts at local control. If a subclinical leak is detected on endoscopy or imaging before ileostomy reversal, local procedures should be undertaken, with direct repair of any leaks and endoanal drainage of any fluid collection. The loop ileostomy should remain in place until complete healing is documented.

Anastomotic Stricture

Stricture is a fairly common complication after IPAA. The literature reports rates ranging from 5 to 38%, depending on follow-up, technique, and series size.[97,98] Some variability may be accounted for by differential definitions of stricture, with some defining it as any narrowing requiring dilations and others defining it as a narrowing, causing mechanical outlet obstruction. Fazio et al studied the outcomes of over 3700 pouches, and using the former definition found a 5% chance of early stricture, which increased to 11% in long-term follow-up.[28] The underlying etiology for stricture formation is believed to be anastomotic tension predisposing to leakage and infection. Poor blood supply is likely another contributing factor, particularly in cases where mesenteric vessels need to be taken to obtain adequate length on the pouch. Most commonly, the stricture is web-like, fracturing easily with gentle finger dilation. Nevertheless, fibrotic strictures can occur and often require multiple dilations in the operating room. Fifty percent of these patients will retain adequate pouch function, although some may require transanal anastomotic resection with pouch advancement.[99]

Pouchitis

Pouchitis, a term referring to inflammation of the pouch, is the most common complication occurring in patients with IPAA with rates as high as 46%.[100] It is observed frequently in patients with underlying UC and is rarely seen in those with familial adenomatous polyposis (FAP). Pouchitis represents a spectrum of disease processes ranging from an acute antibiotic-responsive entity to a chronic antibiotic-refractory type, with possible pathogenetic pathways. Many aspects of pouchitis are challenging in the sense that its etiology and pathogenesis are not entirely clear; there is no consensus on diagnostic criteria or diagnostic instruments for pouchitis.[101] Various placebo-controlled trials and small randomized controlled trials have suggested the efficacy of metronidazole and ciprofloxacin as first-line therapy for acute pouchitis. Comparative studies and a Cochrane review found ciprofloxacin to be superior to metronidazole in terms of symptom score, and endoscopic score. Budesonide enemas are likely as efficacious as metronidazole.[456,465–468] Probiotic therapy may be of benefit for maintenance therapy after resolution of an acute flair, which lends credence to the bacterial overgrowth theory.[102] When unresponsive pouchitis is confirmed, combination therapy using ciprofloxacin and flagyl, steroid enemas, and mesalamine may be considered. Each of these second-line treatments showed a benefit in underpowered studies.[103] Immune modulators and biologic therapies may be utilized as third-line medications. While all studies regarding these alternative medications are lacking in terms of methodology, they have demonstrated the efficacy of cyclosporine enemas, infliximab, and adalimumab in treating intractable pouchitis.

Infertility

Rectal excision with pouch reconstruction is associated with a 30 to 70% reduction in female fecundity.[104] The etiology is presumably pelvic adhesions, although this has not been proven. Given the significant risk of infertility, along with the fact that many women with UC are in their child-bearing years, ileorectal anastomosis or even end ileostomy may be preferred to total proctocolectomy with end ileostomy.

13.4 *Clostridium Difficile* Colitis

Clostridium difficile (C. *difficile*) has been an increasing pathogen to the medical community over the years. Since the 1970's, our understanding of C. *difficile* and its impact on healthcare has changed dramatically. In recent years, we have seen the emergence of hypervirulent strains of C. *difficile* which have increased morbidity and mortality and are resistant to traditional antibiotic therapies.[105] In addition, where C. *difficile* infections (CDI) were once considered exclusively nosocomial, cases are now being seen in the community with increased frequency and virulence.[106,107,108] Based on trends, the incidence, impact, and cost of C. *difficile* on every aspect of healthcare are predicted to markedly increase in the future.[106]

CDI can vary from mildtosevere and can present with many different symptoms. Diarrhea is the most common presenting symptom and reported to be seen in 97% of patients. Nausea and vomiting are also often observed among patients, although much more variable.[109] About one-third of patients are hemoccult positive, but hematochezia is rare.[110] Fever is present in 25% of patients diagnosed with C. *difficile*.[111] Patients with severe disease can have a more dramatic presentation. Diarrhea can be absent, or wax and wane, and in some cases, itself a sign of severe complicated disease.[109,112] In severe cases, patients also commonly have abdominal pain, distention, tenderness, and even peritonitis.[113,114] Finally, severe complicated cases often can lead to dehydration, resulting in tachycardia, electrolyte abnormalities, arrhythmogenic changes, and hypotension.[114,115]

13.4.1 Indications for Operative Intervention

Treatment of the infection depends on the severity of the disease and the symptoms. It can be treated conservatively or with surgery. The most important initial treatment step is to cease administration of the antibiotic that caused the CDI. The continuous administration of antibiotics, which do not treat CDI, not only worsen the patient's condition but may also affect their susceptibility to reinfection.[116] If, due to the primary disease, administration of antibiotics is required, it would be prudent to incorporate antibiotics that are less responsible for extending CDI, such as aminoglycosides, sulfonamides, macrolides, tetracyclines, and vancomycin. In patients with typical symptoms of CDI, such as diarrhea, abdominal pain, nausea and positive stool cultures, antibiotics should be initiated.[117] Empirical therapy is only indicated when there is a very high probability of infection and while awaiting the results of diagnostic tests.[118]

Patients with severe infections may develop systemic failure with copious diarrhea and must be treated in the intensive care unit or surgical ward. If severe CDI is suspected after obtaining the patient's history and performing a physical examination, then radiographic imaging studies are indicated to determine whether ileus, obstruction, perforation, toxic megacolon, colonic-wall thickening, and ascites are present.[119,120] When any of these conditions are present—particularly toxic megacolon, perforation, or colonic-wall thickening—early surgical consultation is indicated, because colectomy can be a life-saving procedure.[121] To decrease morbidity and mortality in patients in particularly high-risk groups such as the elderly or immunocompromised with acute severe colitis, an early surgical intervention should be considered after a joint decision between medical and surgical gastroenterologists.[122]

Surgery successfully eliminates the majority of the disease and the trigger of the systemic inflammatory response.[123] While the majority of CDI are manageable with conservative measures, surgery should be considered without delay in all patients with severe or fulminant CDI. The decision to proceed with surgery is challenging because it requires balancing the risk of proceeding too late with the risk of unnecessarily removing a colon that could have recovered with nonsurgical measures. The mortality rates reported for total colectomy in patients with fulminant CDI have been invariably high in the range of 30 to 50%.[124] The poor outcomes are likely the result of delays in proceeding with surgery but need to be viewed in light of the high overall mortality rate associated with FC in general, estimated to be up to 80%.[125] Earlier surgical intervention and identification of the patient population that will fail medical management are the keys to improving surgical outcomes.[126]

13.4.2 The Role of Minimally Invasive Surgery

Patients who fail medical therapy require surgical management. Traditionally, patients who required surgery underwent emergent subtotal colectomy and end ileostomy formation.[127] Primary anastomosis in the setting of fulminant pancolitis is not considered safe due to the risk of anastomotic failure. Less invasive surgical options are being explored in hopes of improving the morbidity and mortality associated with severe CDI. Recently, an alternative surgical treatment with creation of a diverting loop ileostomy, followed by colonic lavage, has been shown to reduce morbidity and mortality, while preserving the colon. The surgical approach involves the laparoscopic creation of a diverting loop ileostomy. This case-controlled study at the University of Pittsburgh compared cases of FC treated with creation of a loop ileostomy to be used for intraoperative colonic lavage with warmed polyethylene glycol 3350/electrolyte solution and postoperative ante-grade vancomycin flushes to historical controls treated with total colectomy and end ileostomy.[69] This novel treatment strategy, which in the majority of cases was conducted laparoscopically, was performed in 42 patients and compared to 42 immediately preceding historical controls. It resulted in reduced mortality of 19 versus 50%, respectively, and preserved the colon in 39/42 patients; the mean time to resolution of white blood count (WBC) was 6 days. Three patients in the study subsequently required a total abdominal colectomy (▶ Fig. 13.5), either for abdominal compartment syndrome or continued sepsis. The author recommended caution in patients with abdominal compartment syndrome. The impressive series led the authors to state that this approach was beneficial in that the various teams would be less hesitant to proceed with surgery earlier in the disease course due to the lesser invasiveness and higher chance of avoiding a permanent ileostomy. It may represent a future treatment avenue for earlier in the disease course. However, the study warrants a critical examination as it has significant limitations which currently hinder broad application of its conclusions: the small study cohort, retrospective comparison to historical controls, and lack of randomization. As the patients were not randomly assigned, a selection and management bias cannot be ruled out, even though by numbers, the two groups appeared comparable. In fact, the authors themselves admit using this method earlier than colectomy because it is less invasive, suggesting that their cohort of patients was healthier than those undergoing colectomy. The 2015 practice

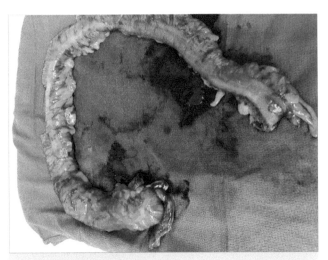

Fig. 13.5 A total abdominal colectomy in a patient with *C. difficile*.

parameter of the American Society of Colon and Rectal Surgeons considers the evidence on this surgical approach weak and recommends caution when contemplating its application.[128] Further studies and longitudinal data are required to validate this approach. In theory, it makes sense as the *Clostridium* spores can be washed away and then antibiotics are delivered topically to the area of concern.

13.4.3 Contraindications to an MIS Approach

Total abdominal colectomy with end ileostomy is the recommended standard approach. There are numerous reasons to perform this in an open rather than laparoscopic fashion: (1) to minimize the duration of the surgery in patients who are often unstable and coagulopathic; (2) because the colon is often enlarged and edematous, making it very heavy and difficult to handle; and (3) because fulminant *C. difficile* colitis and megacolon can prompt abdominal compartment syndrome, which is relieved by an open operation but can be aggravated by gas insufflation. If possible, the operation should aim at an early devascularization of the colon to shut off the systemic inflammatory response—an observation frequently seen but hard to prove in an objective fashion. The major vascular stalks are quickly identified, freed up, and devascularized with clamping and transection. The entire colon is then mobilized from its retroperitoneal attachments starting at the ileocecal junction. The bowel is transected with a linear stapler at the terminal ileum and at the rectosigmoid junction. An end ileostomy is created. The rectal stump may be tagged for later identification. Given that the inflammation commonly also affects the rectum, there is a risk of a rectal stump blowout, that is, leak from the staple line. Efforts to reduce that risk have not been studied but include a rectal washout with povidone–iodine solution or continued decompression of the blind Hartmann pouch for the first few days by means of a larger diameter rectal tube. Alternatively, the proximal end of the rectosigmoid can be brought out as a mucous fistula to the abdominal skin. Vancomycin enemas can be instilled in the rectal tube if there is a concern for continued infection in the rectum.[118]

13.4.4 Open Management Strategies

Currently, about 5% of patients infected with *C. difficile* reach the stage of FC and undergo surgery. The most evidence-based surgical procedure is a subtotal/total abdominal colectomy with end ileostomy and the goal to rapidly eliminate diseased colon without the challenge of a pelvic dissection. The rectal stump typically also harbors disease, but the risks associated with a proctocolectomy outweighs the benefits, and the rectum commonly clears the CDI. Vancomycin in liquid form may be used to perfuse the rectal stump if clinically indicated. Although selected patients are sometimes considered for segmental colectomy, or even defunctioning combined with intensive medical therapy, most authors advocate total or subtotal colectomy and ileostomy as the operation of choice.[129,130] It has been estimated that approximately 15.9% of patients need reoperation after a segmental colectomy to further reduce infected bowel.[131] Earlier surgical intervention is also associated with better results. An emergency colectomy for advanced

forms of *C. difficile* is associated with higher mortality rates. Al-Abed et al operated on 3.7% of his patients with an associated mortality rate of over 40%. The majority of patients who had significant comorbidities (75%) did not survive after an emergency colectomy. The 30-day mortality rate was 45.7%. Therefore, it is crucial to identify infected patients early, before they progress into FC and organ failure.

In the study by Koss et al, the nine patients who underwent total colectomy had a mortality rate of 11.1% compared with 100% in the four patients who underwent left hemicolectomy. One patient who underwent right hemicolectomy survived after a prolonged hospital stay.[127] In their study of 13 patients who underwent colectomy for CDI, Lipsett et al found that all four patients who underwent segmental colectomy died compared with 14% of the remainder who had a subtotal colectomy.[132] The authors emphasize that the external appearance of the colon may be deceptively normal despite severe mucosal disease, and this should not influence the decision to resect the entire colon. In the largest reported series of 73 patients with CDI undergoing colectomy, the mortality rates of patients who underwent segmental (n = 10) or subtotal (n = 63) colectomy was 10 versus 38%, respectively.[132,133]

13.4.5 The Management of Postoperative Complications

Operative consultation should be considered early in the course of severe and complicated CDI, as operative consultation may be beneficial.[134,135,136] High-mortality rates have been reported with operative treatment for CDI, which is likely related to significant delay in operative intervention,[118] but operative therapy for severe CDI can indeed be lifesaving. A systematic review of 510 patients with fulminant *C. difficile* colitis reported decreased mortality compared with operative treatment with medical therapy (RR 0.70, 95% CI 0.49–0.99).[137] Subtotal colectomy and end ileostomy with preservation of rectum has been recommended operative treatment, particularly for FC. A systematic review of 31 studies (n = 1442) of patients undergoing emergency operation for CDI documented that 1.1% of all patients with CDI and 29.9% with severe CDI underwent emergency operation. The most commonly performed operation was total colectomy with end ileostomy in 89% of patients. In patients who underwent partial colectomy, reoperation to resect additional colon was required in 15.9% of patients. Independent risk factors for mortality in patients who underwent colectomy which have been found among multiple studies include: the development of shock (need for vasopressors), increased serum lactate (≥ 5 mM), mental status changes, end organ failure, renal failure, and need for preoperative intubation and ventilation.[127,131,137,138] The more negative prognostic signs a patient has, the earlier surgical consultation and operative management should be considered.

A review of the Nationwide Inpatient Sample 2001–2010 documented over 2.7 million discharges with a diagnosis of CDI in the United States over this decade, and colectomy was performed in 19,374 cases (0.7%), with an associated mortality of 30.7%. Predictors of mortality after colectomy included coagulopathy, age > 60 years, acute renal failure, respiratory failure, sepsis, peripheral vascular disease, and congestive heart failure. Importantly, operative treatment more than 3 days after admission was associated with higher mortality rates.[139] Similarly, a review of the American College of Surgeons National Surgical Quality Improvement Program database from 2005–2010 identified 335 open colectomies for CDI with an overall mortality rate of 33% and a median time to death of 8 days. Risk factors for postoperative mortality included age > 80 years, preoperative shock, preoperative dialysis dependence, chronic obstructive pulmonary disease, thrombocytopenia, coagulopathy, and renal insufficiency.[140]

Recent experience with a minimally invasive, colon-preserving approach as an alternative to total colectomy has proven to be successful in select patients. Diverting loop ileostomy and colonic lavage followed by intravenous metronidazole and vancomycin administered via the efferent limb of the ileostomy (n = 42) is an accepted alternative to total colectomy in the treatment of severe complicated CDI with reduced mortality (19% vs. 50%) compared to a historical total colectomy cohort (n = 42) in a single-institution report.[69] This strategy led to colon preservation in 39/42 patients; three patients subsequently required total colectomy, either for abdominal compartment syndrome or continued sepsis. The advantage of this approach is that it can be considered early if patients are failing medical management, and it can be done laparoscopically in many patients. This approach, however, should not be considered in patients with abdominal compartment syndrome or concern for colonic ischemia, necrosis, or perforation.

The timing of surgical intervention is the key for survival of patients with FC.[135,141] Hall et al reviewed 3,237 consecutive cases of CDI and showed an increased mortality rate when surgical exploration was performed after intubation or the development of respiratory failure and the use of vasopressors. A systematic review and meta-analysis of outcomes following emergency surgery for C. difficile colitis was published by Bhangu et al.[131] Thirty-one studies were included, which presented data for 1433 patients undergoing emergency surgery for C. difficile colitis. It concluded that the strongest predictors for postoperative death were those relating to preoperative physiological status: preoperative intubation, acute renal failure, multiple organ failure, and shock requiring vasopressors. In the Bhangu et al. meta-analysis, the most commonly performed operation for treatment of FC was total colectomy with end ileostomy (89%, 1247/1401). When total colectomy with end ileostomy was not performed, reoperation to resect further bowel was needed in 15.9% (20/126). In the recent meta-analysis by Ferrada et al,[142] 17 studies comparing colectomy versus other procedures or no surgery as treatment for CDI were analyzed. The authors recommended that total colectomy (vs. partial colectomy or other surgery) is the procedure of choice for patients with C. *difficile* colitis.

13.4.6 Conclusion

The incidence and severity of CDI has seen a dramatic increase over the last decade in both the general population as well as in surgical patient populations, and CDI is becoming particularly more prevalent in high-risk groups such as inflammatory bowel disease patients. High-density healthcare, new bacteria strains, and antibiotic resistance may contribute to these trends. Surgical treatment is needed only for a fraction of all patients but should not be delayed when the disease is severe or fulminant. The decision making remains a clinical challenge because of the difficulty in determining the severity of disease and predicting the patient's response to medical versus surgical therapy. There is consensus that early surgical treatment, that is, before evidence of multiorgan failure, is associated with better outcomes, but more studies are needed to determine which patient populations will benefit most from an operation, much less which operation they should have and when they should have it. There are many novel treatment strategies emerging, but sound conclusions about the safety and efficacy of these treatments are limited because they have not been thoroughly studied.

References

[1] Bernell O, Lapidus A, Hellers G. Risk factors for surgery and postoperative recurrence in Crohn's disease. Ann Surg. 2000; 231(1):38–45

[2] Cosnes J, Nion-Larmurier I, Beaugerie L, Afchain P, Tiret E, Gendre JP. Impact of the increasing use of immunosuppressants in Crohn's disease on the need for intestinal surgery. Gut. 2005; 54(2):237–241

[3] Alós R, Hinojosa J. Timing of surgery in Crohn's disease: a key issue in the management. World J Gastroenterol. 2008; 14(36):5532–5539

[4] Bemelman WA, Warusavitarne J, Sampietro GM, et al. ECCO-ESCP Consensus on Surgery for Crohn's Disease. J Crohn's Colitis. 2018; 12(1):1–16

[5] Silverberg MS, Satsangi J, Ahmad T, et al. Toward an integrated clinical, molecular and serological classification of inflammatory bowel disease: report of a Working Party of the 2005 Montreal World Congress of Gastroenterology. Can J Gastroenterol. 2005; 19 Suppl A:5A–36A

[6] Fazio VW, Marchetti F, Church M, et al. Effect of resection margins on the recurrence of Crohn's disease in the small bowel. A randomized controlled trial. Ann Surg. 1996; 224(4):563–571, discussion 571–573

[7] Feagins LA, Holubar SD, Kane SV, Spechler SJ. Current strategies in the management of intra-abdominal abscesses in Crohn's disease. Clin Gastroenterol Hepatol. 2011; 9(10):842–850

[8] Garcia JC, Persky SE, Bonis PA, Topazian M. Abscesses in Crohn's disease: outcome of medical versus surgical treatment. J Clin Gastroenterol. 2001; 32 (5):409–412

[9] Laukoetter MG, Mennigen R, Hannig CM, et al. Intestinal cancer risk in Crohn's disease: a meta-analysis. J Gastrointest Surg. 2011; 15(4):576–583

[10] Cosnes J, Cattan S, Blain A, et al. Long-term evolution of disease behavior of Crohn's disease. Inflamm Bowel Dis. 2002; 8(4):244–250

[11] Muldoon R, Herline AJ. Crohn's disease: surgical management. In: The ASCRS Textbook of Colon and Rectal Surgery. Cham: Springer International Publishing; 2016:843–868

[12] Strong S, Steele SR, Boutrous M, et al. Clinical Practice Guidelines Committee of the American Society of Colon and Rectal Surgeons. Clinical practice guideline for the surgical management of Crohn's disease. Dis Colon Rectum. 2015; 58(11):1021–1036

[13] Ajlouni Y, Iser JH, Gibson PR. Endoscopic balloon dilatation of intestinal strictures in Crohn's disease: safe alternative to surgery. J Gastroenterol Hepatol. 2007; 22(4):486–490

[14] Lian L, Stocchi L, Remzi FH, Shen B. Comparison of endoscopic dilation vs surgery for anastomotic stricture in patients with Crohn's disease following ileocolonic resection. Clin Gastroenterol Hepatol. 2017; 15(8):1226–1231

[15] Lee EC, Papaioannou N. Minimal surgery for chronic obstruction in patients with extensive or universal Crohn's disease. Ann R Coll Surg Engl. 1982; 64 (4):229–233

[16] Yamamoto T, Fazio VW, Tekkis PP. Safety and efficacy of strictureplasty for Crohn's disease: a systematic review and meta-analysis. Dis Colon Rectum. 2007; 50(11):1968–1986

[17] Schwartz DA, Loftus EV, Jr, Tremaine WJ, et al. The natural history of fistulizing Crohn's disease in Olmsted County, Minnesota. Gastroenterology. 2002; 122(4):875–880

[18] Melton GB, Stocchi L, Wick EC, Appau KA, Fazio VW. Contemporary surgical management for ileosigmoid fistulas in Crohn's disease. J Gastrointest Surg. 2009; 13(5):839–845

[19] Poritz LS, Gagliano GA, McLeod RS, MacRae H, Cohen Z. Surgical management of entero and colocutaneous fistulae in Crohn's disease: 17 year's experience. Int J Colorectal Dis. 2004; 19(5):481–485, discussion 486

[20] Young-Fadok TM, Wolff BG, Meagher A, Benn PL, Dozois RR. Surgical management of ileosigmoid fistulas in Crohn's disease. Dis Colon Rectum. 1997; 40(5):558–561

[21] Simillis C, Purkayastha S, Yamamoto T, Strong SA, Darzi AW, Tekkis PP. A meta-analysis comparing conventional end-to-end anastomosis vs. other anastomotic configurations after resection in Crohn's disease. Dis Colon Rectum. 2007; 50(10):1674–1687

[22] Kornbluth A, Sachar DB, Practice Parameters Committee of the American College of Gastroenterology. Ulcerative colitis practice guidelines in adults: American College Of Gastroenterology, Practice Parameters Committee. Am J Gastroenterol. 2010; 105(3):501–523, quiz 524

[23] McIntyre PB, Powell-Tuck J, Wood SR, et al. Controlled trial of bowel rest in the treatment of severe acute colitis. Gut. 1986; 27(5):481–485

[24] Berg DF, Bahadursingh AM, Kaminski DL, Longo WE. Acute surgical emergencies in inflammatory bowel disease. Am J Surg. 2002; 184(1):45–51

[25] Tonelli F, Alemanno G, Di Martino C, Focardi A, Gronchi G, Giudici F. Results of surgical treatment for jejunal Crohn's disease: choice between resection, strictureplasty, and combined treatment. Langenbecks Arch Surg. 2017; 402 (7):1071–1078

[26] Tekkis PP, Purkayastha S, Lanitis S, et al. A comparison of segmental vs subtotal/total colectomy for colonic Crohn's disease: a meta-analysis. Colorectal Dis. 2006; 8(2):82–90

[27] Fazio VW, Ziv Y, Church JM, et al. Ileal pouch-anal anastomoses complications and function in 1005 patients. Ann Surg. 1995; 222(2):120–127

[28] Fazio VW, Kiran RP, Remzi FH, et al. Ileal pouch anal anastomosis: analysis of outcome and quality of life in 3707 patients. Ann Surg. 2013; 257(4): 679–685

[29] Rankin GB, Watts HD, Melnyk CS, Kelley ML, Jr. National Cooperative Crohn's Disease Study: extraintestinal manifestations and perianal complications. Gastroenterology. 1979; 77(4 Pt 2):914–920

[30] Gelbmann CM, Rogler G, Gross V, et al. Prior bowel resections, perianal disease, and a high initial Crohn's disease activity index are associated with corticosteroid resistance in active Crohn's disease. Am J Gastroenterol. 2002; 97(6):1438–1445

[31] Figg RE, Church JM. Perineal Crohn's disease: an indicator of poor prognosis and potential proctectomy. Dis Colon Rectum. 2009; 52(4):646–650

[32] Lewis RT, Bleier JI. Surgical treatment of anorectal crohn disease. Clin Colon Rectal Surg. 2013; 26(2):90–99

[33] Frolkis AD, Lipton DS, Fiest KM, et al. Cumulative incidence of second intestinal resection in Crohn's disease: a systematic review and meta-analysis of population-based studies. Am J Gastroenterol. 2014; 109(11):1739–1748

[34] Reese GE, Nanidis T, Borysiewicz C, Yamamoto T, Orchard T, Tekkis PP. The effect of smoking after surgery for Crohn's disease: a meta-analysis of observational studies. Int J Colorectal Dis. 2008; 23(12):1213–1221

[35] Avidan B, Sakhnini E, Lahat A, et al. Risk factors regarding the need for a second operation in patients with Crohn's disease. Digestion. 2005; 72(4): 248–253

[36] Yamamoto T, Umegae S, Matsumoto K. Impact of infliximab therapy after early endoscopic recurrence following ileocolonic resection of Crohn's disease: a prospective pilot study. Inflamm Bowel Dis. 2009; 15(10): 1460–1466

[37] Milsom JW, Lavery IC, Böhm B, Fazio VW. Laparoscopically assisted ileocolectomy in Crohn's disease. Surg Laparosc Endosc. 1993; 3(2):77–80

[38] Maartense S, Dunker MS, Slors JFM, et al. Laparoscopic-assisted versus open ileocolic resection for Crohn's disease: a randomized trial. Ann Surg. 2006; 243(2):143–149, discussion 150–153

[39] Dasari BV, McKay D, Gardiner K. Laparoscopic versus Open surgery for small bowel Crohn's disease. Cochrane Database Syst Rev. 2011(1):CD006956

[40] Holubar SD, Dozois EJ, Privitera A, et al. Laparoscopic surgery for recurrent ileocolic Crohn's disease. Inflamm Bowel Dis. 2010; 16(8):1382–1386

[41] Milsom JW, Hammerhofer KA, Böhm B, Marcello P, Elson P, Fazio VW. Prospective, randomized trial comparing laparoscopic vs. conventional surgery for refractory ileocolic Crohn's disease. Dis Colon Rectum. 2001; 44(1): 1–8, discussion 8–9

[42] Kirat HT, Pokala N, Vogel JD, Fazio VW, Kiran RP. Can laparoscopic ileocolic resection be performed with comparable safety to open surgery for regional enteritis: data from National Surgical Quality Improvement Program. Am Surg. 2010; 76(12):1393–1396

[43] Aarons CB. Laparoscopic surgery for crohn disease: a brief review of the literature. Clin Colon Rectal Surg. 2013; 26(2):122–127

[44] da Luz Moreira A, Stocchi L, Remzi FH, Geisler D, Hammel J, Fazio VW. Laparoscopic surgery for patients with Crohn's colitis: a case-matched study. J Gastrointest Surg. 2007; 11(11):1529–1533

[45] Umanskiy K, Malhotra G, Chase A, Rubin MA, Hurst RD, Fichera A. Laparoscopic colectomy for Crohn's colitis. A large prospective comparative study. J Gastrointest Surg. 2010; 14(4):658–663

[46] Heimann TM, Swaminathan S, Greenstein AJ, et al. Can laparoscopic surgery prevent incisional hernia in patients with Crohn's disease: a comparison study of 750 patients undergoing open and laparoscopic bowel resection. Surg Endosc. 2017; 31(12):5201–5208

[47] Aytac E, Stocchi L, Remzi FH, Kiran RP. Is laparoscopic surgery for recurrent Crohn's disease beneficial in patients with previous primary resection through midline laparotomy? A case-matched study. Surg Endosc Other Interv Tech. 2012; 26(12):3552–6

[48] Wu JS, Birnbaum EH, Kodner IJ, Fry RD, Read TE, Fleshman JW. Laparoscopic-assisted ileocolic resections in patients with Crohn's disease: are abscesses, phlegmons, or recurrent disease contraindications? Surgery. 1997; 122(4):682–688, discussion 688–689

[49] Hasegawa H, Watanabe M, Nishibori H, Okabayashi K, Hibi T, Kitajima M. Laparoscopic surgery for recurrent Crohn's disease. Br J Surg. 2003; 90(8): 970–973

[50] Holubar SD, Dozois EJ, Privitera A, et al. Laparoscopic surgery for recurrent ileocolic Crohn's disease. Inflamm Bowel Dis. 2010; 16(8):1382–1386

[51] Brouquet A, Bretagnol F, Soprani A, Valleur P, Bouhnik Y, Panis Y. A laparoscopic approach to iterative ileocolonic resection for the recurrence of Crohn's disease. Surg Endosc. 2010; 24(4):879–887

[52] Chaudhary B, Glancy D, Dixon AR. Laparoscopic surgery for recurrent ileocolic Crohn's disease is as safe and effective as primary resection. Colorectal Disease. 2002:(e-pub ahead of print)

[53] Pinto RA, Shawki S, Narita K, Weiss EG, Wexner SD. Laparoscopy for recurrent Crohn's disease: how do the results compare with the results for primary Crohn's disease? Colorectal Dis. 2011; 13(3):302–307

[54] Huang R, Valerian BT, Lee EC. Laparoscopic approach in patients with recurrent Crohn's disease. Am Surg. 2012; 78(5):595–599

[55] Gardenbroek TJ, Verlaan T, Tanis PJ, et al. Single-port versus multiport laparoscopic ileocecal resection for Crohn's disease. J Crohn's Colitis. 2013; 7 (10):e443–e448

[56] Rijcken E, Mennigen R, Argyris I, Senninger N, Bruewer M. Single-incision laparoscopic surgery for ileocolic resection in Crohn's disease. Dis Colon Rectum. 2012; 55(2):140–146

[57] Shaffer VO, Wexner SD. Surgical management of Crohn's disease. Langenbecks Arch Surg. 2013; 398(1):13–27

[58] Rencuzogullari A, Gorgun E, Costedio M, et al. Case-matched comparison of robotic versus laparoscopic proctectomy for inflammatory bowel disease. In: Surgical Laparoscopy, Endoscopy and Percutaneous Techniques. 2016

[59] Steele SR, Hull T, Read TE, Saclarides T, Senagore A, Whitlow C. (Eds.) The ASCRS Textbook of Colon and Rectal Surgery (3ed). Springer Publishing. New York, NY: 2016

[60] Travis SP, Farrant JM, Ricketts C, et al. Predicting outcome in severe ulcerative colitis. Gut. 1996; 38(6):905–910

[61] Bach SP, Mortensen NJ. Ileal pouch surgery for ulcerative colitis. World J Gastroenterol. 2007; 13(24):3288–3300

[62] Moskovitz DN, Van Assche G, Maenhout B, et al. Incidence of colectomy during long-term follow-up after cyclosporine-induced remission of severe ulcerative colitis. Clin Gastroenterol Hepatol. 2006; 4(6):760–765

[63] Campbell S, Travis S, Jewell D. Ciclosporin use in acute ulcerative colitis: a long-term experience. Eur J Gastroenterol Hepatol. 2005; 17(1):79–84

[64] Becker JM. Surgical therapy for ulcerative colitis and Crohn's disease. Gastroenterol Clin North Am. 1999; 28(2):371–390, viii-ix

[65] Parray FQ, Wani ML, Malik AA, et al. Ulcerative colitis: a challenge to surgeons. Int J Prev Med. 2012; 3(11):749–763

[66] Strong SA. Management of acute colitis and toxic megacolon. Clin Colon Rectal Surg. 2010; 23(4):274–284

[67] Cima RR, Pemberton JH. Surgical indications and procedures in ulcerative colitis. Curr Treat Options Gastroenterol. 2004; 7(3):181–190

[68] Rutter MD, Saunders BP, Wilkinson KH, Kamm MA, Williams CB, Forbes A. Most dysplasia in ulcerative colitis is visible at colonoscopy. Gastrointest Endosc. 2004; 60(3):334–339

[69] Neal MD, Alverdy JC, Hall DE, Simmons RL, Zuckerbraun BS. Diverting loop ileostomy and colonic lavage: an alternative to total abdominal colectomy for the treatment of severe, complicated Clostridium difficile associated disease. Ann Surg. 2011; 254(3):423–427, discussion 427–429

[70] Lashner BA, Turner BC, Bostwick DG, Frank PH, Hanauer SB. Dysplasia and cancer complicating strictures in ulcerative colitis. Dig Dis Sci. 1990; 35(3): 349–352

[71] Molodecky NA, Soon IS, Rabi DM, et al. Increasing incidence and prevalence of the inflammatory bowel diseases with time, based on systematic review. Gastroenterology. 2012; 142(1):46–54.e42, quiz e30

[72] Odze RD. Adenomas and adenoma-like DALMs in chronic ulcerative colitis: a clinical, pathological, and molecular review. Am J Gastroenterol. 1999; 94 (7):1746–1750

[73] Gorfine SR, Bauer JJ, Harris MT, Kreel I. Dysplasia complicating chronic ulcerative colitis: is immediate colectomy warranted? Dis Colon Rectum. 2000; 43(11):1575–1581

[74] Maartense S, Dunker MS, Slors JFM, Gouma DJ, Bemelman WA. Restorative proctectomy after emergency laparoscopic colectomy for ulcerative colitis: A case-matched study. Color Dis. 2004:(e-pub ahead of print)

[75] Telem DA, Vine AJ, Swain G, et al. Laparoscopic subtotal colectomy for medically refractory ulcerative colitis: The time has come. Surg Endosc Other Interv Tech. 2010; 24(7):1616–20

[76] Seshadri PA, Poulin EC, Schlachta CM, Cadeddu MO, Mamazza J. Does a laparoscopic approach to total abdominal colectomy and proctocolectomy offer advantages? Surg Endosc. 2001; 15(8):837–842

[77] Watanabe K, Funayama Y, Fukushima K, Shibata C, Takahashi K, Sasaki I. Hand-assisted laparoscopic vs. open subtotal colectomy for severe ulcerative colitis. Dis Colon Rectum. 2009; 52(4):640–645

[78] Marcello PW, Milsom JW, Wong SK, Brady K, Goormastic M, Fazio VW. Laparoscopic total colectomy for acute colitis: a case-control study. Dis Colon Rectum. 2001; 44(10):1441–1445

[79] McAllister I, Sagar PM, Brayshaw I, Gonsalves S, Williams GL. Laparoscopic restorative proctocolectomy with and without previous subtotal colectomy. Color Dis. 2009. DOI: 10.1111/j.1463-1318.2008.01590.x

[80] Holubar SD, Larson DW, Dozois EJ, Pattana-Arun J, Pemberton JH, Cima RR. Minimally invasive subtotal colectomy and ileal pouch-anal anastomosis for fulminant ulcerative colitis: a reasonable approach? Dis Colon Rectum. 2009; 52(2):187–192

[81] Buskens CJ, Sahami S, Tanis PJ, Bemelman WA. The potential benefits and disadvantages of laparoscopic surgery for ulcerative colitis: A review of current evidence. Best Pract Res Clin Gastroenterol. 2014; 28(1):19–27

[82] Geisler DP, Kirat HT, Remzi FH. Single-port laparoscopic total proctocolectomy with ileal pouch-anal anastomosis: Initial operative experience. Surg Endosc Other Interv Tech. 2011; 25:2175

[83] Bulian DR, Knuth J, Krakamp B, Heiss MM. Restorative restproctectomy as single-port surgery through the ostomy site in a three-stage procedure. Surg Endosc Other Interv Tech. 2012; 26(12):3688–90

[84] Gash KJ, Goede AC, Kaldowski B, Vestweber B, Dixon AR. Single incision laparoscopic (SILS) restorative proctocolectomy with ileal pouch-anal anastomosis. Surg Endosc. 2011; 25(12):3877–3880

[85] Pedraza R, Patel CB, Ramos-Valadez DI, Haas EM. Robotic-assisted laparoscopic surgery for restorative proctocolectomy with ileal J pouch-anal anastomosis. Minim Invasive Ther Allied Technol. 2011; 20(4):234–239

[86] Fung AKY, Aly EH. Robotic colonic surgery: is it advisable to commence a new learning curve? Dis Colon Rectum. 2013; 56(6):786–796

[87] Ooi BS, Remzi FH, Fazio VW. Turnbull-Blowhole colostomy for toxic ulcerative colitis in pregnancy: report of two cases. Dis Colon Rectum. 2003; 46 (1):111–115

[88] Crile G, Jr, Thomas CY, Jr. The treatment of acute toxic ulcerative colitis by ileostomy and simultaneous colectomy. Gastroenterology. 1951; 19 (1):58–68

[89] Alves A, Panis Y, Bouhnik Y, Maylin V, Lavergne-Slove A, Valleur P. Subtotal colectomy for severe acute colitis: a 20-year experience of a tertiary care center with an aggressive and early surgical policy. J Am Coll Surg. 2003; 197(3):379–385

[90] Turnbull RB, Jr. Surgical treatment of ulcerative colitis: early results after colectomy and low ileorectal anastomosis. Dis Colon Rectum. 1959; 2(3): 260–263

[91] Parks AG, Nicholls RJ. Proctocolectomy without ileostomy for ulcerative colitis. BMJ. 1978; 2(6130):85–88

[92] Camilleri-Brennan J, Steele RJ. Objective assessment of quality of life following panproctocolectomy and ileostomy for ulcerative colitis. Ann R Coll Surg Engl. 2001; 83(5):321–324

[93] Mortier PE, Gambiez L, Karoui M, et al. Colectomy with ileorectal anastomosis preserves female fertility in ulcerative colitis. Gastroenterol Clin Biol. 2006; 30(4):594–597

[94] Steele SR, Hull T, Read TE, Saclarides T, Senagore A, Whitlow C. (Eds.) The ASCRS Textbook of Colon and Rectal Surgery (3ed). Springer Publishing. New York, NY: 2016

[95] Vignolo Q. Nouveau procede operatoire pour retablir la continuite intestinale dans les resections rectosigmoidiennes etendues. Arch Gen Chir. 1912; 6:621–43

[96] Fazio VW, Kiran RP, Remzi FH, et al. Ileal pouch anal anastomosis: analysis of outcome and quality of life in 3707 patients. Ann Surg. 2013; 257 (4):679–685

[97] Prudhomme M, Dozois RR, Godlewski G, Mathison S, Fabbro-Peray P. Anal canal strictures after ileal pouch-anal anastomosis. Dis Colon Rectum. 2003; 46(1):20–23

[98] Lewis WG, Kuzu A, Sagar PM, Holdsworth PJ, Johnston D. Stricture at the pouch-anal anastomosis after restorative proctocolectomy. Dis Colon Rectum. 1994; 37(2):120–125

[99] Remzi FH, Aytac E, Ashburn J, et al. Transabdominal redo ileal pouch surgery for failed restorative proctocolectomy: lessons learned over 500 patients. In: Annals of Surgery; 2015

[100] Shen B. Acute and chronic pouchitis–pathogenesis, diagnosis and treatment. Nat Rev Gastroenterol Hepatol. 2012; 9(6):323–333

[101] Shen B, Lashner BA. Diagnosis and treatment of pouchitis. Gastroenterol Hepatol (N Y). 2008; 4(5):355–361

[102] Holubar SD, Cima RR, Sandborn WJ, Pardi DS. Treatment and prevention of pouchitis after ileal pouch-anal anastomosis for chronic ulcerative colitis. Cochrane Database Syst Rev. 2010(6):CD001176

[103] Barreiro-de Acosta M, García-Bosch O, Gordillo J, et al. Grupo Joven GETECCU. Efficacy of adalimumab rescue therapy in patients with chronic refractory pouchitis previously treated with infliximab: a case series. Eur J Gastroenterol Hepatol. 2012; 24(7):756–758

[104] Johnson P, Richard C, Ravid A, et al. Female infertility after ileal pouch-anal anastomosis for ulcerative colitis. Dis Colon Rectum. 2004; 47(7):1119–1126

[105] Badger VO, Ledeboer NA, Graham MB, Edmiston CE. Clostridium difficile: Epidemiology, pathogenesis, management, and prevention of a recalcitrant healthcare-associated pathogen. J Parenter Enter Nutr. 2012; 36(6):645–62

[106] Barbut F, Jones G, Eckert C. Epidemiology and control of Clostridium difficile infections in healthcare settings: an update. Curr Opin Infect Dis. 2011; 24 (4):370–376

[107] Cohen SH, Gerding DN, Johnson S, et al. Society for Healthcare Epidemiology of America, Infectious Diseases Society of America. Clinical practice guidelines for Clostridium difficile infection in adults: 2010 update by the Society for Healthcare Epidemiology of America (SHEA) and the Infectious Diseases Society of America (IDSA). Infect Control Hosp Epidemiol. 2010; 31(5):431–455

[108] Clements AC, Magalhães RJS, Tatem AJ, Paterson DL, Riley TV. Clostridium difficile PCR ribotype 027: assessing the risks of further worldwide spread. Lancet Infect Dis. 2010; 10(6):395–404

[109] Jobe BA, Grasley A, Deveney KE, Deveney CW, Sheppard BC. Clostridium difficile colitis: an increasing hospital-acquired illness. Am J Surg. 1995; 169 (5):480–483

[110] Gebhard RL, Gerding DN, Olson MM, et al. Clinical and endoscopic findings in patients early in the course of clostridium difficile-associated pseudomembranous colitis. Am J Med. 1985; 78:45–48

[111] Bartlett JG, Gerding DN. Clinical recognition and diagnosis of Clostridium difficile infection. Clin Infect Dis. 2008; 46 Suppl 1:S12–S18

[112] Stanley JD, Bartlett JG, Dart BW, IV, Ashcraft JH. Clostridium difficile infection. Curr Probl Surg. 2013; 50(7):302–337

[113] Rubin MS, Bodenstein LE, Kent KC. Severe Clostridium difficile colitis. Dis Colon Rectum. 1995; 38(4):350–354

[114] Kyne L, Merry C, O'Connell B, Kelly A, Keane C, O'Neill D. Factors associated with prolonged symptoms and severe disease due to Clostridium difficile. Age Ageing. 1999; 28(2):107–113

[115] Bartlett JG. Clinical practice. Antibiotic-associated diarrhea. N Engl J Med. 2002; 346(5):334–339

[116] Hu MY, Katchar K, Kyne L, et al. Prospective derivation and validation of a clinical prediction rule for recurrent Clostridium difficile infection. Gastroenterology. 2009; 136(4):1206–1214

[117] Drekonja DM, Butler M, MacDonald R, et al. Comparative effectiveness of Clostridium difficile treatments: a systematic review. Ann Intern Med. 2011; 155(12):839–847

[118] Kazanowski M, Smolarek S, Kinnarney F, Grzebieniak Z. Clostridium difficile: epidemiology, diagnostic and therapeutic possibilities-a systematic review. Tech Coloproctol. 2014; 18(3):223–232

[119] Morris JB, Zollinger RM, Jr, Stellato TA. Role of surgery in antibiotic-induced pseudomembranous enterocolitis. Am J Surg. 1990; 160(5):535–539

[120] Olson MM, Shanholtzer CJ, Lee JT, Jr, Gerding DN. Ten years of prospective Clostridium difficile-associated disease surveillance and treatment at the Minneapolis VA Medical Center, 1982–1991. Infect Control Hosp Epidemiol. 1994; 15(6):371–381

[121] Pasic M, Jost R, Carrel T, Von Segesser L, Turina M. Intracolonic vancomycin for pseudomembranous colitis. N Engl J Med. 1993; 329(8):583

[122] Gerding DN, Muto CA, Owens RCJ, Jr. Treatment of Clostridium difficile infection. Clin Infect Dis. 2008; 46 Suppl 1:S32–S42

[123] Kaiser AM, Hogen R, Bordeianou L, Alavi K, Wise PE, Sudan R. Clostridium difficile infection from a surgical perspective. J Gastrointest Surg. 2015; 19(7):1363–77

[124] Dudukgian H, Sie E, Gonzalez-Ruiz C, Etzioni DA, Kaiser AM. C. difficile colitis–predictors of fatal outcome. J Gastrointest Surg. 2010; 14(2):315–322

[125] Butala P, Divino CM. Surgical aspects of fulminant Clostridium difficile colitis. Am J Surg. 2010; 200(1):131–135

[126] Ofosu A. Clostridium difficile infection: a review of current and emerging therapies. Ann Gastroenterol. 2016; 29(2):147–54

[127] Koss K, Clark MA, Sanders DSA, Morton D, Keighley MRB, Goh J. The outcome of surgery in fulminant Clostridium difficile colitis. Colorectal Dis. 2006; 8(2):149–154

[128] Steele SR, McCormick J, Melton GB, et al. Practice parameters for the management of Clostridium difficile infection. Dis Colon Rectum. 2015; 58(1):10–24

[129] Jaber MR, Olafsson S, Fung WL, Reeves ME. Clinical review of the management of fulminant clostridium difficile infection. Am J Gastroenterol. 2008; 103(12):3195–3203, quiz 3204

[130] Byrn JC, Maun DC, Gingold DS, Baril DT, Ozao JJ, Divino CM. Predictors of mortality after colectomy for fulminant Clostridium difficile colitis. Arch Surg. 2008; 143(2):150–154, discussion 155

[131] Bhangu A, Nepogodiev D, Gupta A, Torrance A, Singh P. Systematic review and meta-analysis of outcomes following emergency surgery for Clostridium difficile colitis. Br J Surg. 2012; 99:1501–1513

[132] Lipsett PA, Samantaray DK, Tam ML, Bartlett JG, Lillemoe KD. Pseudomembranous colitis: a surgical disease? Surgery. 1994; 116(3):491–496

[133] Ash L, Baker ME, O'Malley CMJr, Gordon SM, Delaney CP, Obuchowski NA. Colonic abnormalities on CT in adult hospitalized patients with Clostridium difficile colitis: prevalence and significance of findings. AJR Am J Roentgenol. 2006; 186(5):1393–1400

[134] Synnott K, Mealy K, Merry C, Kyne L, Keane C, Quill R. Timing of surgery for fulminating pseudomembranous colitis. Br J Surg. 1998; 85(2):229–231

[135] Osman KA, Ahmed MH, Hamad MA, Mathur D. Emergency colectomy for fulminant Clostridium difficile colitis: striking the right balance. Scand J Gastroenterol. 2011; 46(10):1222–1227

[136] Napolitano LM, Edmiston CE, Jr. Clostridium difficile disease: diagnosis, pathogenesis, and treatment update. Surgery. 2017; 162(2):325–348

[137] Stewart DB, Hollenbeak CS, Wilson MZ. Is colectomy for fulminant Clostridium difficile colitis life saving? A systematic review. Colorectal Dis. 2013; 15(7):798–804

[138] Longo WE, Mazuski JE, Virgo KS, Lee P, Bahadursingh AN, Johnson FE. Outcome after colectomy for Clostridium difficile colitis. Dis Colon Rectum. 2004; 47(10):1620–1626

[139] Halabi WJ, Nguyen VQ, Carmichael JC, Pigazzi A, Stamos MJ, Mills S. Clostridium difficile colitis in the United States: a decade of trends, outcomes, risk factors for colectomy, and mortality after colectomy. J Am Coll Surg. 2013; 217(5):802–812

[140] Lee DY, Chung EL, Guend H, Whelan RL, Wedderburn RV, Rose KM. Predictors of mortality after emergency colectomy for Clostridium difficile colitis: an analysis of ACS-NSQIP. Ann Surg. 2014; 259(1):148–156

[141] Hall JF, Berger D. Outcome of colectomy for Clostridium difficile colitis: a plea for early surgical management. Am J Surg. 2008; 196(3):384–388

[142] Ferrada P, Velopulos CG, Sultan S, et al. Timing and type of surgical treatment of Clostridium difficile-associated disease: a practice management guideline from the Eastern Association for the Surgery of Trauma. J Trauma Acute Care Surg. 2014; 76(6):1484–1493

**Expert Commentary on
Inflammatory/Infectious
Bowel Disease by
Formosa Chen and Clifford Y. Ko

Expert Commentary on Inflammatory/Infectious Bowel Disease

Formosa Chen and Clifford Y. Ko

To Operate or Not to Operate

The indications for surgery in Crohn's disease may be succinctly described as patients who "fail medical management" or "develop complications." However, accepting failure and determining the optimal timing and choice of intervention is more difficult. Less invasive modalities may have high-success rates, but surgical treatment can lead to more durable palliation. The complexity of these decisions is further compounded by the patient's clinical condition, as well as the multidisciplinary expertise and resources available. Consequently, algorithms that are shown to be effective in the literature may not be borne out in the experience of individual surgeons and institutions.

This complexity in decision-making also applies to ulcerative colitis. When patients present with absolute surgical indications—toxic megacolon and generalized peritonitis—the answer is straightforward: stabilize the patient and proceed to emergent surgical exploration. However, when patients are clinically stable or chronically indolent, the decision to operate is less binary. In young patients with physiologic reserve, selecting the surgical procedure is easy. But with increasing numbers of biologic treatment options, surgery can often be overly delayed. On the other hand, in older patients with significant medical comorbidities, how do surgeons balance the likelihood of poor functional outcomes against the patient's desire for intestinal continuity?

In *Clostridium difficile*, colitis mortality is high for emergent surgical intervention, possibly because we proceed to the operating room too late. And yet the very factors that drive the decision toward surgery—the patient's preoperative physiologic status—are the very predictors of mortality. Patients who are not in extremis may have salvageable colons. But patients, who demonstrate through clinical signs the strong need for surgery, are often the ones who are no longer salvageable. The decision to operate is indeed a catch 22 situation.

Unfortunately, even a textbook on surgical decision-making that comprehensively outlines the relevant data about these complex diseases cannot entirely answer the question that all surgical trainees will ask, "when do we operate?" There are no one-size-fits-all answers. However, our decision-making may be optimized in several ways. One, thoughtful discussion with other surgeons to elicit real-time feedback on our thought processes and decisions. This may take the form of a casual discussion with a trusted colleague or seeking guidance from a faculty member to better understand the nuances of their decision-making. Second, timely and open multidisciplinary communication to best understand the patient's clinical context and trajectory. With inflammatory bowel disease, close working relationships with gastroenterologists can often lead to better coordination of care and timely intervention. With critically ill patients, frequent dialogue with infectious disease and critical care specialists can better ensure aggressive antibiotic therapy, adequate resuscitation, as well as improved patient selection for surgery. Third, early engagement and active participation in treatment decision-making, even when there is no clear surgical indication, can often improve outcomes. At times, it is the development of longitudinal relationships with patients that leads to appropriate expectations and increased patient satisfaction. At other times, seemingly minor decisions such as the selection of diagnostic testing, decisions made well before surgical indications are apparent, can influence downstream outcomes. Finally, a patient-centered approach that considers not only the patient's clinical condition but also their values and preferences will help physicians balance the risks and benefits of these challenging decisions.

What trainees need to acquire is an *approach* to complex decision-making. A systematic way to evaluate patients, thoroughly understand their clinical context and surgical candidacy, thoughtfully weigh the risks and benefits of treatment options and, with the aid of multidisciplinary expertise, arrive at patient-centered decisions.

14 Gastroduodenal Ulcers Requiring Surgery

Robert D. Winfield and Marie L. Crandall

Summary

Complicated gastroduodenal ulcers are decreasing in incidence but carry high morbidity and mortality risks. Whether complicated by hemorrhage or perforation, acute care surgeons must be well-versed in management principles, particularly when operative interventions are required and the options that exist. This chapter outlines the pathophysiology of peptic ulcer disease, presentations seen in disease complicated by hemorrhage or perforation, nonoperative, and operative management strategies for complicated disease, and postoperative care. Special attention is paid to endoscopic, vascular interventional radiologic, and minimally invasive surgical approaches for disease management.

Keywords: Peptic ulcer disease, upper gastrointestinal hemorrhage, perforated peptic ulcer

14.1 Introduction

Complicated peptic ulcer disease (PUD; defined for these purposes as a bleeding or perforated gastric or duodenal ulcer) has decreased in incidence over the last three decades.[1] In spite of this, the development of complicated ulcer disease continues to lead to substantial morbidity and mortality.[2] While relatively uncommon in economically developed nations, complicated peptic ulcer disease is frequently seen in low- and middle-income countries, and represents a major contributor to the global burden of surgical disease.[3] Given the ongoing impact of complicated peptic ulcer disease, an understanding of this disease process and surgical remedies is essential for acute care surgeons.

14.2 Risk Factors for Peptic Ulcer Disease

The understanding of PUD changed dramatically in 1982 when Marshall and Warren linked the discovery of *Helicobacter pylori* to the development of gastritis and PUD.[4] This connection and the subsequent ability to treat the disease with antibiotics, along with the discovery of effective gastric acid-blocking agents (selective histamine blockers and proton pump inhibitors,[5,6]), addressed two of the major risk factors for PUD. While *H. pylori* infection and acid secretion are important to the pathophysiology of de novo PUD development and provide good rationale for the medical management of uncomplicated PUD, there are a series of relatively common patient factors that may lead to PUD, including smoking, nonsteroidal anti-inflammatory drug (NSAID) use, steroid use, excessive alcohol consumption, and use of vasoactive illicit drugs (cocaine, methamphetamine).[3] In critically ill patient populations, stress ulcers may manifest in patients who are coagulopathic or require mechanical ventilation, but patients at risk for perturbances of gastric perfusion (hypotensive secondary to burn, sepsis, or trauma) or disruption of vagal input to the stomach (traumatic brain injury) are also at risk. Although rare,

the hypersecretory effects of a gastrinoma (Zollinger–Ellison syndrome) may lead to ulcer development, and should be considered in any patient with recurrent PUD in the setting of optimal medical therapy.[7]

14.3 Disease Presentation

The classic presentation of uncomplicated PUD is that of gnawing epigastric discomfort that improves (duodenal) or worsens (gastric) with food intake. This history may be obtained in patients presenting with complicated PUD, but the most common presentation of perforated PUD is acute onset of severe epigastric pain. Depending on the duration of symptoms, the patient may have progressed to diffuse abdominal pain or generalized peritonitis. Valentino's syndrome is an atypical presentation of perforated PUD in which the patient develops focal right lower quadrant peritonitis secondary to tracking of gastric contents or succus through the retroperitoneum.[8] In addition to the abdominal examination findings, the patients may present with signs of septic shock. Patients with actively bleeding PUD may present with hematemesis or brisk melena, and depending on the rate and duration of hemorrhage, signs of hypovolemic shock include absolute or relative hypotension, tachycardia, oliguria and, in severe cases, obtundation.

14.4 Diagnosis

The diagnosis can frequently be made through the taking of a thorough history and completion of an appropriate physical examination, focusing on the risk factors and classic and atypical presentations of complicated PUD. For perforated PUD, there is a relatively broad differential to include inflammation or perforation of any portion of the gastrointestinal (GI) tract, biliary disease, intra-abdominal vascular catastrophes (aneurysm, occlusion, etc.) and, in less common presentations, renal infection or calculus disease. The differential in hemorrhagic PUD is more straightforward, although obtaining a history of vascular disease and interventions would be of a particularly critical nature, as an aortoenteric fistula would present in a similar fashion. A history of malignancy or cirrhosis has prognostic value, suggesting early need for endoscopy,[9] and also of potential etiology of upper gastrointestinal hemorrhage. Depending on the patient's condition at presentation, additional workup may be a luxury as opposed to a necessity as empiric intervention may be necessary; however, in a patient with relative stability, additional diagnostic testing may help the surgeon in focusing on complicated PUD as the etiology for the patient's state of health.

In general, a complete blood count will provide useful information on the patient with complicated PUD and may point to the need for transfusion of blood or platelets. A metabolic panel can provide some evidence of the patient's severity of illness, with the creatinine possibly showing evidence of acute kidney injury. An arterial or venous pH can point to the degree of resuscitation needed, as can a measurement of base deficit. For patients with signs of sepsis, initiation of the guidelines provided through the

Table 14.1 Surviving sepsis campaign recommendations for care within 1 hour of suspected sepsis

Measure lactate; remeasure if initial lactate is >2 millimoles/liter

Obtain blood cultures prior to administration of antibiotics

Administer broad-spectrum antibiotics

Begin rapid administration of 30 mL/kg crystalloid for hypotension or lactate > 4 mmol/liter.

Apply vasopressors if patient is hypotensive during or after fluid resuscitation to maintain mean arterial pressure ≥ 65 mm Hg.

Adapted from Rhodes et al.[10]

surviving sepsis campaign (SSC)[10] is advised (▶ Table 14.1). From a diagnostic standpoint, this will include a lactate level and blood cultures within one hour of the identification of suspected sepsis. For patients presenting with significant hemorrhage, traditional measures of coagulation can be useful in prognosis, as the presence of coagulopathy (INR > 1.5) has been associated with a five-fold increase in risk of mortality. Viscohemoelastic assay measurements (thromboelastography or rotational thromboelastometry) can be considered for guidance in appropriate blood component resuscitation and may suggest the need for transfusion of plasma, cryoprecipitate, or platelets.

In the case of perforated PUD, an upright chest or abdominal radiograph may demonstrate the presence of free air under the diaphragm, and with a suggestive history and physical examination, this has a diagnostic sensitivity of 75%.[11] Without obvious peritonitis and free air on an upright chest X-ray, many patients will be diagnosed by an abdominal CT scan with a sensitivity of 98%.[11] Abdominal CT findings may include a variety of features pointing to perforated PUD, including retroperitoneal and/or intraperitoneal free air and fluid, as well as inflammation of the stomach or duodenum.

The patient with hemorrhagic PUD will likely be suspected clinically with significant hemorrhage presenting as hematemesis or melena. Placement of a nasogastric (NG) tube may reveal bright red blood in the aspirate, but the absence of blood is not diagnostic, as up to 15% of patients with nonbloody aspirate have subsequently been found to have a significant upper GI lesion.[12] Endoscopy is the gold standard for diagnosis, and as will be discussed subsequently, the first line for management of hemorrhagic PUD. While use of CT angiography has been described in the diagnosis of upper gastrointestinal hemorrhage,[13] its primary role appears to be in patients with presumed lower gastrointestinal hemorrhage, or in those who have undergone upper and lower endoscopy without identification of a source.[14]

14.5 Management of Complicated Peptic Ulcer Disease

As diagnostic and therapeutic modalities evolve and change, it is in many ways appropriate to pursue the least invasive method for caring for patients with diseases traditionally managed surgically. That said, in the setting of complicated PUD, the acute care surgeon will be well-served by an approach that incorporates a healthy skepticism for the role of completely nonoperative management (NOM) and thorough knowledge of the indications and contraindications for minimally invasive and traditional approaches.

For patients with either perforated or hemorrhagic PUD, good general management principles should be employed. Identification of disease and severity should be both prompted by and consist of regular hemodynamic (blood pressure and heart rate) and pulmonary monitoring with pulse oximetry at a minimum. Ensuring adequate intravenous access for fluid and blood products should be an early priority. NG decompression should be employed and bladder catheterization can be utilized to continuously monitor urine output. As before, patients with signs of sepsis (most often perforated PUD) should be managed according to SSC guidelines. Those in hemorrhagic shock (hemorrhagic PUD) may benefit from early activation of institutional massive transfusion protocols and whole blood or balanced component therapy resuscitation guided by viscohemoelastic assay, but the benefits of these maneuvers are as yet unproven in this setting.[15]

Most patients with perforated PUD will require operative intervention. Understanding that this is a case of critical importance, as prompt operative care is critical for patient survival, each hour of delay to operation confers a 2.4% increase in mortality.[3] For patient and family counseling regarding mortality, a series of scoring systems have been developed specific to patients with perforated peptic ulcer.[16] In reviewing these scoring systems, Thorsen et al found that none performed better than an assessment that included age, active malignancy, delay from admission to surgery >24 hours, hyperbilirubinemia, increased creatinine, as well as hypoalbuminemia.[17] The authors further stated that hypoalbuminemia alone was the strongest predictor of 30-day mortality among studied variables and performed nearly as well as existing scoring systems. Although not specific to perforated PUD, the emergency surgery score (ESS) shows high-reliability in prediction of both complication rates and mortality in patients with emergent surgical conditions, and can also be considered for use in preoperative counseling.[18]

Appropriate preoperative setup in coordination with anesthesia providers will help in ensuring as smooth a procedure as possible. Preoperative placement of a footboard to allow the reverse Trendelenburg positioning permits gravity to facilitate exploration. A self-retaining retractor can likewise be helpful, particularly to retract the liver in addition to the abdominal wall. When the diagnosis is unclear, and particularly in the setting of sepsis with shock, exploratory laparotomy through a vertical midline incision would be the approach taken by the majority of surgeons. Rapid identification of the perforation and control of ongoing contamination is the initial goal of surgical intervention. The surgeon will generally first encounter a large amount of bilious or bile-tinged fluid, sometimes with succus or purulence, and occasionally a pneumoperitoneum is found. The most common site for an ulcer is the anterior surface of the duodenum or stomach, but the area should be fully explored, sometimes requiring Kocherization of the duodenum and/or mobilization of the stomach to visualize the posterior surface and greater and lesser curves, to determine the extent of the pathology. Any evidence of chronic inflammation should be noted and the size of the ulcer measured.

Once an ulcer has been identified, the surgeon should be prepared to perform a variety of repair or resective options. The standard approaches in a solitary ulcer of 2 cm diameter or less include primary closure, closure with an omental patch, or placement of an omental patch alone. In patients in whom a pedicled omental patch is not possible, a falciform patch may serve as an alternative.[19] A biopsy is not required on a routine basis in these circumstances; however, if malignancy is suspected (particularly in gastric ulcers), patients should undergo follow-up endoscopy at 6 weeks to evaluate for occult malignancy, which occurs in about 13% of cases.[20] Finally, there is no clear consensus as to whether postoperative drainage is necessary. Pai and colleagues performed a prospective controlled study comparing 44 patients undergoing drainage following duodenal ulcer repair with omental patch to 75 patients not undergoing drainage, finding drains to be ineffective in decreasing abscess formation.[21] More recently, Okumura et al performed a retrospective evaluation of a large Japanese database containing patients undergoing perforated peptic ulcer repair, using propensity score matching to compare patients receiving and not receiving drains.[22] They found that the drain group had a significantly lower risk of postoperative interventions relative to those patients who were undrained at the time of surgery. Depending on the clinical state of the patient, the surgeon may consider placement of a nasojejunal tube past the area of repair to facilitate postoperative nutritional supplementation; however, this is based on anecdotal experience and is not evidence-based practice.

In patients with ulcers larger than 2 cm, or in ulcers that are particularly friable, the surgeon may need to consider resection. Prior to doing this, though, the larger size or friable state of the ulcer should raise suspicion for the presence of malignancy and a biopsy is indicated. The resection performed is frequently dictated by the type and location of the ulcer as well as the relative stability of the patient with regard to sepsis (▶ Fig. 14.1). Type I ulcers occur on or near the lesser curvature. While theoretically, wedge resections are possible, they may be technically challenging due to the presence of the gastroepiploic vessels and resultant distortion of the gastric anatomy on reconstruction, particularly if a resection with margins is required. As such, large Type I ulcers require a distal gastrectomy with Billroth I (BI) or Roux-en-Y (RNY) reconstruction with or without vagotomy, depending on patient factors that will be discussed subsequently. A Billroth II (BII) reconstruction can be performed as well, but this comes with an increase in the risk of bile gastritis development for the patient. Type II ulcers consist of two separate ulcers, with one being near the lesser curvature of the stomach and the second being on the duodenum. In this case, as the duodenum is affected by the disease, a proximal duodenectomy is performed in addition to distal gastrectomy, with RNY reconstruction being the preferred

Ulcer type	Location	Recommended surgical approaches
Type I	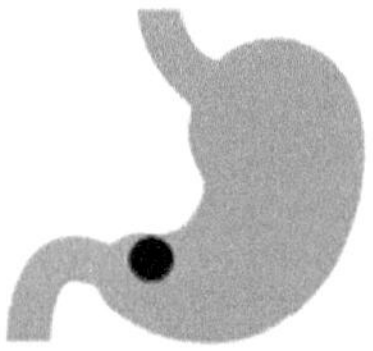	Wedge resection for smaller ulcers, distal gastrectomy with Billroth I or Roux-en-Y reconstruction for larger lesions.
Type II	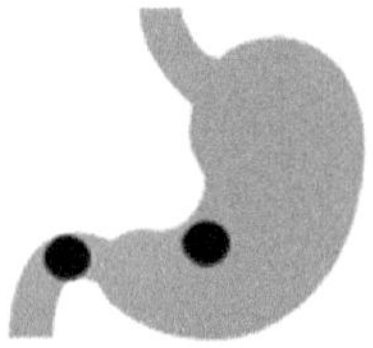	Distal gastrectomy and duodenectomy with Billroth I or Roux-en-Y reconstruction.
Type III	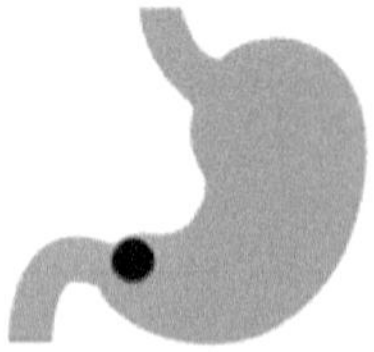	Antrectomy with Billroth I or Roux-en-Y reconstruction.
Type IV	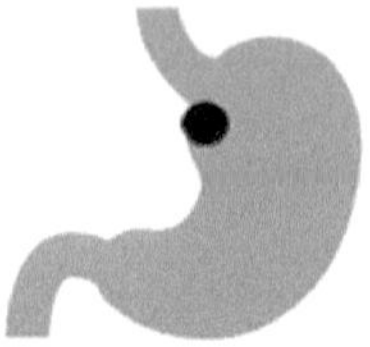	Wedge resection if esophagogastric anatomy permits, otherwise subtotal gastrectomy with Roux-en-Y reconstruction.

Fig. 14.1 Types of peptic ulcer.

method over BII. Type III ulcers are prepyloric in location. These can be managed with wedge resection and closure if possible, but will frequently require antrectomy with BI and RNY reconstructions with or without vagotomy. Type IV ulcers are in the proximal stomach. Once again, wedge resections may be possible, but care must be taken to avoid a closure that occludes the gastroesophageal junction. If this is the case, a subtotal gastrectomy with RNY esophagogastrojejunostomy may be required. Finally, giant duodenal ulcers can be particularly challenging to manage. Omental patch techniques are much more likely to leak in the setting of these large ulcers, occurring up to 12% of the time.[23] If the patient is unstable or has limited reconstruction options secondary to prior surgery or aberrant anatomy, wide external drainage with "triple tube" treatment consisting of Stamm gastrostomy, retrograde duodenostomy, and feeding jejunostomy can be employed. In more stable patients, a series of possibilities exist, including an RNY duodenojejunostomy, pedicled jejunal graft, or jejunal serosal patch. All are subject to significant rates of leakage and, thus, external drainage of the repair is recommended.

For Types I to III ulcers, acid hypersecretion is implicated in the disease pathogenesis and, thus, the surgeon is faced with the question of whether to conduct a procedure to address acid secretion. In the setting of a large, perforated ulcer, this will consist of some form of partial gastrectomy with truncal vagotomy. With a smaller ulcer amenable to primary or patch repair in some form, parietal cell vagotomy can be considered as an adjunct. These procedures should not be performed routinely due to greater associated perioperative morbidity;[24] however, in patients with a known or strongly suspected history of medical noncompliance or failed maximal medical management, it is suggested that these procedures be considered, depending on the comfort and experience of the surgeon with their performance.

Minimally invasive techniques have gained traction in the care of the patient with perforated PUD over the last decade, with up to 46% of patients having been treated with laparoscopy in recent series.[11] The use of laparoscopy has been described since 1996, with Sø et al reporting a series of 53 consecutive patients with perforated duodenal ulcers, 15 of whom were managed with laparoscopic omental patch.[25] The authors reported that 14 patients were successfully managed via the laparoscopic approach and that analgesia was improved relative to patients undergoing open omental patch, albeit at the expense of increased operative time. Katkhouda and colleagues performed a prospective, nonrandomized clinical trial of laparoscopic versus open omental patch repair, finding shorter length of stay and decreased analgesia requirements in patients undergoing laparoscopy, but once again demonstrated a significant increase in operative time.[26] Importantly, the authors reported that five of the 30 patients in the laparoscopic group underwent conversion to open surgery, and that these patients were more likely to have presented with shock or symptoms of greater than 24 hours duration. In a Cochrane review and meta-analysis comparing laparoscopic and open surgery for perforated PUD, results were generally felt to be equivalent, and laparoscopic approaches trended toward reduced septic abdominal complications, but the authors concluded that larger randomized controlled trials were necessary to confirm the findings.[27] A more recent meta-analysis by Cirocchi et al identified laparoscopic surgery as having significant association with decreased perioperative pain (over the first 24 hours) and postoperative wound infection.[28] The authors found no difference in

mortality, reoperation, leak, abscess development, length of stay, or time to return of diet and overall report an equivalence in most outcome parameters. In summary, laparoscopic approach to perforated PUD appears to be as safe as open surgery in experienced hands and may confer some advantages over open repair; however, this field continues to evolve, and new data will continue to clarify the role of laparoscopy in the management of perforated PUD.

While laparoscopy has gained acceptance, it is worth mentioning that natural orifice transluminal endoscopic surgery (NOTES) has also been proposed and examined as a means of treating perforated PUD. Bonin and colleagues reported in a series of 104 patients with perforated PUD treated at the Mayo Clinic that 52% were potential candidates for a NOTES approach based on having undergone omental patch closure of a perforated ulcer and having no contraindications to laparoscopy or endoscopy.[29] Bingener et al followed this with a pilot series of two patients (from 17 consecutive patients presenting with perforated PUD) who were successfully treated using an approach consisting of laparoscopic visualization, accompanied by endoscopic retrieval of an omental pedicle, for plugging of the ulcer.[30] The authors reported negative contrast studies following the procedure and discharge on postoperative days 3 and 4. While this has not gained broad acceptance and needs additional study, this may represent a new way of managing perforated PUD in the future.

When considering patients for laparoscopic management, no clear evidence-based guidance exists regarding selection criteria. In a systematic review, Lunevicius et al point out that prolonged peritonitis may be a more dangerous scenario in which to perform laparoscopy secondary to concerns for increased bacteremia, sepsis, and pulmonary complications; however, the authors point out that this supposition is derived from animal modeling and has not been demonstrated clinically.[31] Urbano et al suggested in their series of six patients treated laparoscopically that open surgery should be used in high-risk patients, but provided no justification for this recommendation.[32] The World Society for Emergency Surgery's 2013 position paper on this topic suggests a series of reasonable recommendations for the use of laparoscopy in the setting of perforated PUD, which is summarized in ► Table 14.2.[33]

Table 14.2 Recommendations from the World Society of Emergency Surgery on the use of laparoscopy in the management of perforated peptic ulcer

We recommend laparoscopic approach to hemodynamically stable patients with free air at X-ray and/or CT for diagnostic purposes.

We suggest laparoscopic repair of PPU in stable patients with PPU < 5 mm in size and in presence of appropriate laparoscopic skills.

We recommend laparoscopy for achieving a better intraperitoneal lavage, even in the presence of diffuse peritonitis.

We suggest that laparoscopy may improve patients' outcome with significantly lower morbidity.

We recommend open surgery in presence of septic shock or in patients with absolute contraindications for pneumoperitoneum.

We suggest open surgery in presence of perforated and bleeding peptic ulcers, unless in stable patients with minor bleeding and in the presence of advanced laparoscopic suturing skills

Abbreviations: CT, computed tomography; PPU, perforated peptic ulcer.
Adapted from Di Saverio et al.[33]

Perioperative planning for a laparoscopic approach is overall similar to the open approach described previously. Positioning may be different depending on the planned placement of trocars and the comfort of the surgeon. Two different trocar positions are depicted in ▶ Fig. 14.2, although these may be modified, depending on patient anatomy or habitus and surgeon comfort. The operating surgeon may choose to stand to the patient's right side, in which case the patient should be positioned supine with a footboard (**2A**), or between the patient's legs, in which case they should be positioned in low lithotomy with the feet in stirrups (**2B**). An additional port may be placed with either configuration to allow use of a fan-blade liver retractor for improved exposure. The choice of entry technique should be based on surgeon comfort, as no difference has consistently been demonstrated in complication rate with either Veress needle insertion or Hasson technique.[34] The patient should be placed in the reverse Trendelenburg position to facilitate visualization of the stomach and duodenum. After a diagnostic laparoscopy is performed to confirm the diagnosis, the surgeon may proceed with identification and management of the ulcer. While sutureless repair with a gelfoam and fibrin glue plug has been described,[35] leak rates are significantly higher with this approach[36] and a sutured repair is generally indicated. A variety of management techniques have been described that generally consist of primary closure with or without omental patch, with proponents and doubters for each.[37,38,39] Lo et al examined laparoscopic primary closure alone

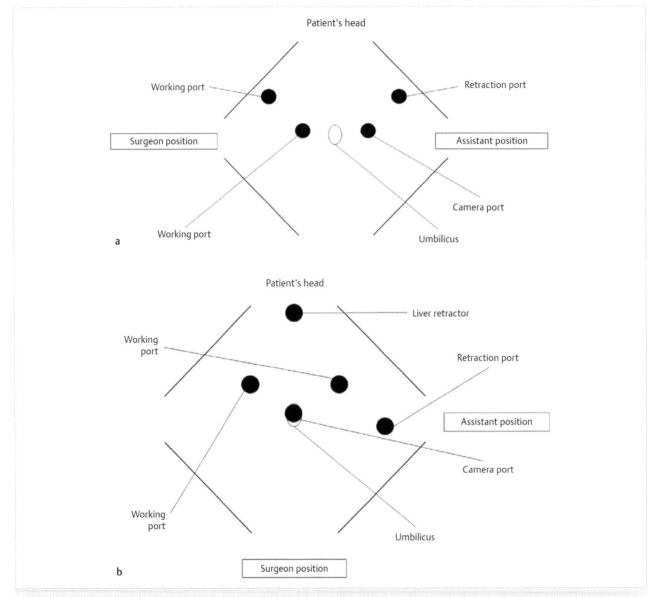

Fig. 14.2 Laparoscopic trocar configurations for the management of perforated peptic ulcer disease. **(a)** The patient is positioned supine with the surgeon to the patient's right and assistant to the left. The surgeon utilizes two working ports in the right upper quadrant, while the assistant operates the camera and retracts with ports in the left upper quadrant. **(b)** The patient is positioned in lithotomy with the surgeon standing between the patient's legs. Working ports are placed in the left and right upper quadrants. The assistant is positioned to the patient's left, operating the camera through a periumbilical port and retracting through a left lower quadrant port. An optional liver retractor may be placed in the epigastrium as needed.

Table 14.3 The Blatchford score for upper gastrointestinal hemorrhage

Variable	Value	Score
Blood urea (millimoles/Liter)	6.5–7.9	2
	8.0–9.9	3
	10.0–25.0	4
	>25.0	6
Hemoglobin (men, grams/Liter)	120–129	1
	100–119	3
	<100	6
Hemoglobin (women, grams/Liter)	100–119	1
	<100	6
Systolic blood pressure (millimeters mercury)	100–109	1
	90–99	2
	<90	3
Other markers	Pulse ≥ 100/minute	1
	Presentation with melena	1
	Presentation with syncope	2
	Hepatic disease*	2
	Cardiac failure**	2

*Known history of or clinical/laboratory evidence of chronic or acute liver disease.
**Known history of or clinical/echocardiographic evidence of cardiac failure.
A score of 6 or more is associated with a greater than 50% risk of needing endoscopic intervention.
Adapted from Blatchford et al.[44]

to primary closure with omental patch, finding no difference in patient outcome.[40] While the data are not complete, the closure technique (if done in a technically sound way) will lead to reasonable outcomes comparable with the variety of other techniques employed. Finally, washout should be performed to complete the procedure prior to closure, and intraoperative cultures sent to guide subsequent antibiotic therapy. As with open intervention, there is no consensus as to whether drainage is required and is up to surgeon discretion.

NOM of perforated PUD is generally not indicated due to the consequences of delayed intervention; however, this may be employed in the correct clinical scenario. A patient with minimal symptomatology and imaging demonstrating a contained perforation is a candidate for NOM, but this should only be considered if the patient is in a setting where he or she can be continuously monitored for signs and symptoms of deterioration and undergo serial abdominal examinations by a surgeon immediately available to intervene. Anecdotally, recommended management would include NG decompression, *nil per os*(NPO), intravenous proton pump inhibitor, and subsequent oral contrast study; however, no published data exists to support the efficacy and timing of these practices. In a single institution retrospective series, Cao et al examined 241 consecutive patients presenting with perforated PUD, finding that 107 were able to be managed nonoperatively using a combination of clinical and radiologic features.[41] Factors associated with successful nonoperative care included age younger than 70, absence of fluid collection detectable by ultrasound, absence of contrast leak on water-soluble contrast study, and APACHE II score of less than 8. Endoscopic stenting of perforated duodenal ulcers has been performed; however, the published data on this method is limited to a single, eight patient series by Bergstrom.[42] It is worth noting that the authors reported successful management in seven of the patients in

their series but, for now, this would be recommended only for unusual circumstances when an experienced and highly skilled endoscopist is available and willing, and would not be considered standard of care for perforated PUD.

14.6 Management of Hemorrhagic Peptic Ulcer Disease

In contradistinction to perforated PUD, the vast majority of hemorrhagic PUD is managed nonoperatively.[43] The primary initial dilemma for the treating provider is to determine the timing of endoscopy for diagnosis and treatment. Patients with severe hemorrhage should undergo immediate endoscopy, while those with less clinically significant hemorrhage may be deferred, even to outpatient management. The Blatchford score (► Table 14.3) can be used to effectively risk stratify patients and can be quickly calculated using standard clinical variables.[44] If a patient is determined to have a clinically significant risk of severe hemorrhage, the immediate addition of proton pump inhibitors to the management principles highlighted previously is indicated secondary to a significant reduction in need for endoscopic therapy, although this has not been conclusively shown to improve other clinically significant outcomes.[45] Overall, the goal for patients with evidence of active hemorrhage and instability should be urgent endoscopy, with early endoscopy (occurring within 24 hours) showing outcome benefit.[46] An area of controversy for the patient undergoing urgent endoscopy is whether prophylactic intubation is indicated to prevent the complication and sequelae of aspiration. The literature is not clear on this matter, with a retrospective series by Rehman and colleagues demonstrating no significant outcome differences in patients receiving and not receiving prophylactic intubation.[47]

Table 14.4 The Forrest classification for endoscopic findings in hemorrhagic peptic ulcer disease

Endoscopic finding	Forrest Classification
Active bleeding	Ia (brisk bleeding)
	Ib (oozing)
Nonbleeding visible vessel	IIa
Adherent clot	IIb
Flat spot	IIc (pigmentation)
Clean base	III
Adapted from Forrest et al.[50]	

A subsequent propensity-matched study by Hayat et al found prophylactic intubation to be associated with an increased risk of cardiopulmonary events.[48] A more recently published series of critically ill patients at Baylor University undergoing upper endoscopy found that aspiration events occurred in 38% of prophylactically intubated patients, suggesting that intubation may not provide the protective effect desired.[49] These conflicting data demonstrate that prophylactic intubation is not clearly beneficial, and should be used at the provider's discretion after considering the specific details of the patient's situation.

On endoscopy, the Forrest classification (▶ Table 14.4) has traditionally been used to guide endoscopic treatment and provides a prognosis for risk of repeat hemorrhage.[50] Forrest III lesions are considered low-risk, and require no endoscopic intervention.[51] Forrest I and II lesions are moderate to high risk for repeat hemorrhage without intervention, and endoscopic therapy is indicated. In general, endoscopic therapy can be classified as injection, thermal, and mechanical. Endoscopist discretion is generally used to guide the method chosen; however, clear evidence exists demonstrating that injection monotherapy is inadequate to prevent repeat hemorrhage, and that use of injection plus a second modality has a beneficial effect on mortality.[52] A recent Cochrane analysis suggests that mechanical therapy is the most appropriate second modality but that thermal methods are also effective.[53] That said, no benefit has been shown for dual therapy in this manner when compared to thermal or mechanical monotherapy.

While endoscopic methods are highly effective when carried out by expert endoscopists, repeat hemorrhage rates are not inconsequential, with recurrent hemorrhage occurring in up to 10% of patients treated with endoscopy and postprocedural proton pump inhibition.[54,55] While routine reevaluation with endoscopy is not indicated,[56] repeat endoscopy may be performed in patients with recurrent hemorrhage with good success rates.[57,58] In a randomized, controlled trial, patients with ulcers larger than 2 cm or repeat hemorrhage with hypotension suggested probable failure for additional endoscopic treatments.[58] Coagulopathy and hemoglobin of less than 10 mg/dL have also been shown to correlate with endoscopic failure.[59] For those patients with ongoing hemorrhage, where the technology and expertise are available, arterial embolization may be considered as an alternative to surgery. An audit of the 2007 United Kingdom National Health Service database conducted in 2012 evaluated cases of acute upper GI hemorrhage, assessing 163 cases of recurrent hemorrhage undergoing surgery or transcatheter embolization, finding an overall mortality of 23.2% but a decrease in mortality for embolization (10%) when compared to surgery (29%).[59] A more recent meta-analysis comparing these two techniques showed a trend toward improved mortality and significant reduction in complications for embolization, somewhat tempered by a worsened rate of rebleeding, and greater requirement for further intervention in this group.[60] It should be noted that the existing literature on the role of transcatheter embolization is limited to one prospective cohort study and a variety of retrospective series, so the role of embolization relative to the standard of surgical management for refractory hemorrhage is still yet to be determined. Nonetheless, current data suggests that embolization is reasonable in this scenario, providing a less-invasive option with equivalent, if not improved, effects on mortality.

Whether due to failure of, or unavailability of, less-invasive forms of management, surgery remains an effective means of treating hemorrhagic PUD. Minimally invasive techniques are generally not recommended for patients with hemorrhage due to difficulties with lesion identification as well as poor visualization in the setting of ongoing hemorrhage. As such, operative management is generally done via laparotomy. As with perforated PUD, supine positioning of the patient with a footboard to allow the reverse Trendelenburg positioning is advised. In these cases, it is further recommended that an endoscope be available in the room to aid in identification of the lesion, although this is not mandatory. Resection is the mainstay of treatment for hemorrhagic gastric ulcers, as malignancy is a significant concern, even in the setting of a benign-appearing lesion.[61] Resections are carried out based on location, as described above, for perforated PUD. In the event that resection is not an option, gastrotomy may be performed and the bleeding vessel oversewn. Again, due to the risk of malignancy, it is critical that biopsies are taken of the ulcer if this approach is utilized.

For hemorrhagic duodenal ulcers, the standard approach is to perform a longitudinal duodenotomy that includes division of the pylorus. This will expose the posterior wall of the duodenum, where the vessel can be identified. The primary culprit vessel is the gastroduodenal artery (GDA). The GDA is controlled by utilizing suture ligation proximally and distally (recalling that there is extensive collateral blood flow to the duodenum, and backbleeding can be an issue) along with a U-stitch deep to the ulcer to control transverse pancreatic branches. The longitudinal enterotomy is then closed transversely, completing a Heineke-Mikuliczpyloroplasty. As covered in the discussion of perforated PUD, in patients with a known or strongly suspected history of medical noncompliance or who have previously failed maximal medical management, a vagotomy should be considered. Furthermore, in this patient population, vagotomy may be associated with a decrease in mortality.[24]

14.7 Postoperative Management of Complicated Peptic Ulcer Disease

As these patients frequently present in a compromised state, it is not unusual that they will have ongoing critical care needs; however, intensive care unit placement should be at the discretion of the treating providers and based on the patient's perioperative and postoperative state. Sepsis should be treated according to SSC guidelines with ongoing anti-infective therapy guided by cultures. While concern frequently exists for the presence of fungal species (present in up to 63% of intraoperative cultures[62]), the role for antifungal therapy appears to be limited to those who are critically ill or are otherwise immune suppressed. In a retrospective review of 107 patients with perforated ulcer, Horn et al showed that Candida species were isolated in 52% of peritoneal cultures, but that the addition of antifungal therapy in the perioperative period made no difference in patient outcome[63] regardless of fungal isolate. Likewise, Li and colleagues looked at 133 patients of whom 57 patients received antifungal treatment postoperatively, and regardless of the presence of Candida in intraoperative cultures, no outcome differences were seen between those patients and patients not receiving antifungal therapy.[64] Given the known role of *Helicobacter pylori* in ulcer pathogenesis, all patients should undergo testing for *H. pylori* antigen as per their institutional regimen. A positive test should lead to therapy with a regimen consisting of acid suppression and appropriate eradicative antibiotic administration (▶ Table 14.5).

Frequently, physicians will perform postoperative upper gastrointestinal series to assess for leak. While this is common practice, no data that we are aware of support the routine use of this imaging study, and as such it may be used (or not used) at the surgeon's discretion. As mentioned previously, upper endoscopy should be performed at 6 weeks following surgery in the setting of gastric ulcers in which biopsies have not been performed due to the risk of malignancy.[20]

In select patients with perforated PUD, an enhanced recovery after surgery (ERAS) pathway may be used. Mohsina and colleagues performed a prospective randomized, controlled trial of 149 patients with perforated PUD, comparing patients enrolled in an ERAS pathway to those receiving standard care.[65] Patients were excluded for refractory shock, American Society of Anesthesiologists (ASA) class ≥ 3, and perforation ≥ 1 cm. Fifty patients were randomized to ERAS (components in ▶ Table 14.6), and

Table 14.5 FDA-approved treatment options for H. pylori infection

Omeprazole 40 mg daily + clarithromycin 500 mg three times daily × 14 days, then omeprazole 20 mg daily × 14 days

Ranitidine 400 mg twice daily + clarithromycin 500 mg three times daily × 14 days, then ranitidine 400 mg twice daily × 14 days

Bismuth subsalicylate 525 mg four times daily + metronidazole 250 mg four times daily + tetracycline 500 mg four times daily × 14 days + H$_2$-receptor antagonist therapy × 28 days

Lansoprazole 30 mg twice daily + amoxicillin 1 gram twice daily + clarithromycin 500 mg three times daily × 10 days

Lansoprazole 30 mg three times daily + amoxicillin 1 gram three times daily × 14 days

Ranitidine 400 mg twice daily + clarithromycin 500 mg twice daily × 14 days, then ranitidine 400 mg twice daily × 14 days

Omeprazole 20 mg twice daily + clarithromycin 500 mg twice daily + amoxicillin 1 gram twice daily × 10 days

Lansoprazole 30 mg twice daily + clarithromycin 500 mg twice daily + amoxicillin 1 gram twice daily × 10 days

Adapted from https://www.cdc.gov/ulcer/files/hpfacts.pdf

Table 14.6 Components of adapted ERAS pathway following surgery for perforated peptic ulcer

Component	Treatment
Preoperative care	Nonopioid multimodal analgesia (IV acetaminophen andlumbar epidural analgesia)
	Opioids for breakthrough pain
Intraoperative care	Avoidance of benzodiazepines, morphine, and nitrous oxide
	Short acting opioids and anesthetic agents when necessary
	Epidural lidocaine in patients with epidural catheters
Postoperative care	Nonopioid multimodal analgesia
	POD#0– IV diclofenac 75 mg IV BID
	POD#1– IV diclofenac 75 mg IV PRN
	POD#2– oral acetaminophen 500 TID
	POD#3– oral acetaminophen prn and break through opioids PRN
	Epidural bupivacaine infusion for 24 hours postoperatively
	Opioids for breakthrough pain
Adjuvant medication	POD#0 and 1–IV metoclopramide 10 mg TID
	PPI–IV or oral
Antibiotics	IV ceftriaxone and metronidazole x 5 days (oral if discharged prior to POD#5)
Mobilization	Ambulate POD#0
Tubes and drains	Urinary catheter withdrawn when urine output 1 mL/kg/hr for 24 hours
	Drains– when drainage ≤ 100 mL/day
	NG tube– when drainage ≤ 300 mL/day
Resumption of oral feeds	NPO until ileus resolution (based on presence of bowel sounds), then liquid diet to be advanced as tolerated within 24 hours

Abbreviations: NG, nasogastric, NPO, nil per os.
Adapted from Mohsinaet al.[65]

these individuals were found to have a shorter time to flatus, bowel movement, diet initiation, and hospital length of stay. Outcomes were notable for an ERAS group reduction in superficial surgical site infection (SSI), postop nausea and vomiting, and pulmonary complications. The confirmation of the benefits of this pathway and the development of standard perioperative management for patients with complicated PUD is an area in need of further investigation.

14.8 Conclusion

While the incidence of complicated PUD has decreased with improvements in medical management, the morbidity and mortality of this condition has remained unaffected by these advancements. Because of this, the acute care surgeon must be familiar with the management of patients with bleeding or perforated peptic ulcers. While medical management of these conditions can be utilized during appropriate scenarios, prompt surgical attention remains a critical element in the care of these patients, and it is crucial that the acute care surgeon be prepared to perform a variety of interventions based on preoperative planning and intraoperative findings. Minimally invasive techniques show promise in the care of patients with perforated PUD, but the indications must be known and carefully considered, and the surgeon embarking on minimally invasive management of a perforation must be sound in both judgment and technical ability.

References

[1] Bashinskaya B, Nahed BV, Redjal N, Kahle KT, Walcott BP. Trends in peptic ulcer disease and the identification of helicobacter pylori as a causative organism: population-based estimates from the US nationwide inpatient sample. J Glob Infect Dis. 2011; 3(4):366–370

[2] Sonnenberg A. Time trends of ulcer mortality in Europe. Gastroenterology. 2007; 132(7):2320–2327

[3] Søreide K, Thorsen K, Harrison EM, et al. Perforated peptic ulcer. Lancet. 2015; 386(10000):1288–1298

[4] Marshall BJ, Warren JR. Unidentified curved bacilli in the stomach of patients with gastritis and peptic ulceration. Lancet. 1984; 1(8390):1311–1315

[5] Deakin M, Williams JG. Histamine H2-receptor antagonists in peptic ulcer disease. Efficacy in healing peptic ulcers. Drugs. 1992; 44(5):709–719

[6] Lin HJ. Role of proton pump inhibitors in the management of peptic ulcer bleeding. World J GastrointestPharmacolTher. 2010; 1(2):51–53

[7] Epelboym I, Mazeh H. Zollinger-Ellison syndrome: classical considerations and current controversies. Oncologist. 2014; 19(1):44–50

[8] Amann CJ, Austin AL, Rudinsky SL. Valentino's syndrome: a life-threatening mimic of acute appendicitis. ClinPract Cases Emerg Med. 2017; 1 (1):44–46

[9] Adamopoulos AB, Baibas NM, Efstathiou SP, et al. Differentiation between patients with acute upper gastrointestinal bleeding who need early urgent upper gastrointestinal endoscopy and those who do not. A prospective study. Eur J GastroenterolHepatol. 2003; 15(4):381–387

[10] Rhodes A, Evans LE, Alhazzani W, et al. Surviving sepsis campaign: International Guidelines for Management of Sepsis and Septic Shock: 2016. Intensive Care Med. 2017; 43(3):304–377

[11] Thorsen K, Glomsaker TB, von Meer A, Søreide K, Søreide JA. Trends in diagnosis and surgical management of patients with perforated peptic ulcer. J GastrointestSurg. 2011; 15(8):1329–1335

[12] Aljebreen AM, Fallone CA, Barkun AN. Nasogastric aspirate predicts high-risk endoscopic lesions in patients with acute upper-GI bleeding. GastrointestEndosc. 2004; 59(2):172–178

[13] Miyaoka Y, Amano Y, Ueno S, et al. Role of enhanced multi-detector-row computed tomography before urgent endoscopy in acute upper gastrointestinal bleeding. J GastroenterolHepatol. 2014; 29(4):716–722

[14] Geffroy Y, Rodallec MH, Boulay-Coletta I, Jullès MC, Ridereau-Zins C, Zins M. Multidetector CT angiography in acute gastrointestinal bleeding: why, when, and how. Radiographics. 2011; 31(3):E35–E46

[15] Sommer N, Schnüriger B, Candinas D, Haltmeier T. Massive transfusion protocols in nontrauma patients: A systematic review and meta-analysis. J Trauma Acute Care Surg. 2019; 86(3):493–504

[16] Thorsen K, Søreide JA, Søreide K. Scoring systems for outcome prediction in patients with perforated peptic ulcer. Scand J Trauma ResuscEmerg Med. 2013; 21:25

[17] Thorsen K, Søreide JA, Søreide K. What is the best predictor of mortality in perforated peptic ulcer disease? A population-based, multivariable regression analysis including three clinical scoring systems. J GastrointestSurg. 2014; 18 (7):1261–1268

[18] Nandan AR, Bohnen JD, Sangji NF, et al. The Emergency Surgery Score (ESS) accurately predicts the occurrence of postoperative complications in emergency surgery patients. J Trauma Acute Care Surg. 2017; 83(1): 84–89

[19] Boshnaq M, Thakrar A, Martini I, Doughan S. Utilisation of the falciform ligament pedicle flap as an alternative approach for the repair of a perforated gastric ulcer. BMJ Case Rep. 2016:2016

[20] Kumar P, Khan HM, Hasanrabba S. Treatment of perforated giant gastric ulcer in an emergency setting. World J GastrointestSurg. 2014; 6(1):5–8

[21] Pai D, Sharma A, Kanungo R, Jagdish S, Gupta A. Role of abdominal drains in perforated duodenal ulcer patients: a prospective controlled study. Aust N Z J Surg. 1999; 69(3):210–213

[22] Okumura K, Hida K, Kunisawa S, et al. Impact of drain insertion after perforated peptic ulcer repair in a Japanese nationwide database analysis. World J Surg. 2018; 42(3):758–765

[23] Jani K, Saxena AK, Vaghasia R. Omental plugging for large-sized duodenal peptic perforations: A prospective randomized study of 100 patients. South Med J. 2006; 99(5):467–471

[24] Schroder VT, Pappas TN, Vaslef SN, De La Fuente SG, Scarborough JE. Vagotomy/drainage is superior to local oversew in patients who require emergency surgery for bleeding peptic ulcers. Ann Surg. 2014; 259(6): 1111–1118

[25] Sø JB, Kum CK, Fernandes ML, Goh P. Comparison between laparoscopic and conventional omental patch repair for perforated duodenal ulcer. SurgEndosc. 1996; 10(11):1060–1063

[26] Katkhouda N, Mavor E, Mason RJ, Campos GM, Soroushyari A, Berne TV. Laparoscopic repair of perforated duodenal ulcers: outcome and efficacy in 30 consecutive patients. Arch Surg. 1999; 134(8):845–848, discussion 849–850

[27] Sanabria A, Villegas MI, Morales Uribe CH. Laparoscopic repair for perforated peptic ulcer disease. Cochrane Database Syst Rev. 2013(2):CD004778

[28] Cirocchi R, Soreide K, Di Saverio S, et al. Meta-analysis of perioperative outcomes of acute laparoscopic versus open repair of perforated gastroduodenal ulcers. J Trauma Acute Care Surg. 2018; 85(2):417–425

[29] Bonin EA, Moran E, Gostout CJ, McConico A, Zielinski M, Bingener J. Natural orifice transluminal endoscopic surgery for patients with perforated peptic ulcer. SurgEndosc. 2012; 26(6):1534–1538

[30] Bingener J, Loomis EA, Gostout CJ, et al. Feasibility of NOTES omental plug repair of perforated peptic ulcers: results from a clinical pilot trial. SurgEndosc. 2013; 27(6):2201–2208

[31] Lunevicius R, Morkevicius M. Systematic review comparing laparoscopic and open repair for perforated peptic ulcer. Br J Surg. 2005; 92(10):1195–1207

[32] Urbano D, Rossi M, De Simone P, Berloco P, Alfani D, Cortesini R. Alternative laparoscopic management of perforated peptic ulcers. SurgEndosc. 1994; 8 (10):1208–1211

[33] Di Saverio S, Bassi M, Smerieri N, et al. Diagnosis and treatment of perforated or bleeding peptic ulcers: 2013 WSES position paper. World J EmergSurg. 2014; 9:45

[34] Ahmad G, Baker J, Finnerty J, Phillips K, Watson A. Laparoscopic entry techniques. Cochrane Database Syst Rev. 2019; 1:CD006583

[35] Lau WY, Leung KL, Kwong KH, et al. A randomized study comparing laparoscopic versus open repair of perforated peptic ulcer using suture or sutureless technique. Ann Surg. 1996; 224(2):131–138

[36] Lee FY, Leung KL, Lai PB, Lau JW. Selection of patients for laparoscopic repair of perforated peptic ulcer. Br J Surg 2001; 88(1):133–136

[37] Siu WT, Leong HT, Li MK. Single stitch laparoscopic omental patch repair of perforated peptic ulcer. J R CollSurgEdinb. 1997; 42(2):92–94

[38] Song KY, Kim TH, Kim SN, Park CH. Laparoscopic repair of perforated duodenal ulcers: the simple "one-stitch" suture with omental patch technique. SurgEndosc. 2008; 22(7):1632–1635

[39] Ates M, Sevil S, Bakircioglu E, Colak C. Laparoscopic repair of peptic ulcer perforation without omental patch versus conventional open repair. J LaparoendoscAdvSurg Tech A. 2007; 17(5):615–619

[40] Lo HC, Wu SC, Huang HC, Yeh CC, Huang JC, Hsieh CH. Laparoscopic simple closure alone is adequate for low risk patients with perforated peptic ulcer. World J Surg. 2011; 35(8):1873–1878

[41] Cao F, Li J, Li A, Fang Y, Wang YJ, Li F. Nonoperative management for perforated peptic ulcer: who can benefit? Asian J Surg. 2014; 37(3):148–153

[42] Bergström M, Arroyo Vázquez JA, Park PO. Self-expandable metal stents as a new treatment option for perforated duodenal ulcer. Endoscopy. 2013; 45(3): 222–225

[43] Wang YR, Richter JE, Dempsey DT. Trends and outcomes of hospitalizations for peptic ulcer disease in the United States, 1993 to 2006. Ann Surg. 2010; 251(1):51–58

[44] Blatchford O, Murray WR, Blatchford M. A risk score to predict need for treatment for upper-gastrointestinal haemorrhage. Lancet. 2000; 356(9238): 1318–1321

[45] Sreedharan A, Martin J, Leontiadis GI, et al. Proton pump inhibitor treatment initiated prior to endoscopic diagnosis in upper gastrointestinal bleeding. Cochrane Database Syst Rev. 2010(7):CD005415

[46] Barkun AN, Bardou M, Kuipers EJ, et al. International Consensus Upper Gastrointestinal Bleeding Conference Group. International consensus recommendations on the management of patients with nonvariceal upper gastrointestinal bleeding. Ann Intern Med. 2010; 152(2):101–113

[47] Rehman A, Iscimen R, Yilmaz M, et al. Prophylactic endotracheal intubation in critically ill patients undergoing endoscopy for upper GI hemorrhage. GastrointestEndosc. 2009; 69(7):e55–e59

[48] Hayat U, Lee PJ, Ullah H, Sarvepalli S, Lopez R, Vargo JJ. Association of prophylactic endotracheal intubation in critically ill patients with upper GI bleeding and cardiopulmonary unplanned events. GastrointestEndosc. 2017; 86(3): 500–9–.–e1

[49] Perisetti A, Kopel J, Shredi A, Raghavapuram S, Tharian B, Nugent K. Prophylactic pre-esophagogastroduodenoscopy tracheal intubation in patients with upper gastrointestinal bleeding. ProcBaylUniv Med Cent. 2019; 32(1):22–25

[50] Forrest JA, Finlayson ND, Shearman DJ. Endoscopy in gastrointestinal bleeding. Lancet. 1974; 2(7877):394–397

[51] Holster IL, Kuipers EJ. Management of acute nonvariceal upper gastrointestinal bleeding: current policies and future perspectives. World J Gastroenterol. 2012; 18(11):1202–1207

[52] Marmo R, Rotondano G, Piscopo R, Bianco MA, D'Angella R, Cipolletta L. Dual therapy versus monotherapy in the endoscopic treatment of high-risk bleeding ulcers: a meta-analysis of controlled trials. Am J Gastroenterol. 2007; 102(2):279–289, quiz 469

[53] Shi K, Shen Z, Zhu G, Meng F, Gu M, Ji F. Systematic review with network meta-analysis: dual therapy for high-risk bleeding peptic ulcers. BMC Gastroenterol. 2017; 17(1):55

[54] Lau JY, Sung JJ, Lee KK, et al. Effect of intravenous omeprazole on recurrent bleeding after endoscopic treatment of bleeding peptic ulcers. N Engl J Med. 2000; 343(5):310–316

[55] Sung JJ, Barkun A, Kuipers EJ, et al. Peptic Ulcer Bleed Study Group. Intravenous esomeprazole for prevention of recurrent peptic ulcer bleeding: a randomized trial. Ann Intern Med. 2009; 150(7):455–464

[56] Chiu PW, Joeng HK, Choi CL, et al. High-dose omeprazole infusion compared with scheduled second-look endoscopy for prevention of peptic ulcer rebleeding: a randomized controlled trial. Endoscopy. 2016; 48(8):717–722

[57] Saeed ZA, Cole RA, Ramirez FC, Schneider FE, Hepps KS, Graham DY. Endoscopic retreatment after successful initial hemostasis prevents ulcer rebleeding: a prospective randomized trial. Endoscopy. 1996; 28(3):288–294

[58] Lau JY, Sung JJ, Lam YH, et al. Endoscopic retreatment compared with surgery in patients with recurrent bleeding after initial endoscopic control of bleeding ulcers. N Engl J Med. 1999; 340(10):751–756

[59] Jairath V, Kahan BC, Logan RF, et al. National audit of the use of surgery and radiological embolization after failed endoscopic haemostasis for nonvariceal upper gastrointestinal bleeding. Br J Surg. 2012; 99(12):1672–1680

[60] Tarasconi A, Baiocchi GL, Pattonieri V, et al. Transcatheter arterial embolization versus surgery for refractory non-variceal upper gastrointestinal bleeding: a meta-analysis. World J EmergSurg. 2019; 14:3

[61] Hopper AN, Stephens MR, Lewis WG, et al. Relative value of repeat gastric ulcer surveillance gastroscopy in diagnosing gastric cancer. Gastric Cancer. 2006; 9(3):217–222

[62] Shan YS, Hsu HP, Hsieh YH, Sy ED, Lee JC, Lin PW. Significance of intraoperative peritoneal culture of fungus in perforated peptic ulcer. Br J Surg. 2003; 90(10):1215–1219

[63] Horn CB, ColeoglouCenteno AA, Rasane RK, et al. Pre-operative anti-fungal therapy does not improve outcomes in perforated peptic ulcers. Surg Infect (Larchmt). 2018; 19(6):587–592

[64] Li WS, Lee CH, Liu JW. Antifungal therapy did not improve outcomes including 30-day all-cause mortality in patients suffering community-acquired perforated peptic ulcer-associated peritonitis with Candida species isolated from their peritoneal fluid. J Microbiol Immunol Infect. 2017; 50(3): 370–376

[65] Mohsina S, Shanmugam D, Sureshkumar S, Kundra P, Mahalakshmy T, Kate V. Adapted ERAS pathway vs. standard care in patients with perforated duodenal ulcer-a randomized controlled trial. J GastrointestSurg. 2018; 22 (1):107–116

Expert Commentary on Gastroduodenal Ulcers Requiring Surgery by *L. D. Britt*

Expert Commentary on Gastroduodenal Ulcers Requiring Surgery

L. D. Britt

In this comprehensive review of the evaluation process and management of acute and chronic peptic ulcer disease, the authors cover the entire spectrum of pathology that the acute care surgeon will likely encounter, particularly gastroduodenal ulcer diseases that necessitate surgical intervention. For this chapter, the authors defined "complicated peptic ulcer disease" as a "bleeding or perforated gastric or duodenal ulcer." However, there are actually five basic indications for surgical management of gastroduodenal ulcers which are as follows: 1. refractory bleeding, 2. perforation, 3. obstruction, 4. intractable pain, and 5. evidence or documentation of a malignancy. Certainly, in an emergency setting, the acute care surgeon needs to have the requisite clinical acumen (and be technically proficient) in the management of the first three, including an ulcer diathesis resulting in an obstruction.

In addition to having a more chronic presentation, gastric outlet obstruction can occur in the acute setting in patients with duodenal ulcer disease. The inflammatory process, with the associated edema, can cause obstruction in both the pyloric channel and the bulb (or first portion) of the duodenum. The associated symptoms are frank emesis, nausea, and dehydration, with the patient sometimes presenting with a hypochloremic alkalosis, secondary to hydrochloric acid depletion. Fortunately, acute gastric outlet obstruction usually resolves with intravascular volume reexpansion, nasogastric suction, and the utilization (intravenous) of antisecretory medication (e.g., antimuscarinic drugs, H_2 receptor antagonists, and proton-pump inhibitors). However, because of recurrent episodes, scarring and stenosis can result, giving the patient a fixed outlet obstruction. After ruling out (with endoscopic interrogation) an obstruction due to malignancy, the definitive surgical management should be a truncal vagotomy and antrectomy. While there are many advocates for performing a parietal cell vagotomy (with an accompanying gastrojejunostomy), time/effort efficiency usually makes the former recommendation the preferred option Two major stimuli for acid secretions are eliminated when a vagotomy and antrectomy are performed–acetylcholine (vagus) and gastrin (antrum).

After a successful truncal vagotomy and antrectomy, gastrointestinal continuity should be established by a Billroth II reconstruction, with a gastrojejunal anastomosis being performed, although there is support for a Billroth I reconstruction, anastomosing the duodenum to the gastric remnant. In performing the antrectomy and ensuring that there is no retained antrum after the resection, the antrum should be divided along a line that connects an area just above the incisura of the stomach with the point on the greater curvature, where the gastroepiploic vessels disappear. As it has been reported that the antial tissue occasionally extends upward along the lesser curvature, resecting the antrum along a line extending from a position just below the gastroesophageal junction to a point along the greater curvature–midway between the fundus and the pylorus. Knowledge of these anatomical boundaries is key in order to perform a complete anatomical antrectomy. In addition to an incomplete vagotomy, a retrained remnant of the antrum is one of the etiologies that must be considered in a patient with persistent ulcer diathesis, after he or she has undergone a truncal vagotomy and antrectomy for definitive management of a gastric outlet obstruction.

With respect to gastric perforation, there are advocates for performing a wedge resection of that gastric area where the perforated site is located and subsequently performing either a primary closure or a Graham patch or serosal (small intestine) buttress. However, this should be reserved for patients who run a very high risk with significant comorbidities. The caveat that always needs to be considered is that a perforated gastric ulcer is a malignancy until proven otherwise. For those patients who have been on antisecretory agents and have undergone *H. pylori* eradication, a formal gastric respective procedure should be performed, with removal of the acid-producing parietal cells and the performance of vagotomy, if possible. Finally, choosing a nonoperative management for patients presenting with a documented acute gastrointestinal perforation should not be overemphasized for there are very few indications for such an approach.

15 Intestinal Bowel Obstruction

Bishwajit Bhattacharya and Adrian A. Maung

Summary

Patients with bowel obstruction, both small and large, are commonly referred to acute care surgeons. Although not all patients require surgical interventions, minimally invasive options are being increasingly utilized with several apparent advantages. However, proper patient selection as well as recognition of the available surgical skill set are crucial in optimizing outcomes.

Keywords: Intestinal obstruction, laparoscopy

15.1 Introduction

Bowel obstruction is a common problem encountered by acute care surgeons. Optimal management requires not only prompt and accurate diagnosis but also selection of an *appropriate* therapeutic strategy. Although dependent on etiology as well as the location in the intestinal tract, many patients can be successfully managed without an operation. Yet some patients will require urgent surgery while others will not resolve without an eventual operation. It is therefore important to understand and *identify key features that guide the management strategy.*

This chapter will begin by discussing evidence-based management strategies, including the initial evaluation and the decision regarding operative or nonoperative pathways. Although exploratory laparotomy had been the default operation for many years, minimally invasive surgery is now a viable and, perhaps preferred, option for many patients and surgeons. In addition, some patients with large bowel obstruction may be managed appropriately with endoscopic endolumenal therapies. This chapter will therefore review the current evidence for both open and minimally invasive surgical options for both small and large bowel obstruction.

15.2 Background

Bowel obstruction represents a significant burden for the healthcare system. It is estimated that approximately 20% of admissions for abdominal pain in the United States are secondary to intestinal obstruction.[1] This equates to more than 300,000 patients admitted with small bowel obstruction (SBO) each year, 30–40% of whom will require an operative intervention.[2,3] In 1994, this was estimated to cost more than one billion dollars annually.[4]

Although majority of obstructions occur in the small bowel, up to 25% can be in the large intestine.[5] Adhesive disease represents the most common etiology for SBO (approximately 65–80%),[1,2] with hernias, inflammatory bowel disease, strictures, tumors, and volvulus representing other common causes. In the large intestine, colon cancer is the most common cause of obstruction while volvulus represents the most common benign etiology.[6,7] Other etiologies for large bowel obstruction (LBO) include hernias, strictures from diverticular or inflammatory bowel disease, adhesions, and other malignancies including lymphoma, ovarian, and pancreatic cancer.

Prior abdominal surgery is the most common risk factor for bowel obstruction due to adhesions, as they are estimated to develop in over 90% of patients who undergo abdominal surgery.[3] For example, in a study using the Scottish National Health Service Database, a cohort of 12,584 patients who underwent lower abdominal surgery was followed for 10 years. A third of patients were readmitted for potential adhesion-related problems over that period.[8] Adhesions, however, can also occur from inflammatory processes such as appendicitis or diverticulitis; some of which may not have been formally diagnosed. This is an important consideration, which will be discussed further, especially in patients presenting with SBO but without prior abdominal surgery.

15.3 Diagnostic Workup

The initial evaluation of patients with suspected bowel obstruction should not only strive to confirm the diagnosis and determine the possible etiology but also delineate certain elements that may help decide the need for and timing of operative intervention.[9] An appropriate history and physical examination should be performed. Specific elements that should be elicited from the history include prior abdominal operations or other pertinent abdominal disorders such as inflammatory bowel disease, diverticulitis, cancer, or prior radiation. Physical examination should especially seek signs suggestive of bowel ischemia including systemic toxicity and peritonitis. In an era of widely available imaging, an unfortunately neglected but still crucial part involves examination to detect the presence of hernias. Laboratory studies can also provide additional information and should evaluate for presence of metabolic abnormalities, acidosis and leukocytosis, all which may also suggest bowel ischemia but have low specificity.[9]

Imaging has an important role in the diagnostic workup of patients with suspected bowel obstruction. The Eastern Association for Surgery of Trauma (EAST) guideline for the evaluation and management of SBO made a Level I recommendation that CT scan of abdomen and pelvis should be performed in all patients with suspected SBO as it "provides incremental information over plain films in differentiating grade, severity, and etiology of SBO that may lead to changes in management."[9] (▶ Fig. 15.1) CT scan can determine the cause in 80 to 91% of SBO and has been shown to have 85 to 100% sensitivity in detection of bowel ischemia. Furthermore, water-soluble contrast studies, specifically using Gastrografin which is ionic and highly osmolar, have been shown to both accurately predict the need for surgery and reduce the need for operative intervention.[10,11]

15.4 Small Bowel Obstruction

15.4.1 Indications for Operative Intervention

Since the management of SBO is dependent on the inciting cause of the blockage, this chapter will primarily focus on

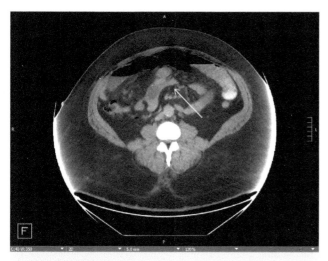

Fig. 15.1 Identification of the transition point and etiology of obstruction using CT scan.

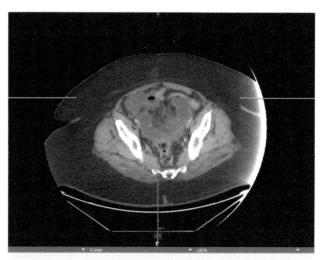

Fig. 15.2 Small bowel mesenteric congestion and mucosal hyperenhancement suggestive of ischemia.

discussing the management of the most common etiology of SBO, that is, adhesions. Management of inflammatory bowel disease and incarcerated hernias are reviewed, respectively, in Chapters 13 and 16. Historically, the management of adhesive SBO could be broadly generalized by the often-quoted dictum that "the sun should never set or rise on a complete SBO." In the 21st century, although nonoperative management (NOM) can be successful in a majority (60–80%) of patients, a portion of the patients still require urgent surgery and others will require surgery if the obstruction does not improve after the period of nonoperative management.[9] Selection of patients can be aided by certain evidence-based considerations.

Early operative management should be pursued in patients with suspected bowel ischemia as delays have been linked to both increased morbidity and mortality. Clinical signs and symptoms, which include fever, tachycardia, continuous pain and peritonitis, as well as laboratory studies (leukocytosis, metabolic acidosis, lactic acidosis) can correctly identify bowel ischemia in only approximately 40 to 50% of cases. The addition of cross-sectional imaging increases the sensitivity to 70 to 96%.[9] CT findings suggestive of ischemia include reduced bowel wall enhancement, wall thickening, mesenteric venous congestion, mesenteric fluid and ascites (▶ Fig. 15.2).

Patients without suspected bowel ischemia can safely undergo a trial of NOM as patients will improve within 2 to 5 days. Although failure to regain bowel function within 3 to 5 days is commonly used as an indicator for the need for an operation, a retrospective study of 293 admissions for SBO demonstrated that a significant proportion of patients may resolve even after 5 days.[12] There are currently significant limitations of the existing literature, including lack of randomized studies as well as selection bias, to define an optimal duration of NOM.

In patients who are selected for initial NOM, the need for eventual surgery may be elucidated using water-soluble contrast. A protocol in which Gastrografin was administered via

nasogastric tube (NGT) and followed by serial X-rays at 8 and 24 hours was demonstrated to decrease hospital length of stay as the presence of contrast in the cecum within 24 hours correctly identified patients whose SBO was resolved, thus allowing earlier removal of NGT and advancement of diet.[13] Conversely, operative intervention was recommended in patients in whom contrast failed to reach the cecum with in 24 hours.

Timely operative intervention has also been historically recommended in patients without previous abdominal surgery (PAS). One cited reason which was a concern was that in the absence of adhesions from prior surgeries, there would be a higher likelihood of malignant obstruction. The validity of this surgical dogma has been recently challenged. Several studies have demonstrated the presence of adhesive SBO in patients without PAS. In a retrospective review of 62 patients, adhesions were the etiology of obstruction in 75% despite no PAS.[14] In another series of 72 patients without PAS, adhesions were the cause of obstruction in 66.7%, and 40% were successfully underwent NOM.[15] Both studies had comparable rates of adhesive-related obstruction in patients with and without PAS. Furthermore, in a posthoc analysis of prospectively collected multicenter data on 101 patients with no PAS, only three patients had a malignant etiology for the obstruction.[16] In this study, the use of Gastrografin test also led to a decrease in the rate of operative interventions such that there was no difference in operative exploration rates between patients with and without PAS who underwent a contrast study.

15.4.2 Minimally Invasive Surgery for Small Bowel Obstruction

Over the past three decades, laparoscopy has been increasingly utilized in the treatment of various surgical diseases. Prior to the publications of two case reports of laparoscopic management of SBO in the early 1990s, one which involved the division of a single adhesive band, surgical therapy for adhesive SBO was synonymous with open laparotomy.[17,18] Over the subsequent decades, the use of minimally invasive surgery (MIS) has increased such that in 2010 about 15% of SBO cases were managed laparoscopically and its use has continued to increase.[19] Although numerous studies have investigated the use of MIS for the management of adhesive SBO, there are unfortunately still no randomized controlled trials comparing MIS to open surgery. Although one such trial has been proposed and was originally scheduled to be completed in 2018, the results have not been published at this point.[20] The current literature is therefore limited to retrospective analyses, nonrandomized comparative studies, and meta-analyses.

Overall, laparoscopic surgery has been shown to be safe in appropriate situations. Potential benefits include shorter length of stay, improved analgesia with lower narcotic medication requirements, shorter duration of ileus, and reduced morbidity.[1] In a systematic review of 11 nonrandomized studies, the use of laparoscopy was associated with decreased mortality and overall morbidity.[21] Specifically, patients in the MIS group had lower rates of pneumonia, wound infection, and length of hospital stay. The rates of bowel injury and reoperation were not significantly different between the open and laparoscopic group, but the operative time was longer in the MIS group. However, a different study, utilizing an administrative database, demonstrated a higher incidence of bowel-related complications (53.5 vs. 43.4%) with laparoscopic procedures.[22]

Laparoscopy can also be utilized as a diagnostic tool to confirm the diagnosis and etiology as well as evaluate bowel viability, need for resection, and complexity of the intra-abdominal adhesions that might require conversion to open surgery. This initial diagnostic evaluation, even if it subsequently requires conversion to open surgery, does not appear to significantly prolong the operation.[23] Furthermore, preemptive conversion (due to anticipated difficulty) after diagnostic laparoscopy is associated with lower morbidity compared to conversion due to intraoperative complications such as bowel injury.[24] Overall, conversion to open surgery is relatively common, estimated to occur in at least 1/3rd of all laparoscopically initiated operations.[22]

15.4.3 Technical Considerations in Minimally Invasive Surgery for Small Bowel Obstruction

The decision to intervene laparoscopically on SBO is typically made with consideration of both objective and subjective factors. Subjective considerations include the experience, technical skill set and comfort level of the individual surgeon and how it matches with the anticipated complexity of the disease process to be encountered. Laparoscopic intervention is most likely to be successful in instances where there is a single or few adhesive bands[25] and can be more challenging in an abdomen with very distended loops of bowel and/or complex adhesions.[26] Preoperative CT imaging may be able to aid the surgeon in this decision-making process.[27] Absolute and relative contraindications to laparoscopy in general should also be considered, including inability to tolerate pneumoperitoneum due to cardiovascular instability, severe chronic obstructive pulmonary disease

(COPD), uncorrectable hypercarbia or high peak pressures, and uncorrectable coagulopathy. The presence of prior intra-abdominal mesh is a relative contraindication. Both portal hypertension, which can lead to abdominal wall varices, and history of multiple prior surgeries or abdominal radiation may make obtaining port access challenging.

Preoperative considerations should include insertion of an NGT to aid in decompressing the stomach and proximal bowel as well as Foley catheter to decompress the bladder. Perioperative antibiotics should cover not only skin flora but also enteric organisms in the event of enteric spillage and/or bowel resection. The patient is typically placed in a supine position. The arms can be out at 90 degrees, although tucking them at the side of the patient may improve the ergonomics of the operation and allow the surgeon and assistant to stand on the same side. Video monitors should be positioned based on the surgeon's preference and a 5 mm, 30-degree angled scope is typically selected. Using a smaller scope allows the surgeon to interchange the camera between different ports, thus more easily achieving different view perspectives.

It is advisable to place the initial port in a location which is less likely to have adhesions and thus, if possible, avoid previous surgical scars.[28] There is considerable surgeon variability in entrance technique, for example, open cut down approach and Veress needle insufflation have been described. The use of ultrasound has been described as a potential method of identifying safe entry points.[29] Ultimately, the optimal approach is likely the method the surgeon is most experienced in using.[27]

Sometimes, the initial port ends up not being utilized during the surgery and is used only to insufflate the abdomen and help guide the placement of the subsequent, more optimally located, ports under direct visualization. It is preferable to place working ports in an area furthest away from the zone of interest to create a viable working space as well as help with triangulation. The port sizes can range from 5 to 12 mm, depending on the need for endoscopic stapling or auto suturing devices. Many cases that require only lysis of adhesions can be completed with 5 mm ports. Furthermore, ports can be upsized to accommodate larger instruments as needed.

Preoperative imaging can aid in not only identifying an area for the initial port placement but also localizing the transition point to a specific quadrant. The transition point can be found by looking for decompressed loops of bowel and following them back more proximally to a transition zone using atraumatic, nonlocking graspers (▶ Fig. 15.3). Alternatively, one can identify the ligament of Treitz by grasping the epiploic appendices of the transverse colon to retract it cephalad and identifying the base of the colon mesentery. The small bowel can then be run toward the terminal ileum, although this may be more challenging with very dilated proximal bowel. Some studies suggest a higher incidence of bowel injury in laparoscopic interventions.[22] This risk can be decreased by manipulating the mesentery of the bowel and avoiding the grasping the bowel itself, especially the dilated and thin-walled proximal bowel (▶ Fig. 15.4). Adhesions can be lysed with scissors, electrocautery, harmonic scalper or bipolar tissue sealing system, as appropriate (▶ Fig. 15.5).

In cases of dense adhesive disease, laparoscopic intervention is less likely to be successful and dense adhesions is the most

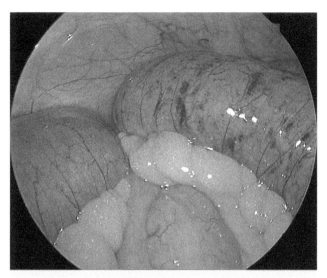

Fig. 15.3 Decompressed and dilated loops of small bowel.

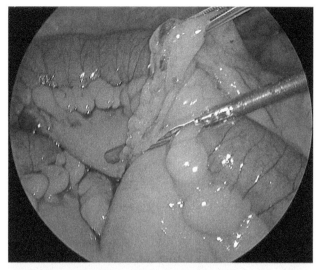

Fig. 15.4 Use of atraumatic graspers and avoidance of manipulating dilated bowel directly. In this case, an omental adhesion was causing an internal hernia.

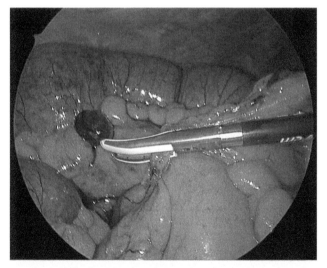

Fig. 15.5 Division of adhesion with bipolar tissue sealing system.

common reason for conversion (27.7%) followed by need for bowel resection (23.1%).[30] Preoperative CT scan imaging showing thickened bowel walls, reduced bowel wall enhancement, mesenteric venous congestion, mesenteric fluid and ascites have been shown to correlate with bowel ischemia. Laparoscopic exploration has been demonstrated to be a safe and effective technique to assess bowel viability and the need for resection.[23] Intraoperatively, the viability of bowel can be assessed using clinical findings such as visual color inspection, presence of peristalsis, and arterial pulsation. The presence of blood flow can be determined by Doppler ultrasound or the use of fluorescence techniques.[31] Bowel that is necrotic or not viable must be resected, and continuity reestablished with an anastomosis. If technically feasible and within the skill set of the surgeon, laparoscopic bowel resection and intracorporal anastomosis can be performed. Even in cases when it is deemed

necessary to convert to an open procedure, laparoscopy may still permit for a smaller, less-invasive "mini-laparotomy" by helping in localizing the segment of the small bowel which requires resection. Other common reasons to convert are inability to locate the region or zone of obstruction, iatrogenic injury, and inadequate visualization.[30] If carcinomatosis is encountered, laparoscopic intervention should be aborted or converted to open if a palliative intervention is deemed feasible. If the clinical scenario does not permit safe laparoscopic exploration, the surgeon should also exercise flexibility in converting to open. A surgeon should view conversion of the case to open not as a failure but as good judgement.

15.4.4 Early Postoperative Obstruction

Early postoperative obstruction is another dilemma encountered by surgeons. The time frame defining this entity is variable but usually refers to a period up to 6 weeks after the index operation.[32,33] Distinguishing between early postoperative ileus and mechanical obstruction can be challenging. Dense, inflammatory adhesions typically form within 10 to 14 days after open exploration. Operative intervention in a recently intervened abdomen faces the risk of encountering these adhesions and may cause more harm than good. The etiology for obstruction is usually adhesions, edema, or inflammatory tissues; bowel ischemia is usually not encountered. In the absence of signs of bowel compromise, NOM with nasogastric decompression is the favored approach for 1 to 14 days beyond which it is unlikely to resolve without an intervention.[33,34,35] A Gastrografin challenge has not been shown to have a beneficial effect in the case of early postoperative SBO.[36] Patients who have undergone laparoscopic exploration as the index operation may have less adhesions and, in such patients, earlier reexploration may be safer compared to instances where the index case was an open exploration.[37]

15.5 Large Bowel Obstruction

15.5.1 Operative Intervention for Large Bowel Obstruction

Large bowel obstruction (LBO) can occur secondary to several different etiologies. In the United States, colonic malignancy is the most common cause for LBO followed by benign causes from diverticular disease or sigmoid volvulus.[6,7] The optimal management approach depends upon the location and etiology of the obstruction as well as the presentation of the individual patient. LBO can cause a closed loop obstruction between the ileocecal valve and the obstruction site, resulting in dilation of the proximal colon, venous congestion, ischemia, and ultimately perforation. The most common location for perforation is the cecum; this is believed to occur due to the larger diameter in this region and consequent greatest wall tension.[38] Patients presenting with signs of perforation or ischemic bowel require emergent surgery. In the absence of hard signs, an operation can be delayed, giving time for resuscitation but should not be delayed beyond 12 to 24 hours.

Right-sided colonic obstructions are treated with right hemicolectomy which is associated with up to a 10% risk of anastomotic leak in the obstructed patient; patients with risk factors for a leak can be treated with a protective diverting loop or end ileostomy.[39] More distal obstructions can be treated by a host of techniques, depending upon patient's risk factors and surgeon's comfort with emergency colorectal surgery. Definitive treatment involves performing a resection of the lesion. Traditionally, a two-staged approach has been advocated for emergency colonic surgery due to concern for an anastomotic leak. However, a Hartman's reversal is not a benign intervention and is associated with up to a 30% complication rate.[40] In recent decades, this paradigm has been questioned, as data suggests lower mortality when a primary anastomosis is performed in the index operation.[41,42] If there is concern for viability of the anastomosis, a diverting loop ileostomy can be utilized. Current trends indicate Hartman's procedure is increasingly reserved for patients with poor physiology where an end colostomy is likely to be permanent.[40]

Another benign cause for LBO is volvulus, most commonly involving the sigmoid but can also occur in the cecum or transverse colon. In the United States, colonic volvulus is a relatively rare cause of intestinal obstruction, accounting for about 1.9% of such cases; however, in endemic areas such as Africa, the Middle East and South America, the incidence is much higher, ranging from 10 to 50%.[43,44,45] Sigmoid volvulus is more commonly seen in elderly males (over 70 years), diabetics, and patients with neuropsychiatric disorders. Cecal volvulus is relatively more common in younger women. The overall mortality for sigmoid volvulus in the United States is about 9.4% and 6.6% for cecal volvulus.[43] In cases of sigmoid volvulus, the initial treatment, in the absence of signs of bowel ischemia or perforation, involves decompressing the volvulus with endoscopy. The rate of recurrence ranges from 20 to 70% and definitive treatment involves performing resection of the redundant colon with or without a primary anastomosis.[46,47,48] Historically, a Hartman's procedure has been the intervention of choice in this frail patient population, due to the difficulty in creating an anastomosis between proximally dilated colon and normal caliber distal bowel. However, the demographics of the patient population has shifted to a younger healthier population and performing a primary anastomosis at the index operation is a safe option in select patients.[43]

Some patients with sigmoid volvulus are at high-risk for major surgical interventions and less-invasive procedures can be considered. These include loop sigmoid colostomy or percutaneous endoscopic colostomy as an effective alternative in patients too frail to tolerate more aggressive operative intervention.[49,50,51,52] Both techniques are based upon the principal of anchoring the colon to the anterior abdominal wall. Endoscopic procedures are associated with risk of complications ranging from chronic wound healing, leakage, tube migration, and fecal peritonitis but may be comparable to the mortality risk with operative intervention in frail and elderly patients.[53,54] Patients with an unresectable malignant obstruction can also be treated with a decompressive loop ostomy or endoluminal stent if feasible.

15.5.2 Minimally Invasive Surgery for Large Bowel Obstruction

As with other fields of general surgery, advances in laparoscopic techniques have allowed for the use of a laparoscopic approach to the management of LBO. In the elective setting, numerous studies have identified several advantages of laparoscopic over open colon resection, including decreased pain, narcotic requirements, wound and pulmonary complications, length of stay, and earlier return of bowel function regardless of location of the colonic resection.[55,56,57,58] In the hands of surgeons with the appropriate technical skills, laparoscopic intervention for large bowel obstruction is feasible and safe.[59] Contraindications to MIS approach for LBO are like those for SBO. Furthermore, the surgeon should be well-versed in elective laparoscopic colon surgery. In recent years, robotic surgery has also been increasingly used for elective colorectal surgery with favorable results, especially in aiding the pelvic dissection of key structures. This technology has however not been evaluated in the emergent setting.

15.5.3 Technical Considerations in Minimally Invasive Surgery for Large Bowel Obstruction

Various techniques have been described in the elective setting, including laparoscopic and hand-assisted laparoscopic approaches with both intra and extracorporeal anastomoses. The location of the obstruction, and thus the extent of the resection, can be identified using preoperative imaging. Patient can be positioned supine for right-sided resections or lithotomy for extended right- or left-sided resections. In either case, the patient should be well-secured to the operating table as steep positioning is often necessary to allow gravity to facilitate the exposure. Port placement is dependent on the type of planned resection but generally ports are placed in the midline or opposite the side of resection. A 12 mm port is typically required to accommodate a stapling device and an angled 5 or 10 mm camera should be utilized. Considerations of the method of entry, open cut down or Veress needle, are like those discussed previously for SBO. Once the peritoneal cavity is entered, the key is to create adequate working space. This can sometimes be achieved by decompressing the colon by percutaneously aspirating the gaseous content of the colon, thus making the colon more mobile and easier to manipulate.

15.5.4 Endoscopic Management of Large Bowel Obstruction

With advances in endoscopic technology, operative intervention can be avoided in certain cases. Distal large bowel obstructions that are accessible with endoscopy may be potentially alleviated with an endoluminal stent. In cases of unresectable malignant obstruction, this can serve as a preferred palliative option with faster return to diet, shorter length of postprocedural stay, and improved quality of life compared to surgical intervention.[60,61] Shorter malignant strictures with less angulation to the obstruction are more likely to be successfully stented compared to benign longer strictures.[62] Some studies suggest that endoscopic stenting may be the initial treatment of choice in resectable distal colonic obstructions, serving as a bridge to elective resection with better long-term outcomes and higher likelihood of primary anastomosis.[60,63,64] However, stenting has also been associated with a significant risk of clinical and subclinical perforation.[65]

References

[1] Sajid MS, Khawaja AH, Sains P, Singh KK, Baig MK. A systematic review comparing laparoscopic vs open adhesiolysis in patients with adhesional small bowel obstruction. Am J Surg. 2016; 212(1):138–150

[2] Davies SW, Gillen JR, Guidry CA, et al. A comparative analysis between laparoscopic and open adhesiolysis at a tertiary care center. Am Surg. 2014; 80(3):261–269

[3] Jafari MD, Jafari F, Foe-Paker JE, et al. Adhesive small bowel obstruction in the united states: has laparoscopy made an impact? Am Surg. 2015; 81(10):1028–1033

[4] Diamond MP, Freeman ML. Clinical implications of postsurgical adhesions. Hum Reprod Update. 2001; 7(6):567–576

[5] Markogiannakis H, Messaris E, Dardamanis D, et al. Acute mechanical bowel obstruction: clinical presentation, etiology, management and outcome. World J Gastroenterol. 2007; 13(3):432–437

[6] Greenlee HB, Pienkos EJ, Vanderbilt PC, et al. Proceedings: acute large bowel obstruction. Comparison of county, veterans administration, and community hospital populations. Arch Surg. 1974; 108(4):470–476

[7] Sawai RS. Management of colonic obstruction: a review. Clin Colon Rectal Surg. 2012; 25(4):200–203

[8] Parker MC, Ellis H, Moran BJ, et al. Postoperative adhesions: ten-year follow-up of 12,584 patients undergoing lower abdominal surgery. Dis Colon Rectum. 2001; 44(6):822–829, discussion 829–830

[9] Maung AA, Johnson DC, Piper GL, et al. Eastern Association for the Surgery of Trauma. Evaluation and management of small-bowel obstruction: an Eastern Association for the Surgery of Trauma practice management guideline. J Trauma Acute Care Surg. 2012; 73(5) Suppl 4:S362–S369

[10] Branco BC, Barmparas G, Schnüriger B, Inaba K, Chan LS, Demetriades D. Systematic review and meta-analysis of the diagnostic and therapeutic role of water-soluble contrast agent in adhesive small bowel obstruction. Br J Surg. 2010; 97(4):470–478

[11] Trésallet C, Lebreton N, Royer B, Leyre P, Godiris-Petit G, Menegaux F. Improving the management of acute adhesive small bowel obstruction with CT-scan and water-soluble contrast medium: a prospective study. Dis Colon Rectum. 2009; 52(11):1869–1876

[12] Shih SC, Jeng KS, Lin SC, et al. Adhesive small bowel obstruction: how long can patients tolerate conservative treatment? World J Gastroenterol. 2003; 9(3):603–605

[13] Azagury D, Liu RC, Morgan A, Spain DA. Small bowel obstruction: a practical step-by-step evidence-based approach to evaluation, decision making, and management. J Trauma Acute Care Surg. 2015; 79(4):661–668

[14] Beardsley C, Furtado R, Mosse C, et al. Small bowel obstruction in the virgin abdomen: the need for a mandatory laparotomy explored. Am J Surg. 2014; 208(2):243–248

[15] Ng YY, Ngu JC, Wong AS. Small bowel obstruction in the virgin abdomen: time to challenge surgical dogma with evidence. ANZ J Surg. 2018; 88(1–2):91–94

[16] Collom ML, Duane TM, Campbell-Furtick M, et al. EAST SBO Workgroup. Deconstructing dogma: Nonoperative management of small bowel obstruction in the virgin abdomen. J Trauma Acute Care Surg. 2018; 85(1):33–36

[17] Clotteau JE, Premont M. [Treatment of severe median abdominal cicatricial eventrations by an aponeurotic plastic procedure (author's transl)]. Chirurgie. 1979; 105(4):344–346

[18] Bastug DF, Trammell SW, Boland JP, Mantz EP, Tiley EH, III. Laparoscopic adhesiolysis for small bowel obstruction. Surg Laparosc Endosc. 1991; 1(4):259–262

[19] Kelly KN, Iannuzzi JC, Rickles AS, Garimella V, Monson JR, Fleming FJ. Laparotomy for small-bowel obstruction: first choice or last resort for adhesiolysis? A laparoscopic approach for small-bowel obstruction reduces 30-day complications. Surg Endosc. 2014; 28(1):65–73

[20] Sallinen V, Wikström H, Victorzon M, et al. Laparoscopic versus open adhesiolysis for small bowel obstruction - a multicenter, prospective, randomized, controlled trial. BMC Surg. 2014; 14:77

[21] Wiggins T, Markar SR, Harris A. Laparoscopic adhesiolysis for acute small bowel obstruction: systematic review and pooled analysis. Surg Endosc. 2015; 29(12):3432–3442

[22] Behman R, Nathens AB, Byrne JP, Mason S, Look Hong N, Karanicolas PJ. Laparoscopic surgery for adhesive small bowel obstruction is associated with a higher risk of bowel injury: a population-based analysis of 8584 patients. Ann Surg. 2017; 266(3):489–498

[23] Johnson KN, Chapital AB, Harold KL, et al. Laparoscopic management of acute small bowel obstruction: evaluating the need for resection. J Trauma Acute Care Surg. 2012; 72(1):25–30; discussion 30–1; quiz 317

[24] Dindo D, Schafer M, Muller MK, Clavien PA, Hahnloser D. Laparoscopy for small bowel obstruction: the reason for conversion matters. Surg Endosc. 2010; 24(4):792–797

[25] Lujan HJ, Oren A, Plasencia G, et al. Laparoscopic management as the initial treatment of acute small bowel obstruction. JSLS. 2006; 10(4):466–472

[26] Ten Broek RPG, Krielen P, Di Saverio S, et al. Bologna guidelines for diagnosis and management of adhesive small bowel obstruction (ASBO): 2017 update of the evidence-based guidelines from the world society of emergency surgery ASBO working group. World J Emerg Surg. 2018; 13:24

[27] Vettoretto N, Carrara A, Corradi A, et al. Italian Association of Hospital Surgeons (Associazione dei Chirurghi Ospedalieri Italiani-ACOI). Laparoscopic adhesiolysis: consensus conference guidelines. Colorectal Dis. 2012; 14(5):e208–e215

[28] Nagle A, Ujiki M, Denham W, Murayama K. Laparoscopic adhesiolysis for small bowel obstruction. Am J Surg. 2004; 187(4):464–470

[29] Borzellino G, De Manzoni G, Ricci F. Detection of abdominal adhesions in laparoscopic surgery. A controlled study of 130 cases. Surg Laparosc Endosc. 1998; 8(4):273–276

[30] Ghosheh B, Salameh JR. Laparoscopic approach to acute small bowel obstruction: review of 1061 cases. Surg Endosc. 2007; 21(11):1945–1949

[31] Karakaş BR, Sırcan-Küçüksayan A, Elpek OE, Canpolat M. Investigating viability of intestine using spectroscopy: a pilot study. J Surg Res. 2014; 191(1):91–98

[32] Stewart RM, Page CP, Brender J, Schwesinger W, Eisenhut D. The incidence and risk of early postoperative small bowel obstruction. A cohort study. Am J Surg. 1987; 154(6):643–647

[33] Miller G, Boman J, Shrier I, Gordon PH. Readmission for small-bowel obstruction in the early postoperative period: etiology and outcome. Can J Surg. 2002; 45(4):255–258

[34] Sajja SB, Schein M. Early postoperative small bowel obstruction. Br J Surg. 2004; 91(6):683–691

[35] Pickleman J, Lee RM. The management of patients with suspected early postoperative small bowel obstruction. Ann Surg. 1989; 210(2):216–219

[36] Khasawneh MA, Ugarte ML, Srvantstian B, Dozois EJ, Bannon MP, Zielinski MD. Role of gastrografin challenge in early postoperative small bowel obstruction. J Gastrointest Surg. 2014; 18(2):363–368

[37] Goussous N, Kemp KM, Bannon MP, et al. Early postoperative small bowel obstruction: open vs laparoscopic. Am J Surg. 2015; 209(2):385–390

[38] Lopez-Kostner F, Hool GR, Lavery IC. Management and causes of acute large-bowel obstruction. Surg Clin North Am. 1997; 77(6):1265–1290

[39] Phillips RK, Hittinger R, Fry JS, Fielding LP. Malignant large bowel obstruction. Br J Surg. 1985; 72(4):296–302

[40] Garber A, Hyman N, Osler T. Complications of Hartmann takedown in a decade of preferred primary anastomosis. Am J Surg. 2014; 207(1):60–64

[41] Constantinides VA, Tekkis PP, Athanasiou T, et al. Primary resection with anastomosis vs. Hartmann's procedure in nonelective surgery for acute colonic diverticulitis: a systematic review. Dis Colon Rectum. 2006; 49(7):966–981

[42] Maher M, Caldwell MP, Waldron R, et al. Staged resection or primary anastomosis for obstructing lesions to the left colon. Ir Med J. 1996; 89(4):138–139

[43] Halabi WJ, Jafari MD, Kang CY, et al. Colonic volvulus in the United States: trends, outcomes, and predictors of mortality. Ann Surg. 2014; 259(2):293–301

[44] Oncü M, Pískín B, Calik A, Yandi M, Alhan E. Volvulus of the sigmoid colon. S Afr J Surg. 1991; 29(2):48–49

[45] Påhlman L, Enblad P, Rudberg C, Krog M. Volvulus of the colon. a review of 93 cases and current aspects of treatment. Acta Chir Scand. 1989; 155(1):53–56

[46] Brothers TE, Strodel WE, Eckhauser FE. Endoscopy in colonic volvulus. Ann Surg. 1987; 206(1):1–4

[47] Atamanalp SS, Ozturk G. Sigmoid volvulus in the elderly: outcomes of a 43-year, 453-patient experience. Surg Today. 2011; 41(4):514–519

[48] Larkin JO, Thekiso TB, Waldron R, Barry K, Eustace PW. Recurrent sigmoid volvulus - early resection may obviate later emergency surgery and reduce morbidity and mortality. Ann R Coll Surg Engl. 2009; 91(3):205–209

[49] Bhatnagar BN, Sharma CL. Nonresective alternative for the cure of nongangrenous sigmoid volvulus. Dis Colon Rectum. 1998; 41(3):381–388

[50] Cubas V, Adedeji O. The insertion of a percutaneous endoscopic sigmoidostomy tube. Tech Coloproctol. 2016; 20(6):413

[51] Baraza W, Brown S, McAlindon M, Hurlstone P. Prospective analysis of percutaneous endoscopic colostomy at a tertiary referral centre. Br J Surg. 2007; 94(11):1415–1420

[52] Mullen R, Church NI, Yalamarthi S. Volvulus of the sigmoid colon treated by percutaneous endoscopic colostomy. Surg Laparosc Endosc Percutan Tech. 2009; 19(2):e64–e66

[53] Tun G, Bullas D, Bannaga A, Said EM. Percutaneous endoscopic colostomy: a useful technique when surgery is not an option. Ann Gastroenterol. 2016; 29(4):477–480

[54] Frank L, Moran A, Beaton C. Use of percutaneous endoscopic colostomy (PEC) to treat sigmoid volvulus: a systematic review. Endosc Int Open. 2016; 4(7):E737–E741

[55] Veldkamp R, Kuhry E, Hop WC, et al. Colon cancer Laparoscopic or Open Resection Study Group (COLOR). Laparoscopic surgery versus open surgery for colon cancer: short-term outcomes of a randomised trial. Lancet Oncol. 2005; 6(7):477–484

[56] Yamamoto S, Inomata M, Katayama H, et al. Japan Clinical Oncology Group Colorectal Cancer Study Group. Short-term surgical outcomes from a randomized controlled trial to evaluate laparoscopic and open D3 dissection for stage II/III colon cancer: Japan Clinical Oncology Group Study JCOG 0404. Ann Surg. 2014; 260(1):23–30

[57] Lorenzon L, La Torre M, Ziparo V, et al. Evidence based medicine and surgical approaches for colon cancer: evidences, benefits and limitations of the laparoscopic vs open resection. World J Gastroenterol. 2014; 20(13):3680–3692

[58] Salem JF, Gummadi S, Marks JH. Minimally invasive surgical approaches to colon cancer. Surg Oncol Clin N Am. 2018; 27(2):303–318

[59] Gash K, Chambers W, Ghosh A, Dixon AR. The role of laparoscopic surgery for the management of acute large bowel obstruction. Colorectal Dis. 2011; 13(3):263–266

[60] Tan CJ, Dasari BV, Gardiner K. Systematic review and meta-analysis of randomized clinical trials of self-expanding metallic stents as a bridge to surgery versus emergency surgery for malignant left-sided large bowel obstruction. Br J Surg. 2012; 99(4):469–476

[61] van Hooft JE, van Halsema EE, Vanbiervliet G, et al. European Society of Gastrointestinal Endoscopy. Self-expandable metal stents for obstructing colonic and extracolonic cancer: European Society of Gastrointestinal Endoscopy (ESGE) Clinical Guideline. Endoscopy. 2014; 46(11):990–1053

[62] Boyle DJ, Thorn C, Saini A, et al. Predictive factors for successful colonic stenting in acute large-bowel obstruction: a 15-year cohort analysis. Dis Colon Rectum. 2015; 58(3):358–362

[63] Jiménez-Pérez J, Casellas J, García-Cano J, et al. Colonic stenting as a bridge to surgery in malignant large-bowel obstruction: a report from two large multinational registries. Am J Gastroenterol. 2011; 106(12):2174–2180

[64] Amelung FJ, de Beaufort HW, Siersema PD, Verheijen PM, Consten EC. Emergency resection versus bridge to surgery with stenting in patients with acute right-sided colonic obstruction: a systematic review focusing on mortality and morbidity rates. Int J Colorectal Dis. 2015; 30(9):1147–1155

[65] Gianotti L, Tamini N, Nespoli L, et al. A prospective evaluation of short-term and long-term results from colonic stenting for palliation or as a bridge to elective operation versus immediate surgery for large-bowel obstruction. Surg Endosc. 2013; 27(3):832–842

Expert Commentary on Intestinal Bowel Obstruction by *Andrew B. Peitzman*

Expert Commentary on Intestinal Bowel Obstruction

Andrew B. Peitzman

Fastidious decision-making is critical in the management of the patient with acute intestinal obstruction. Admit the patient to a surgical service to facilitate close observation and prompt operation if necessary. The key decisions in the management of the patient with bowel obstruction are: which patient needs emergent operation and which patient can be safely observed; large bowel obstruction versus small bowel obstruction; and initial open versus laparoscopic approach when operation is required.

Although most patients with small bowel obstruction (SBO) can be managed nonoperatively, early intervention is critical in patients at risk of intestinal infarction. Computed tomography (CT) provides vital information in the management of patients with intestinal obstruction. Findings on initial assessment which mandate emergent operation include hemodynamic instability, peritonitis, pneumoperitoneum, incarcerated hernias, closed loop obstruction, cecal volvulus, and sigmoid volvulus with systemic toxicity or peritoneal signs.

Several caveats must be remembered in the assessment of the patient with bowel obstruction. The patient with previous bariatric surgery must be approached with a more aggressive approach toward operative intervention. Colonic pseudo-obstruction (Ogilvie's syndrome) must be included in the discussion of diagnosis of possible bowel obstruction. Other uncommon but difficult to diagnose etiologies include obturator, Spigelian, and paraduodenal hernias.

Much of the chapter concentrates on laparoscopic management of intestinal obstruction. The literature on the role of laparoscopy in SBO is heavily biased by case selection and lack of detail in patient selection. Only 15% of patients with SBO are approached laparoscopically, with a 30% conversion rate in most series. Do the outcomes reflect the advantages of laparoscopy or a different patient population from those initially managed open? Adhesiolysis is a high-risk operation; a recognized enterotomy has significant morbidity and disastrous consequences. Thus, the need for preemptive rather than reactive conversion from laparoscopy to laparotomy when dense adhesions are encountered. To expand on the observations from the Dindo paper,[1] complications resulted in operations completed laparoscopically (8.3%), preemptive conversion (20%), and reactive conversion (48.6%). Small bowel injury occurred in 4.7% and was missed at index operation in 33%.

Table 15.1.1 Odds ratio for bowel injury based on number of previous laparotomies[2]

Previous laparotomies	Odds ratio for bowel injury
None (reference)	1.0
1	2.27
2 or 3	10.03
≥4	15.8

As TenBroek et al stated, "the most important predictor of unplanned enterotomy is the number of previous laparotomies (▶ Table 15.1.1)."[2] Bowel injury resulted in 6.3 to 26.9% of patients undergoing laparoscopic adhesiolysis. The authors concluded that "when simple operative treatment is required, a laparoscopic approach might improve results for simple cases of adhesive SBO."

The authors referenced the Sallinen study,[3] which is a randomized, controlled trial of 100 patients of open versus laparoscopic adhesiolysis after failure of observation. This was a highly select group of patients, with extensive exclusion criteria, intending to generate a pool of patients with high-likelihood of a single adhesive band. Results in laparoscopy versus open adhesiolysis were as follows: postoperative length of stay (LOS), 4.2 versus 5.5 days; time to bowel function, 41 versus 63 hours; complications, 43% versus 31%–quicker recovery with laparoscopy. However, even in this highly selected population, conversion from laparoscopy to laparotomy was necessary in 25%. Importantly, bowel injury occurred equally in each group (22–24%). If more complex patients were included, such figures would likely be higher.

Thus, what is accurate regarding laparoscopy for SBO–if the operation can be performed *safely* laparoscopically, the patient incurs less physiologic perturbations, less pain, and shorter LOS. Patient selection and early conversion to laparotomy are critical factors.

References

[1] Dindo D, Schafer M, Muller MK, Clavien PA, Hahnloser D. Laparoscopy for small bowel obstruction: the reason for conversion matters. SurgEndosc. 2010; 24(4):792–797

[2] Ten Broek RPG, Krielen P, Di Saverio S, et al. Bologna guidelines for diagnosis and management of adhesive small bowel obstruction (ASBO): 2017 update of the evidence-based guidelines from the world society of emergency surgery ASBO working group. World J EmergSurg. 2018; 13:24

[3] Sallinen V, DiSaverio S, Haukijarvi E, et al. Laparoscopic versus open adhesiolysis for adhesive small bowel obstruction (LASSO): an international, multicentre, randomised, open-label trial. Lancet GastroenterolHepatol. 2019; 4(4):278–286.

16 Surgical Management of Incarcerated Hernias

Jessica Koller Gorham and William S. Richardson

Summary

Asking medical students the names and anatomy of abdominal wall hernias is a favorite surgical topic. Although this is interesting information, equally important is how to identify complications and surgically repair them. In this chapter we have discussed anatomy and treatment of incarcerated abdominal wall hernias.

Keywords: Incarceration, inguinal hernia, umbilical hernia, epigastric hernia, incisional hernia, ventral hernia, spigelian hernia, diaphragmatic hernia, Morgagni hernia, Bochdalek hernia, paraesophageal hernia, internal hernia, flank hernia, pelvic hernia, obturator hernia

16.1 Introduction

Abdominal wall hernias are a common consult for the general surgeon. They occur when intra-abdominal contents protrude through a defect in the tissue meant to contain them. There remains a lot of debate on when to perform elective repairs on hernias. Most surgeons would agree that incarceration is an indication for hernia repair. The urgency of repair would depend on symptoms and other signs that would suggest ischemia or infarction, also called strangulation.

Hernias occur in many parts of the abdominal wall: the navel, inguinal area, diaphragm, flank, pelvis, and then there are internal hernias as well. All of these have different risks for symptoms, growth, and strangulation, as well as nuances regarding proper repair.

In this chapter, we will start with a general overview of hernias, and then go into specific types, with examples of incarcerated hernias highlighting our approach to their repair.

16.2 Epidemiology

Incarcerated hernias of the abdominal wall present as masses. Risk factors for incarceration include female gender, femoral hernia, history of prior hernia repair, internal hernia, and obturator hernia. Tenderness, erythema or associated fever, tachycardia, or bowel obstruction may indicate strangulation or perforation and warrant emergent surgical intervention. Strangulated hernias increase the risk of infection and mortality, especially with advanced patient age (>65), American Society of Anesthesiologists (ASA) > II, and acute incarcerated >24 hours duration.[1] The incidents of emergent hernia repair seem to be increasing from 2001 to 2010 but with the increase of minimally invasive approaches to the abdomen and increased use of complex hernia repair that may decrease rate of recurrence, we expect that rates will start to decrease.[2]

16.3 Differential Diagnosis

Incarcerated hernias of the abdominal wall frequently present as discreate masses with or without tenderness. Other diagnoses to consider are musculoskeletal disorders, abscess, lymphadenopathy, and other benign or malignant masses. In the groin, varicocele and hydrocele should be considered. Pelvic hernias may be difficult to palpate and are often found on computed tomography (CT). Diaphragmatic hernias typically have no findings on chest or abdominal physical examination. Many internal hernias are found on CT but may be missed on all preoperative workup. For most of these, there is a prior history of surgery.

16.4 Diagnosis

The history of a patient with an incarcerated hernia typically includes intermittent symptoms at the hernia site prior to acute incarceration, unless they have some sort of high Valsalva-inducing event prior to the onset. Some incarcerated hernias are asymptomatic; however, most patients experience pain or associated symptoms of ischemia or bowel obstruction such as nausea, vomiting, or peritonitis, or signs of pending infarction of herniated contents or perforation such as hemodynamic abnormalities or free air on imaging. At a minimum, complete blood count (CBC) and basic metabolic panel (BMP) should be obtained to identify inflammatory signs or dehydration (in cases of bowel obstruction and vomiting), and CT may be indicated if history and physical examination are not sufficiently diagnostic. Some hernias are not identified until abdominal exploration.

16.5 Treatment

Generally, operative treatment is indicated for all incarcerated hernias and urgent or emergent procedures for strangulated, ischemic, or infarcted hernias. Based on history, vital signs and labs, fluid resuscitation is initiated prior to surgery. Antibiotics, ulcer, and deep vein thrombosis (DVT) prophylaxis is initiated. Open operation, minimally invasive, and robotic surgery have all been used with good success, and we will discuss more about this as we get into individual hernia types.[3]

Predictors of mortality from National Surgical Quality Improvement Program (NSQIP) database in one study included increasing age, history of congestive heart failure or peripheral vascular disease, presence of ascites, elevated blood urea nitrogen (BUN), and elevated white cell count (WBC).[1] Mesh closure has been shown to decrease reoperations for recurrent hernias. Mesh use in emergent ventral hernia repair may not increase morbidity or mortality; however, there was no indication of when permanent or absorbable mesh was used in associated studies,[4] World Society of Emergency Surgery (WSES) guidelines for emergent hernia repair recommend primarily closing defects less than or equal to 3 cm, and avoiding use of permanent mesh in clean contaminated, contaminated, and dirty cases.[3]

Frequently, emergent or urgent hernia repair is considered in patients with significant comorbidities. Control of comorbidities to the greatest extent possible prior to repair is ideal, but in the case of acute strangulation, emergent intervention should not be delayed when the decision to pursue an operation is made. In particular, in patients with uncompensated cirrhosis and ruptured

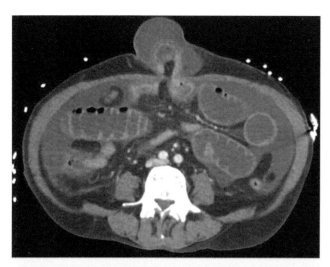

Fig. 16.1 Incarcerated umbilical hernia, resulting in small bowel obstruction in patient with liver failure and uncontrolled ascites.

umbilical hernias, there is an associated 30% risk of complete liver failure, leading to liver transplant or death (▶ Fig. 16.1).[5] This might suggest that hernia repair be considered early on. Tense ascites is frequently the cause of symptomatic hernias in the patients, and any modalities successful in decreasing ascites will also decrease symptoms. Once ascites management is maximized, elective repair should be considered. The perioperative risk of liver decompensation can be estimated with model for end-stage liver disease (MELD) scoring. If ascites is not well managed, the postoperative risk of hernia recurrence and spontaneous bacterial peritonitis are significantly increased. Postoperative ascites can be managed with intermittent drainage either with needle aspiration or permanent type of drainage catheter such as peritoneal dialysis catheter.

16.6 Inguinal Hernia

There are three types of inguinal hernias: direct, indirect, and femoral. About 1 in 10 men will develop an inguinal hernia. Although inguinal hernias are much less common in women, these hernias are at higher risk of incarceration, particularly in the case of femoral hernias.[6]

Generally, mesh infections are rare after inguinal hernia repair, but general guidelines should be followed, as for other hernia repairs, with regard to mesh use. Murky fluid frequently develops as part of an acute incarceration process, and it may be difficult to tell if this is a true infection at the time of surgery. Certainly, in cases of gangrene, cellulitis or clinical signs of infection, permanent mesh should not be used.

Several articles have shown safety of laparoscopic and open approaches to incarcerated inguinal hernias, with decreased wound infection rates in the laparoscopic groups and similar recurrence rates when mesh was used.[7,8] Further quality studies evaluating the efficacy, safety, and cost of robotic inguinal hernia repairs are warranted. The hernia contents must be carefully viewed for possible ischemia and gangrene, regardless of approach, and care must be used when reducing these hernias to prevent bleeding or bowel perforation. Opening of the internal inguinal ring or direct hernia defect may be required. This is usually done with cautery from an anterior approach. In direct hernias, it should be done in the cephalad direction. In indirect hernias, it can be performed laterally along the direction of the transversalis, taking care to avoid unrecognized injury to the ilioinguinal nerve. In femoral hernias, the ilioinguinal ligament may have to be partially sacrificed, which can make an open repair more difficult. If the contents of the hernia reduce spontaneously during induction of anesthesia, intra-abdominal contents must still be evaluated. This can be done through a lower midline incision, using a laparoscope through the hernia defect, or laparoscopically or robotically from a transabdominal approach. If a totally extraperitoneal (TEP) repair is being performed, a defect in the peritoneum is necessary to evaluate the bowel. Another helpful tool in minimally invasive cases is bimanual reduction, where the bowel is pulled with traction internally, and concomitant manual manipulation at the level of the hernia externally.

16.6.1 Examples

The first example is an 87-year-old woman with chronic obstructive pulmonary disease (COPD) on home O2, hyperlipidemia (HLD), hypertension (HTN), arthritis, osteoporosis, and emphysema. She had a known right inguinal hernia for 25 years but prior to coming to the emergency room (ER), it acutely enlarged and she began to experience lower abdominal pain, nausea with vomiting, and increased shortness of breath. She was afebrile, with heart rate 100, blood pressure 149/67, and O2 saturation 100%. On physical examination, the hernia was only mildly tender with no erythema and was partially reduced in the ER with mild pressure. Her WBC was 14 and the rest of her labs unremarkable. No radiologic testing was done. She was stable overnight and was taken to the operating room (OR) the next day for an open repair. In the OR, an incarcerated direct hernia was found. The direct hernia sac was opened, and the incarcerated omentum was viable and resected with the hernia sac. The repair was done with mesh. The patient was discharged the next day and was doing well in follow-up. In this case, the patient did not have an acute need for operation but an urgent one. Despite the comorbidities of the patient, the urgent procedure was well-tolerated.

The second example is a 77-year-old with acute right lower quadrant (RLQ) abdominal pain, starting 12 hours prior to presentation and which was associated with nausea and vomiting. Her past medical history was unremarkable. A firm, tender femoral hernia was palpated on examination, which was nonreducible. WBC was 14, but she was not acidotic. CT confirmed a femoral hernia (▶ Fig. 16.2). She was urgently taken to the OR for open repair. There was black, necrotic bowel which was not reducible through the defect. Exploratory laparotomy was performed, and bimanual manipulation reduced the bowel without rupture after dividing the ilioinguinal ligament. A small bowel resection was performed through the laparotomy and the bowel repaired with a side-to-side anastomosis. The hernia was fixed with the help of Cooper's ligament repair. She developed ileus after surgery and spent 10 days in the hospital. At follow-up, she was doing well.

The third example is a 67-year-old man's status post right inguinal hernia repair five times with obesity (body mass index [BMI] 33) and smoking habit. He had a known recurrence of

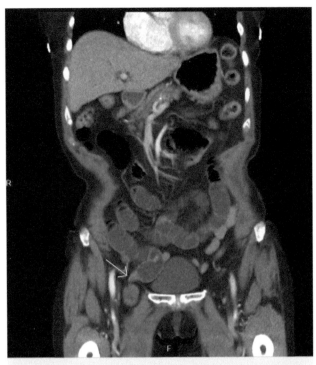

Fig. 16.2 CT image of strangulated femoral hernia in a 77-year-old woman. CT, computed tomography.

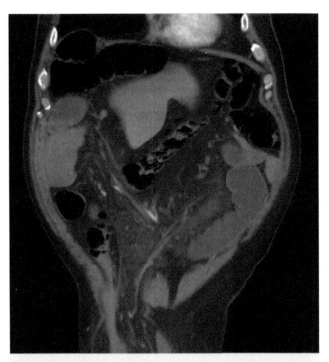

Fig. 16.3 CT image of large incarcerated right inguinal hernia. CT, computed tomography.

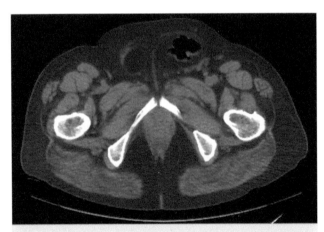

Fig. 16.4 CT image of incarcerated left inguinal hernia containing colon. CT, computed tomography.

hernia. He developed a bad cough 2 days prior to admission and secondarily developed right groin pain, nausea, and vomiting. His past medical history is otherwise unremarkable. He had a large, tender, scrotal hernia on examination, dehydration on labs, WBC 14, and CT showed bowel obstruction secondary to large scrotal hernia with fluid in the hernia (▶ Fig. 16.3). After volume resuscitation, the patient was taken urgently to the OR where open hernia repair was performed. A large inguinal incision was made. After the sac was entered, the small bowel, colon and omentum appeared viable and was reduced back into the abdomen. There was 1 liter of straw-colored fluid in the sac. The sac was amputated and closed. An absorbable mesh was used to repair the defect, and the tissues it was attached to

were considered weak and attenuated. The patient was discharged 4 days later after an unremarkable postop course.

In the fourth example, a 55-year-old male presented with acute pain in his left groin and irreducible bulge on examination. CT imaging revealed bilateral inguinal hernias, the left containing incarcerated colon, of which he had no prior knowledge of diagnosis (▶ Fig. 16.4). This patient's case was approached robotically via transabdominal preperitoneal (TAPP), in order to allow for intra-abdominal inspection of bowel, delicate reduction under visualization, and confirmation of complete reduction of bilateral hernia defects. As the colon was viable, these were both repaired with preperitoneal placement of permanent light-weight mesh. He was discharged home as an outpatient and was doing well at his 2-week postoperative visit.

16.7 Umbilical Hernia

The umbilical cord is formed around the fourth week of gestation, consisting of the umbilical vein, two umbilical arteries, and vitelline duct, covered by amnion. The defect in the linea alba that comprises the umbilical ring occurs where the cephalic, caudal, and right and left lateral embryologic folds come together and involute into the coelomic cavity. During development, the intestinal tract outgrows this cavity and between weeks 5 to 10 protrudes through the umbilicus; once it recedes, the umbilical ring starts to close. About 20% of neonates are born with an umbilical hernia, the vast majority of which close spontaneously over the first few years of life. While generally asymptomatic, incarceration can occur during this time period, which warrants open primary repair. Elective repair is often pursued if the hernia is present after 5 years of age, or if the child undergoes general anesthesia for another reason earlier.

In adults, this area of natural weakness is a common location for abdominal wall defects to occur; umbilical hernia remains the most common type of ventral hernia with an estimated prevalence of 2%. Small, asymptomatic umbilical hernias can generally be safely watched; however, up to 10% of umbilical hernias will require urgent or emergent intervention for incarceration. A recent Swiss study suggests that hernias with an increased hernia-neck-ratio, defined as the greatest diameter of the hernia sac parallel to the abdominal wall fascia measured on sagittal CT imaging, and divided by the maximum fascial defect on sagittal view, of >2.5 have a greater risk of incarceration or strangulation and should thus be repaired regardless of symptoms with 91% sensitivity and 84% specificity.[9] Notably, the median size of the hernia defect was not a predictor of incarceration on its own.

Incarcerated umbilical hernias can be repaired in both open and minimally invasive fashion. When performed open, a skin incision is made at a position directly overlying the hernia sac, and dissection carried circumferentially around the sac to the fascial neck. The herniated contents are reduced and the hernia sac resected. Posterior adhesions are carefully taken down if the mesh is going to be used. Inspection of the bowel to assess for viability is essential. If performed laparoscopically or robotically, an orogastric tube should be placed to decompress the stomach, and access is typically gained in the left upper quadrant, using the surgeon's preferred technique, with placement of further trocars on the left lateral abdomen; if additional assistant ports are required, the right lateral abdomen as well. The herniated contents and sac should be reduced in their entirety and efforts made to close the fascial defect. The mesh can be placed in an intraperitoneal or preperitoneal location. Multiple studies have demonstrated the safety of laparoscopy in emergent ventral hernia repair, as well as decreased rates of postoperative wound infection and shorter hospital length of stay.[10,11] There is less data available regarding a robotic approach; however, this is likely to translate to a similar outcome. The cost, although, may prove to be higher with robotics.

16.8 Epigastric, Ventral, and Incisional Hernias

Epigastric hernias are frequently found as upper midline firm masses, associated with the fascia, and frequently incarcerated but not strangulated. They otherwise are rubbery and feel like a lipoma. They are rarely present in the lower midline. They are congenital and are frequently symptomatic due to emanating from a very small defect in the linea alba. Although they can contain bowel, it is most common that they contain the falciform ligament or omentum. Since they may not be easily palpated after anesthesia, a careful description of the location should be given on preoperative examination, so they can be easily found at operation. They may be repaired by open midline incision over the hernia or laparoscopically. Mesh may not be indicated if the defect is small.

The incidence of incisional hernias should be decreasing as minimally invasive procedures are becoming more common.

Certainly, the repair of a trocar site hernia is generally easier than larger incisional hernias and less likely to recur because of the smaller fascial incision. The high-incidence of recurrent ventral hernias has led to increasingly complex methods of hernia repair that allow primary closure of fascia with preperitoneal mesh to reinforce the closure, so that bowel will not be able to adhere to mesh and provide added strength. In acute situations, these repairs may be inadvisable as they may lead to increased operative time and risk of infection through a larger operative field and infect several abdominal wall layers. Outcomes of transversus abdominis release in the nonelective hernia repair has been shown to have increased wound morbidity and requires more interventions than after elective hernia repair.[12] Certainly, in nonelective hernia repair, it may be impossible to primarily close the fascia due to loss of domain. If primary repair is attempted in these circumstances, increased abdominal pressure can lead to abdominal compartment syndrome and increased difficulty of breathing or ventilation due to increased peak inspiratory pressure. There are several options in this case: spanning mesh, either permanent dual mesh, absorbable mesh, or placement of a wound vac on the bowel or on over a mesh. With class II through class IV wounds, primary repair (generally for defects less than 3 cm) is advisable, but otherwise a spanning absorbable mesh should be used.[3] In a patient where second-look operations, like a patient with bowel left in discontinuity, a wound vac or Bogota bag is a good option, followed by spanning absorbable mesh when further operative interventions appear unlikely.[13]

In a multi-institutional study, laparoscopic versus open emergent ventral hernia repair demonstrated a lower length of hospital stay in the laparoscopic group with a slight increase in missed enterotomy.[14] Greater care has to be taken with laparoscopic lysis of adhesions, and excising mesh or peritoneum with the attached bowel can be considered. A larger study involving the American College of Surgeons National Surgical Quality Improvement Program Database showed that laparoscopic repair not only had lower length of hospital stay but also lower infection rates and no difference in major complications, reoperations and mortality.[10] One criticism of this type of study is that the groups are not equivalent; among other things, there are increased rates of contaminated or dirty wounds and sepsis in the open group.

As an example, a 66-year-old morbidly obese male with HTN, HLD, uncontrolled insulin-dependent diabetes and BMI 44.5 kg/m2 presented following multiple failed attempts at ventral hernia repair, with a surgical history of 15 abdominal procedures, including ileostomy with reversal and partial small bowel resection for obstruction. He was briefly admitted to an outside hospital for bowel obstruction but discharged after tolerating a diet. One week later, he presented with worsening abdominal pain, tachycardia with heart rate of 100 bpm, leukocytosis with left shift, and thrombocytosis. CT abdomen/pelvis was obtained, showing multiple bowel-containing ventral hernias, with interval development of a fluid collection containing a small amount of free air in the left lower quadrant hernia sac, which is concerning for perforation of herniated small bowel (▸ Fig. 16.5). Exploratory laparotomy was performed; adhesiolysis took 3 hours. Resection of perforated ischemic small bowel was performed and he was left in discontinuity (▸ Fig. 16.6). Multiple drains were placed. A negative pressure wound device was placed at the open

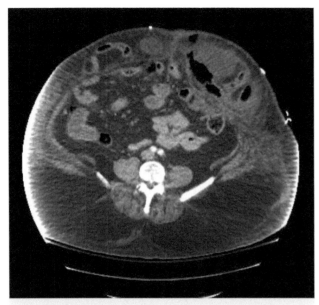

Fig. 16.5 Representative image from the preoperative CT of an incarcerated incisional hernia. CT, computed tomography.

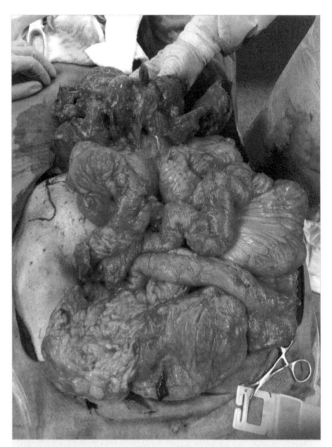

Fig. 16.6 Intraoperative findings of strangulated intestine in an incisional hernia.

abdomen. He was brought back to the OR 4 days later at which time an additional 5 hours of adhesiolysis was performed and his bowel put back into continuity. Again, a negative pressure wound vac was placed, which required replacement during washout 3 days later. He was extubated the following day and ultimately closed with bridging biologic mesh and a negative pressure device 6 days thereafter. He tolerated sequential diet progression and was discharged to a long-term acute care facility 1 week later.

16.9 Spigelian Hernia

Spigelian hernias are relatively rare and uncommonly become incarcerated. They occur medially and below the semilunar line and laterally to the rectus. They are just lateral to the internal ring of an indirect inguinal hernia. They are usually below the external oblique, making them difficult to palpate the hernia defect. If palpable, the contents of the hernia are felt just medial to the anterior superior iliac spine (ASIS). They can be just peritoneal fat but if they include bowel, there is almost always a peritoneal sac. In case reports, many pelvic organs and the appendix have been described in the hernia. Like any incarcerated hernia, they can be repaired with either an open or minimally invasive approach. Recurrence is common after open surgery, but since the hernia is rare, there is no significant literature comparing outcomes to robotic and laparoscopic repairs. A laparoscopic preperitoneal repair with mesh repair allows a larger, more greatly overlapped repair than open repair, without sutures in the expected area of the ilioinguinal nerve if the hernia is not large.

16.10 Diaphragmatic Hernia

Herniation through the crura of the hiatus is the most common type of diaphragmatic hernia, which is also known as paraesophageal hernia. Type 1, or sliding hiatal hernia, occurs when the esophagogastric junction and proximal stomach herniate through the hiatus, but keep their normal anatomic configuration; incarceration in this setting is extremely unlikely. Type 2, or a true paraesophageal hernia, occurs when the fundus of the stomach herniates through the hiatus, but the esophagogastric junction remains in its intraabdominal location; this has the highest risk of incarceration. This is not to be confused with a parahiatal hernia, in which the stomach herniates through a diaphragmatic defect located just outside of the crural musculature, rather than the hiatus. Type 3 paraesophageal hernia occurs when both the esophagogastric junction and stomach herniate through the hiatus, but the configuration is such that the stomach lays cephalad to the lower esophageal sphincter. This accounts for most of the large hiatal hernia and can be associated with organoaxial or mesoaxial volvulus, with rotation around the long-axis of the stomach or around its mesentery, respectively. The latter is at much higher risk of strangulation or infarction. Type 4 paraesophageal hernias include other organs such as colon, pancreas, spleen or liver, and generally occur with very large hiatal defects.

Patients with incarcerated paraesophageal hernias present with severe substernal chest pain, and in light of this, they are often worked up for acute cardiac events. Emesis and oral intolerance are often associated. If patients are hemodynamically normal, nasogastric decompression should

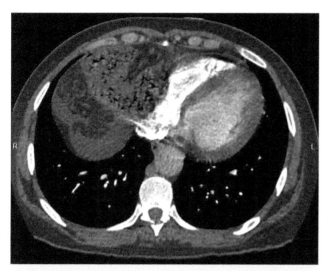

Fig. 16.7 Axial CT image of incarcerated Morgagni hernia. CT, computed tomography.

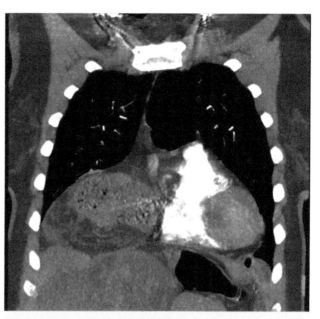

Fig. 16.8 Coronal CT image of incarcerated Morgagni hernia. CT, computed tomography.

be attempted, and Gastrograffin CT or upper gastrointestinal tract radiography (GI) performed to evaluate for obstruction. If the patient is hemodynamically unstable or upper GI series is consistent with gastric outflow obstruction, emergent intervention is warranted. These patients are at higher risk of aspiration during intubation, and the anesthesia team should be aware.

Incarcerated paraesophageal hernia repair can be approached minimally invasively, as would elective repair. Typically, five to six upper abdominal trocars are used, and the surgeon positions him or herself on the patient's right or between split legs. Care should be taken during reduction of the herniated contents, as the stomach or other organs may be friable and congested if the vascular supply was compromised. Very large hernia sacs should be resected and removed following reduction or at least be detached fully around the crura to prevent recurrence. It can be difficult to identify the vagus nerves, as they frequently are attached to the sac and no longer run along the esophagus. The right gastric vascular pedicle is also important to spare. Significant necrosis or gastric perforation warrants exploratory laparotomy and damage control surgery with resection of nonviable tissues. The patient may be left in discontinuity with planned return for a second look and reconstruction when hemodynamically normalized. Bioabsorbable mesh may be used during hiatal repair if the defect is adequately significant and closure cannot be done under tension but primary repair with mesh reinforcement is more common. Making a separate incision in the diaphragm on the left lateral side may allow primary closure of the hiatus, but then this defect will have to be repaired with a spanning permanent mesh. As in other cases, permanent meshes should be used with caution in cases where there is possible infection. Gastropexy may be utilized in the emergent setting rather than fundoplication.

There has been much debate regarding elective repair of asymptomatic paraesophageal hernias. Recent studies suggest that watchful waiting is not only safe, but that elective repair also results in lower quality of life results than most asymptomatic patients who do not undergo surgery.[15] A large population-based study in the United States found the

postoperative mortality rate following emergent paraesophageal hernia repair versus elective paraesophageal hernia repair to be 3.2% and 0.37%, respectively.[16] Given the overall infrequency of emergent paraesophageal hernia repair, and the potential morbidity and recurrences associated with elective repair, this may argue against elective repair in asymptomatic patients.

Morgagni hernias occur in the anterior diaphragm, between the sternum and costal diaphragmatic attachments, with contents protruding through the right or left sternocostal triangle (just below the costal margin on the right or left of the falciform ligament). It is also called the foramen of Morgagni which is where the superior epigastric arteries perforate the diaphragm. These hernias are rare, comprising only 3% of congenital diaphragmatic hernias, and may include omentum, stomach, colon, or other intraabdominal structures. Most of these have a peritoneal lining. Patients with symptomatic incarcerated Morgagni hernias present with severe retrosternal pain, like incarcerated paraesophageal hernias, and may also have associated nausea and vomiting. Reduction and repair can successfully be done in a minimally invasive approach.

For example, a 45-year-old African-American female with HTN, anxiety, and depression with current 1-ppd smoking history presented to the Emergency Department (ED) with severe, crushing retrosternal chest pain. Computed tomography angiography (CTA) without oral contrast was obtained to evaluate for cardiovascular abnormalities. Cardiac workup was negative, however the CTA did reveal a large Morgagni hernia with herniated stomach, transverse colon, omentum, and fluid posterior to the sternum (▶ Fig. 16.7 and ▶ Fig. 16.8). The patient was taken urgently to the OR for urgent laparoscopic repair, which provided excellent visualization of the defect and inspection of the herniated contents to assess for viability. A 12 mm optical trocar was used to get access 18 cm inferior to the xiphoid and three 5 mm working subcostal trocars. Following reduction, the hernia sac was dissected from the mediastinum and removed; it should be noted that great care is taken during this dissection to avoid injury to the pericardium and pleura. The falciform ligament was taken down to allow for proper mesh overlap. The defect was closed with interrupted 0-permanent pledgeted suture, and dual type of mesh placed over the closure with 3 cm overlap in all directions. She was discharged home on postoperative day 1, tolerating a diet and doing well. She was seen at 1-month postop and was symptom-free.

Bochdalek hernias are congenital diaphragmatic hernias that occur posteriorly when the posterolateral diaphragmatic foramina fail to close properly and contain retroperitoneal structures such as retroperitoneal fat or kidneys and, more rarely, bowel or other organs. These hernias generally do not have a peritoneal lining. They are generally identified in infancy (called congenital diaphragmatic hernias or CDH) and are thus quite rare in adulthood. Whereas respiratory symptoms are common in children, symptomatic adults tend to present acutely with complaints consistent with gastrointestinal obstruction.[17] Autopsy and imaging studies have found incidence ranging from as low as .17% to as high as 6%.[18,19] When considering operative approaches for repair, minimally invasive techniques can be employed pending imaging findings and surgeon skill level. Generally, a transabdominal approach is recommended when patients present with concern of stomach or bowel incarceration to evaluate for viability. Adhesions of abdominal contents in the chest are rare. When gastrointestinal integrity is not of concern, a transthoracic approach can be considered. If the contents of the hernia cannot be reduced safely through the abdomen, a chest approach can be added. Large defects may require the use of a permanent mesh product.

Traumatic diaphragmatic hernias are rare but can occur following both penetrating and blunt trauma, and deliberate attention should be paid to not miss a traumatic defect at the time of damage-control laparotomy. Iatrogenic injuries can also occur during upper abdominal or thoracic operations, and care should be taken to avoid this occurrence. Delayed presentation of traumatic diaphragmatic hernias can result in respiratory compromise, incarceration, or strangulation of intra-abdominal organs, which rarely result in intraperitoneal or intrathoracic perforation. It is generally accepted that most late-presentations of incarceration or strangulation were missed smaller injuries at a prior date, highlighting the importance of initial recognition. Significant respiratory compromise more commonly occurs from a left-sided injury, as herniation of contents on the right may be somewhat limited do to the liver. Patients may present with shock secondary to tension viscerothorax, for which correct diagnosis is of particular importance, as treatment requires nasogastric decompression and insertion of thoracostomy tubes can result in gastrointestinal perforation.[20] Approach to repair again depends on the patient's clinical state and sequelae from herniated contents. A transabdominal approach allows for assessment of stomach and bowel and resection when required.

16.11 Flank Hernia

Most flank hernias are due to flank incisions and many are merely diastasis caused by those incisions. These rarely strangulate; although, they can cause bowel obstructions due to adhesions from the prior surgery. There are upper and lower congenital defects. These are easily palpated on physical examination of the flank. Incarceration has only been described in case reports and open, laparoscopic and robotic repairs have been utilized.[21,22]

Primary repair can be used but it appears that recurrence is frequent, so underlay mesh may improve outcomes.

16.12 Pelvic Hernia

The most common of these is the obturator hernia which accounts for less than 1% of hernias and less than 0.5% of bowel obstructions (▸ Fig. 16.9). Incarcerated bladder, ovary and fallopian tube have also been described. It is far more common among older women.[23]

Frequently, no mass is palpated on physical examination because the hernia is small and below the pectineal fascia, but there may be tenderness of the adductor muscles due to pressure on the obturator nerve. In this case, hip extension, adduction or internal rotation will increase the pain. It is usually identified on preoperative CT. It must be carefully looked for if no other cause of obstruction is found on diagnostic laparoscopy or exploratory laparotomy. An open approach can be taken through a transabdominal or preperitoneal approach. If a preperitoneal approach is performed, an overlay mesh can be used; otherwise, the defect can be sutured after reduction of the hernia sac with careful attention to avoid the obturator nerve and vessels. Laparoscopic total extraperitoneal (TEP) repair, with careful evaluation of the hernia contents and bowel, is possible but may have a conversion rate of 25%.[24]

Sciatic hernias account for less than 0.1% of all hernias and are typically not incarcerated on presentation. When larger, they bulge at the gluteal fold.[25] Ureteral obstruction has also been described.[26]

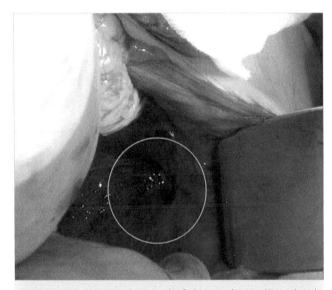

Fig. 16.9 Intraoperative photograph of obturator hernia. (Reproduced with permission of the Journal of the Louisiana State Medical Society.)

16.13 Internal Hernia

Internal hernias occur when bowel protrudes through a mesenteric, intraperitoneal or retroperitoneal defect. Most of these are acquired, due to postoperative or traumatic changes; however, rare congenital internal hernias such as paraduodenal, pericecal, and transmesenteric or transomental hernias can occur. Common surgeries after which internal hernias may occur include small bowel or colonic resections, or those during which intestines are mobilized and reanastomosed such as pancreaticoduodenectomy or roux-en-y gastric bypass. Adhesions in and of themselves can create spaces for internal hernias, which can be sequelae of prior surgery or significant trauma. Internal hernias after liver transplantation have also been well-described.[27]

Much like those of external hernias, patients with internal hernias may be asymptomatic, or present with symptoms of intermittent abdominal cramping, nausea, vomiting, diarrhea, or severe abdominal pain with or without obstipation, and the latter may indicate obstruction, strangulation or. The incidence of internal hernias may be < 1%; however, they cause up to 5.8% of all small-bowel obstructions, and patients who present in extremis carry a mortality rate as high as 50%, emphasizing the importance of early recognition and surgical correction.[28,29] CT scan is the preferred imaging modality for diagnosis, with various signs that can reliably indicate internal herniation.[30] For paraduodenal hernias, a circumscribed mass of small-bowel loops will be noted in the left upper quadrant of the abdomen, lateral to the ascending colon if on the left, or inferior and lateral to the descending duodenum if on the right. If through the foramen of Winslow, loops of small bowel will be noted medial and posterior to the stomach. Pericecal hernia findings show clustered distal small-bowel loops posterior and lateral to the cecum in the right paracolic gutter. CT findings consistent with internal hernia, particularly following roux-en-y, include "swirling" of mesenteric vessels, clustered loops of small bowel, "mushroom" shape of herniated mesenteric root with crowding of the vessels, tubular or round shape of distal mesenteric fat closely surrounded by bowel loops, presence of small bowel other than duodenum passing posterior to the superior mesenteric artery, and right-sided location of jejunojejunostomy.[30] Internal hernias can be dynamic, however, particularly in patients with colicky symptoms, which can be missed during a moment of transient reduction. As such, exploration, which we recommend be done laparoscopically if possible, is warranted if symptoms continue despite negative imaging studies in high-risk patients. This can often be conducted in an elective or semi-urgent fashion in stable patients with minimal symptoms. Physical examination may note a palpable area of fullness with associated tenderness, in which case exploration should not be delayed. Signs or symptoms of peritonitis or imaging revealing pneumoperitoneum require emergent intervention. The bowel should be run in its entirety and should start at a fixed point such as the terminal ileum, so as not to exacerbate the herniated bowel (although this is not fixed when there is malrotation).

References

[1] Chung PJ, Lee JS, Tam S, et al. Predicting 30-day postoperative mortality for emergent anterior abdominal wall hernia repairs using the American college of surgeons national surgical quality improvement program database. Hernia. 2017; 21:322–333

[2] Beadles CA, Meagher AD, Charles AG. Trends in emergent hernia repair in the United States. JAMA Surg. 2015; 150(3):194–200

[3] Birindelli A, Sartelli M, Di Saverio S, et al. 2017 update of the WSES guidelines for emergency repair of complicated abdominal wall hernias. World J EmergSurg. 2017; 12:37

[4] Haskins IN, Amdur RL, Lin PP, Vaziri K. The use of mesh in emergent ventral hernia repair: effects on early patient morbidity and mortality. J GastrointestSurg. 2016; 20(11):1899–1903

[5] Malespin M, Moore CM, Fialho A, et al. Case series of 10 patients with cirrhosis undergoing emergent repair of ruptured umbilical hernias: natural history and predictors of outcomes. Exp Clin Transplant. 2019; 17 (2):210–213

[6] Dahlstrand U, Wollert S, Nordin P, Sandblom G, Gunnarsson U. Emergency femoral hernia repair: a study based on a national register. Ann Surg. 2009; 249(4):672–676

[7] Tastaldi L, Krpata DM, Prabhu AS, et al. Emergent groin hernia repair: a single center 10-year experience. Surgery. 2019; 165(2):398–405

[8] Pechman DM, Cao L, Fong C, Thodiyil P, Surick B. Laparoscopic versus open emergent ventral hernia repair: utilization and outcomes analysis using the ACSNSQIP database. SurgEndosc. 2018; 32(12):4999–5005

[9] Fueter T, Schäfer M, Fournier P, Bize P, Demartines N, Allemann P. The hernia-neck-ratio (HNR), a novel predictive factor for complications of umbilical hernia. World J Surg. 2016; 40(9):2084–2090

[10] Azin, et al. Emergency laparoscopic and open repair of incarcerated ventral hernias: a multi-institutional comparative analysis with coarsened exact matching. SurgEndosc. 2018. DOI: 10.1007/s00464-018-6573-6

[11] Landau O, Kyzer S. Emergent laparoscopic repair of incarcerated incisional and ventral hernia. SurgEndosc. 2004; 18(9):1374–1376

[12] Alkhatib H, Tastaldi L, Krpata DM, et al. Outcomes of transversus abdominis release in non-elective incisional hernia repair: a retrospective review of the Americas Hernia Society Quality Collaborative (AHSQC). Hernia. 2019; 23(1): 43–49

[13] Rodriguez-Unda N, Soares KC, Azoury SC, et al. Negative-pressure wound therapy in the management of high-grade ventral hernia repairs. J GastrointestSurg. 2015; 19(11):2054–2061

[14] Kao AM, Huntington CR, Otero J, et al. Emergent laparoscopic ventral hernia repairs. J Surg Res. 2018; 232:497–502

[15] Jung JJ, Naimark DM, Behman R, Grantcharov TP. Approach to asymptomatic paraesophageal hernia: watchful waiting or elective laparoscopic hernia repair? SurgEndosc. 2018; 32(2):864–871

[16] Jassim H, Seligman JT, Frelich M, et al. A population-based analysis of emergent versus elective paraesophageal hernia repair using the Nationwide Inpatient Sample. SurgEndosc. 2014; 28(12):3473–3478

[17] Hamid KS, Rai SS, Rodriguez JA. Symptomatic Bochdalek hernia in an adult. JSLS. 2010; 14(2):279–281

[18] Salaçin S, Alper B, Cekin N, Gülmen MK. Bochdalek hernia in adulthood: a review and an autopsy case report. J Forensic Sci. 1994; 39(4):1112–1116

[19] Gale ME. Bochdalek hernia: prevalence and CT characteristics. Radiology. 1985; 156(2):449–452

[20] Wakai S, Otsuka H, Aoki H, Yamagiwa T, Nakagawa Y, Inokuchi S. A case of incarcerated and perforated stomach in delayed traumatic diaphragmatic hernia. Tokai J Exp Clin Med. 2017; 42(2):85–88

[21] Kapur SK, Liu J, Baumann DP, Butler CE. Surgical outcomes in lateral abdominal wall reconstruction: a comparative analysis of surgical techniques. J Am CollSurg. 2019; 229(3):267–276–; epub ahead of print

[22] Zhou DJ, Carlson MA. Incidence, etiology, management, and outcomes of flank hernia: review of published data. Hernia. 2018; 22(2):353–361

[23] Otsuki Y, Konn H, Takeda K, Koike M. Midline extraperitoneal approach for obturator hernia repair. Keio J Med. 2018; 67(4):67–71

[24] Carter T, Ballard DH, Bhargava P, et al. Obturator hernia, 'the little old lady hernia'. J La State Med Soc. 2017; 169:96–98

[25] Losanoff JE, Basson MD, Gruber SA, Weaver DW. Sciatic hernia: a comprehensive review of the world literature (1900–2008). Am J Surg. 2010; 199(1):52–59

[26] Speeg JS, Vanlangendonck RM, Jr, Fusilier H, Richardson WS. An unusual presentation of a sciatic hernia. Am Surg. 2009; 75(11):1139–1141

[27] Blachar A, Federle MP. Bowel obstruction following liver transplantation: clinical and ct findings in 48 cases with emphasis on internal hernia. Radiology. 2001; 218(2):384–388

[28] Ghahremani GG. Abdominal and pelvic hernias. In: Gore RM, Levine MS, eds. Textbook of Gastrointestinal Radiology. 2nd ed. Philadelphia, PA: Saunders; 2000:1993–2009

[29] Newsom BD, Kukora JS. Congenital and acquired internal hernias: unusual causes of small bowel obstruction. Am J Surg. 1986; 152(3):279–285

[30] Martin LC, Merkle EM, Thompson WM. Review of internal hernias: radiographic and clinical findings. AJR Am J Roentgenol. 2006; 186(3): 703–717

Expert Commentary on Surgical Management of Incarcerated Hernias by *Brent Matthews*

Expert Commentary on Surgical Management of Incarcerated Hernias

Brent Matthews

The heterogeneity of inguinal, epigastric, umbilical, ventral, incisional, flank, Spigelian, diaphragmatic and internal hernias and varied clinical scenarios for presentation of the patient with an incarcerated hernia requires that the acute care surgeon possess a broad-based understanding of the technical aspects of damage control surgery with regard to definitive hernia repair, utilizing minimally invasive techniques. This chapter by Drs. Gorham and Richardson provides an excellent overview of the different types of incarcerated hernias, anatomical approaches to surgical repair with pertinent technical pearls, critical review of clinical outcomes for acute repair as well as the use of biomaterials. Several clinical case examples and images highlight the information provided. The authors provide a reference to the World Society of Emergency Surgery (WSES) Guidelines from 2017 for emergency repair of complicated abdominal wall hernias. This publication outlines recommendations for the laparoscopic approach to repair of incarcerated hernias, and the use of synthetic mesh in cases without bowel strangulation or requiring concurrent intestinal resection.

Incarcerated hernias are likely to be a more common clinical condition cared for by the acute care surgeon. The rate of emergent ventral hernia repair in the United States is on the rise, particularly in patients >65 years of age. Both race and socioeconomic status have been associated with increased risk of presenting with an acute hernia complication requiring emergent surgery. Therefore, future healthcare policy decisions affecting access or coverage could alter the incidence of incarcerated hernias in certain patient populations. The American Society for Metabolic and Bariatric Surgery (ASMBS) estimate of bariatric surgery numbers 2011 to 2017 published in 2018 estimated that 362,000 Roux-en-Y gastric bypass procedures were performed during that 7-year period. Based on historical rates of 2 to 3% for internal hernias, it would be expected that between 7,240 to 10,860 patients will develop this postoperative complication. Although the rates of gastric bypass surgery are decreasing, there is still a significant number of patients exposed to this potential complication. As Prehabilitation, a program to preoperatively optimize patients prior to elective hernia repair to minimize the postoperative risk of preoperative morbidities such as diabetes, obesity, tobacco use, sarcopenia, and anemia, becomes more ubiquitous, the likelihood of patients presenting with incarcerated hernias may increase as these patients are delaying repair by either being in the optimization program or electing not to comply with programmatic standard, thus deferring repair. This clinical scenario is an unintended consequence of optimization programs that may take months to complete. The acute care surgeon could ultimately be responsible for the management of patients in all these illustrations. Ultimately, patient outcomes are optimized when the acute care surgeon is aware of the variety of options for management and how to choose the best strategy for each unique patient and clinical situation.

17 Mesenteric Ischemia

James Becker, Todd W. Costantini, and Joseph M. Galante

Summary

Acute mesenteric ischemia (AMI) causes hypoperfusion of the intestine and can be the result of embolic, thrombotic, veno-occlusive or non-occlusive etiologies. While AMI is somewhat rare, it represents a potential surgical emergency that the acute care surgeon will be called upon to evaluate. Optimal treatment of AMI requires a high index of suspicion, prompt diagnosis and timely intervention to prevent bowel necrosis and even death. This chapter will review the presentation, diagnostic tests, imaging modalities, and treatment options to manage AMI.

Keywords: Bowel ischemia, gut, thrombosis, embolism

17.1 Introduction

Broadly, the diagnosis of mesenteric ischemia refers to decreased perfusion of the mesenteric vessels, which fails to meet the metabolic demands of the hollow viscera. This diagnosis most frequently describes hypoperfusion of the jejunum and ileum, while ischemic colitis is a separate clinical entity. Mesenteric ischemia can be categorized by chronicity (acute versus chronic) and etiology of hypoperfusion (embolic, thrombotic, nonocclusive, and veno-occlusive) (▶ Table 17.1). This represents an important diagnostic distinction, as the recommended treatment depends on the etiology of the mesenteric ischemia.

Acute mesenteric vascular occlusive disease is somewhat rare, accounting for less than 7 per 100,000 hospital admissions, but represents a potentially devastating condition with a mortality rate greater than 50%.[1] It is primarily a disease of the elderly, most commonly affecting patients in their 60s and 70s. There is a disproportionately high prevalence in women, with a rate almost three times that of men. Typically, patients with acute mesenteric ischemia (AMI) will suffer from multiple cardiovascular comorbidities, and commonly have a history of tobacco use.

Embolic mesenteric ischemia is the most commonly encountered form of AMI, accounting for 40 to 50% of cases. Most of these cases are cardioembolic in nature, and a careful history and physical examination may reveal the inciting event. Recent myocardial infarction, atrial fibrillation or flutter, ventricular aneurysm, congestive heart failure, cardiac valvular disease, recent catheter-based interventions, and prior embolic events are all risk factors for embolic mesenteric ischemia. The rate of embolic mesenteric ischemia appears to be declining, and it is hypothesized that this may be due to improved anticoagulation of patients with known atrial arrhythmias. The mortality rate with embolic mesenteric ischemia is documented as ranging from 30 to 50%, and has remained consistent over time, despite improving resuscitative strategies and the advent of endovascular approaches to therapy.

Thrombotic mesenteric ischemia is the second most common type of mesenteric ischemia, accounting for about 25 to 30% of cases. It typically occurs in the setting of preexisting mesenteric vascular atherosclerosis, with acute plaque rupture and thrombosis. There is frequently a history of weight loss and/or food avoidance, which is consistent with chronic mesenteric vascular stenosis. Some series demonstrate a higher mortality rate (upward of 75%) associated with thrombotic mesenteric ischemia. This is presumed to be due to the fact that the thrombosis occurs near the ostium of the superior mesenteric artery (SMA), as opposed to more heterogeneous and distal emboli, resulting in longer, confluent segments of bowel necrosis.

Nonocclusive mesenteric ischemia (NOMI) is less common, causing about 5 to 15% of cases. It results from an acute decrease in mesenteric vascular blood flow.[2] It has been demonstrated that periods of reduced mesenteric perfusion result in reactive mesenteric vasoconstriction which may further compound the ischemic insult.[3] This effect may, similarly, be precipitated by the use of vasoconstricting agents in the management of shock. Unlike thrombotic mesenteric ischemia, in nonocclusive disease, the mesenteric vasculature remains patent, but there is an acute decrease in blood flow through the narrowed vessels. This is often due to hypovolemia, resulting in reduced cardiac output and hypoperfusion. Other risk factors include acute myocardial infarction, sepsis resulting in shock, congestive heart failure, and known visceral arterial atherosclerosis. Pancreatitis may also precipitate NOMI, reportedly in about 6.7% of cases, due to the proximity of the pancreas and SMA.[4] The mortality rate from NOMI is very high, on the order of 50%, likely because of the high-rate of concurrent medical conditions (shock, CHF, MI, etc.).[5]

Mesenteric venous thrombosis (MVT) also accounts for between 5 and 15% of cases of AMI. Obstruction of outflow from the intestines leads to venous congestion, ultimately

Table 17.1 Causes of acute mesenteric ischemia

Cause	Incidence	Clinical presentation	Risk factors
Embolic	40–50%	Acute diffuse abdominal pain, out of proportion to examination findings	Arrhythmia (atrial fibrillation), recent myocardial infarction, recent heart catheterization, valvular disease, cardiomyopathy
Thrombotic	25–30%	Chronic pain, weight loss, acute worsening	Atherosclerosis (chronic mesenteric ischemia), hypercoagulable states
Veno-occlusive	5–15%	Subacute, progressive abdominal pain	Hypercoagulable states, pancreatitis, portal hypertension (cirrhosis, right-heart failure), recent abdominal surgery, intraabdominal infection
Nonocclusive	5–15%	Acute abdominal pain or unexplained deterioration in critically ill patient	Hypovolemia, use of vasoconstrictors, low cardiac output

compromises microvascular circulation, and causes bowel necrosis. Factors that increase the risk of venous thrombosis in general also increase the risk for venous mesenteric ischemia. Conditions leading to intraabdominal inflammation, such as pancreatitis, inflammatory bowel disease, recent abdominal operations, and intra-abdominal infections increase risk. Obesity, portal hypertension, increased intraabdominal pressure, and congestive heart failure lead to increased intraabdominal pressure and venous congestion. Inherited and acquired thrombophilic conditions such as Factor V Leiden, protein C and S deficiency, thrombocytosis, heparin-induced thrombocytopenia, and malignancies also increase risk of MVT. Overall, the mortality rate from MVT is similar to other etiologies, ranging from 20 to 50%, and more likely in patients with comorbid obesity, portal vein thrombosis, and systemic venous thromboembolism.[6,7]

Chronic mesenteric ischemia is, as the name implies, a gradual process of atherosclerotic narrowing of the mesenteric vasculature. It is associated with aortoiliac atherosclerosis and has a strong link with smoking history. Clinical features classically include a fear of eating due to the severe pain that accompanies the increased and unmet metabolic demands of the bowel after eating. Due to the progressive nature of the disease, there are typically robust collateral vessels that form and prevent frank bowel necrosis. While chronic mesenteric ischemia is typically not a disease managed by the acute care surgeon, it is important to recognize the role it may play in predisposing patients to other forms of AMI, particularly thrombotic and non-occlusive mesenteric ischemia. As such, it is important for the acute care surgeon to recognize chronic mesenteric ischemia and consider it as a risk factor when evaluating patients in the acute setting.

Early recognition of AMI remains a challenge faced by acute care surgeons, requiring a high-degree of suspicion, familiarity with vascular and gastrointestinal surgical techniques, and expeditious management, which is critical to optimize patient survival.[8]

17.2 Anatomy of Mesenteric Circulation

The abdominal hollow viscera derive their blood supply from segmental branches of the primitive ventral aorta, which persist throughout embryogenesis and develop into the celiac trunk, SMA, inferior mesenteric artery (IMA), and the collateral circulation between these vessels. The celiac axis is the first major branch of the abdominal aorta, arising at the level of T12–L1, just below the diaphragmatic hiatus. It is bounded superiorly by the median arcuate ligament and inferiorly by the superior border of the pancreas. It classically gives rise to three branches: the splenic artery, left gastric artery, and common hepatic artery, although multiple variations to this scheme are seen in practice. The celiac artery has collateral circulation with the SMA around the head of the pancreas and through the gastroduodenal and pancreaticoduodenal vessels.

The SMA typically arises about 1 centimeter caudal to the celiac axis, around the inferior border of L1, and courses posterior to the neck of the pancreas. The SMA emerges anterior to the uncinate process of the pancreas and lies anterior to the course of the left renal vein and the third portion of the duodenum. Multiple visceral branches arise from the SMA and are responsible for the perfusion of most of the bowel, from the proximal jejunum through the splenic flexure of the colon. The SMA first gives off the inferior pancreaticoduodenal arteries, then the middle colic artery, followed by the jejunal and ileal arcades, right colic, and ileocolic vessels. The SMA supplies blood to the majority of the intestines, from the duodenum to the distal transverse colon. The SMA has collateral flow with the IMA through the meandering mesenteric artery (also called the arc of Riolan) and the marginal artery of Drummond around the level of the splenic flexure (Griffith's point).

The IMA arises from the aorta, slightly to the left of midline, about 4 centimeters proximal to the aortic bifurcation, and around the level of the L3 vertebra. It gives rise to the left colic and sigmoidal arteries and terminates in the superior rectal artery. The IMA provides perfusion from the distal transverse colon to the proximal rectum. The superior rectal (from the IMA) and middle/inferior rectal arteries (from branches of the internal iliac artery) form collaterals in the pelvis around the rectum at Sudak's point.

17.3 Diagnosis of Acute Mesenteric Ischemia

Mesenteric ischemia is rare but has a very high mortality rate, requiring expeditious diagnosis and treatment to optimize chances of survival. Due to the devastating nature of the disease, a high-index of suspicion is necessary when evaluating the patient with abdominal pain. In order to differentiate AMI from the myriad conditions that can cause abdominal pain, a careful history, physical examination, laboratory analysis, and imaging workup is required. Sometimes, the diagnosis may be made in the operating room (OR) in a patient who presents with peritonitis and instability.

17.3.1 History and Physical Examination

The classic description of patients with AMI is one of pain out of proportion to their physical examination findings. The physical findings reflect the degree of bowel injury, with the initial presentation of pain without tenderness progressing to peritonitis as the bowel ischemia becomes transmural, and the parietal peritoneum is exposed to inflammatory mediators. Patients may develop abdominal distention fairly early in the course of their illness. As the bowel mucosa becomes ischemic and sloughs, there may be evidence of gastrointestinal bleeding. There is frequently associated tachycardia and, as the disease progresses to frank bowel necrosis, patients may develop fever, oliguria, hypotension, and altered mental status.

AMI resulting from embolic occlusion of the SMA results in the rapid onset of severe abdominal pain. As these patients have not frequently developed collateral circulation, the pain is rapidly progressive, and there are typically no antecedent symptoms. There may be a history of associated nausea and vomiting and/or diarrhea that came on shortly after the pain began. In patients with thrombotic occlusion of the SMA, there is frequently underlying atherosclerosis of the mesenteric vessels, resulting in the development of collateral circulation. As such, the pain from an SMA thrombus may be a bit more insidious, with some degree of discomfort and nausea for many days prior to the acute worsening that prompts medical evaluation. NOMI typically arises in patients who are already hospitalized. There is frequently a history of shock and multiorgan failure, requiring vasopressor use, with an abrupt worsening of the patient's condition as the bowel begins to infarct. In the ambulatory population, there may be a history of progressive shortness of breath and pedal edema, consistent with heart failure exacerbation, which is complicated by abdominal pain due to cardiogenic shock and hypoperfusion of the gut. MVT is difficult to diagnose on history alone. There is typically a report of diffuse abdominal pain, of varying duration, prior to the patient presenting for evaluation. There is often a history of nausea and vomiting, and lower gastrointestinal symptoms such as diarrhea are relatively less common. Patients with MVT may be younger than those with other types of mesenteric ischemia, and there is more likely to be a history of DVT or another hypercoagulable event.

As stated previously, there are a number of risk factors that might be elucidated from a careful history. While not always obtainable due to alterations in mental state, efforts should be made to elicit any history of cardiac disease, especially atrial fibrillation, and breaks in the use of anticoagulants, as these are clues as to a possible embolic source. A history of chronic mesenteric ischemia certainly increases the concern for both thrombotic and nonocclusive disease, and a careful assessment of concomitant illness that might predispose the patient to NOMI is mandatory. Finally, a history of hypercoagulability, both personal and familial, raise suspicion for mesenteric venous occlusion.

17.3.2 Laboratory Analysis

While there are no laboratory studies that are specific for SMA occlusion or MVT, studies that reflect a systemic inflammatory state and end-organ hypoperfusion may be abnormal. Accordingly, blood counts may demonstrate leukocytosis and

thrombocytosis, and a basic metabolic panel may show an elevated serum creatinine and an elevated anion gap. Measured L-lactate may be elevated (86% sensitivity), especially later in the course of the disease, but represents a nonspecific (44%) marker. Elevated D-dimers are fairly sensitive (96%) but not specific (40%) to AMI either.

The novel biomarkers such as intestinal fatty acid-binding protein (I-FABP), ischemia modified albumin, α-glutathione S-transferase (α-GST), and citrulline are under investigation for the diagnosis of acute intestinal ischemia but are not yet widely used. In a recent meta-analysis, the most promising candidates appeared to be ischemia-modified albumin (sensitivity 95%, specificity 86%) and I-FABP by the Uden kit (sensitivity 79%, specificity 91%). Both tests were noted to be suitable for rapid performance and had early elaboration in the disease process, allowing for timely diagnosis. The authors concluded that while promising, these data required further confirmation to identify the ideal role for ischemia-modified albumin and I-FABP assays in diagnosing mesenteric ischemia.[9]

17.3.3 Imaging

Abdominal angiography has been considered the gold standard imaging study for mesenteric ischemia until recently. It is sensitive (74–100%) and specific (100%) for AMI and allows for therapeutic intervention in the hands of an experienced endovascular surgeon. In the last decade, the improved quality and availability of multidetector computed tomography (CT) has changed the paradigm of imaging for mesenteric ischemia. CT arteriography (CTA) is widely available, rapidly obtainable, and highly accurate (sensitivity 93%, specificity 100%), and has supplanted conventional angiography as the recommended initial imaging study[10] (▶ Fig. 17.1). The presence of ostial thromboses or more distal embolic disease within the SMA confirms the diagnosis. While as many as 25% of patients with NOMI may present without classical findings on CT scan,[11] SMA vasospasm is present in 66% of patients, confirming the diagnosis. In addition, 76% patients showed signs of intestinal ischemia in the absence of mesenteric vascular occlusion.[12]

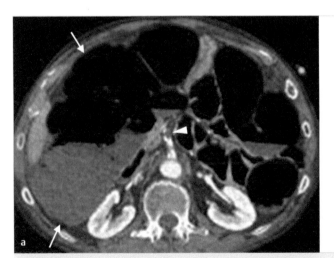 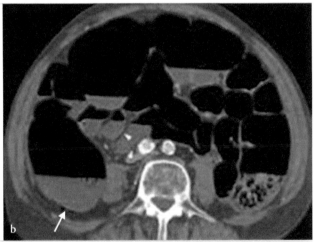

Fig. 17.1 (a, b) Embolic mesenteric ischemia seen on CT angiography of the abdomen. *Arrowhead* demonstrates clot in the superior mesenteric artery. Source: Claire K. Sandstrom: Pathophysiology and imaging diagnosis of acute mesenteric ischemia. Digestive Disease Interventions 2018; 02(03): 195-209.

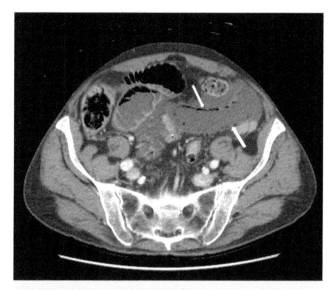

Fig. 17.2 Pneumatosisintestinalis. Small intestinal pneumatosis (*arrows*) seen on CT scan of the abdomen.

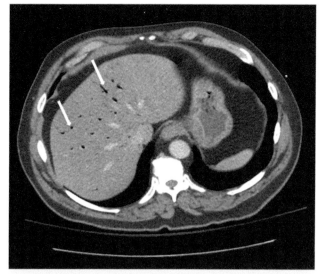

Fig. 17.3 Portal venous gas (*arrows*) on CT scan of the abdomen.

Table 17.2 CT findings of acute mesenteric ischemia

Vascular

- Arterial atherosclerosis, stenosis, vasospasm, occlusion, dissection; portal venous or mesenteric venous occlusion, portal venous gas

Bowel

- Bowel wall thickening with acute injury or thinning with irreversible injury, hypoattenuation with edema, hyperattenuation with hemorrhage hypoperfusion, pneumatosisintestinalis; luminal dilation

Peritoneal cavity

- Mesenteric edema, gas bubbles; ascites, pneumoperitoneum

Abbreviation: CT, computed tomography.

Conventional catheter-based angiography has, as a result, become less common as a diagnostic modality, although it has seen increased use as a therapeutic modality with the advent of catheter-directed therapies.[13]

While CT angiography is the test of choice when diagnosing mesenteric ischemia, there may exist evidence of mesenteric ischemia, seen on other imaging modalities and obtained when mesenteric ischemia is not being considered. Series with contrast in the portal venous phase may demonstrate signs of mesenteric ischemia as well. In addition to detecting MVT, portal venous phase CT scans may show bowel wall thickening, pneumatosis (▶ Fig. 17.2), mesenteric stranding, portal venous gas (▶ Fig. 17.3), and decreased mucosal enhancement suggestive of mesenteric ischemia (▶ Table 17.2).

Plain abdominal films are both insensitive and nonspecific, frequently only contributing to the diagnosis of mesenteric ischemia after it has progressed to frank bowel necrosis and perforation. Earlier in the course of the disease, an ileus may be identified on plain radiographs, and occasionally pneumatosis or "thumbprinting" may be seen prior to bowel perforation, although neither finding is specific to mesenteric ischemia.

Duplex ultrasonography may be used in the diagnosis of chronic mesenteric ischemia but plays a small role in the evaluation of a patient, who is thought to have AMI. In stable, fasting patients, ultrasonography can accurately identify lesions in the celiac and SMAs. Accuracy, however, varies with provider capability and is diminished by patient discomfort and bowel distention seen in cases of AMI. Mesenteric duplex may be useful in monitoring vascular patency after intervention for AMI.

Magnetic resonance angiography (MRA) is an alternative modality for assessing the mesenteric vessels. While appealing due to the lack of ionizing radiation and iodinated contrast, it is limited by availability, longer image acquisition times, and decreased spatial resolution of these images compared to CT scans. Even with gadolinium contrast-enhancement, MRA is not currently sensitive enough to detect more distal emboli or ischemia secondary to low-flow states. For these reasons, MRA is less widely used than CT for the diagnosis of mesenteric ischemia.[14,15]

Diagnostic laparoscopy has recently been proposed as a minimally invasive diagnostic modality for cases in which other imaging studies are either inconclusive or unavailable. The current experience with laparoscopy suggests that it is not sensitive for the detection of the early phase of AMI, when findings may be limited to the mucosal layer of the bowel wall. In this setting, missed mucosal ischemia may progress to full thickness necrosis despite negative initial laparoscopy.[16] There have been porcine series and human case reports successfully combining laparoscopy with fluorescence angiography to evaluate the serosal surface of the bowel for areas of hypoperfusion[17,18,19,20] (▶ Fig. 17.4). These techniques may also be employed in open explorations. There is no adequate experience to date in terms of this technique's ability to quantitate and the value it adds to diagnosing AMI, nor is there a well-defined false negative rate to assess the risk this technique may expose patients to. If laparoscopy is used for the diagnosis of AMI, results should be interpreted in the context of the lack of high-quality data supporting this approach, and a low-threshold for repeat evaluation should be maintained.

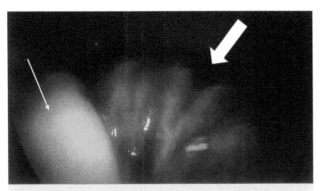

Fig. 17.4 Intra-operative fluorescence imaging to detect small bowel ischemia. Intravenous Indocyanine Green (ICG) used to evaluate perfusion of the small bowel. Normally perfused bowel appears green (*thin arrow*) while an adjacent section of small bowel demonstrates poor uptake of the ICG dye (*wide arrow*) indicating bowel ischemia.

While less commonly performed, exploratory laparotomy remains a useful tool in the evaluation of a patient presenting with peritonitis. In the setting of gangrenous bowel at laparotomy, evaluation of the mesenteric vasculature is mandatory. Palpation of the mesenteric arteries, intraoperative ultrasonography, and on-table angiography may reveal the source of ischemia if not previously identified.

17.4 Treatment of Acute Mesenteric Ischemia

17.4.1 Resuscitation

The appropriate treatment of AMI is dependent on accurate and timely diagnosis of the etiology of the ischemia, and the recognition of nonviable bowel if present. Irrespective of the cause, many patients with AMI present in a state of hypovolemia and frequently experience electrolyte disturbances that should be corrected to avoid hemodynamic collapse on induction of anesthesia. Initial resuscitation should proceed with isotonic crystalloid solution, and careful attention should be paid to the correction of hyperkalemia resultant from underlying bowel infarction.[21] We recommend bladder catheterization, central venous access, and arterial pressure monitoring, in order to guide resuscitation, and ongoing hemodynamic monitoring postoperatively. Many patients with AMI have other cardiovascular comorbidities and are at risk for pulmonary edema from the required volume resuscitation. While we recommend against the routine use of vasopressors in the treatment of AMI, if patients remain hypotensive after adequate volume resuscitation, then low doses of dopamine or epinephrine may be useful. Pure alpha-agonists should be avoided as the resultant vasoconstriction may worsen intestinal ischemia. Inotropic agents such as dobutamine and milrinone may increase cardiac output without compromising intestinal perfusion.[22] A therapeutic intravenous heparin infusion should be started promptly, with a goal-activated partial thromboplastin time of 60 to 80 seconds (antifactorXa level 0.3–0.7 IU/mL), to prevent propagation of clot. Broad-spectrum antibiotics should be administered during the initial resuscitation, as the risk of bacterial translocation due to the failure of gut barrier function from ischemia is high.[22]

17.4.2 Operative Exposure of the Mesenteric Vessels

The celiac artery can be approached anteriorly via a midline laparotomy. The left lobe of the liver is mobilized by incising the left triangular ligament and is retracted to the right. The stomach is gently retracted caudally and the gastrohepatic ligament incised to expose the retroperitoneum at the level of the diaphragmatic hiatus. The phrenoesophageal ligament is divided to expose the crura of the diaphragm and the celiac trunk which lies just posteriorly. The abdominal esophagus is then retracted to the left and the retroperitoneum overlying the celiac axis incised for exposure of the vessel and the supraceliac aorta. The median arcuate ligament may be incised longitudinally to gain additional exposure of the supraceliac aorta.

Alternatively, the celiac axis may be approached via a left flank retroperitoneal approach. This approach is beneficial in patients who underwent prior abdominal surgery and/or abdominal wall stomas, and in patients with truncal obesity. The patient is placed on a bean bag with the left chest rolled over to the right side, and the hips square on the operating table. The iliac crest is centered over the break in the bed to allow for increased distance between the costal margin and iliac crest as the bed is placed in the jackknife position. An oblique incision is made in the 10th intercostal space, parallel to the course of the rib, and carried from the posterior axillary line to the midline of the abdomen about 1 cm below the umbilicus. This incision is then deepened through the layers of the abdominal wall, taking care to control the inferior epigastric vessels during this dissection. The exposed peritoneum is then swept away from the abdominal wall. This plane is more easily developed at the posterolateral extent of the dissection and proceeds medially from there. Care must be taken to avoid peritoneal disruption at the posterior aspect of the rectus muscle, where it is frequently adherent. The left kidney is then medially rotated, and the large lumbar vein draining into the left renal vein is divided to facilitate exposure of the aorta. The left diaphragmatic crus may be divided to gain greater access to the supraceliac segment of the abdominal aorta.

The SMA may also be approached anteriorly, with the patient flat and in the supine position. This is most commonly through the posterior parietal peritoneum at the base of the transverse mesocolon. The transverse colon is reflected cephalad, and the small bowel retracted to the right shoulder of the patient. The middle colic artery is identified and may be followed back to its origin from the SMA. To gain more proximal access to the SMA, the ligament of Treitz may be incised and the fourth portion of the duodenum mobilized. The inferior border of the pancreas is then retracted cephalad to expose the proximal SMA.

The IMA is similarly exposed through a midline incision, with the transverse colon retracted cephalad and the small bowel retracted to the right shoulder. The ligament of Treitz and retroperitoneal duodenal attachments are divided, and the duodenum reflected to the right along with the small bowel. The periaortic tissues are then incised and the periadventitial plane entered. This dissection is carried caudally from the level of the left renal vein down to the aortic bifurcation, proceeding along the right anterior surface of the aorta in order to avoid inadvertent injury to the IMA. The IMA is identified about 3 to 4 centimeters cephalad to the aortic bifurcation, arising from the left anterior surface of the aorta. Proximal control should be obtained close to the origin of the IMA in order to avoid injury to the early branches of the vessel.

17.4.3 Thromboembolic Mesenteric Ischemia

After diagnosis of acute thrombotic or embolic mesenteric ischemia, the next critical step is to determine whether the patient has necrotic bowel at the time of presentation. Because patients with embolic AMI are less likely to have the vascular collateralization seen in more chronic ischemic states, the likelihood of underlying bowel infarction is higher at the time of presentation to medical care. Thrombotic mesenteric ischemia is frequently associated with a degree of chronic ischemia from ostial stenosis and may have a more insidious onset. If a patient presents with peritonitis, the role of endovascular treatment is limited as bowel resection is required. In patients who present early in the course of illness, without frank peritonitis, endovascular treatment with mechanical aspiration embolectomy, angioplasty and stenting, or catheter-directed thrombolytic infusion may play a role.[23]

Endovascular Treatment

The precise role or endovascular interventions for AMI is still being defined; however, multiple investigators have published series of successful endovascular revascularization. In one retrospective review of 21 patients with thromboembolic AMI,[24] 76% were able to be managed with endovascular treatment alone, although about 69% of these patients had either >–30% residual stenosis of the SMA or residual distal emboli after revascularization. Despite partial revascularization, only two of these patients had complaints of abdominal pain during the follow-up period of the study (median 28 months). The 30-day mortality rate was 9.5% in this series, and only one patient suffered from short-bowel syndrome after laparotomy.

Similarly, Arthurs et al[25] evaluated 70 patients with AMI of either thrombotic or embolic etiology, 81% of whom were treated primarily with an endovascular approach. The technical success rate of endovascular intervention in this study was 87%, with no difference in success rate based on etiology or location of the lesion. There was a higher likelihood of success in partial vascular occlusions (100%) compared with complete occlusions (82%). The authors found that the mortality rate of patients treated with an endovascular approach was less than those treated with initial laparotomy (36 vs. 50%).

While meta-analyses of retrospective studies are encouraging,[26,27] to our knowledge there are no prospective randomized evaluations of endovascular versus open treatment for AMI, and the reported success with endovascular therapy remains subject to the risk of confounding inherent in retrospective analyses. It is critically important to recognize the main drawback of endovascular therapy for AMI, namely, the lack of ability to evaluate the bowel. In patients presenting with peritonitis or radiographic suggestion of necrotic bowel, endovascular therapy alone is not sufficient. Even with complete revascularization, threatened bowel may progress to frank necrosis, and a low-threshold for exploration must be maintained.[28] The addition of

diagnostic laparoscopy to endoluminal revascularization is controversial.[21,29] Unless frankly necrotic, the serosal surface of the intestine is not a reliable indicator of perfusion status, and there lies the risk of missing subtle ischemia.[20] This is not mitigated by laparotomy; however, it does simplify repeated examinations of the bowel if the abdomen is managed with a temporary closure. Further, due to the patchy nature of the bowel ischemia in embolic disease, complete evaluation of the intestine requires a degree of laparoscopic expertise that is not always available. Fluorescent perfusion imaging intraoperatively may assist with recognizing poorly perfused bowel, but measurable benefit remains to be proven. While there may be a role for endovascular treatment in early AMI or partial SMA occlusions, it is our preference that these patients be monitored in the intensive care unit (ICU) and taken expeditiously to the OR for open exploration if they should develop persistent or worsening abdominal pain or physiology suggestive of untreated inflammation.

Endovascular treatment of AMI also requires the availability of a skilled endovascular surgeon and is not typically present in the skill set of the acute care surgeon. A full description of endovascular approaches to mesenteric embolectomy are beyond the scope of this chapter and are best performed by a vascular subspecialist.

Open Treatment

Open abdominal exploration with mesenteric revascularization remains a viable alternative to endovascular therapy and is preferred in cases where laparotomy is necessary for treatment of peritonitis. Open approaches to mesenteric embolectomy have the benefit of being rapid and definitive, and they simplify repeated evaluation of the bowel by the use of an initial damage-control strategy with a planned second-look operation to reassess bowel viability. Further, abdominal exploration and open embolectomy are within the scope of practice of the acute care surgeon and may be a life-saving procedure, as timeliness is paramount in the treatment of AMI.

As described above, the preferred exposure of the mesenteric vessels happens by way of midline laparotomy, which also grants access to the full peritoneal cavity for careful inspection of the bowel and resection of necrotic areas. After the root of the mesentery is exposed, the treatment options vary depending on the etiology of the ischemia and the location of the vascular obstruction.

The preferred management of embolic mesenteric ischemia at laparotomy is the rapid reperfusion of threatened bowel by balloon embolectomy. Mesenteric emboli tend to affect the SMA preferentially, due to the oblique angle that arises from the aorta. These emboli lodge distal to the origin of the SMA, sparing the ileocolic and middle colic vessels, and may not involve the transverse colon or proximal jejunum. Typically, this produces a patchy pattern of bowel necrosis, and care must be taken to evaluate the entire length of the small bowel and colon. The distal location of emboli usually results in a preserved pulse in the relatively healthy proximal SMA, providing a point of access for balloon embolectomy. After obtaining proximal and distal control with vessel loops, systemic heparin is administered and a transverse arteriotomy is made on the anterior wall of the SMA. A #2 or #3 Fogarty balloon catheter is passed proximally and distally, withdrawing while the balloon is slowly inflated. This process is repeated until no further embolus is evacuated, and then once more. Distal vessels unable to accommodate the balloon catheter may be addressed by manual expression of the clot and/or administration of intra-arterial thrombolytics. After successful embolectomy, the arteriotomy closed in interrupted fashion with 6-0 or 7-0 polypropylene suture. Restoration of flow is confirmed by palpation of the mesenteric artery, and the presence of Doppler signals in the distal SMA and on the antimesenteric surface of the bowel.

Thrombotic occlusion of the SMA more commonly occurs at the origin of the vessel, at the site of atherosclerotic narrowing, and extends into the first few centimeters of the artery. Due to the location of thrombosis, this has traditionally required operative bypass to restore flow to the gut. After exposure of the superior mesenteric artery, proximal and distal control is obtained similar to the exposure for an embolectomy. With a mesenteric bypass, the aorta and iliac vessels must also be exposed. We recommend dividing the retroperitoneum adjacent to the ligament of Treitz, onto the anterior surface of the aorta, and following it down to the iliac bifurcation. The inflow vessel for bypass is typically chosen based on the lie of the graft and the degree of calcification of the vessel. CT scans can be helpful in choosing the ideal graft site.

Proximal and distal control of the inflow vessel is also obtained. Again, systemic heparin is administered if it has not yet been given. The proximal SMA is addressed by making a longitudinal anterior arteriotomy that allows for endarterectomy prior to bypass. After removing the plaque from the recipient vessel, the SMA is proximally transected and ligated. Care must be taken to preserve all of the branches from the SMA in the preparation of the recipient vessel.

If possible, we recommend retrograde end-to-end beveled bypass from the right common iliac artery with the graft in a "lazy C" orientation. This has the benefits of a comfortable graft lie, avoids the need to clamp the aorta for any period of time, and is potentially less devastating to address should it become infected. If this is not feasible due to atherosclerotic burden of the right common iliac, a similar bypass may be performed with the left common iliac artery or the distal infrarenal aorta as the inflow vessel. Unfortunately, many patients with thrombotic mesenteric arterial occlusion have a large volume of atherosclerosis of the distal aorta and iliac vessels, and it may be necessary to use the more proximal aorta for inflow. A short, wide (8–10 millimeter), and end-to-side graft may be fashioned at the portion of the aorta immediately below the renal vessels but carries an increased risk of kinking. It may even be necessary to create an antegrade bypass from the supraceliac aorta. This is more technically demanding and time consuming and carries with it the physiologic insult of supraceliac clamping in a group of patients who are typically ill to begin with.

In the absence of gross peritoneal contamination, we recommend the use of 7- or 8 millimeter externally supported (ringed) polytetrafluoroethylene (PTFE) grafts to avoid kinking. In cases of significant soilage, great saphenous vein is the preferred conduit, although this is more susceptible to kinking and care must be taken to ensure patency after release of the retractors. In either case, we recommend sequestering the graft from the rest of the peritoneal cavity by the application of a pedicledomental flap as described by Kazmers.[30]

An alternative approach to revascularization with retrograde open mesenteric stenting (ROMS) was described by Milner et al in 2004,[31] and has since been proposed as a rapid and simple method of mesenteric revascularization that still allows for adequate assessment of the bowel[32,33] (▶ Fig. 17.4). In this approach, the SMA is exposed and controlled at the base of the transverse mesocolon and a thromboendarterectomy performed. Next, a patch angioplasty is performed, and the vessel cannulated with a flexible sheath in a retrograde fashion. Balloon-expandable stents are used to treat the lesion, frequently requiring more than one due to the length of occlusion (about 4 cm on average),[34] and a retrograde arteriogram is performed to document the resolution of the stenosis. The data supporting this approach is limited, with no randomized trials to clarify the comparative efficacy of ROMS and open bypass or a pure endovascular approach. Retrospective analyses suggest that it is generally feasible, with a high-technical success rate (93–98%), and short-term mortality is similar to open bypass (20–45%).[34,35] This approach is complicated by the risk of restenosis, and patients must be followed with serial mesenteric duplex USG to detect lesions prior to the onset of symptoms. The primary patency of ROMS at 12-month ranges is 76 to 83% and the primary-assisted patency is 91 to 93%. Secondary patency is 97 to 100% over the first 12 months after intervention.[34,35] Open mesenteric bypass techniques have reported primary patency of 82 to 97% over the initial 12 months after surgery and have long-term follow-up reporting patency as high as 89% at 72 months postoperatively.[36,37,38]

We recommend that, unless there is bowel perforation and gross contamination of the peritoneal cavity, mesenteric revascularization precede bowel resection. After perfusion is restored to the bowel, resection of frankly necrotic segments should follow. We recommend a period of 30 minutes for bowel reperfusion prior to resection, if the patient's physiology allows. Note should be taken of any areas of poor perfusion, as almost 40%[39] of patients with marginally viable bowel will subsequently go on to require resection at reoperation. Questionably viable areas of bowel should be left in situ, and a temporary abdominal closure placed with a "second-look" procedure planned for 12 to 24 hours later. This allows for expeditious return to the ICU for continued resuscitation and provides time for questionably viable bowel to either recover or infarct, such that the minimal amount of bowel necessary is resected.

17.4.4 Veno-occlusive Mesenteric Ischemia

After resuscitation, the mainstay of therapy for mesenteric ischemia caused by MVT consists of therapeutic anticoagulation with a heparin infusion. In stable patients with partial occlusions or collateral flow, anticoagulation may be sufficient treatment, and anticoagulation alone has been reported to have about 90% success in this population.[40,41] Repeated abdominal examinations and close monitoring are required to detect bowel necrosis and need for operative intervention. Peritonitis, bowel perforation, and uncontrolled gastrointestinal bleeding warrant surgical exploration. If surgery is required in the course of treatment for these patients, the aim is to resect areas of necrosis and plan for a second-look operation. Bowel should be resected to viable tissue without any clot burden in the small mesenteric veins, and primary anastomosis delayed ensuring healthy tissue.

Less invasive methods have been devised for clearance of mesenteric venous clot burden, with increasing use of thrombolytics and endovascular therapies in recent years. While there are no prospective studies to identify the specific population that might benefit from these techniques, there have been small series documenting efficacy in patients without indication for laparotomy. Local thrombolysis can be delivered by Thrombolysis ImPlementation in Stroke (TIPS) by percutaneous cannulation of the intrahepatic portal system, or by instillation into the SMA. Percutaneous transhepatic thrombolysis appears to be rather successful, with 75 to 88.5% of patients achieving restoration of flow in retrospective studies.[42,43,44] There was no difference in mortality at 30 days, when compared to a similar cohort of 14 patients treated with anticoagulation instead of thrombolysis, although fewer patients who underwent thrombolysis progressed to require bowel resection (5.5 vs. 35.7%). Followed-up for up to 3 years, the thrombolysis group did have a lower incidence of portal hypertension (11.1 vs. 50%). Di Minno identified hemorrhagic complications in only 1/18 patients treated with thrombolytics,[42] although Hollingshead et al saw hemorrhagic complications in 60% of their patients.[43] This may be attributable to the higher doses of thrombolytics in the latter study and the small sample sizes of the studies.

Mechanical thrombectomy has also been described, with aspiration catheters and by angioplasty, to disrupt more tenacious thromboses.[45,46,47] This may have the advantage of more rapid recanalization of large vein thromboses, however, it cannot remove clot from more distal veins. While the literature consists primarily of case reports, most authors advocate combining mechanical thrombectomy with thrombolysis. Surgical thrombectomy is rarely indicated, although there are case reports describing successful revascularization with this approach.[48,49] Given the high likelihood of significant morbidity with surgical thrombectomy, we do not recommend it as a standard therapy.

Postoperatively, patients should be kept on bowel rest until return of bowel function. In the absence of anticoagulation, MVT has a high-recurrence rate, between 30 and 36%.[50,51] Most of these recurrences are documented during the first 30 days after hospitalization, but there are reports of recurrences many years later. While no randomized trials have evaluated the effect of anticoagulation after MVT, retrospective studies showed that the cumulative risk of major thrombotic events continued to increase over the duration of follow-up, and rose sharply upon discontinuation of anticoagulation.[52,53] The rate of major bleeding in these studies was less than that of thrombotic events, and no deaths in either series were attributable to hemorrhage in anticoagulated patients. Anticoagulation with an oral vitamin K antagonist or low-molecular weight heparin should be started when the patient is stable postoperatively, and probably be continued for life in patients without absolute contraindications.[54]

17.4.5 Non-Occlusive Mesenteric Ischemia

Generally, NOMI is secondary to shock from another source, and treatment is primarily directed at supporting perfusion and controlling the primary illness. Systemic pharmacologic therapies directed at mesenteric vasodilation lack convincing data to support their routine use. There are case series of patients who were treated with intravenous prostaglandin E(1) early in the course of NOMI, although this has not been widely accepted as standard therapy.[55,56] There are also case reports describing the use of the phosphodiesterase inhibitor cilostazol to inhibit platelet aggregation and induce vasodilation for the treatment of NOMI; however, this has not been evaluated in a prospective fashion.[57] Large animal studies have demonstrated increased mesenteric blood flow with the administration of intra-arterial captopril, prostacyclin derivatives, and gastric inhibitory peptide; however, these have not been translated to human trials.[58]

As described previously, mesenteric vasospasm is thought to contribute to continued hypoperfusion in NOMI, and intra-arterial infusion of papaverine or prostaglandin E(1) has been described with some encouraging findings in retrospective analyses.[5,55,59,60,61] These techniques may be employed independent of laparotomy and may reduce the amount of bowel requiring resection. Generally, the infusions are continued for several days, until the patient improves, or complications are encountered. The vasodilator infusions are generally well-tolerated, so long as the catheter remains in the SMA; however, migration of the catheter into the systemic circulation may produce profound vasodilation and hypotension.

Operative interventions are not indicated for revascularization, as there is generally no mechanical obstruction of the main mesenteric vessels. Surgery is reserved for peritonitis, in which case there are usually large segments of necrotic bowel requiring excision. As with other forms of mesenteric ischemia, treatment with bowel resection and temporary abdominal closure is advisable. Multiple resections may be required, depending on the ability to control the original illness. Intestinal perfusion may be evaluated with fluorescein dyes, as previously described, in an effort to preserve marginal but viable bowel.[62,63,64,65,66]

17.5 Ischemic Colitis

Ischemic colitis is the most common cause of intestinal ischemia and is caused by diminished blood flow to the colon, resulting in mucosal ischemia and inflammation.[67] Ischemic colitis is predominantly a disease of the elderly with most cases occurring in patients over age 65. There is wide variation in severity at clinical presentation for patients with ischemic colitis, ranging from mild, self-limiting mucosal ischemia to severe transmural necrosis. Most cases of ischemic colitis are caused by nonocclusive etiologies with impaired microcirculation in the colon wall, leading to hypoperfusion. Despite collateral circulation within the colon, areas where the circulation from the major, named arteries meet (SMA, IMA, rectal arteries) are more susceptible to ischemia. These "watershed regions" include the splenic flexure (Griffith's point) and the rectosigmoid junction (Sudek's point). Risk factors for ischemic colitis include heart failure, peripheral arterial occlusive disease, coronary artery disease, and inflammatory bowel disease.[68] For patients who develop ischemic colitis while in the inpatient setting, factors such as heart failure, hypotensive episodes, and recent vasopressor use may compromise perfusion to the colon. Postoperative ischemic colitis can be seen after surgery for abdominal aortic aneurysm due to lack of adequate collateral blood flow, following ligation of the IMA or after cardiac surgery due to low-flow state.[69]

Patients presenting with ischemic colitis frequently experience sudden onset abdominal pain that is frequently associated with nausea and vomiting. Patients often develop mild hematochezia beginning within 24 hours of developing abdominal pain. Bleeding associated with ischemic colitis is often minor and usually self-limited. Patients often undergo an extensive imaging workup due to their nonspecific presentation and symptoms. Plain X-rays may demonstrate colonic dilation and "thumbprinting" of the colon wall, which is suggestive of submucosal edema. CT scan may demonstrate bowel wall thickening and stranding of the pericolonic fat that is suggestive of acute inflammation.[70] CT imaging is also important to help localize the site of colon ischemia. Evidence of colon wall pneumatosis is suggestive of more severe, transmural ischemia. The gold standard for the diagnosis of ischemic colitis is flexible endoscopy to visualize the mucosa for evidence of ischemia or ulceration. Endoscopy, while useful in making a diagnosis, does not enable one to assess if the ischemia is transmural, merely if it is present or not. Severity of disease relies upon present disease and the patient hemodynamic status.

Treatment for ischemic colitis depends on the severity of ischemia at the time of diagnosis. A majority of patients presenting with ischemic colitis will response to nonsurgical therapy that consists of bowel rest, aggressive fluid hydration if dehydration exists, and empiric treatment with broad-spectrum antibiotics to cover bother aerobic and anaerobic bacteria. Serial abdominal examinations should be followed to ensure clinical improvement. For patients that present with advanced colon ischemia and/or necrosis, and those who have progression of disease despite nonoperative management, should undergo prompt surgical intervention. Ischemic colitis should be managed operatively with a segmental colon resection, and frequently requires diverting end ileostomy or colostomy in the urgent setting due to the presence of a potentially tenuous blood flow to the newly created anastomosis.[71] Since ischemic colitis often occurs in "watershed areas," an anatomic colon resection should be performed to ensure that the remaining colon is supplied by sufficient arterial flow. A second-look operation may be needed to reassess bowel perfusion and viability.[71]

17.6 Conclusion

Mesenteric ischemia is associated with significant morbidity and mortality. Clinicians must have a high-index of suspicion for the diagnosis of mesenteric ischemia, as a delayed diagnosis can be catastrophic. Initial treatment should be focused on fluid resuscitation, and interventions aimed at restoring perfusion to the bowel, if possible. Ischemic and nonviable bowel should be promptly resected, usually with a second-look operation to assess the viability of the remaining bowel. Ongoing studies are needed to define the role of endovascular options to restore perfusion and evaluate the use of fluorescence in order to assess bowel perfusion and viability.

References

[1] Sise MJ. Acute mesenteric ischemia. SurgClin North Am. 2014; 94(1):165–181

[2] Bassiouny HS. Nonocclusive mesenteric ischemia. SurgClin North Am. 1997; 77(2):319–326

[3] Siegelman SS, Sprayregen S, Boley SJ. Angiographic diagnosis of mesenteric arterial vasoconstriction. Radiology. 1974; 112(3):533–542

[4] Hirota M, Inoue K, Kimura Y, et al. Non-occlusive mesenteric ischemia and its associated intestinal gangrene in acute pancreatitis. Pancreatology. 2003; 3 (4):316–322

[5] Trompeter M, Brazda T, Remy CT, Vestring T, Reimer P. Non-occlusive mesenteric ischemia: etiology, diagnosis, and interventional therapy. EurRadiol. 2002; 12(5):1179–1187

[6] Blumberg SN, Maldonado TS. Mesenteric venous thrombosis. J VascSurg Venous LymphatDisord. 2016; 4(4):501–507

[7] Hedayati N, Riha GM, Kougias P, et al. Prognostic factors and treatment outcome in mesenteric vein thrombosis. Vasc Endovascular Surg. 2008; 42 (3):217–224

[8] Eslami MH, Rybin D, Doros G, McPhee JT, Farber A. Mortality of acute mesenteric ischemia remains unchanged despite significant increase in utilization of endovascular techniques. Vascular. 2016; 24(1):44–52

[9] Montagnana M, Danese E, Lippi G. Biochemical markers of acute intestinal ischemia: possibilities and limitations. Ann Transl Med. 2018; 6(17):341

[10] Cudnik MT, Darbha S, Jones J, Macedo J, Stockton SW, Hiestand BC. The diagnosis of acute mesenteric ischemia: a systematic review and meta-analysis. AcadEmerg Med. 2013; 20(11):1087–1100

[11] Bourcier S, Oudjit A, Goudard G, et al. Diagnosis of non-occlusive acute mesenteric ischemia in the intensive care unit. Ann Intensive Care. 2016; 6 (1):112

[12] Pérez-García C, de Miguel Campos E, Fernández Gonzalo A, et al. Non-occlusive mesenteric ischaemia: CT findings, clinical outcomes and assessment of the diameter of the superior mesenteric artery. Br J Radiol. 2018; 91(1081): 20170492

[13] Oliva IB, Davarpanah AH, Rybicki FJ, et al. ACR Appropriateness Criteria imaging of mesenteric ischemia. Abdom Imaging. 2013; 38(4):714–719

[14] Laissy JP, Trillaud H, Douek P. MR angiography: noninvasive vascular imaging of the abdomen. Abdom Imaging. 2002; 27(5):488–506

[15] Gilfeather M, Holland GA, Siegelman ES, et al. Gadolinium-enhanced ultrafast three-dimensional spoiled gradient-echo MR imaging of the abdominal aorta and visceral and iliac vessels. Radiographics. 1997; 17(2):423–432

[16] Zamir G, Reissman P. Diagnostic laparoscopy in mesenteric ischemia. SurgEndosc. 1998; 12(5):390–393

[17] Paral J, Ferko A, Plodr M, et al. Laparoscopic diagnostics of acute bowel ischemia using ultraviolet light and fluorescein dye: an experimental study. SurgLaparoscEndoscPercutan Tech. 2007; 17(4):291–295

[18] McGinty JJ, Jr, Hogle N, Fowler DL. Laparoscopic evaluation of intestinal ischemia using fluorescein and ultraviolet light in a porcine model. SurgEndosc. 2003; 17(7):1140–1143

[19] Cocorullo G, Mirabella A, Falco N, et al. An investigation of bedside laparoscopy in the ICU for cases of non-occlusive mesenteric ischemia. World J EmergSurg. 2017; 12:4

[20] CocorulloG, MirabellaA, GulottaG, MandalàV. Laparoscopy in acute mesenteric ischemia. In: Mandalà V, ed. The Role of Laparoscopy in Emergency Abdominal Surgery. Milano: Springer Milan; 2012:117–28

[21] Tilsed JVT, Casamassima A, Kurihara H, et al. ESTES guidelines: acute mesenteric ischaemia. Eur J Trauma EmergSurg. 2016; 42(2):253–270

[22] Bala M, Kashuk J, Moore EE, et al. Acute mesenteric ischemia: guidelines of the World Society of Emergency Surgery. World J EmergSurg. 2017; 12(1):38

[23] Branco BC, Montero-Baker MF, Aziz H, Taylor Z, Mills JL. Endovascular therapy for acute mesenteric ischemia: an NSQIP analysis. Am Surg. 2015; 81(11): 1170–1176

[24] Jia Z, Jiang G, Tian F, et al. Early endovascular treatment of superior mesenteric occlusion secondary to thromboemboli. Eur J VascEndovascSurg. 2014; 47(2):196–203

[25] Arthurs ZM, Titus J, Bannazadeh M, et al. A comparison of endovascular revascularization with traditional therapy for the treatment of acute mesenteric ischemia. J VascSurg. 2011; 53(3):698–704, discussion 704–705

[26] El Farargy M, Abdel Hadi A, AbouEisha M, Bashaeb K, Antoniou GA. Systematic review and meta-analysis of endovascular treatment for acute mesenteric ischaemia. Vascular. 2017; 25(4):430–438

[27] Beaulieu RJ, Arnaoutakis KD, Abularrage CJ, Efron DT, Schneider E, Black JH, III. Comparison of open and endovascular treatment of acute mesenteric ischemia. J VascSurg. 2014; 59(1):159–164

[28] Wyers MC. Acute mesenteric ischemia: diagnostic approach and surgical treatment. SeminVascSurg. 2010; 23(1):9–20

[29] Sauerland S, Agresta F, Bergamaschi R, et al. Laparoscopy for abdominal emergencies: evidence-based guidelines of the European Association for Endoscopic Surgery. SurgEndosc. 2006; 20(1):14–29

[30] Kazmers A. Operative management of acute mesenteric ischemia. Part 1. Ann VascSurg. 1998; 12(2):187–197

[31] Milner R, Woo EY, Carpenter JP. Superior mesenteric artery angioplasty and stenting via a retrograde approach in a patient with bowel ischemia: a case report. Vasc Endovascular Surg. 2004; 38(1):89–91

[32] Moyes LH, McCarter DHA, Vass DG, Orr DJ. Intraoperative retrograde mesenteric angioplasty for acute occlusive mesenteric ischaemia: a case series. Eur J VascEndovascSurg. 2008; 36(2):203–206

[33] Stout CL, Messerschmidt CA, Leake AE, Veale WN, Stokes GK, Panneton JM. Retrograde open mesenteric stenting for acute mesenteric ischemia is a viable alternative for emergent revascularization. Vasc Endovascular Surg. 2010; 44(5):368–371

[34] Oderich GS, Macedo R, Stone DH, et al. Low Frequency Vascular Disease Research Consortium Investigators. Multicenter study of retrograde open mesenteric artery stenting through laparotomy for treatment of acute and chronic mesenteric ischemia. J VascSurg. 2018; 68(2):470–480.e1

[35] Blauw JTM, Meerwaldt R, Brusse-Keizer M, Kolkman JJ, Gerrits D, Geelkerken RH, Multidisciplinary Study Group of Mesenteric Ischemia. Retrograde open mesenteric stenting for acute mesenteric ischemia. J VascSurg. 2014; 60(3): 726–734

[36] McMillan WD, McCarthy WJ, Bresticker MR, et al. Mesenteric artery bypass: objective patency determination. J VascSurg. 1995; 21(5):729–740, discussion 740–741

[37] Scali ST, Ayo D, Giles KA, et al. Outcomes of antegrade and retrograde open mesenteric bypass for acute mesenteric ischemia. J VascSurg. 2019; 69(1): 129–140

[38] Roussel A, Castier Y, Nuzzo A, et al. Revascularization of acute mesenteric ischemia after creation of a dedicated multidisciplinary center. J VascSurg. 2015; 62(5):1251–1256

[39] Kougias P, Lau D, El Sayed HF, Zhou W, Huynh TT, Lin PH. Determinants of mortality and treatment outcome following surgical interventions for acute mesenteric ischemia. J VascSurg. 2007; 46(3):467–474

[40] Acosta S, Alhadad A, Svensson P, Ekberg O. Epidemiology, risk and prognostic factors in mesenteric venous thrombosis. Br J Surg. 2008; 95(10): 1245–1251

[41] Brunaud L, Antunes L, Collinet-Adler S, et al. Acute mesenteric venous thrombosis: case for nonoperative management. J VascSurg. 2001; 34(4): 673–679

[42] Di Minno MN, Milone F, Milone M, et al. Endovascular thrombolysis in acute mesenteric vein thrombosis: a 3-year follow-up with the rate of short and long-term sequaelae in 32 patients. Thromb Res. 2010; 126(4): 295–298

[43] Hollingshead M, Burke CT, Mauro MA, Weeks SM, Dixon RG, Jaques PF. Transcatheter thrombolytic therapy for acute mesenteric and portal vein thrombosis. J VascIntervRadiol. 2005; 16(5):651–661

[44] Zhou W, Choi L, Lin PH, Dardik A, Eraso A, Lumsden AB. Percutaneous transhepaticthrombectomy and pharmacologic thrombolysis of mesenteric venous thrombosis. Vascular. 2007; 15(1):41–45

[45] Goldberg MF, Kim HS. Treatment of acute superior mesenteric vein thrombosis with percutaneous techniques. AJR Am J Roentgenol. 2003; 181(5): 1305–1307

[46] Nakayama S, Murashima N, Isobe Y. Superior mesenteric venous thrombosis treated by direct aspiration thrombectomy. Hepatogastroenterology. 2008; 55(82–83):367–370

[47] Rosen MP, Sheiman R. Transhepatic mechanical thrombectomy followed by infusion of TPA into the superior mesenteric artery to treat acute mesenteric vein thrombosis. J VascIntervRadiol. 2000; 11(2 Pt 1):195–198

[48] Demertzis S, Ringe B, Gulba D, Rosenthal H, Pichlmayr R. Treatment of portal vein thrombosis by thrombectomy and regional thrombolysis. Surgery. 1994; 115(3):389–393

[49] Bergentz SE, Ericsson B, Hedner U, Leandoer L, Nilsson IM. Thrombosis in the superior mesenteric and portal veins: report of a case treated with thrombectomy. Surgery. 1974; 76(2):286–290

[50] Jona J, Cummins GM, Jr, Head HB, Govostis MC. Recurrent primary mesenteric venous thrombosis. JAMA. 1974; 227(9):1033–1035

[51] Rhee RY, Gloviczki P, Mendonca CT, et al. Mesenteric venous thrombosis: still a lethal disease in the 1990s. J VascSurg. 1994; 20(5):688–697

[52] Ageno W, Riva N, Schulman S, et al. Long-term clinical outcomes of splanchnic vein thrombosis: results of an international registry. JAMA Intern Med. 2015; 175(9):1474–1480

[53] Dentali F, Ageno W, Witt D, et al. WARPED consortium. Natural history of mesenteric venous thrombosis in patients treated with vitamin K antagonists: a multi-centre, retrospective cohort study. ThrombHaemost. 2009; 102(3):501–504

[54] Bergqvist D, Svensson PJ. Treatment of mesenteric vein thrombosis. SeminVascSurg. 2010; 23(1):65–68

[55] Kamimura K, Oosaki A, Sugahara S, Mori S. Survival of three nonocclusive mesenteric ischemia patients following early diagnosis by multidetector row computed tomography and prostaglandin E1 treatment. Intern Med. 2008; 47(22):2001–2006

[56] Mitsuyoshi A, Obama K, Shinkura N, Ito T, Zaima M. Survival in nonocclusive mesenteric ischemia: early diagnosis by multidetector row computed tomography and early treatment with continuous intravenous high-dose prostaglandin E(1). Ann Surg. 2007; 246(2):229–235

[57] Murthy KA, Kiran HS, Cheluvaraj V, Bhograj A. Non-occlusive mesenteric ischemia and the role of cilostazol in its management. J Pharmacol Pharmacother. 2012; 3(1):68–70

[58] Kozuch PL, Brandt LJ. Review article: diagnosis and management of mesenteric ischaemia with an emphasis on pharmacotherapy. Aliment PharmacolTher. 2005; 21(3):201–215

[59] Boley SJ, Sprayregan S, Siegelman SS, Veith FJ. Initial results from an agressiveroentgenological and surgical approach to acute mesenteric ischemia. Surgery. 1977; 82(6):848–855

[60] Sommer CM, Radeleff BA. A novel approach for percutaneous treatment of massive nonocclusive mesenteric ischemia: tolazoline and glycerol trinitrate as effective local vasodilators. Catheter CardiovascInterv. 2009; 73(2):152–155

[61] Ogi K, Sanui M, Iizuka Y, et al. Successful treatment of nonocclusive mesenteric ischemia after aortic valve replacement with continuous arterial alprostadil infusion: A case report. Int J Surg Case Rep. 2017; 35:8–11

[62] Karampinis I, Keese M, Jakob J, et al. Indocyaninegreen tissue angiography can reduce extended bowel resections in acute mesenteric ischemia. J GastrointestSurg. 2018; 22(12):2117–2124

[63] Ishizuka M, Nagata H, Takagi K, et al. Usefulness of intraoperative observation using a fluorescence imaging instrument for patients with nonocclusive mesenteric ischemia. IntSurg. 2015; 100(4):593–599

[64] Nakagawa Y, Kobayashi K, Kuwabara S, Shibuya H, Nishimaki T. Use of indocyanine green fluorescence imaging to determine the area of bowel resection in non-occlusive mesenteric ischemia: a case report. Int J Surg Case Rep. 2018; 51:352–357

[65] Irie T, Matsutani T, Hagiwara N, et al. Successful treatment of non-occlusive mesenteric ischemia with indocyanine green fluorescence and open-abdomen management. Clin J Gastroenterol. 2017; 10(6):514–518

[66] Nitori N, Deguchi T, Kubota K, et al. Successful treatment of non-occlusive mesenteric ischemia (NOMI) using the HyperEye Medical System for intraoperative visualization of the mesenteric and bowel circulation: report of a case. Surg Today. 2014; 44(2):359–362

[67] Moszkowicz D, Mariani A, Trésallet C, Menegaux F. Ischemic colitis: the ABCs of diagnosis and surgical management. J ViscSurg. 2013; 150(1): 19–28

[68] Halaweish I, Alam HB. Surgical management of severe colitis in the intensive care unit. J Intensive Care Med. 2015; 30(8):451–461

[69] Paterno F, Longo WE. The etiology and pathogenesis of vascular disorders of the intestine. RadiolClin North Am. 2008; 46(5):877–885, v

[70] Trotter JM, Hunt L, Peter MB. Ischaemic colitis. BMJ. 2016; 355:i6600

[71] Schneider TA, Longo WE, Ure T, Vernava AM, III. Mesenteric ischemia. Acute arterial syndromes. Dis Colon Rectum. 1994; 37(11):1163–1174

**Expert Commentary on
Mesenteric Ischemia by
*David Spain***

Expert Commentary on Mesenteric Ischemia

David Spain

For mesenteric ischemia, the classic presentation of the sudden onset of pain out of proportion to the physical examination in a patient with either preexisting postprandial pain and food fear or atrial fibrillation is, in my experience, an uncommon occurrence. But in these cases, the path is clear: the patient needs rapid resuscitation and evaluation and an expeditious trip to the operating room for assessment of bowel viability and reestablishment of arterial inflow.

More commonly, the acute care surgeon is called to evaluate a patient in one of two settings. The first is the patient with acute mesenteric venous thrombosis, either *de novo* (often due to an undiagnosed thrombophilia) or postoperatively (most commonly after colorectal surgery or splenectomy). These patients may respond quickly to volume resuscitation and systemic anticoagulation. The second is the patient in the intensive care unit (ICU), often on pressors, who experiences a clinical deterioration and has a CT scan of the abdomen which shows some areas of bowel hypoenhancement concerning for ischemia but without frank necrosis. Occasionally, these patients may be candidates for endovascular therapy. However, in both situations, clinical examination for signs of peritonitis can be very challenging.

I believe patients who have had perfusion sufficiently restored, either by medical management (resuscitation, anticoagulation, thrombolytic therapy, etc.) or intervention (endovascular procedure), can benefit from diagnostic laparoscopy. The acute care surgeon should be facile enough to run the entire small bowel laparoscopically (assume no prior laparotomies) and assess viability. Also, a laparoscopic approach is an excellent option for a second-look procedure. Gaining access and reestablishing pneumoperitoneum should be very straightforward. In addition, if there are areas that have progressed to require resection, laparoscopy can assist in making a strategically placed smaller incision for that limited area. Thus, there should be a low threshold for using diagnostic laparoscopy in patients with possible or confirmed mesenteric ischemia that do not require open revascularization.

Another common scenario facing the acute care surgeon is the patient with ischemic colitis. Occasionally, these patients present *de novo* to the emergency department with abdominal pain and get a CT scan to confirm the diagnosis. But more often, we're consulted to attend to a critical ill patient in the ICU who is deteriorating, usually on pressors and has an abdominal examination that is difficult to interpret. CT imaging with intravenous contrast combined with flexible endoscopy will usually make the diagnosis. Diagnostic laparoscopy can also be helpful in determining transmural ischemia. One challenge that remains is whether to perform a colostomy or restore GI continuity after segmental colectomy. An increasing amount of data suggest that colonic anastomosis can be performed in many adverse conditions. However, these patients are usually quite fragile and may not tolerate another physiological insult. On the other hand, their current critical illness on top of their underlying comorbidities often makes them poor candidates for stoma reversal in the future. In the case of ischemic colitis, the key step to making this decision (stoma or not) involves assessing the patient's overall stability and perfusion of the bowel.

18 Esophageal Emergencies: Emergency Management of Paraesophageal Hernias and Esophageal Perforations

Geoffrey P. Kohn

Summary

Esophageal emergencies are some of the most challenging problems which the acute care surgeon may need to manage. Two of the most common of these emergent conditions are obstructed paraesophageal hernias and perforations of the esophagus. Management is time critical, complex, and frequently multi-modal. The decision of when to operate is as important as the details of any operation. A trend has developed towards less invasive treatment of both conditions, and new endoscopic and radiologically-guided percutaneous options are increasingly useful tools in the management of esophageal perforations.

Keywords: Hiatal hernia, paraesophageal hernia, esophageal perforation, self expandable stents, negative pressure wound therapy

18.1 Introduction

Disorders of the esophagus and gastroesophageal junction are very common. Many of these are manageable on an outpatient basis, such as the management of gastroesophageal reflux disease. Frequently, elective surgery is required for their management. The acute care surgeon may encounter less common life-threatening conditions of this area, of which the most likely are the acute gastric obstruction of a strangulated paraesophageal hernia or perforation of the esophagus. The diagnosis and management of these conditions are considered below.

18.2 Paraesophageal Hernias

Hiatal hernias result from an enlargement of the esophageal hiatus of the diaphragm. The most common Type I hiatal hernia, also known as a sliding hiatal hernia, occurs when the gastroesophageal junction herniates into the thoracic cavity.

Often associated with gastroesophageal reflux disease, Type I hiatal hernias are distinct from other types of hiatal hernia (Type II–IV) (▶ Fig. 18.1); these other types are known as paraesophageal hernias and occur when the gastroesophageal junction lies below other parts of the stomach. In such hernias, the gastric fundus, and often a greater portion of the stomach, is displaced into the chest and may be accompanied by other abdominal viscera. Like hernias elsewhere in the body, the clinical significance of paraesophageal hernias lies in the possibility of obstruction, incarceration, and strangulation of the hernia contents.

Paraesophageal hernias are a consequence of the widening of the esophageal hiatus, which lies between the left and right crural pillars of the diaphragm. This permits passage of the abdominal contents into the posterior mediastinum. Paraesophageal hernias often develop over many years and the slow progression of symptoms often leads to an under appreciation of the severity of symptoms.[1] Frequently, the severity of the symptoms is only fully appreciated in their absence after paraesophageal hernia repair. These symptoms include obstructive symptoms such as dysphagia, regurgitation, and heartburn. Early satiety, vomiting, and postprandial pain are common. Poor emptying of the stomach may cause reflux of gastric contents into the esophagus and, in addition to the typical heartburn and regurgitation symptoms, it may also manifest as the atypical reflux symptoms of cough, wheeze, aspiration, and dysphonia. Symptoms may also be due to the volume of stomach in the chest, which is likely larger in the full, postprandial state. By displacing lung volume or even causing cardiac chamber compression,[2] such symptoms may include reduction in forced vital capacity,[3] postprandial or exertional dyspnea, as well as substernal chest pain.[4] Anemia is common with paraesophageal hernias[5] and may be attributable to the development of ulceration or erosions at the level of the diaphragm, which are known as Cameron's ulcers that when present are often on the lesser curve of the stomach. Chronic vomiting may cause erosions, which might be the cause of anemia, as might gastric mucosal ischemia in cases of chronic incarceration.

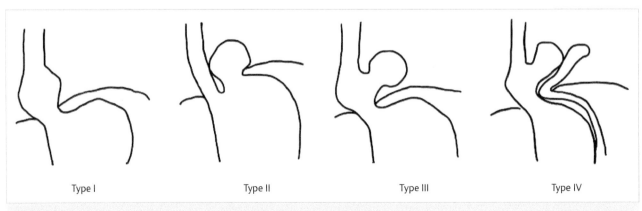

Type I   Type II   Type III   Type IV

Fig. 18.1 Classification of hiatal hernia.

18.2.1 Etiology

Paraesophageal hernias tend to occur more frequently in older patients, and perhaps in those with persistently higher intra-abdominal pressures such as the obese population. Most hernias are acquired, probably being present for a long time prior to diagnosis in a majority of patients.[6] Women develop more paraesophageal hernias than men. Paraesophageal hernias more frequently develop toward the left side of the esophageal hiatus.

18.2.2 Classification

Traditionally, hiatal hernias have been classified into Types I to IV. Type I hernias, also called "sliding hernias," are defined by the gastroesophageal (GE) junction lying above the diaphragm. Often associated with gastroesophageal reflux, these hernias are exceedingly unlikely to obstruct or strangulate, and management tends to be directed toward control of the associated reflux rather than targeted toward the hernia itself.[1] In contradistinction, hernias of Types II to IV may cause complications, and are often grouped together by the term paraesophageal hernias or "rolling" hernias. Although these can be associated with gastroesophageal reflux, management of these hernias is usually directed toward the hernia itself. Type II hernias have a normally located GE junction with herniation of the gastric fundus into the chest. Type III hernias combine features of type I and II in that they have proximally displaced GE junction together with herniation of the stomach, usually the fundus. Type IV hiatal hernias contain other abdominal viscera, such as the spleen, colon, small bowel or pancreas, and symptoms such as small bowel obstruction may arise.

The most common hiatal hernia is the Type I, making up approximately 85% of all hiatal hernias. Of the paraesophageal hernias, Type III is the most common, followed by Type IV and finally by the rare type II.

Although these types of hernias have comprised the traditional classification system, the type of paraesophageal hernia is probably less important than other factors. The size of the hernia, whether measured by vertical dimension or area of the diaphragmatic defect, probably correlates more closely with the development of symptoms and complications. The term "giant" paraesophageal hernia is often found in the literature, but this has no strictly defined definition.[7,8,9,10] It is often taken to mean a situation where greater than 50% of the volume of the stomach resides intrathoracically, or where the vertical height of the hernia is greater than 5 cm, or when a transverse measurement of the diaphragmatic hiatus is greater than 8 cm.

Also, importantly correlated with symptoms is the anatomic orientation of the herniated stomach. Any significant bend or twist in the stomach may impede emptying. The entire stomach can fold on itself, which is described as a gastric volvulus.

18.2.3 Incarceration and Strangulation

Strangulation of a paraesophageal hernia is the most feared complication and can lead to gastric obstruction, ischemia, necrosis, and perforation. The sequalae to these complications will be severe and may result in death of the patient.

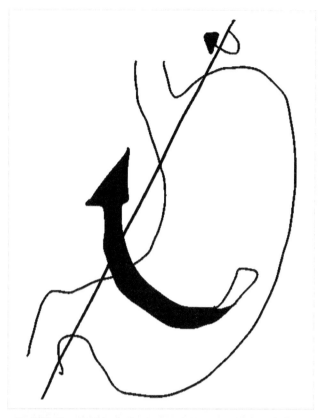

Fig. 18.2 Organoaxial volvulus.

Incarceration is not necessarily a major issue, although it is more frequently associated with symptomatic hernias and may progress to strangulation.

The stomach can turn on one of two axes, which will have a large effect on emptying; when the stomach turns about its longitudinal axis, it is called organoaxial volvulus (▶ Fig. 18.2), and when it turns on its short axis, it is termed mesenteroaxial volvulus (▶ Fig. 18.3). These conditions may be chronic in nature but can also be acute in presentation, leading to acute gastric obstruction. Symptoms of an acute gastric volvulus include chest pain or epigastric pain, retching but without vomiting, inability to tolerate fluids or even the patient's own secretions, and often inability to pass a nasogastric tube. Not all symptoms are present for all cases. Such a condition is a true surgical emergency.

18.2.4 Diagnosis

Many patients with paraesophageal hernia report being asymptomatic, and many indeed are so. However, due to the slow development of symptoms over the many years of this condition, symptoms may be underappreciated and not really noticed until their resolution postoperatively. Thus, a very careful history must be taken. Physical examination is often normal, although bowel sounds can be often heard on chest auscultation. Many patients have their paraesophageal hernias diagnosed during investigations for gastroesophageal reflux or chest pain. Radiologic imaging of the chest performed for other reasons might incidentally detect a hiatal hernia.

Radiological Studies

Plain chest radiographs can diagnose hiatal hernia but are not very sensitive. The pathognomonic feature is the presence of an air/fluid level in the posterior mediastinum. This cannot necessarily distinguish between hernias protruding through the esophageal hiatus as distinct to traumatic diaphragmatic hernias or congenital defects of the diaphragm such as Morgagni or Bochdalek hernias. Cross-sectional imaging with computed tomography (CT) or magnetic resonance imaging (MRI) may be helpful in these cases.

Contrast esophagram can be very useful in diagnosis. The location of the hernia is identified as well as the anatomy of the stomach and esophagus (▶ Fig. 18.4). This accurately differentiates between hiatal hernias and other diaphragmatic defects. When performed as a dynamic study, information is also obtained regarding gastric emptying and, to a lesser degree, esophageal motility. Care should be taken in the choice of contrast medium; obstruction of the stomach will increase the risk of aspiration, and when ionic media have been used, a potential fatal chemical pneumonitis may develop. Barium, or non-ionic media, may be safer in these situations.

Upper Endoscopy

Upper endoscopy will usually, but not always, confirm the presence of a paraesophageal hernia. As endoscopic diagnosis often depends on assessment of the location of the stomach and GE junction compared to the endoscopic landmark of the diaphragmatic impression, this can often be difficult when the crura are separated widely enough, so as not to demonstrate a clear point of reference. Endoscopy will also detect ulceration, evidence of reflux esophagitis or Barrett's esophagus, or mucosal lesions.

Upper endoscopy is particularly important in acute gastric volvulus. While is it often difficult to pass a nasogastric tube blindly into the stomach, passage of the gastroscope under direct visualization is usually successful. Mucosal viability can be assessed, and the stomach can be decompressed. This decompression may convert a surgical emergency into a more elective situation. If the gastric mucosa is viable and nonischemic, then it is unlikely that the stomach is at immediate risk. Conversely, mucosal ischemia does not guarantee full-thickness gastric ischemia but certainly increases the risk thereof.

Esophageal Physiology Studies–Esophageal Manometry and pH Monitoring

These play no role in the emergency management of paraesophageal hernias. In the more elective situations, they may however be of use. Manometry will demonstrate esophageal body motility, and many surgeons will alter the subsequent repair operation based on these results. However, there is little data in the literature to support such "tailoring" of the operation to manometry findings.[1] In addition, motility often improves after reduction of the hernia, thereby increasing the false positive rates of manometry for motility disorders in these patients. However, when preoperatively normal esophageal function is

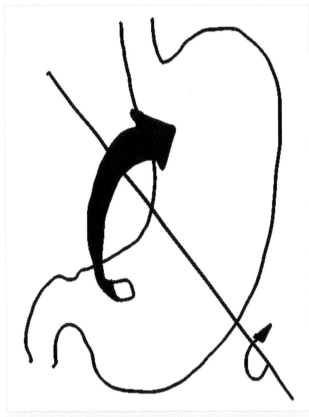

Fig. 18.3 Mesenteroaxial volvulus.

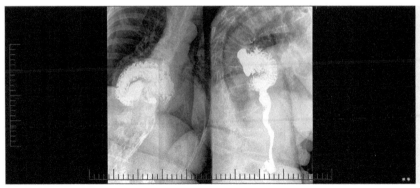

Fig. 18.4 PEH with organoaxial volvulus. PEH, paraesophageal.

demonstrated, this may facilitate postoperative management, particularly during the early phases when postoperative dysphagia regularly is present. pH-metry is less important for paraesophageal hernias than it is for the management of Type I hernias. In the latter, management is often dependent on the objective demonstration of gastroesophageal reflux, but for paraesophageal hernias, treatment is often guided by symptoms of obstruction or volume displacement.

18.2.5 Indications for Repair

The determination of suitable indications for elective repair of paraesophageal hernias is often difficult. This disease tends to occur in older patients and therefore consideration must be given to often extensive medical comorbidities. Elective repair in the asymptomatic elderly or infirm is usually contraindicated. Elective repair in the young and otherwise healthy should be considered and may prevent future complications of the hernia. The mortality rate for an elective paraesophageal hernia repair should be well less than 1%, but emergent repair after strangulation and gastric necrosis approaches 50% mortality.[1]

Elective repair in symptomatic patients is more strongly indicated. Once symptoms are present, risk of emergency presentation, and the possibility of strangulation that it entails, can approach 14% chance per year.[11]

Strangulation, acute gastric obstruction, and gastric ischemia must be considered separately—some form of treatment is always indicated.

18.2.6 Management of Acute Gastric Obstruction

This must be recognized as a surgical emergency. History and examination are undertaken. Appropriate resuscitative measures are implemented. Other causes for the presenting symptoms should be considered, and when chest pain is present, a cardiac cause should be ruled out. Chest X-ray should be performed.

Early decompression of the stomach is extremely important. If it can be achieved by bedside placement of a large-bore nasogastric tube, then this is preferable. However, the tube frequently cannot be placed into the stomach due to associated gastric volvulus. If the nasogastric is thought to have passed, it must be confirmed radiologically. Decompression improves gastric mucosal blood flow and decreases gastric volume, perhaps allowing the hernia to reduce. The quality of any aspirated fluid should be examined; if blood-stained, mucosal ischemia is more likely. With decompression of the stomach, time is available for stabilization of the patient's physiology and detailed discussions can be held regarding the patient's wishes for surgery.

If gastric decompression is unable to be achieved by nasogastric tube, then prompt upper endoscopy should be performed. In an unwell patient, this should be performed in the operating room rather than an endoscopy suite, in order to allow for progression to operation if decompression is impossible or gastric ischemia is found.

After decompression, priority then turns to assessment of the state and viability of the stomach. If mucosal ischemia is identified, then examination of the entire stomach is required,

preferably laparoscopically if the patient can tolerate pneumo-peritoneum. Resection of necrotic or perforated stomach is required, and the surgeon's experience and skillset will determine whether such resection can be performed laparoscopically or if conversion to open operation is necessary. Respiratory and wound complications increase for open operations as compared to laparoscopic.[1]

Operation requires reduction of the hernia and examination of the stomach and any other herniated organs. If the patient remains hemodynamically stable on the operating table, then the hiatal defect should be closed and a fundoplication performed. The ideal degree of wrap of the fundoplication is controversial, but this author believes that a partial wrap is preferable. These patients who are frequently elderly and infirm are, in the author's opinion, more likely to suffer from prolonged dysphagia and bloating after a 360-degree fundoplication rather than a partial fundoplication, although this is not necessarily supported in the limited available literature.[12]

Occasionally, the hernia defect is too large to successfully close. This is frequently the case when the crura are very attenuated and therefore do not hold sutures well without tearing through. A variety of surgical techniques have been tried to address this issue, including right-sided diaphragmatic relaxing incision, left-sided relaxing incisions,[13] combining anterior and posterior crural repair, or augmented closure with mesh. This is a difficult problem to overcome, and most options are reasonable except for placement of a bridging piece of absorbable mesh, which never provides a long-term solution. To minimize mesh infection, synthetic nonabsorbable mesh should not be placed if gastrectomy is required.

Rarely, the patient may be too physiologically unstable to tolerate the short extra time required to achieve diaphragmatic crural approximation. Under these circumstances, the operation can be abbreviated and the stomach can be reduced and then affixed to the anterior abdominal wall, either by sutures or via a gastrostomy tube.[14] This achieves resolution of the gastric obstruction, but recurrence of the hernia is likely.

Even after successful crural closure, gastrostomy placement should sometimes be considered. A bruised stomach with blood supply having been restored only recently may not function very well in the immediate postoperative period and acute gastric distension can result. The prophylactic placement of a gastrostomy would in these circumstances allow venting of the stomach until function returns.

18.2.7 Operative Technique

After establishment of pneumoperitoneum, ports are placed and a liver retractor is inserted. Repair of paraesophageal hernias requires dissection of the hernia sac and not of the stomach itself. By grasping the sac, traction injuries to the stomach are avoided. The is particularly the case when handling tissue in elderly patients. By gradually reducing the sac, the hernia is nearly always able to be successfully reduced. Blunt dissection is usually effective, with this author preferring advanced energy devices such as ultrasonic shears to control the small vessels present in this relatively avascular plane outside of the hernia sac. The sac should be reduced in its entirety[15] with wide mediastinal mobilization of the esophagus, and at least 3 cm of intrabdominal esophageal length achieved.[16,17] This is nearly always possible, but in the uncommon case that it is not, esophageal lengthening procedures such as gastric wedge fundectomy or Collis gastroplasty can be performed.[18]

At this time, the stomach must be inspected. If nonviable, gastrectomy is required. If, as is usually the case, more than a simple wedge gastrectomy is needed to excise the nonviable area, then reconstruction will be necessary and management should follow damage control principles. If the patient's current physiological states permits immediate reanastomosis, then this is preferably carried out, otherwise the patient can be returned to the intensive care unit for delayed restoration of gastrointestinal continuity. Appropriate management of any perforation and soiling of either the chest or abdomen will be required, with placement of drains or leaving of a laparostomy. These salvage procedures are very difficult with frequently poor outcomes.

18.3 Esophageal Perforation

Esophageal trauma is infrequently encountered by the acute care surgeon and due to this and the difficult anatomic location of the organ and its unusual blood supply, management of esophageal trauma can be quite challenging. Due to a lack of a serosal lining, the esophagus is more prone to leaks which are less likely to spontaneously close than those in other parts of the gastrointestinal tract. Trauma to the esophagus includes foreign body impaction, caustic injuries, and variceal bleeding. Only the former has been included in the remit of this chapter.

Perforation of the esophagus can result from many causes. Iatrogenic causes are the most common, particularly in an era of an increasing number of therapeutic endoscopic interventions to the gastrointestinal (GI) tract. Spontaneous perforation of the esophagus—Boerhaave's syndrome—occurs occasionally. Penetrating injuries to the esophagus can also occur and, to a lesser frequency, blunt injuries as well.

18.3.1 Etiology

Iatrogenic perforation: As a direct result of the large number of flexible endoscopic procedures being performed on the upper GI tract, this remains the most common cause of iatrogenic esophageal perforation. Although less likely to cause a perforation than the previously common rigid esophagoscopy, the flexible endoscope certainly can still cause injury. Increasingly, therapeutic interventions are being performed through the endoscope, such as dilation of upper gastrointestinal strictures, endoscopic mucosal resection, submucosal dissection and endoluminal stenting, all of which increase the risk over a diagnostic procedure. Varying types of esophageal intubation can cause perforations, with nasogastric tubes,[19,20] bougies,[21,22] manometry catheters and transesophageal echocardiogram probes all incurring risk.[23] Certain "natural orifice" surgical techniques, namely, per-oral endoscopic myotomy (the POEM procedure) aim to perforate, and then to close the esophagus as part of the planned therapy. Other causes of perforation also occur when operations are performed in proximity to the esophagus, such as hiatal hernia repairs, lung surgery, and pharyngeal diverticuloplasty.

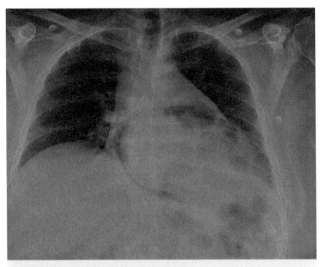

Fig. 18.5 Boerhaave's syndrome—esophageal perforation into the pericardium. (This image is provided courtesy of Dr. Dean C. Spilias, Monash Medical Centre, Melbourne, Australia.)

Spontaneous perforation: Boerhaave's syndrome is characterized by barotrauma to an otherwise normal esophagus.[24] Sudden increases in intra-abdominal pressure are responsible, usually related to vomiting. As this often occurs after a meal with a full stomach, gross soiling of the mediastinum occurs sometimes with extension into the pleura. This perforation may also occur secondary to an underlying pathology such as malignancy or inflammation. The most common location for such a perforation is in the left posterolateral position, and either the thoracic or the abdominal esophagus may be affected. The perforation specifically occurs at the margin of the contact between "clasp" and oblique esophageal fibers.[25] It is important to note that the mucosal side of the perforation is usually longer than the adventitial side with implications for repair as detailed below. The perforation may drain into the mediastinum, abdomen, pleura, lung, or pericardium (▶ Fig. 18.5).

Traumatic perforations: Penetrating injuries to the esophagus are rare, particularly to the thoracic esophagus, and almost never isolated to the single organ. When concurrent vascular, cardiac, or pulmonary injuries are present, the esophageal injury may be initially missed. After addressing the more time-critical injuries, such an injury should be actively sought, as delayed recognition can have life-threatening consequences. Penetrating injuries can also occur from the luminal aspect following ingestion of sharp objects such as fish, or meat bones, or needles (▶ Fig. 18.6).

Access to the cervical esophagus is relatively straightforward. Many perforations in this area cause little in the way of systemic symptoms as any leak may be confined to local structures. Extension into the mediastinum is however possible and if it occurs, severe systemic consequences may result. Local exploration, repair, and/or drainage can be instituted even when there has been a significant delay prior to treatment.

Blunt trauma perforations of the esophagus are rare and are almost universally associated with the enormous forces experienced in motor vehicle accidents. These injuries are almost certain to be associated with other intrathoracic and

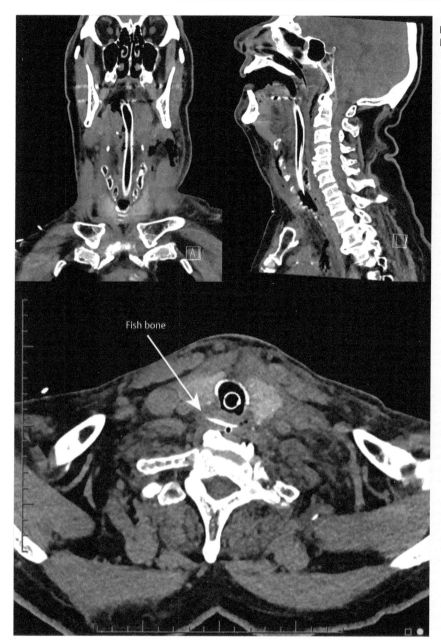

Fig. 18.6 Perforation of the cervical esophagus by a fish bone.

Fish bone

intra-abdominal injuries. The fixed points of the esophagus at the cricoid cartilage, carina, and phrenoesophageal junction are the most susceptible to trauma due to rapid deceleration.[24]

18.3.2 Investigations

Plain chest radiographs are often performed early in the assessment of trauma. Esophageal injury may be detected, although with a rather low sensitivity, and these images will identify large pleural effusion or large amount of mediastinal air.

CT scan is more sensitive in the detection of mediastinal air. If oral contrast is given, the extravasation may be identified, but usually the diagnosis can be made without this. It should be noted that a frequent presenting symptom of spontaneous esophageal perforation is *abdominal* pain. Unless perforation is considered,

then an abdominal CT scan alone may be performed, and an intra-thoracic esophageal perforation may be missed.

Fluoroscopic Contrast Video Esophagram

These can be very useful in a stable patient. False-negative rates are approximately 10 to 38%[26,27] and therefore probably higher than that of CT,[28] but when performed as a complementary study, additional information can be obtained. Demonstration of ongoing free contrast leak as well as information regarding drainage of the perforation are important. Mucosal irregularities (such as due to malignancy) may be seen. Barium studies may be the most sensitive in detection of a leak, but there are problems if this material accumulates in the pleural or peritoneal cavities. Therefore, aqueous media are preferred as the initial diagnostic contrast media. If no perforation is demonstrated, and if a repeat contrast study is thought necessary, some surgeons perform esophagram with dilute barium. The esophagram should be performed in both left lateral and right lateral decubitus positions as this might increase the sensitivity of the study.[27]

Upper Endoscopy

Endoscopy can be very helpful in ruling out perforation as a normal endoscopy has a very high negative-predictive value. It can be performed on patients too unwell for transfer to the radiology department. These procedures can be therapeutic if it is decided that the perforation may be managed endoscopically or if enteral access need be established for nutritional support via placement of a nasojejunal tube. The endoscopist must be mindful not to overly insufflate the esophagus or cause more trauma. Carbon dioxide insufflation is probably preferred over air insufflation, and an experienced endoscopist is favored over others.

18.3.3 Management

The major risks of esophageal perforation are sepsis and death, resulting from leakage of enteric contents. Accordingly, the focus of treatment should be the timely delivery of appropriate systemic antibiotics; elimination of the source of infection by repairing, occluding, diverting or exteriorizing the leak; adequate drainage of extraluminal fluid collections; and provision of nutritional support.[27] The leaked enteric contents can cause extensive corrosion and damage to the surrounding tissues and large fluid shifts can occur, exacerbating the hypotension of sepsis. Fluid volume resuscitation is paramount. Broad-spectrum antibiotic cover is required to target gastrointestinal organisms, and antifungal cover is often needed, particularly if a period of premorbid obstruction was present or if the patient has been taking acid-suppressant medications (particularly proton pump inhibitors), both of which increases the frequency of fungal colonization of the esophagus.[29] Intercostal drainage by tube thoracostomy of large collections should occur early while plans are underway for more definitive management.

Nonoperative Management

Until recently, it was believed that all esophageal perforation needed urgent surgical management to prevent major morbidity and death. It was often taught that operative drainage was mandated within the first 24 hours of perforation.[30] Mortality rates in the setting of treatment occurring after 24 hours are quoted to be double of those recognized and managed earlier.[31] Of course, surgical management can cause major morbidity too and there has emerged a consensus that highly selected patients can be managed nonoperatively.[32,33] An increasingly nonoperative approach to the problem is being employed, although it remains true that the individual cases must be highly selective, closely observed, and resources must be available to escalate management rapidly if required.

To aid in selection of patients for nonoperative therapy, criteria have been developed,[24,32,33,34,35,36] which rely on both clinical and radiologic assessment. An example of such criteria is given below (▶ Table 18.1). These criteria have been combined into various scoring systems. Although widely utilized,

Table 18.1 Criteria for assessing suitability of nonoperative management of esophageal perforation

- Age < 75 years
- Perforation contained by mediastinal pleura
- No solid food contamination of mediastinal or pleural spaces
- Drainage of contrast back into esophagus on contrast swallow
- No symptoms or signs of mediastinitis (e.g., leukocytosis, fever, or tachypnea)
- Tolerance to pleural or mediastinal contamination with appropriate drainage
- Absence of esophageal pathology (e.g., malignancy) or distal obstruction (e.g., stricture) which will impair healing

these scores do not reliably predict the outcome of nonoperative management.[37]

Nonoperative management includes the use of broad-spectrum antibiotics and bowel rest. Repeat contrast studies should be performed to demonstrate healing prior to the initiation of *per os* alimentation. Nutritional support with parenteral nutrition may be indicated. The patient should be carefully observed to assure that their clinical course does not deteriorate. Patients should be converted to other management strategies should clinical deterioration occur.

Endoscopic Management

Advances in technology and product development have now permitted novel endoscopic techniques to be used in the management of esophageal perforation. Endoscopic procedures can now be performed to close or exclude the defect in the esophageal wall. Options include endoscopic clips (either mucosal only or full-thickness closure), endoscopic suturing, or endoluminal stent placement. It should be again be emphasized that such closure techniques do nothing to treat the soiling of the mediastinum, chest or peritoneal cavity, and must be accompanied by additional drainage procedures such as tube thoracostomy or CT-guided drain placement.

Endoscopic through-the-scope (TTS) mucosal clips are frequently successfully deployed for esophageal closure in the POEM procedure. In this very specific indication, and in fasted patients, there is no soiling outside the esophagus even when there is clear evidence of full-thickness perforation (▶ Fig. 18.7). There is no inflammation from the recently surgically created esophageal mucosotomy, and a mucosal flap is fashioned to prevent direct communication of the lumen with the mediastinum. These clips have been used to achieve closure of esophageal perforations due to other causes.[38,39,40]

Over-the-scope clips (OTSC) (e.g., OTSC System; Ovesco Inc., Tübingen, Germany) have been used with the idea being that these strengthen the closure of the wall of the esophagus and provide more full-thickness closure.[40,41] The larger diameter of this type of clips also allows for closure of larger perforations.

Self-expanding metallic stents have been available since the 1990's and are made of materials such as nitinol (nickel and titanium) or elgiloy (cobalt, nickel, and chromium). They can be bare metal, partially covered, or fully covered by a plastic sleeve. Bare metals stents with large spaces between the metallic strands are not useful for closure of perforations as leak will persist through the gaps. The covering sleeve must be

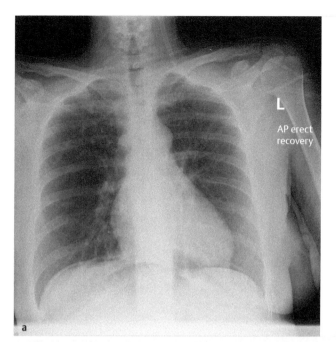
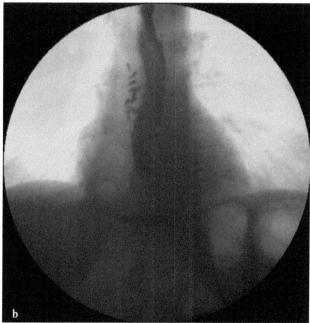

Fig. 18.7 (**a, b**) Imaging after POEM procedure, with the subdiaphragmatic air of full-thickness perforation, and confirmation of successful closure by through-the-scope clips. POEM, per-oral endoscopic myotomy.

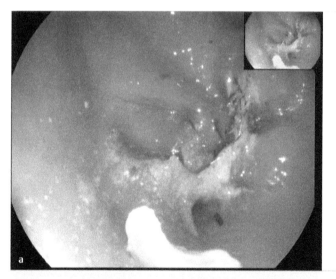
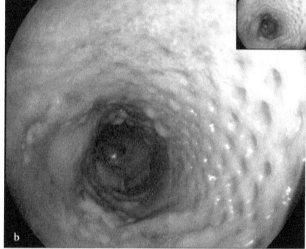

Fig. 18.8 (**a, b**) Tissue ingrowth into uncovered portion of stent.

present to achieve closure but the more covered the stent, the less securely it adheres to the esophageal wall and the more susceptible it is to migration. The corollary is that fully covered stents are easier to remove once healing has occurred. If left in place for an extended period, partially covered stents can be extremely difficult to retrieve due to tissue ingrowth (▶ Fig. 18.8) between the uncovered fibers, and caution should be used before using them in patients with perforations due to anything other than end-stage malignancy. More recently, expandable plastic stents have been developed. These are far easier to remove after the patient recovers, but migration remains an issue.

Stents are usually placed by a semi-rigid delivery system under fluoroscopic and/or endoscopic guidance. Placement of these stents can be difficult and possible complications include deployment of the stent through the perforation rather than into the native lumen, or further tearing of the esophageal wall. Migration of the stent can occur, causing distal obstruction or erosion (▶ Fig. 18.9). Some endoscopists secure the stent to prevent migration, using clips or sutures. Pain can be a problem for some patients. Not all stents will completely control the leak. Stents cannot be used high in the esophagus near the cricopharyngeus muscle where the sensation will be intolerable to the patient. Stents across the gastroesophageal function will

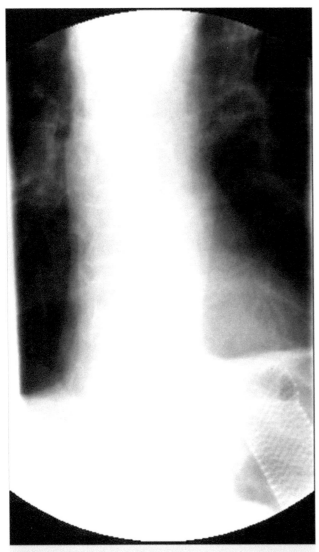

Fig. 18.9 Stent migration.

cause severe reflux. A collection which is draining back into the esophagus (which can be identified on preoperative contrast esophagram) will be converted to a problematic undrained collection if the return path is occluded by the stent. Small contained cavities can be drained by endoscopically placed drain tubes such as pigtail catheters or even nasogastric tubes.

A novel therapy is the endoscopic vacuum device. Based on the successful experience with similar devices in contaminated superficial wounds, these devices consist of a polyurethane sponge on the end of a catheter, which is placed either into, or adjacent to, the perforation. Suction is applied through the catheter and hopefully healing slowly occurs, with some degree of control of extraluminal contamination at the same time.[42,43,44] These devices should be changed frequently, perhaps every 48 to 72 hours, with a decrease in the size of the sponge, leading to the consequent large utilization of resources.

Operative Management

Prior to the advent of the endoscopic therapies, primary repair of the esophagus was widely advocated. Repair was emergently undertaken with the belief that after delay of more than 24 hours the tissues would become too friable from the surrounding inflammation and primary repair would have to be abandoned. Esophageal fistulae were frequent complications of perforation managed by drainage alone. With increasing experience, this practice has slowly changed, and primary repair is likely still possible well beyond the first day.[30]

Primary repair is best performed in two layers, the first layer incorporating the "strength" layer of the submucosa and mucosa, and the second layer incorporating the muscular coat of the esophagus. A key principle of repair is to obtain adequate visualization of the mucosal layer; the perforation of this layer often extends further than the defect in the muscle, and muscle often must be divided to identify the edges of the mucosal defect with any certainty. Nonviable mucosa should be debrided, so that the repair is through health tissue. Care should be taken not to cause luminal narrowing, and some surgeons advocate performing the repair over a bougie, although placement of the bougie has been occasionally known to extend the perforation.

Access to the perforation site depends on its location. The cervical esophagus is usually accessed through the left neck with an incision being made anterior to the sternocleidomastoid muscle. Primary surgical repair of the perforated cervical esophagus is not often required with outcomes no better than those obtained simply by achieving adequate drainage.[45,46] Perforation of the abdominal esophagus must be accessed from the abdomen. Proximal or midesophageal perforations are probably easiest to access through the right chest, often by open thoracotomy at a level between the 4th and 6th interspace. Distal esophageal perforations can be reached most easily from a low left-sided thoracic approach performed around the 7th interspace. Occasionally, a transabdominal approach can reach lower esophageal perforations. The primary repair can be reinforced by buttressing with healthy pleura, pericardium, or peritoneum. At the time of repair, washout with decortication, debridement, and drainage of the contaminated spaces is also important. A drain should be placed near the esophageal suture line.[27] If the repair is tenuous despite best attempts, then some will insert a large bore T-tube through the defect in addition to para-esophageal drains.[24] This commits the patient to an esophagocutaneous fistula, which hopefully will be controlled and so is inferior to a successful primary repair.

Thoracoscopic and laparoscopic access can be reasonable in selected patients, but principles of contamination control by esophageal closure and drainage must still be observed. When present, a large volume of contamination is difficult to adequately evacuate with minimally invasive techniques and, with very little margin for error in these often desperately ill patients, open operation is often preferred. However, perforations of the abdominal esophagus and of the esophagus immediately adjacent to the diaphragmatic hiatus are sometimes easier to access and repair laparoscopically, particularly among obese patients.

It is essential to plan for postoperative nutritional support as the patient will be prevented from taking oral intake for a significant period. Enteral feeding is preferable as it protects mucosal integrity of the gut and prevents complications associated with parenteral feeding. Access can be through either the stomach or the jejunum. If future esophagectomy is conceivable, the gastric conduit should be protected and operative jejunostomy preferred. If tube gastrostomy is the preferred access, this should be placed operatively rather than endoscopically to avoid pulling the tube past the esophageal repair site.

Consideration must be given to the underlying esophageal pathology, which may influence choice of repair and other aspects of treatment. Iatrogenic perforations due to dilatation in achalasia is a prime example. Here, consideration must be given to treatment of the underlying condition, to not only aid in subsequent control of dysphagia but also relieve obstruction at the lower esophageal sphincter which otherwise would inhibit healing. In this case, an esophageal cardiomyotomy should be performed, usually performed at a different location on the esophageal circumference.

In certain cases, the esophagus may be deemed unsalvageable after a perforation, usually due to preexisting diseases such as end-stage achalasia with esophageal dilatation, and an esophagectomy may offer the best functional outcome. This usually includes a transthoracic approach to permit synchronous debridement and drainage of the chest. Consideration should be given to the current physiologic state of the patient; if transthoracic approach with the requirement for single-lung ventilation is not able to be tolerated, then a transhiatal approach may be the only option, with adjuncts of percutaneous thoracic drainage required.

After esophagectomy, the patient may be too unwell for anastomosis to be undertaken amid concerns for sepsis-related hypotension and hypoperfusion adversely affecting the reconstruction. Postoperative edema from severe hypoalbuminemia will also affect any anastomosis. In these circumstances, the construction of a cervical esophagostomy is very helpful in achieving diversion of secretions. A left neck incision is employed which provides best protection to the recurrent laryngeal nerve that is in the operative field. The esophagus should be divided as distally as feasible to facilitate subsequent delayed reconstruction after stabilization of the patient.

A particularly difficult situation is that of the perforation of an esophageal malignancy, regardless of it being spontaneous or iatrogenic (for example, during placement of a stent to relieve dysphagia). It is believed that perforation of an esophageal cancer renders the cancer incurable,[24,47] although currently accepted staging systems do not specifically refer to perforation[48,49] as a prognosticator. Management depends not only on the clinical state of the patient and the specifics of the perforation (especially if the perforation is at a site different to the location of the tumor) but also on the stage of the cancer and the prognosis of the patient. If an esophagectomy was to be likely in the patient's future, such as for an early stage adenocarcinoma, then in highly selected cases, an esophagectomy should be expedited, but the likely palliative nature of this treatment should be known to all. Although there are supporters of esophagectomy to palliate symptoms of incurable cancer,[50,51,52] this author is extremely hesitant to consider such a major operation with a likely poor short- to medium-term outcome. It remains unclear what the cancer-related survival is for these patients, even if the esophagectomy is uncomplicated. Certainly, a rapid demise of the patient is likely with no treatment. If the patient is deemed not likely to have been an operative candidate due to the extent of the cancer, then alternative methods of management should be employed, such as endoscopic stenting[53] or simply palliative measures.

18.3.4 Outcomes

Overall mortality rates for perforated esophagus remain high at approximately 13%,[54] which probably represents a slight improvement from approximately 18%[31] reported a couple of decades ago. Mortality following spontaneous perforations (36%) is almost double of that from iatrogenic injuries (19%), presumably due to the later diagnosis of the former and the fact that iatrogenic injuries usually occur in a fasted patient with less gastric contents to contaminate the mediastinum.[27,31]

Analyses of the surgical treatment of esophageal perforation have shown widely varied results from variable quality studies of heterogenous patient cohorts,[55] with mortality rates of 4 to 80% reported. In a 2017 meta-analysis of 379 patients from 12 studies, healing of the perforation occurred in 87%.[54] Comparison between the different treatment modalities is fraught with problems due to the paucity of comparative data and the complete absence of well-controlled or randomized data.

Most reported perforation sites are of the thoracic esophagus (73%), but this may reflect reporting bias.[54] Iatrogenic perforations are more commonly reported (47%) than spontaneous perforations (38%).

Since the introduction of esophageal stents, enthusiasm for their application in the treatment of esophageal perforation has been increasing.[27] Results from cohorts treated endoscopically compare favorably to surgical repair. A meta-analysis published in 2015 of 643 patients (81% postoperative leaks and 19% perforations or fistulae) treated with esophageal stenting found a clinical success rate of 77%.[56] These values seem reasonably reproducible in the literature with an earlier systematic review reporting clinical success rate of 85% regardless of type of stent (fully covered, partially covered, or plastic), with highest rates of stent migration being observed, as expected, in plastic self-expanding stents (31%), followed by fully covered stents (26%) and finally partially covered metallic stents (12%), despite earlier removal of the metallic stents.[57] While successful stent placement may seal the perforation, any extraluminal collection will still require drainage. This review reported that 59% percent of patients require concurrent drainage of extraesophageal fluid collections. Mortality for stented patients was 13%, which is similar to patients undergoing surgical repair. Surgical intervention for incomplete occlusion or stent-related complications was necessary in 13% of patients. Patients at increased risk for failure of endoscopic management include those with a perforation of the cervical esophagus or gastro-esophageal junction, and those with esophageal injuries longer than 6 cm.[58]

The role of endoscopic clipping as therapy for esophageal perforation using either TTS clips or OTSC clips was assessed in a recent literature review.[40] The analysis included 194 patients from nine articles, with four of these articles using the larger OTSC. Success rates for closure of the perforations were achieved in up to 92% of cases. They concluded that TTS clips are effective in the treatment of early perforations (<24 hours old) with limited contamination and lengthless than 10 mm, whereas lesions up to 20 mm could be treated with OTS clipping.[59]

A recent systematic review of endoscopic vacuum therapy of esophageal defects assessed data on approximately 180 patients, with success rates ranging from 83 to 100%.[60]

18.3.5 Conclusion

Management of an esophageal perforation is challenging. The treating surgeon must be well-versed in various treatment modalities. Most importantly, early diagnosis, rapid initiation of treatment, and frequent review must be employed. If improvement stalls at any stage, or if there is deterioration of the patient, then there must be flexibility in the planning of the surgeon to adopt different measures. Frequently, management requires utilization of multiple modalities, and there would seem to be benefits in the early employment of a multidisciplinary approach. Mortality rates have improved significantly over the years, but esophageal perforation remains a difficult, life-threatening, and complex problem even today.

References

[1] Kohn GP, Price RR, DeMeester SR, et al. SAGES Guidelines Committee. Guidelines for the management of hiatal hernia. SurgEndosc. 2013; 27 (12):4409–4428

[2] van der Linde RA, Lases SS, Buist TJ, van Westreenen HL, Nieuwenhuijs VB. A decreased preload due to a loaded stomach: a rare presentation of a paraesophageal hernia. Ann ThoracSurg. 2017; 104(6):e451–e453

[3] Low DE, Simchuk EJ. Effect of paraesophageal hernia repair on pulmonary function. Ann Thorac Surg. 2002; 74(2):333–337, discussion 337

[4] Awais O, Luketich JD. Management of giant paraesophageal hernia. Minerva Chir. 2009; 64(2):159–168

[5] Carrott PW, Markar SR, Hong J, Kuppusamy MK, Koehler RP, Low DE. Iron-deficiency anemia is a common presenting issue with giant paraesophageal hernia and resolves following repair. J GastrointestSurg. 2013; 17(5): 858–862

[6] Hill LD, Tobias JA. Paraesophageal hernia. Arch Surg. 1968; 96(5):735–744

[7] Martin TR, Ferguson MK, Naunheim KS. Management of giant paraesophageal hernia. Dis Esophagus. 1997; 10(1):47–50

[8] Leese T, Perdikis G. Management of patients with giant paraesophageal hernia. Dis Esophagus. 1998; 11(3):177–180

[9] Antonoff MB, D'Cunha J, Andrade RS, Maddaus MA. Giant paraesophageal hernia repair: technical pearls. J Thorac CardiovascSurg. 2012; 144(3): S67–S70

[10] Falk GL. Giant paraesophageal hernia repair and fundoplication: a timely discussion. J Am CollSurg. 2016; 222(3):329–330

[11] Treacy PJ, Jamieson GG. An approach to the management of para-oesophageal hiatus hernias. Aust N Z J Surg. 1987; 57(11):813–817

[12] Tedesco P, Lobo E, Fisichella PM, Way LW, Patti MG. Laparoscopic fundoplication in elderly patients with gastroesophageal reflux disease. Arch Surg. 2006; 141(3):289–292, discussion 292

[13] Greene CL, DeMeester SR, Zehetner J, Worrell SG, Oh DS, Hagen JA. Diaphragmatic relaxing incisions during laparoscopic paraesophageal hernia repair. SurgEndosc. 2013; 27(12):4532–4538

[14] Boerema WJ. Anterior gastropexy: a simple operation for hiatus hernia. Aust N Z J Surg. 1969; 39(2):173–175

[15] Edye M, Salky B, Posner A, Fierer A. Sac excision is essential to adequate laparoscopic repair of paraesophageal hernia. SurgEndosc. 1998; 12(10):1259–1263

[16] Oelschlager BK, Pellegrini CA, Hunter J, et al. Biologic prosthesis reduces recurrence after laparoscopic paraesophageal hernia repair: a multicenter, prospective, randomized trial. Ann Surg. 2006; 244(4):481–490

[17] Cohn TD, Soper NJ. Paraesophageal hernia repair: techniques for success. J Laparoendosc Adv Surg Tech A. 2017; 27(1):19–23

[18] DeMeester SR. Laparoscopic paraesophageal hernia repair: critical steps and adjunct techniques to minimize recurrence. Surg Laparosc Endosc Percutan Tech. 2013; 23(5):429–435

[19] Jackson RH, Payne DK, Bacon BR. Esophageal perforation due to nasogastric intubation. Am J Gastroenterol. 1990; 85(4):439–442

[20] Mileder LP, Müller M, Reiterer F, et al. Esophageal perforation with unilateral fluidothorax caused by nasogastric tube. Case Rep Pediatr. 2016; 2016: 4103734

[21] Kim ES, Kang JY, Cho IS, Rhee GW. Traumatic esophageal perforation by a self bougienage. J Thorac Dis. 2017; 9(5):E408–E411

[22] Lowham AS, Filipi CJ, Hinder RA, et al. Mechanisms and avoidance of esophageal perforation by anesthesia personnel during laparoscopic foregut surgery. SurgEndosc. 1996; 10(10):979–982

[23] Shapira MY, Hirshberg B, Agid R, Zuckerman E, Caraco Y. Esophageal perforation after transesophageal echocardiogram. Echocardiography. 1999; 16(2): 151–154

[24] Wahed S, Griffin SM. Oesophageal emergencies. In: Griffin SM, Lamb PJ, eds. Oesophagogastric Surgery: A Companion To Specialist Surgical Practice. 6th ed./ed.2019:xiv, 351 pages

[25] Korn O, Oñate JC, López R. Anatomy of the Boerhaave syndrome. Surgery. 2007; 141(2):222–228

[26] Swanson JO, Levine MS, Redfern RO, Rubesin SE. Usefulness of high-density barium for detection of leaks after esophagogastrectomy, total gastrectomy, and total laryngectomy. AJR Am J Roentgenol. 2003; 181(2):415–420

[27] Watson TJ, Peyre CG. Etiology and management of esophageal perforation. In: Yeo CJ, ed. Shackelford's Surgery Of The Alimentary Tract. 8th edition. ed. Philadelphia, PA: Elsevier; 2018

[28] Fadoo F, Ruiz DE, Dawn SK, Webb WR, Gotway MB. Helical CT esophagography for the evaluation of suspected esophageal perforation or rupture. AJR Am J Roentgenol. 2004; 182(5):1177–1179

[29] Elsayed H, Shaker H, Whittle I, Hussein S. The impact of systemic fungal infection in patients with perforated oesophagus. Ann R Coll SurgEngl. 2012; 94 (8):579–584

[30] Wang N, Razzouk AJ, Safavi A, et al. Delayed primary repair of intrathoracic esophageal perforation: is it safe? J Thorac Cardiovasc Surg. 1996; 111(1): 114–121, discussion 121–122

[31] Brinster CJ, Singhal S, Lee L, Marshall MB, Kaiser LR, Kucharczuk JC. Evolving options in the management of esophageal perforation. Ann ThoracSurg. 2004; 77(4):1475–1483

[32] Cameron JL, Kieffer RF, Hendrix TR, Mehigan DG, Baker RR. Selective nonoperative management of contained intrathoracic esophageal disruptions. Ann ThoracSurg. 1979; 27(5):404–408

[33] Altorjay A, Kiss J, Vörös A, Bohák A. Nonoperative management of esophageal perforations. Is it justified? Ann Surg. 1997; 225(4):415–421

[34] Wahed S, Dent B, Jones R, Griffin SM. Spectrum of oesophageal perforations and their influence on management. Br J Surg. 2014; 101(1): e156–e162

[35] Griffin SM, Lamb PJ, Shenfine J, Richardson DL, Karat D, Hayes N. Spontaneous rupture of the oesophagus. Br J Surg. 2008; 95(9):1115–1120

[36] Schweigert M, Sousa HS, Solymosi N, et al. Spotlight on esophageal perforation: A multinational study using the Pittsburgh esophageal perforation severity scoring system. J Thorac CardiovascSurg. 2016; 151(4): 1002–1009

[37] Wigley C, Athanasiou A, Bhatti A, et al. Does the Pittsburgh severity score predict outcome in esophageal perforation? Dis Esophagus. 2019; 32(2)

[38] Sriram PV, Rao GV, Reddy ND. Successful closure of spontaneous esophageal perforation (Boerhaave's syndrome) by endoscopic clipping. Indian J Gastroenterol. 2006; 25(1):39–41

[39] Siddiqi S, Schraufnagel DP, Siddiqui HU, et al. Recent advancements in the minimally invasive management of esophageal perforation, leaks, and fistulae. Expert Rev Med Devices. 2019; 16(3):197–209

[40] Yılmaz B, Unlu O, Roach EC, et al. Endoscopic clips for the closure of acute iatrogenic perforations: where do we stand? Dig Endosc. 2015; 27(6): 641–648

[41] Robotis J, Karabinis A. Esophageal perforation due to transesophageal echocardiogram: new endoscopic clip treatment. Case Rep Gastroenterol. 2014; 8(2):235–239

[42] Goenka MK, Goenka U. Endotherapy of leaks and fistula. World J GastrointestEndosc. 2015; 7(7):702–713

[43] Heits N, Bernsmeier A, Reichert B, et al. Long-term quality of life after endovac-therapy in anastomotic leakages after esophagectomy. J Thorac Dis. 2018; 10(1):228–240

[44] Ooi G, Burton P, Packiyanathan A, et al. Indications and efficacy of endoscopic vacuum-assisted closure therapy for upper gastrointestinal perforations. ANZ J Surg. 2018; 88(4):E257–E263

[45] Brewer LA, III, Carter R, Mulder GA, Stiles QR. Options in the management of perforations of the esophagus. Am J Surg. 1986; 152(1):62–69

[46] Wilson SE, Stone R, Scully M, Ozeran L, Benfield JR. Modern management of anastomotic leak after esophagogastrectomy. Am J Surg. 1982; 144(1):95–101

[47] Adam DJ, Thompson AM, Walker WS, Cameron EW. Oesophagogastrectomy for iatrogenic perforation of oesophageal and cardia carcinoma. Br J Surg. 1996; 83(10):1429–1432

[48] Rice TW, Patil DT, Blackstone EH. 8th edition AJCC/UICC staging of cancers of the esophagus and esophagogastric junction: application to clinical practice. Ann CardiothoracSurg. 2017; 6(2):119–130

[49] Japan Esophageal Society. Japanese Classification of Esophageal Cancer, 11th Edition: part II and III. Esophagus. 2017; 14(1):37–65

[50] MacGillivray DC, Etienne HB, Snyder DA. Transhiatal esophagectomy in the management of perforated esophageal cancer. Mil Med. 1991; 156(11):634–636

[51] Yeo CJ, Lillemoe KD, Klein AS, Zinner MJ. Treatment of instrumental perforation of esophageal malignancy by transhiatal esophagectomy. Arch Surg. 1988; 123(8):1016–1018

[52] Grewal N, El-Badawi K, Nguyen NT. Minimally invasive Ivor Lewis esophagectomy for the management of iatrogenic esophageal perforation in a patient with esophageal cancer. Surg TechnolInt. 2009; 18:82–85

[53] Ferri L, Lee JK, Law S, Wong KH, Kwok KF, Wong J. Management of spontaneous perforation of esophageal cancer with covered self expanding metallic stents. Dis Esophagus. 2005; 18(1):67–69

[54] Sdralis EIK, Petousis S, Rashid F, Lorenzi B, Charalabopoulos A. Epidemiology, diagnosis, and management of esophageal perforations: systematic review. Dis Esophagus. 2017; 30(8):1–6

[55] Bayram AS, Erol MM, Melek H, Colak MA, Kermenli T, Gebitekin C. The success of surgery in the first 24 hours in patients with esophageal perforation. Eurasian J Med. 2015; 47(1):41–47

[56] van Halsema EE, van Hooft JE. Clinical outcomes of self-expandable stent placement for benign esophageal diseases: A pooled analysis of the literature. World J GastrointestEndosc. 2015; 7(2):135–153

[57] van Boeckel PG, Sijbring A, Vleggaar FP, Siersema PD. Systematic review: temporary stent placement for benign rupture or anastomotic leak of the oesophagus. Aliment PharmacolTher. 2011; 33(12):1292–1301

[58] Freeman RK, Ascioti AJ, Giannini T, Mahidhara RJ. Analysis of unsuccessful esophageal stent placements for esophageal perforation, fistula, or anastomotic leak. Ann Thorac Surg. 2012; 94(3):959–964, discussion 964–965

[59] Paspatis GA, Dumonceau JM, Barthet M, et al. Diagnosis and management of iatrogenic endoscopic perforations: European Society of Gastrointestinal Endoscopy (ESGE) Position Statement. Endoscopy. 2014; 46(8):693–711

[60] Newton NJ, Sharrock A, Rickard R, Mughal M. Systematic review of the use of endo-luminal topical negative pressure in oesophageal leaks and perforations. Dis Esophagus. 2017; 30(3):1–5

Expert Commentary on Esophageal Emergencies by *Steven DeMeester*

Expert Commentary on Esophageal Emergencies

Steven DeMeester

This chapter is an excellent overview of the management and diagnosis of emergent surgical problems in the esophagus, including perforation and incarcerated, obstructed paraesophageal hernias. As with many emergent surgical situations, there is a role for laparoscopic, thorascoscopic, or endoscopic management in some of these patients which may decrease the postoperative morbidity.[1]

This chapter also highlights the benefits of surgeons being able to carry out advanced endoscopy. While this is not historically in the general surgeon's skill set, there exists data that suggests that advanced endoscopy skills are desirable for practicing surgeons.[2] These skills augment the surgeon's armamentarium in the management of both elective and emergent problems, particularly since not every hospital will have an advanced endoscopist readily available. Increasingly, surgical graduates are completing their residency with training in advanced endoscopy skills.

Placing a stent for an esophageal perforation or controlling an upper gastrointestinal bleed would not only allow for resuscitation but also prevent the need for an emergent procedure that is likely to be more complicated. Since most esophageal perforations occur as a consequence of an iatrogenic injury, the ability to deploy clips or suture endoscopically may allow closure of the mucosal defect endoscopically prior to significant contamination or infection. Using endoscopy to place a decompressing nasogastric tube in the case of a gastric volvulus allows for the edema of the herniated fundus to dissipate and converts an urgent case into an elective repair. Finally, placing a stent across a near obstructing esophageal cancer would allow for oral alimentation and palliation of dysphagia.

Emergent diseases of the esophagus are not common, but management is complicated. Open surgical approaches in many instances are being replaced by endoscopic and minimally invasive approaches that can limit the surgical stress or allow for a more definitive, staged operation after the patient has been resuscitated. Familiarity with these options and understanding their risks and benefits allows the clinician to best manage these potentially catastrophic emergencies.

References

[1] Freeman RK, Herrera A, Ascioti AJ, Dake M, Mahidhara RS. A propensity-matched comparison of cost and outcomes after esophageal stent placement or primary surgical repair for iatrogenic esophageal perforation. J Thorac CardiovascSurg. 2015; 149(6):1550–1555

[2] Deal SB, Cook MR, Hughes D, et al. Training for a career in rural and nonmetropolitan surgery-a practical needs assessment. J SurgEduc. 2018; 75(6): e229–e233

Index

Note: 't' denotes table and 'f' denotes figure.

A

ABCDEF Bundle 19
– in Intensive Care Unit 20f
abdominal anatomy
– penetrating abdominal trauma 63
Abdominal Aortic Aneurysm (AAA) 15
abdominal closure
– blunt abdominal trauma 56
abdominal stab wounds
– Western Trauma Association algorithm 67f
acalculous cholecystitis 135
Accreditation Council for Graduate Medical Education (ACGME) 3
acute appendectomy
– and conservative management 121f
Acute Care Surgery (ACS) 1, 14
– care delivery models 4
– components 2f
– cost modeling analysis 3
– definition of 1–6
– drivers for 1–3
– vs. Emergency General Surgery 1
– fellowship training 3
– implementation 3
– patient throughput improvements 3–4
– patients in shock 14
– preoperative critical care 14–18
– surgeon satisfaction with 3
– and vasopressors 16
acute cholecystitis 133
– diagnostic evaluation 131
– expert commentary 147
– indications and timing for operative intervention 132–133
– management of complications 139–140
– Minimally Invasive Surgery 136–138
– nonoperative management 139
– symptomatic gallbladder disease 133
acute diverticulitis 148
– contraindications to MIS 151–152
– damage control 152
– Diverting Loop Ileostomy (DLI) 152
– emergent operation 149
– expert commentary 159
– Hartmann's procedure 152
– management of postoperative complications 153–154
– and Minimally Invasive Surgery (MIS) 150–151
– nonemergent surgery 149–150
– nonoperative management 149
– open management strategies 152
– operative intervention 148–149
– postoperative morbidity, mortality, and complications 154t
– Primary Anastomosis (PA) 152
acute gastric obstruction
– management 245
– operative technique 245–246
acute kidney injury 28
acute myocardial infarction 18
Acute Respiratory Distress Syndrome (ARDS) 14, 16
– epidemiology and outcomes 24–25

– mechanical ventilation algorithm 26f
– mechanical ventilation in adult patients 27t
– net FiO$_2$ and PEEP titration 27t
– rescue strategies 25–27, 25f
acute respiratory failure 24
ADRENAL trial 24
airway management 15–16
Airway Pressure Release Ventilation (APRV) 16
alternative minimal invasive techniques 121–122
American Association for the Surgery of Trauma (AAST) 1, 3
– grade III splenic injury on CT scan 48f
– grade IV liver injury on CT scan 49f
– grade IV splenic injury on CT scan 48f
– grading of solid organ injuries 47t
American Association of Blood Banks (AABB) 21
– RBC transfusion thresholds and storage 21t
American Association of Medical Colleges 1
American College of Surgeons 1
American Hospital Association (AHA) 4
anastomotic stricture 181
anatomy
– of mesenteric ischemia 229
anemia
– management in ICU 20, 22
anterior abdominal
– CT scan 65f
– selective nonoperative management 65–69
– stab wound 65f
antibiotics
– vs. appendectomy 121–122
appendectomy
– vs. antibiotics 121–122
appendicitis
– with abscess formation 116f
– alvarado score 115f
– with appendix 116f
– complicated 123
– Computed Tomography 116–117
– diagnosis 114–115
– in elderly 123–124
– epidemiology 112–113
– expert commentary 131
– Iatrogenic 114f
– laparoscopic vs. open appendectomy 118–121
– Magnetioc Resonance Imaging (MRI) 118
– pathogenesis 113–114
– with perforation and phlegmon formation 117f
– phlegmon 117f
– pregnancy 124–125
– treatment 118
– ultrasound 115–116
– uncomplicated 122–123
appendix
– appendicitis with 116f
argyle shunt
– brachial artery 106f
APROCCHSS trial 24

B

Blatchford score
– gastrointestinal hemorrhage 197t
blood gases 15
blunt abdominal trauma 46
– abdominal closure 56
– complications 50
– diagnosis 47–48
– diaphragm injuries 55–56
– expert commentary 61
– Gastroesophageal (GE) junction injuries 51–53
– general approach to 46–47
– hollow viscus injuries 50–51
– major vascular injuries 54–55
– management of specific injuries after 47–50
– pancreatic injuries 53–54
– solid organ injuries 47
– surgical techniques 48–50
Blunt Cerebrovascular Injury (BCVI) 34
– grading scale for 40t
– screening criteria 40t
blunt neck trauma
– Blunt Cerebrovascular Injury (BCI) Management 39–40
Boerhaave's syndrome 246f
brachial artery 98
– argyle shunt 106f
– transection 97f
brachial disruption
– Computed Tomography Angiography (CTA) 96f
broad-spectrum IV antibiotics 18
bronchoscopy 16

C

cancer prophylaxis 178
cardiac injuries 87
– and mediastinal injuries 83
– treatment 88
cardiac trauma
– presentation and evaluation 87–88
cardiogenic shock 14, 15
– management 18
care delivery models 4
carotid artery 98
celiac artery 99
cellular hypoxia 14
cervical esophagus
– injury 36
– perforation 247f
cervical trauma 34
– carotid artery and 37–38
– cervical esophageal injury 36
– cervical vascular injury 36–37
– expert commentary on 45
– penetrating neck trauma 34–35
– subclavian artery and 38–39
– vertebral artery and 38
cervical vascular injury 36–37
chest
– physiotherapy 16
cholangitis 134
cholecystectomy program
– sages safe 137f

cholecystenteric fistula 135
cholecystitis
– older population 136
– in pregnancy 136
choledocholithiasis 133–134
cirrhosis 136
clamshell incision 84f
clamshell thoracotomy 84f
clinical manifestations
– colonic perforation 178
– contraindications to mis approach 179
– emergent indications 177
– Inflammatory/Infectious Bowel Disease 176–177
– life-threatening severe colitis 177
– massive hemorrhage 178
– minimally invasive surgery 178–179
– open management strategies 179
– subtotal colectomy with end ileostomy 179
– total proctocolectomy and end ileostomy 179–180
– turnbull-blowhole colostomy 179
clostridium difficile colitis 181–182
– contraindications to an MIS approach 183
– management of postoperative complications 183–184
– minimally invasive surgery 182
– open management strategies 183
– operative intervention 182
– total abdominal colectomy 182f
colectomy
– with ileostomy 179
colo-ovarian fistula
– Crohn's disease (CD) 176f
colon
– Gastroesophageal (GE) junction injuries 52
– and rectum 174–175
colonic perforation 178
Combined Mechanism (CM) 95
Common Bile Duct 135
Common Femoral Artery (CFA)
– and vein 100
complicated biliary disease
– acalculous cholecystitis 135
– cholangitis 134
– choledocholithiasis 133–134
– diaphragm injuries 56
– gallstone pancreatitis 134
– gangrenous cholecystitis 134–135
Computed Tomography (CT)
– abdomen gunshot wound 70f
– anterior abdominal 65f
– appendicitis 116–117
– femoral hernia 218f
– Grade 4 splenic injury 105
– grade III and IV splenic injury 49f
– grade IV liver injury 49f
– left and right inguinal hernia 218f
– preoperative critical care 15
– Western Trauma Association algorithm 71f
Computed Tomography Angiography (CTA)

– brachial disruption 96f
congestive cardiomyopathy 14–15
conservative management
– and acute appendectomy 121f
cost modeling analysis 3
Crohn's disease (CD) 172
– colo-ovarian fistula 176f
– colon and rectum 174–175
– fat wrapping 172f
– fistulizing/penetrating disease 173–174
– ileocolic disease 174
– indications for operative intervention 172–173
– laparoscopic resection 172f
– Minimally Invasive Approaches (MIA) 175–176
– perianal disease 175
– recurrent disease 175
– stricturing/obstructing disease 173
– toxic colitis 174
– upper gastrointestinal tract and duodenal disease 174
crystalloid boluses
– shock and 16
CT-tractography 66

D

Damage Control Surgery (DCS)
– acute diverticulitis 152
– operative principles 74t
– penetrating abdominal trauma 73–75
– resuscitation 75
diagnosis
– alvarado score for appendicitis 115f
– appendicitis 114–115
– diaphragm injuries 55
– major vascular injuries 54
diaphragm injuries
– blunt abdominal trauma 55–56
– blunt injury 56f
– complications 56
– diagnosis 55
– management strategy 55
– surgical techniques 55–56
diaphragmatic hernia 220–222
diaphragmatic injury 83
Distal SFA 101
distributive shock 14
diverticulitis
– Hinchey scoring system 148
Diverting Loop Ileostomy (DLI) 152
dopamine 16
duodenal disease
– and upper gastrointestinal tract 174
duodenum
– Gastroesophageal (GE) junction injuries 52

E

Eastern Associationfor the Surgeryof Trauma (EAST) 66
elective
– thoracic trauma 82
electrocardiograph (EKG) 17
electrolytes
– and sepsis 15
Emergency Department (ED). see Intensive Care Unit (ICU)

Emergency Department Thoracotomy (EDT) 106
Emergency General Surgery
– vs. Acute Care Surgery (ACS) 1
– burden of disease for 2f
– and common public health concerns 6f
– patient outcomes 4–6
– volume and adjusted cost per hospitalization 5f
empyema 83
End-tidal capnography 17
endoscopic management
– large bowel obstruction 211
endoscopic necrosectomy 165f
endoscopic transgastric debridement 164–165
Enhanced Recovery After Surgery (ERAS) pathway
– perforated peptic ulcer 199t
enterotomy 180f
epidemiology
– Acute Respiratory Distress Syndrome (ARDS) 24–25
– appendicitis 112–113
– incarcerated hernias 216
– penetrating abdominal trauma 62–63
epigastric hernias 219–220
Erythropoiesis-stimulating Agent (ESA) 22
esophageal perforations
– endoscopic management 248–250
– etiology 246
– expert commentary 257
– nonoperative management 248t
– operative management 250–251
– and paraesophageal hernias 242
physiology studies 244–245
Esophageal Pressure-guided Positive End-expiratory Pressure (PEEP) 14
etiology
– esophageal perforation 246
– hiatal hernia 243
etomidate 15
expert commentary
– appendicitis 131
– penetrating abdominal trauma 79
Extracorporeal Membrane Oxygenation (ECMO) 14, 16, 27
extremity injuries 101
– considerations after repair of 101
extremity vascular 111

F

fellowship training 3
femoral hernia
– CT image 218f
flank hernia 222
fluid resuscitation 16
Fluoroscopic Contrast Video Esophagram 247–248
– management 248
– nonoperative management 248
– upper endoscopy 248
Focused Assessment with Sonography for Trauma (FAST) 15, 80
foreign body removal 83
forrest classification

– hemorrhagic peptic ulcer disease 198t

G

gallstone ileus. see porcelain gallbladder
gallstone pancreatitis 134
gangrenous cholecystitis 134–135
gastroduodenal ulcers
– expert commentary 205
– Peptic Ulcer Disease (PUD) risk factors 192
– requiring surgery 192
Gastroesophageal (GE) junction injuries
– blunt abdominal trauma 51–53
– complications 53
– duodenum 52
– rectum 52–53
– small bowel and colon 52
– stomach 51–52
– surgical techniques in trauma 51f
gastrointestinal hemorrhage
– Blatchford score 197t
gelfoam 103
General Surgery Service(GSS) model
– grading systems 4
geriatric patients
– laprascopy 12
Glasgow coma scale (GCS) 65
great vessels
– and thoracic aorta 96–98
gunshot wounds
– evaluation and management 69–73
– operative principles 72–73

H

hard signs 64–65, 69–70
Helicobacter pylori
– FDA-approved treatment 199t
hemodynamic effects
– laprascopy 9t
hemopericardium 61f
hemorrhagic peptic ulcer disease
– forrest classification 198t
– management 197–198
hemorrhagic shock 14
– management 17–18
hemostatic resuscitation 14
hemothorax 15, 16
hiatal hernia
– classification of 242f
– etiology 243
Hinchey scoring system
– diverticulitis 148
hollow viscus injuries 50–51
– blunt abdominal trauma 50–51
– diagnosis 50
– management strategy 51
– surgical techniques 51
Hospital-based emergency care 1
hydrops 135
hypercarbia
– physiologic effects 10, 11f
hyperchloremia 16
hypotension 14
hypothermia
– lethal triad 15
hypoventilation 16
hypovolemia 15

hypovolemic shock 14, 15
hypoxemia 16
– rescue strategies 25f

I

Iatrogenic appendicitis 114f
Ileal Pouch-anal Anastomosis (IPAA) 174, 180
ileorectal anastomosis 180
incarcerated hernias
– diagnosis 216
– differential diagnosis 216
– epidemiology 216
– epigastric, ventral, and incisional hernias 219–220
– expert commentary 227
– inguinal hernia and 217
– and strangulation 243
– treatment 216–217
– umbilical hernia and 218–219
incarcerated morgagni hernia
– axial and coronal Computed Tomography (CT) 221
incisional hernia
– computed tomography 220f
Indocyanine Green (ICG) 138–139
infection
– and necrosis 160–161
Inferior Mesenteric Artery (IMA) 99–100
Inferior Vena Cava (IVC) 9
– and abdominal aorta 99
infertility 181
Inflammatory/Infectious Bowel Disease
– clinical manifestations 176–177
– Crohn's disease (CD) 172
– expert commentary on 191
inguinal hernia 217
– CT image 218f
injuries
– cardiac 87
– pulmonary vascular 87
Intensive Care Unit (ICU)
– ABCDEF Bundle in 20f
– acute respiratory failure 24
– admission, discharge, and triage guidelines 18–19
– anemia management 20
– NUTRIC score 29f
– pain, agitation, and delirium 28
– physician staffing standard 19
intensivist
– and surgical team 18–19
intercostal injuries
– and internal mammary injuries 86–87
internal hernia 223
internal mammary injuries
– and intercostal injuries 86–87
intestinal bowel obstruction
– diagnostic workup 206
– expert commentary 215
– small bowel obstruction 206–209
intra-abdominal pressure
– physiologic effects 9, 10f
intractable colorectal inflammation 178
Intraoperative Cholangiogram(IOC) 138–139
Intraoperative Ultrasound 138–139

intrathoracic hemorrhage 83
ischemic colitis 235–236

K

ketamine 15
kidney
– surgical techniques 48–49

L

laboratory analysis
– mesenteric ischemia 230
laparoscopic approach
– vs. open appendectomy 118–121
laparoscopic cholecystectomy 136
– laparoscopic subtotal 138f
laparoscopic debridement 161
laparoscopic resection
– Crohn's disease (CD) 172f
laparoscopic transgastric
   necrosectomy 165–166, 166f
Laparoscopic trocar configurations
– Peptic Ulcer Disease (PUD) 196f
laparoscopy
– penetrating abdominal trauma 73
large bowel obstruction 210–211
– endoscopic management 211
– minimally invasive surgery 210
– operative intervention 210
left innominate artery
– pseudoaneurysm of 103
Left Subclavian Artery (LSCA) 104
Lemmel Syndrome 135
lethal triad
– hypothermia 15
life-threatening severe colitis 177
liver
– surgical techniques 49–50
lung
– injury 86
LUNG-SAFE study 25

M

major vascular injuries
– blunt abdominal trauma 54–55
– complications 55
– diagnosis 54
– management strategy 54
– surgical techniques 54–55
management strategy
– diaphragm injuries 55
– major vascular injuries 54
Mannheim peritonitis index 150t
massive hemorrhage 178
Mean Arterial Pressure (MAP) 17
mediastinal injuries
– and cardiac injuries 83
mesenteric ischemia
– anatomy of 229
– causes of 228t
– CT angiography 230f
– diagnosis 229
– expert commentary 241
– laboratory analysis 230
– non-occlusive 235
– operative exposure 232–233
– resuscitation 232
– thromboembolic 233
– treatment 229
– veno-occlusive 234–235

Mesenteroaxial volvulus 244f
Michigan Surgical Quality 4
Minimally Invasive Approaches (MIA)
– Crohn's disease (CD) 175–176
– recurrent disease 177f
Minimally Invasive Retroperitoneal
   Pancreatectomy (MIRP) 161–162
Minimally Invasive Surgery (MIS)
– and acute diverticulitis 150–151
– contraindications to 179
– future 12
– large bowel obstruction 210
– large bowel obstruction technical
   considerations 210–211
– physiological considerations 12
– small bowel obstruction 207–208
– small bowel obstruction technical
   considerations 208–209
Mirizzi's syndrome 135
Multidetector Computed Tomography
   (MDCT) 116
Multidetectorcomputed Tomographic
   Angiography (MD-CTA) 35
Myocardial Ischemia And Transfusion
   (MINT) 21t

N

neck exposure 82
neck trauma
– penetrating 34–35
– tracheal injury 35
necrosis
– and infection 160–161
necrotizing fasciitis 15
neurogenic shock 14
non-occlusive mesenteric ischemia 235
nonhemorrhagic shock 16
noninvasive ventilatory strategies 24
norepinephrine 16
NUTRIC score
– Intensive Care Unit (ICU) 29f
nutrition 28

O

obstruction 178
obstructive shock 14, 15
older population
– cholecystitis 136
open appendectomy
– vs. laparoscopic 118–121, 119f, 120f
open cholecystectomy 139
open management strategies 179
– Ileal Pouch-Anal Anastomosis
   (IPAA) 180
– ileorectal anastomosis 180
– management of postoperative
   complications 181
– total abdominal colectomy 180
– total proctocolectomy 180
open necrosectomy 161
open thoracic surgery 83–87
open transgastric necrosectomy 166
operating room
– transport 18
operative exposure 83–85, 94
operative intervention
– intractable colorectal
   inflammation 178
– nonemergent indications 178
operative management

– esophageal perforation 250–251
operative principles
– gunshot wounds 72–73
operative techniques 86–87
– arterial injuries 86
– intercostal and internal mammary
   injuries 86–87
– lung injury 86
– pulmonary vascular injuries 87
– vascular injury 86
– venous injuries 86
optimal fluid 16
organ function
– and preoperative intravascular
   volume 14
organoaxial volvulus 243

P

pancreatic injuries
– blunt abdominal trauma 53–54
– complications 54
– diagnosis 53
– management strategy 53
– surgical techniques 53
paraesophageal hernias 244f
– diagnosis 243
– and esophageal perforations 242
– indications for repair 245
– radiological studies 244
– upper endoscopy 244
pathogenesis
– appendicitis 113–114
patient populations
– laprascopy 11–12
pediatric patients 11
pelvic hernia 222
pelvic sepsis 181
penetrating abdominal trauma
– abdominal anatomy 63
– anterior abdominal stab wound 65f
– basic operative principles 64
– basic principles of 63–64
– brief history 62
– damage control surgery 73–75
– Damage Control Surgery (DCS)
   73–75
– EAST practice management
   guidelines 68t
– epidemiology 62–63
– evaluation and management 64–69
– expert commentary 79
– initial evaluation 63
– laparoscopy 73
– mechanisms of injury 63
– pregnancy 73
Penetrating Neck Trauma (PNT) 34–35
– hard signs 34t
– soft signs 34t
Peptic Ulcer Disease (PUD)
– diagnosis 192–193
– disease presentation 192
– Laparoscopic trocar
   configurations 196f
– management of complicated
   193–197
– management of hemorrhagic
   197–198
– postoperative management of
   complicated 198–200
– risk factors 192
– types 194f

– World Society of Emergency
   Surgery 195t
percutaneous cholecystostomy 139
perforated cholecystitis
– with hepatic abscess 139
perforated peptic ulcer
– adapted ERAS components 199t
Perianal disease 175
peripancreatic collections 160
– alcoholic pancreatitis 167f
– endoscopic transgastric
   debridement 164–165
– expert commentary 171
– indications for intervention 161
– laparoscopic debridement 161
– necrosis and infection 160
– open necrosectomy 161
– retroperitoneal debridement 161
– transgastric debridement 164
persistent pneumothorax 61f
phenylephrine 16
physiological effects
– minimally invasive surgery 12
physiological effects
– hypercarbia 10, 11f
– laprascopy 9–10
physiotherapy
– chest 16
Plateletpheresis 16
pnecrotizing fasciitis 15
pneumatosisintestinalis 231f
pneumomediastinum 61f
pneumothorax 15, 16, 82–83
Point Of Care Ultrasonography
   (POCUS) 14–15
Polytetrafluoroethylene (PTFE) 101
Popliteal Artery 101
porcelain gallbladder 136
Portal Vein (PV)
– and Superior Mesenteric Vein
   (SMV) 100
portal venous gas 231f
Positive end-expiratory Pressure
   (PEEP) 15
Postanesthesia Care Unit (PACU) 19
postoperative critical care 18–30
– resuscitation goals 19–20
– surgical team and intensivist 18–19
– transfusion strategies 20–22
Postoperative management
– of complicated Peptic Ulcer Disease
   (PUD) 198–200
pouchitis 181
pregnancy
– appendicitis 124–125
– cholecystitis in 136
– penetrating abdominal trauma 73
pregnant patients
– laprascopy 11–12
preoperative critical care
– acute care surgery 14–18
– airway management 15–16
– initial resuscitation 16–17
– monitoring 17
– optimizing respiratory function 16
– organ function and preoperative
   intravascular volume 14
– resuscitation goals 19–20
– timing of surgery 14–15
preoperative intravascular volume
– and organ function 14
Pressure Controlled Inverse Ratio
   Ventilation (PCIRV) 16

Primary Anastomosis (PA) 152
proctocolectomy 180
Profunda Femoral Artery (PFA)
– and Proximal SFA 101
prophylaxis
– prevention of complications 30
proximal coil 104
Proximal SFA
– and Profunda Femoral Artery (PFA) 101
pseudoaneurysm
– of left innominate artery 103f
– overed stent–graft repair 103f
pseudocyst
– walled-off necrosis (WON) 160f
pulmonary vascular injuries 87
pulmonary vasoconstriction 10

R

radiological studies
– paraesophageal hernias 244
Randomized Control Trials(RCTs) 21
rectum
– and colon 174–175
– Gastroesophageal (GE) junction injuries 52–53
recurrent disease 175
– Minimally Invasive Approaches (MIA) 177f
Red Blood Cell (RBC) 20
– American Association of Blood Banks (AABB) guidelines 21t
refractory shock 18
renal artery
– and vein 100
renal replacement therapy
– Mean Arterial Pressure (MAP) 17
respiratory function 16
resuscitation 14, 19–20, 232
– preoperative critical care 16–17
Resuscitative endovascular balloon occlusion of the aorta (REBOA) 106–107, 107f
retained hemothorax 61f, 82
retrograde intubation 85
retroperitoneal debridement 161
– primary percutaneous drainage 164
– two trocar technique 163f
rib fractures 16

S

saphenous vein 101
sepsis
– 6-hour bundle 24t
– acute kidney injury and 28
– definitions 22
– and electrolytes 15
– guidelines and bundles 22
– management of 22
– new vs. prior definitions 23
– surviving sepsis campaign 1-hour bundle 24t

septic shock 14–15, 22
– management 18
– vasopressors in 16
Serial Clinical Examinations (SCEs) 66
shock
– Acute Care Surgery (ACS) patients 14
– cardiogenic 14, 15, 18
– crystalloid boluses and 16
– distributive 14
– hypovolemic 15
– hypovolemic and hemorrhagic 14
– neurogenic 14
– nonhemorrhagic 16
– obstructive 14, 15
– septic 14, 22
shunts 105
simultaneous resuscitation
– surgery and 14–15
small bowel obstruction 206–209
– decompressed and dilated loops 209f
– division of adhesion 209f
– early postoperative 209
– etiology 207f
– Gastroesophageal (GE) junction injuries 52
– ischemia 207f
– minimally invasive surgery 207–208
– omental adhesion 209f
– operative intervention 206–207
– resection 52f
Society of Critical Care Medicine (SCCM) 19
soft signs 34t
solid organ injuries 47
– American Association for the Surgery of Trauma (AAST) grading of 47t
– blunt abdominal trauma 47
– management strategy 48
spigelian hernia 220
spleen
– surgical techniques 48–49
stab wounds
– operative principles 69
– profunda femoral artery 103f
stent
– migration 250
– tissue ingrowth 249
stent–graft repair 103f
sternotomy 97
steroids
– septic shock 24
stoma reversal
– timing of 153
stomach
– Gastroesophageal (GE) junction injuries 51–52
strangulation
– and incarceration 243
subclavian artery 38–39
subcutaneous emphysema 10
Superior Mesenteric Artery (SMA) 99
Superior Mesenteric Vein (SMV)
– and Portal Vein (PV) 100
surgeon satisfaction 3

surgery
– immediate vs. delayed 15
– simultaneous resuscitation and 14–15
– timing 14–15
surgical team
– and intensivist 18–19
surgical techniques
– diaphragm injuries 55–56
– liver 49–50
– major vascular injuries 54–55
– pancreatic injuries 53
– spleen and kidney 48–49
surgical transgastric necrosectomy 165
Surviving Sepsis Campaign (SSC) 22
symptomatic gallbladder disease 133
– acute cholecystitis 133
– chronic cholecystitis 133
– percutaneous cholecystostomy 133
synthetic colloids 16
Systemic Inflammatory Response Syndrome (SIRS) 22
Systemic Vascular Resistance (SVR) 11

T

thoracic aorta
– and great vessels 96–98
thoracic duct ligation 83
thoracic trauma
– airway management 85
– elective 82
– expert commentary 93
– initial evaluation 80
– open thoracic surgery 83–87
– operative intervention 80–82
– thoracic damage control 82
thromboembolic mesenteric ischemia 233
– endovascular treatment 233
– opentreatment 233–234
total abdominal colectomy 180
total proctocolectomy
– and end ileostomy 179–180
tourniquets 105–106
toxic colitis 174
tracheal injury 35
tracheal repair 85
transfusion strategies
– anemia management 22
– restrictive 20–21
transgastric debridement 164
turnbull-blowhole colostomy 179
two trocar technique 163–164

U

ultrasound
– appendicitis 115–116
– diagnosis of appendicitis 116f
umbilical hernia
– incarcerated hernias and 218–219
upper endoscopy

– Fluoroscopic Contrast Video Esophagram 248
upper gastrointestinal tract
– and duodenal disease 174

V

vascular injury 86, 94
vascular trauma 94
– diagnostic testing 94–96
– endovascular interventions 102–105
– expert commentary 111
– incisions/exposures 111
– operative considerations and approaches 96–101
vasopressors 16
– in septic shock 16
vein
– and Common Femoral Artery (CFA) 100
– and renal artery 100
venous injuries 86, 102
ventral hernias 219–220
vertebral artery 94
vertebral artery exposure 98
Vertical Shear (VS) 95
Video-assisted Retroperitoneal Debridement (VARD) 162–163
Video-assisted Thoracoscopic Surgery (VATS) 82
– advantages and indications 82
– cardiac and mediastinal injuries 83
– contraindications and complications 83
– diaphragmatic injury 83
– empyema 83
– foreign body removal 83
– history 82
– indications 82–83
– intrathoracic hemorrhage 83
– operative technique 82
– pneumothorax 82–83
– retained hemothorax 82
– thoracic duct ligation 83

W

walled-off necrosis (WON)
– pseudocyst 160f
Western Trauma Association algorithm
– Computed Tomography (CT) 71f
wide pulse pressure 14
work Relative Value Unit (wRVU) 3
World Society of Emergency Surgery
– peptic ulcer 195t
World Society of Emergency Surgery (WSES) 95
– Pelvic trauma algorithm 95f
wounds
– anterior abdominal stab 65f
– evaluation and management of gunshot 69–73
– hard signs to operate 69–70